BY THE EDITORS OF
CONSUMER GUIDE®
with Ira J. Chasnoff, M.D.,
Jeffrey W. Ellis, M.D.
and Zachary S. Fainman, M.D.

FAMILY MEDICAL GUIDE

The Illustrated Medical and Health Advisor

WILLIAM MORROW AND COMPANY, INC.

Medical Consultants:
Ira J. Chasnoff, M.D., Pediatrics
Jeffrey W. Ellis, M.D., Obstetrics and Gynecology
Zachary S. Fainman, M.D., Internal Medicine
Consultant for Prescription Drugs:
Nicola Giacona, Doctor of Pharmacology, Director,
Drug Information Center, University of Utah Hospital

Cover Design: Linda Snow Shum
Book Design: Ingeborg Jakobson
Illustrations: Teri J. McDermott, M.A., Medical Illustrator

Notice:
In this book, the authors and editors have done their best to outline the indicated general treatment for various conditions, injuries, diseases, ailments, and their symptoms. Also, recommendations are made regarding certain drugs, medications, and preparations; and descriptions of certain medical tests and procedures are offered.

Different people react to the same treatment, medication, preparation, test, or procedure in different ways. This book does not attempt to answer all questions about all situations that you may encounter.

Neither the Editors of CONSUMER GUIDE® and Publications International, Ltd., nor the authors or publisher take responsibility for any possible consequences from any treatment, procedure, test, action, or application of medication or preparation by any person reading or following the information in this book. The publication of this book does not constitute the practice of medicine, and this book does not attempt to replace your physician. The authors and publisher advise the reader to check with a physician before administering any medication or undertaking any course of treatment.

Library of Congress Cataloging in Publication Data
Main entry under title:
Family medical guide.
Includes index.
1. Medicine, Popular. 2. Health. I. Consumer guide.
RC81.F24 1983 616.02'4 83-13105
ISBN 0-688-02210-3

Printed in the United States of America

First Edition
1 2 3 4 5 6 7 8 9 10

Contents

Introduction

The *Family Medical Guide* is designed to help the one person who is responsible for your health and the health of your family—*you*. You are the only one who can observe your health and regulate your personal health habits on a daily basis. You are the one who decides what you eat, how you exercise, when you sleep, and where you go when a medical problem occurs. You are the one who wants to protect your good health and prevent illness. You are the one who wishes to avoid unnecessary trips to the doctor while at the same time becoming informed about when you should see a physician and what the field of medicine can do. How can you intelligently fulfill these goals?

This *Family Medical Guide* provides the answers. Its wide coverage of health and medical topics shows you how to design and plan your health care and that of your family. As medical costs continue to rise and medical testing becomes both more sophisticated and more expensive, average people in need of medical care often find it impossible to keep up with what needs to be known to assure good health for themselves and their families. This book provides a guide to medical care and health practices that will help you make the right decisions about what you and your family need.

The *Family Medical Guide* is not a substitute for your doctor. Rather, it gives you the information you need to make the best use of modern medical care—whether you are trying to select the right doctor for your family, decide on which specialist you need to see, or simply make sure that you and your family stay healthy.

You will find advice on how to find a doctor and how to make certain that he or she is the best doctor for you. You will also find an explanation of all of the specialties in medicine—from anesthesiology (the study of painkilling substances used in surgery) to urology (the study of disorders of the urinary tract).

You will learn the difference between clinical and laboratory tests and be able to familiarize yourself with the commonly administered tests. If you have to have tests done, you will know what to expect, how to prepare yourself for as little discomfort as possible, and what the results may indicate.

If your doctor prescribes a medication, you will learn how to read the prescription and interpret the directions. You can read about buying drugs—and saving money on your prescriptions—as well as about storing and administering your medications. You will learn how your medication works and how to anticipate and, if necessary, cope with any possible side effects of your medicine. Most important, you'll find out how to work with your doctor in developing the best medication program for you.

The heart of the *Family Medical Guide* is a comprehensive medical encyclopedia arranged in alphabetical order for easy and fast reference. This A to Z section covers diseases, disorders, conditions, syndromes, symptoms, diagnostic procedures, treatments, and medical terms. Each entry is presented in clear, easy-to-understand language with practical advice about when to treat a problem at home, when to consult a doctor, and when to administer emergency first aid or to seek immediate emergency care. Since this section is a reference manual, each entry is designed to be self-contained; for example, terms that may not be a part of everyday vocabulary are defined where they occur, even if they have been defined elsewhere. On the other hand, if another entry or section of the book naturally expands or complements a topic, there is a cross reference for you to find the additional information. Furthermore, to make the Medical Guide as useful as possible, numerous detailed illustrations have been included. These illustrations are designed to clarify the information and expand your knowledge about the topics.

In those entries that discuss a disease or disorder, the description of the problem, the cause (if known), the symptoms, the treatment, the prognosis, and the risk factors are discussed. In addition, preventive action is outlined, if appropriate or possible. In those entries that define a term or discuss a procedure, the explanation includes examples to illustrate the concept or idea. In short, each entry attempts to be as inclusive as possible without being technical and hard to understand.

In addition to diseases and other abnormal problems the A to Z medical guide includes descriptions of body systems (for example, the nervous system) and organs (the heart) as they function normally in a healthy body. These entries give you a reference point for becoming familiar with the way your body should work; to understand disease as a departure from the normal healthy state of an organ or system, you should understand what is normal and healthy.

Finally, the A to Z medical guide is followed by an Emergency first aid action guide. These illustrated step-by-step instructions cover life-threatening emergencies when seconds count as well as emergency situations when minutes count. You will be able to see at a glance the emergency procedures for choking, heatstroke, bleeding, shock, and other circumstances that require immediate action. Read this section before an emergency arises.

The aim of the *Family Medical Guide* is to help you take charge of your health care and that of your family. This book will help you develop a personal health plan that fits your life as well as meets your health and medical needs. Equally important, this family health guide will help you communicate with your doctor as he or she diagnoses your ailments and prescribes treatment for them. It will help you describe your problem more accurately, thus enabling the doctor to help you with greater understanding.

Maintaining good health is a team effort between you, your doctor, and the other members of your family who need medical care. Remember, however, that the final responsibility for your health is yours—you are the one in charge of your health on a day-to-day basis. The best way to help yourself and your family is to be informed about your medical needs. You can gain that knowledge by reading the *Family Medical Guide.*

And if you need medical care, see your doctor. This book will tell you when and why.

How to choose a doctor

Most people never think about how to choose a doctor until they need one in a hurry. When a person is injured or suddenly becomes ill, finding a good doctor is a necessity, and there is often no time to spare in finding one.

If a person does not have a family doctor, injury or sudden illness means a quick visit to an emergency room or outpatient section of the nearest hospital, where staff physicians who know nothing about the patient's personal medical history must treat him or her symptomatically and, more often than not, on an urgent basis. This is usually not a good way to establish a lasting physician-patient relationship.

A better way to assure yourself of medical care is to have a personal physician who is familiar with you and your family's medical history and who is available (or has associates who are available) when you need care. This way, your health needs are being met by someone who knows you and whom you know.

The best time, then, to choose a doctor is when you don't need one. You should never wait until you have no choice about the doctor you see. How do you choose a doctor? Here are some guidelines on making an informed choice.

Choosing a family doctor

Many families want a doctor who is familiar both with family members as individuals and with the family as a group. Doctors who have specialized in family medicine are called family practitioners. They have evolved from what used to be called "general practitioners," and their education and training have been expanded to enable the family practitioner not only to provide medical care, but also to recognize and handle the social, emotional, and psychological factors that affect the health and well-being of their patients and their families. Whereas in the past, general practitioners usually had only one year of internship (postgraduate clinical hospital training usually divided among several branches of medicine) before entering general practice, today's family practitioner completes the one-year rotating internship and a two-year residency in family practice, during which he or she receives more intensive training in general surgery, internal medicine, obstetrics-gynecology, and pediatrics among other fields.

Family practitioners care for all the members of a family so that there is often no need for a different specialist for each individual. A family practitioner is well equipped to handle routine care such as Pap smears, uncomplicated pregnancies, immunizations, and routine physicals. A family practitioner can diagnose and treat all of the common ailments as well as many of the uncommon ones and can also guide you and your family to the right specialist when you need one.

In addition to comprehensive medical care for all family members, today's family practitioner is interested in maintaining your good health and preventing illness. He or she is as interested in preventing disease as in curing or treating it. This interest is part of the family practitioner's overall goal to view and treat the patient and the family as an individual or an entity with physical, emotional, and social needs as well as medical requirements.

How can you find a family practitioner who is right for your family? You can call the county medical society or your local chapter of the American Medical Association. These organizations have uniform requirements for physicians to be admitted to their lists, for example, board certification, level of training, and so forth. They also can tell you where you can find a specialist. However, these societies do not offer an opinion on the overall quality of a physician. This is something you must assess for yourself, and the questions listed below will help you make this assessment.

You should also ask people in your neighborhood about the doctor they see. They may be able to offer suggestions based on their personal experience with local physicians. In addition, if you live in a city, you may find that there is a local organization that evaluates the medical profession on behalf of the consumer. Neighborhood consumer groups often will make medical referral information available to you at no charge and will steer you toward physicians who have a proven record of treating their patients with respect and concern.

In the process of selecting a family physician, you should draw up a list of basic questions to ask the doctor:

- Will the doctor treat all family members?
- Does the doctor provide care during pregnancy and perform deliveries?
- Does the doctor have staff privileges at a nearby accredited hospital?
- Does the doctor perform surgery and, if so, what types of surgery?
- Does the doctor encourage preventive medicine, such as routine checkups, immunizations, and follow-up tests?
- Does the doctor make emergency house calls for bedridden family members?
- Does the doctor have office hours that are convenient for your family, especially for those who work or attend school?
- What arrangement does the doctor have for a substitute when he or she is unavailable?
- What are the fees for the various services?
- Is the doctor certified by the American Board of Family Practice (or a specialty board of another area)?

The answers to these questions, along with the recommendations of friends and neighbors, will help you select the right doctor for you and your family.

How to choose a specialist

In approaching the problem of finding a specialist, you should remember that most specialists receive their patients through referrals from family doctors or from other specialists. Many have a policy of not accepting a patient who has not first been examined and referred by a family doctor. This is a method of making sure that those who really need specialists see them, and those who do not need them do not incur the expense that seeing a specialist would entail.

Whether or not you should see a specialist, then, is usually a medical decision: it is a decision made by your doctor about whether your medical complaint needs the attention of somebody who specializes in that particular area. For example, if you have a mild inflammation of the ear (perhaps as a result of a fungus infestation of the ear canal from swimming in the ocean), your family doctor is more than capable of treating it, prescribing for it, and assuring you of complete recovery in a short time. On the other hand, if you have a chronic inflammation of the ear canal, have suffered a partial loss of hearing, or your doctor has discovered a large abscess along the mastoid bone under the ear, he or she will probably refer you to an otologist or ear specialist.

You must also remember that difficulties in one area of the body affect other areas, so it is not always a specialist who is needed to find out what is wrong. For example, visual problems may be limited to abnormalities in the eye itself, but they may also be the result of a wide variety of causes, including diabetes, arteriosclerosis (hardening of the arteries), strokes, or even a brain tumor in that part of the brain that controls vision. The human body is an organic system. Changes in one part of that system affect other parts of the system. No part of the system functions in isolation. Consequently, the first task in diagnosing an illness is to discover the real causes of the ailment. When the culprit is found, *then* you may be referred to a specialist who deals with the specific area of the body that is causing the problem.

So the first line of action in selecting a specialist is to follow your family doctor's advice. He or she will know whether or not you need a specialist. However, you can always ask for a second opinion or seek out a specialist on your own. If for no other reason than knowing that you did all that you were able to do, you should always try to get as much information as possible about your family or a family member's illness. You may even find something that one of the doctors missed.

If your family doctor refers you to a specialist, or if you seek one on your own, you should know what each specialty consists of and what to expect when you see each specialist. The following section gives you a brief description of each of over 30 medical and surgical specialties. As you read about each one, remember that an internship is the period, immediately after a doctor graduates from medical school, during which he or she receives supervised practical experience in a hospital setting. A residency, also supervised in a hospital setting, follows an internship, and it is a period of advanced training in a doctor's chosen medical specialty. The length of a residency varies, depending on the specialty. Board certification means that a doctor is certified as meeting the professional standards of a medical specialty organization called a board, which usually requires a residency in an accredited institution (hospital); a rigorous set of examinations; and, in some fields, a year or two of clinical experience.

Allergy and immunology

This branch of medicine is concerned with the study, diagnosis and treatment of disorders related to immunity (the body's ability to resist disease or other threatening substances) and to the body's immune system. The body's immune system fights against the intrusion of outside forces, whether they be in the form of irritating substances that cause allergic reactions or of microorganisms that cause infection. This is the system that helps us fight off illness every day of our lives. Modern immunological research indicates that many infections can be as much a result of defects in a person's immune system as they are a result of exposure to viruses or bacteria.

Immunologists are also studying the role of the immune system in cancer growth. It may someday be possible to prevent cancer by modifying the immune system to reject the introduction of cancerous growth in the body.

In addition, immunologists are interested in the opposite effect of the immune system: the rejection of foreign substances at times when it would be better for the body if they were not rejected. The most obvious examples are the rejections of organ transplants. Immunologists are seeking to find ways to effect *selective* operation of the immune system: to reject cancer, but to accept a new heart, kidney, or liver.

The best-known branch of immunology deals with allergies, which are responses of the body's immune system to an irritating environmental substance. Doctors who practice as allergists are involved in identifying environmental irritants causing symptoms and formulating a plan of treatment. Allergists may treat allergies by suggesting environmental modifications to eliminate the offending substance, by the use of drugs to relieve the symptoms, or by a program of desensitization. Desensitization involves injecting minute amounts of the offending agent to make the immune system less sensitive to it. Once this program is set up, your family doctor can often give the injections. Allergists also serve as consultants in the management of difficult cases of diseases such as asthma.

An immunologist will complete a residency in internal medicine or pediatrics after graduating from medical school. After this residency he or she completes a two-year fellowship program of training in allergy and immunology. Specialty board examinations are also required.

Anesthesiology

Modern surgery is done without pain during the procedure. While many minor procedures may be done with a local anesthetic—a painkiller that is usually injected into or rubbed onto the affected area—other more complex procedures require that the patient be unconscious — in short, "put to sleep."

An anesthesiologist is a specialist in those drugs that cause a cessation of the experience of pain. The word "anesthesia" is derived from two Greek roots: *ana*, meaning the loss or lack of something; and *esthesia*, the act or process of sensing. Hence, "anaesthesia" means, literally, a lack of sensation.

Anesthesiologists, like other medical specialists, have completed medical school, an internship, and a residency in their specialty — anesthesiology — before starting their practice. They may also receive some training in a field other than anesthesiology, such as internal medicine, pediatrics, or obstetrics. Some of them also do tours of surgical residency, in order to broaden and deepen their knowledge of surgical techniques and needs.

Bariatrics

Bariatrics is a relatively new field in medicine, brought into popularity by the public's keen interest in the problems of being overweight.

Bariatricians have been making advances in what is known about being over- or underweight, by dispelling myths and substituting hard scientific evidence. Their training usually involves an internship in internal medicine, with a special residency in bariatrics. In addition, bariatricians are certified by their specialty group, the American Society of Bariatric Physicians, which issues its own standards of practice.

Cardiology

Cardiology is a branch of internal medicine that deals with the diagnosis and treatment of diseases of the heart. It covers the entire field of heart and circulatory system difficulties that may stem from birth abnormalities, childhood diseases, or advancing age.

Cardiology and heart surgery complement each other. Over the years, doctors in each of these fields have worked closely together in the treatment of heart diseases. For example, the cardiologist may determine that a child has been born with a hole between the chambers of the heart. The heart surgeon, also called a cardiovascular surgeon, is the one who will repair this hole through open heart surgery.

Cardiologists may take care of a variety of heart conditions such as rheumatic heart disease in children and congestive heart failure and heart attacks in adults.

There have been many medical advances in the last few years in both the medical treatment and surgical treatment of heart disease. All of this means that a cardiologist must be acquainted not only with anatomy and physiology, but also with modern computerized diagnostic equipment as well. As research progresses in the field of artificial or mechanical hearts, we can expect even more to be demanded of the cardiologist.

Training in cardiology involves a residency in internal medicine followed by at least two years of specialized training in cardiology.

Cardiovascular surgery

The cardiovascular surgeon performs surgery on the heart and blood vessels of the body. Open heart surgery came into its own during the 1950s and underwent further refinement in the 1960s and 1970s. It has been nearly two decades since the first heart transplant. In 1983, a successful implantation of an artificial heart took place.

The cardiovascular surgeon performs many different types of surgery on the heart that include the replacement of heart valves and bypasses of blocked coronary arteries.

Training in cardiovascular surgery involves the completion of a general surgery residency followed by two or three years of specialized training in all aspects of heart and blood vessel surgery.

Dentistry

Dentistry is the prevention, diagnosis, and treatment of diseases, disorders, and malformations of the teeth, mouth, and jaws. Most people select a dentist with a general practice who can provide routine dental care and, if necessary, recommend a dental specialist for those needing specialized treatment. Some of the dental specialties include:

- orthodontia–straightening of teeth
- periodontia—treatment of gums
- endodontia—root canal treatment
- exodontia—extraction of teeth

A dentist planning to establish a general practice will complete four years of dental school and perhaps an optional one-year general residency. Dental specialists will have specific training in their specialty.

Finding a family dentist is much like finding a family doctor. You should ask friends and neighbors for recommendations or contact your local dental society. Often, too, your family doctor can suggest a dentist that will meet the needs of your family.

Dermatology

Dermatology is the diagnosis and treatment of skin diseases. This is another relatively recent addition to the specialties of medicine. All dermatologists will have had training in allergies, since over the years many skin conditions have been recognized as allergic reactions instead of skin diseases.

Other skin disorders diagnosed and treated by dermatologists range from acne and contact dermatitis (skin inflammation caused by contact with irritating substances) to psoriasis (drying and scaly skin) and skin cancer.

As with all specialists, the dermatologist must also be completely knowledgeable about all of the diseases, disorders, and conditions involving other parts of the body that may have some bearing on the condition of the skin.

Dermatologists are required to do an internship, usually in internal medicine, followed by at least a three-year residency in dermatology.

Endocrinology

When we think of "messages" being sent throughout the body, we usually think of the nervous system. But there is another communication system in the body, called the endocrine system. It is made up of the ductless glands including the pituitary gland, the adrenal glands, the thyroid gland, the parathyroid glands, the islet cells in the pancreas, the ovaries (in women), and the testes (in men). These glands secrete hormones that travel as messengers throughout the body to direct and integrate a vast number of bodily functions.

An endocrinologist is a specialist in the diagnosis and treatment of disorders of the endocrine system. He or she must know the symptoms that such disorders exhibit and the specific treatment that such symptoms call for. This means an internal medicine internship and residency, with solid competency in biochemistry, followed by two years of training in endocrinology.

Epidemiology

This medical field deals with the outbreak, frequency, distribution, and control of communicable diseases in the human community. The unofficial headquarters of this activity is the Center for Disease Control (once the Communicable Disease Center) in Atlanta, Georgia.

Epidemiology not only deals with disease communication in general, but also with the specific conditions under which certain diseases seem to flourish. For example, the relatively new field of Urban Epidemiology specifically addresses itself to those diseases and conditions peculiar to city settings. In addition, epidemiologists work to devise ways of preventing disease, such as developing vaccines against the contraction and spread of disease.

In addition to diseases, epidemiology also studies other causes of illness. For example, lead poisoning in children as a result of eating lead-base paint was a major cause of brain damage among children before epidemiologists ferreted out the cause. Epidemiologists have led the medical field in seeking environmental causes for a host of disorders once attributed to bacteria or other sources. Lead poisoning is only one of these causes. Air and water pollution, toxic substances in foods, toxic substances used in the manufacture of a variety of products—all of these subjects come under the scrutiny of the modern epidemiologist.

Epidemiology attracts physicians not only from internal medicine, but from other fields as well, such as immunology, occupational medicine, pediatrics, and others. An epidemiologist will usually have completed three years of specialized training and a year of independent research or teaching.

Gastroenterology

A gastroenterologist specializes in the diagnosis and treatment of diseases and disorders of the esophagus, the stomach, and the intestines. The word comes from two Greek words: *gastro* meaning stomach or belly; *entero* meaning inner tubular structure. A gastroenterologist also specializes in related organs that help in the digestive process such as the liver or pancreas. Gastritis (inflammation of the stomach), enteritis (inflammation of the intestinal tract), ulcers, inability to digest certain foods, constipation, diarrhea, hyperacidity, "heartburn," and a host of other disorders make up the gastroenterologist's diagnostic and treatment arena.

Gastroenterologists are the specialists who do the procedure called endoscopy. Endoscopy is the technique of directly viewing hollow organs, such as the esophagus, stomach, and colon, through flexible tubes. Diagnosis and treatment of many conditions, such as ulcers and polyps, are done with this procedure. Biopsies (gathering tissue samples for testing) are also carried out with these instruments.

These specialists are trained as internists or pediatricians with an additional two-year residency in gastroenterology.

Hematology

Hematology is the study of blood and diseases and disorders of the blood and the blood-forming organs such as the bone marrow and the spleen. A hematologist is proficient in a wide range of diagnostic techniques in which blood samples are used to shed light on disorders in the rest of the body. Blood analyses can aid a diagnostician in developing treatment for a patient. The hematologist's primary concern, however, is the host of diseases and disorders of the blood itself: inability to carry oxygen, inability to help in the fight against invading microorganisms, and the inability of the body to produce normal blood levels. The first set of problems centers around the function of red blood cells, the second centers around the disease-fighting characteristics of white blood cells, and the last centers around the manufacture of blood cells by bone marrow. The hematologist is also an expert in cancers of the blood (leukemia) and in blood clotting problems (hemophilia).

The hematologist must be firmly grounded not only in internal medicine, anatomy, and physiology, but in biochemistry as well. Today this means a sound knowledge of computerized diagnostic equipment associated with biochemical analyses.

A hematologist completes an internship and a residency in internal medicine plus two years of training in hematology. Many, if not most, hematologists today are also trained as and practice as oncologists (cancer specialists).

Internal medicine

Internal medicine is the branch of medicine that deals with the diagnosis and treatment of diseases of adults except for those conditions that require a surgeon or obstetrician. Along with the family practitioner, the internist is trained to handle a wide range of illnesses; in fact, many people select an internist as their family doctor. The internist is specifically trained to deal with chronic (long-term) illnesses, such as diabetes or high blood pressure and acute (short-term) diseases, such as infections. In addition, an internist has both the range and depth to diagnose illnesses that might escape a specialist if they lay outside his or her special field. For this reason, internists are often called diagnosticians because they make diagnoses, treat the patient, and then route patients to other specialists if necessary.

After graduating from medical school an internist completes one year of internship, followed by two years of residency in internal medicine. Internal medicine is also the basis for many of the specialties mentioned here (for example, cardiology, endocrinology, gastroenterology, hematology, and nephrology). This is the reason that these branches are often referred to as subspecialties and the doctors as subspecialists. In order to become a subspecialist, the internist does at least two years of additional training, referred to as a fellowship, in his or her chosen subspecialty and is then eligible for subspecialty board certification.

Nephrology

Nephrologists treat kidney disorders. Their patients are usually referred to them by internists, as kidney problems become evident and are diagnosed as needing special care. While many nephrologists are associated with hospitals (where they perform diagnoses, treatment, research, and teaching), many are associated also with dialysis centers, located outside hospitals.

In treating kidney disorders, the nephrologist may make use of medicines or dialysis (in which machines take over the kidney's function). Referral for surgery (for example, if a transplant is indicated) is also initiated by a nephrologist. In addition, nephrologists perform kidney biopsies that are used to diagnose, treat, and follow a number of kidney diseases other than cancer.

Nephrologists are thoroughly grounded in internal medicine, with special attention to the physiological processes performed by the kidneys. These specialists must be equally well-grounded in biochemistry and the tools of modern biochemical analysis, because of the complex nature of kidney functions. An internship and residency in internal medicine is the required procedure, followed by a two-year training period in nephrology plus specialty board exams. A nephrologist will be more than familiar with all of the latest computerized testing equipment, as well as the latest in dialysis machines.

Neurology

Neurology is the field of medical science that studies the nervous system—the brain, the spinal cord, and the body's complex network of nerves. Clinical neurology concerns itself with the diagnosis and treatment of diseases of the nervous system. When a physician calls himself or herself a neurologist, that person usually means a clinical neurologist.

In order for a neurologist to do diagnostic work, he or she must be aware of the entire range of physical and psychological causes of human behavior and symptoms. Diseases and disorders of other parts of the body can affect the nervous system, and diseases of the nervous system can affect the functioning of other parts of the body. The neurologist must draw these two ends of the diagnostic spectrum together in order to get at the root of the patient's problems.

Training in neurology involves a one-year internal medicine internship followed by a three-year residency in neurology.

Obstetrics/gynecology

The fields of obstetrics and gynecology are closely related, and physicians generally practice these specialties together. While gynecology involves the diagnosis and treatment of disorders of the female reproductive system, obstetrics specifically deals with pregnancy and childbirth.

Many obstetricians are members of a group practice. Most obstetric groups make sure that every doctor in the group either has seen or is familiar with each patient during the pregnancy period. Thus, when it comes time for delivery, the mother will generally be taken care of by a doctor that she knows.

After medical school, an obstetrician/gynecologist completes a four-year residency. During this time, he or she will also receive some training in internal medicine, general surgery, and care of the newborn infant.

The obstetrician/gynecologist often acts as the primary care giver for women. He or she will also work closely with other medical specialists if specific problems occur that do not directly involve the reproductive system.

Occupational medicine

This is a relatively new field of medicine, not to be confused with "occupational therapy" in which patients are given tasks to help them overcome the aftereffects of disease or trauma. Occupational medicine began with industrial and business clinics, which were usually staffed with a physician (who may have only visited the clinic periodically, if the business or industry was small) and an industrial nurse (one who has specialized in the care of patients within a working environment).

As more is discovered about the effects of the working environment on employees, occupational medicine has grown to include the study, diagnosis, and treatment of a vast range of illnesses caused by the industrial environment itself. Asbestos-induced cancer, "black lung" (in which coal dust literally turns the inside of the lung black, with accompanying damage to the lung), allergic reactions to industrial fibers, eye damage from welding arcs, and injury to the feet from jobs that require standing are but a few of the hundreds of disorders treated by occupational medicine physicians.

People in the field have a strong background in internal medicine, with special training in the causes of industrially-related illnesses. In many cases, these specialists have completed a public health training program. Often, these doctors will finish medical school and an internship and then complete a public health program before going on to their specialty residency.

Oncology

Oncology is the study of tumors, particularly cancer. This is a relatively new field and is often associated with hematology (the study of the blood). The reason for this association is that, strictly speaking, oncology deals only with solid tumors and not with cancers of the blood, such as leukemia. Today, however, many in the field are now trained as hematologist-oncologists so that they are certified to deal with both types of cancer.

Oncology embraces a large number of medical and technical disciplines, from surgery to nutrition, from immunology to biochemistry, from diagnosis of symptoms to treatment with nuclear radiation. A thorough knowledge of modern computerized diagnostic instruments is also required of the oncologist. The oncologist may also coordinate other specialists in the management of cancer, such as radiotherapists, gynecologists, and surgeons.

There are many subdivisions of oncology. The medical oncologist is primarily responsible for prescribing and implementing chemotherapy, along with diagnosing and treating complications unique to cancer. Surgical oncologists perform cancer surgery. Pediatric oncologists diagnose and treat cancer in children. Gynecological oncologists deal with cancer in the female reproductive system.

After graduating from medical school, a medical oncologist completes an internship and residency in internal medicine, followed by an additional training program in oncology, which includes training in hematology and chemotherapy. Surgical oncologists are usually general surgeons who have completed a subspecialty fellowship in cancer surgery. Pediatric and gynecological oncologists are certified first in their respective fields and then go on to oncology fellowships in their fields.

Ophthalmology

An ophthalmologist is a medical doctor who diagnoses and treats diseases and injuries of the eyes. Most ophthalmologists are also eye surgeons. They perform a variety of operations, some of which include the reattachment of detached retinas, removal of cataracts, repairing injuries, relieving pressure caused by glaucoma, repairing blood vessel ruptures, and removing eyes that have been injured beyond repair.

An ophthalmologist may have a background in both internal medicine and surgery. This specialty requires an additional three-year residency in ophthalmology after a one-year internship, either rotating (through many specialties) or in internal medicine, and specialty board examinations. (To clarify the roles of various eye specialists: an *optometrist* tests the eyes for the purpose of properly fitting a person with glasses or contact lenses. An *optician* is a person who makes or fits glasses. Most ophthalmologists test the eyes to determine the proper lens prescription if their patients need glasses. An optometrist, however, is not a medical doctor and therefore is not permitted to treat diseases of the eye or to prescribe drugs. An optician takes the ophthalmologist's or the optometrist's recommendations and fits glasses. An *ocularist* fits artificial eyes.)

Orthopedics

Orthopedics is the branch of surgery that specializes in the diagnosis and treatment of diseases or disorders of the bones and joints. The orthopedist treats broken bones, disorders of the bones and joints that can be corrected surgically, and bone tumors, as well as other problems of the skeletal system. In addition, because of his or her knowledge of the functioning of the skeletomuscular system, the orthopedist often treats sports injuries and may serve as the physician for amateur and professional athletic teams.

The orthopedist is required to complete four years of training in orthopedic surgery along with a one-year internship in general surgery, followed by a year of independent practice before specialty board examinations.

Otorhinolaryngology

This specialty combines the study of the ear (*oto*), the nose (*rhino*), and the throat (*laryngo*) into a single discipline called *otorhinolaryngology*, often referred to as "ENT" (ear, nose, and throat) for short. Years ago, before ophthalmology became fully established as a separate discipline, eye doctors also did ENT work.

The ear and throat are connected by the eustachian tube, which leads from the inner ear to the throat. The nose leads directly into the part of the throat referred to as the nasopharynx. Inflammations of the nose may spread to the throat and vice versa. Inflammations of the throat often spread through the eustachian tube to the ears. Consequently, any infection in any of these areas could result in an infection in all of them.

Ear, nose, and throat specialists are primarily surgeons. They perform such varied procedures as rhinoplasty ("nose job"); removal of tumors from the oral, nasal, and neck areas; reconstructive ear surgery; and sinus surgery. They also function as diagnosticians of diseases of the head and neck excluding the brain and eyes.

Medical school is followed by a one-year residency in general surgery and a four-year residency in otorhinolaryngology.

Pathology

Pathology is the study of the intrinsic nature of diseases: the changes in tissue brought about by disease and the ways in which these changes in tissue provide clues not only to the causes of disease or death, but also to ways in which the spread of disease may be checked.

There are a variety of specializations within pathology, including the following:

- Cellular pathology, in which cells themselves are the focus of study
- Clinical pathology, in which laboratory methods are used to aid clinical diagnoses
- Comparative pathology, in which human diseases are compared to those of the lower animals
- Experimental pathology, in which artificially-induced diseases or disorders are studied in order to shed light on naturally-induced diseases and disorders
- General pathology, which is the study of the processes that may occur in various diseases
- Forensic pathology, in which the results of pathologic examinations (such as autopsies, tissue samples, and chemical analyses) are used as evidence in legal proceedings.

Much of the pathologist's work is done with the microscope, preparing and interpreting biopsies (tissue samples). Pathologists are charged with deciding whether a tissue specimen is malignant or not. They also perform autopsies to determine the cause(s) of death. The pathologist is knowledgeable both in the cause and course of disease.

Pathologists ordinarily do work in both internal medicine and surgery during their training. A strong laboratory background is a necessity, with extensive training in modern instrumentation. Three- to four-year residencies in pathology are required, depending on the particular subspecialty.

Pediatrics

Pediatricians specialize in the diagnosis and treatment of diseases of children. They care for a child immediately upon birth through adolescence.

A pediatrician treats childhood illnesses and administers the appropriate immunizations to prevent disease. In addition, pediatricians perform other important tasks: they watch for any abnormalities that may appear during the growth of the child and they advise parents about the child's social and psychological needs, as well as the physical needs.

Pediatricians have at least two years of training in general pediatrics plus an additional year of training in a pediatric subspecialty or in a field other than pediatrics. This is followed by another two-year period of further training or practice and finally an examination by the specialty board.

Peripheral vascular diseases

In addition to cardiovascular (heart and circulatory) diseases, there are many diseases of the vascular (circulatory) system alone, outside of the heart and its vessels. Physicians who specialize in peripheral vascular diseases treat the following disorders:

- Arteriosclerosis, in which the normal artery walls become abnormally thickened or hardened (in advanced cases, the arteries may become partially or completely blocked)
- Arterial occlusion and embolism, in which undissolved material in the bloodstream (such as clumps of clotted blood, bacteria, or tissue fragments) block or occlude the flow of blood in the artery causing a loss of blood to and possibly the death (gangrene) of the tissue beyond the blockade (when flow in a vessel is blocked, there is said to be an "occlusion"; when that block is made up of clotted blood, it is called a "thrombus"; when small bits of material break off the main clump and travel to other parts of the body, they are referred to as "emboli" or an "embolism")
- Carotid occlusive disease, in which the carotid arteries (the arteries in the neck that supply the brain with blood) become blocked (this is one cause of stroke)
- Aortic and femoral artery occlusive disease, in which the aorta (the main artery from the heart going through the chest and abdomen) and/or the femoral artery (a tributary artery of the aorta carrying blood to the legs) become blocked
- Venous thrombosis, in which the veins become clogged, usually with blood clots, with resulting pain and swelling of the affected extremity (when venous thrombosis occurs, it is often associated with inflammation, and this is called thrombophlebitis; if the vein becomes inflamed without thrombosis, it is referred to as phlebitis)
- Pulmonary embolism, in which clots travel to the lungs

Specialists in this area can be internists with extensive cardiovascular training. For the most part, they are vascular surgeons.

Physical medicine and rehabilitation

The field of physical medicine and rehabilitation is concerned with the diseases and disorders of the neuromuscular (nerves/muscles) system. This specialist is skilled in using heat, cold, water, electricity, massage, and exercise to help patients regain use and function of those parts of the body damaged by problems such as injuries, stroke, severe arthritis, or spinal cord injury.

The physical medicine and rehabilitation specialist is required to complete at least three years of training in the specialty, followed by two years of independent practice. Specialty board examinations are required.

Podiatry

Podiatrists concentrate on diseases in and injuries to the feet. Only recently have all the states recognized podiatry as a legitimate healing field. Doctors in this area have degrees in podiatric medicine, but not M. D. degrees; they have not attended medical school. Many podiatrists have joined the ranks of sports medicine practitioners, since many foot injuries result from popular sports activities.

Many podiatrists are qualified to perform surgery on the feet when it is indicated. They also fit a variety of orthotic devices (corrective devices inserted into shoes) to correct foot problems. The boom in jogging and running that has characterized the fitness movement has increased the demand for the services of podiatry.

Preventive medicine

The relatively new field of preventive medicine seeks to prevent illnesses from happening, in addition to diagnosing and treating them after they occur. Physicians from every field have made contributions to preventive medicine. Practitioners range from immunologists (who seek to prevent illness by inoculations) to urban epidemiologists (who search out the causes of widespread illnesses—such as childhood lead poisoning—and try to alter the environment so that the illnesses can be prevented).

Preventive medicine advocates often recommend regular or periodic physical examinations, prescribe certain regimens, and warn against toxic environments. Critics of the field claim that there are no safeguards against some types of illnesses. Advocates of the field point out that the same was said of infections before antibiotics.

Occupational medicine and public health specialists are important members of this field of medicine. In addition, preventive medicine is concerned with reviewing present health services and anticipating and planning future medical needs.

Preventive medicine specialists complete at least three years of specialized training, one year of research or teaching, and examinations by their specialty board.

Proctology

The proctologist specializes in diseases and disorders of the end of the digestive tract: the anus and rectum. The rectum is the last portion of the large intestine; the anus is the opening to the outside from the rectum. Some of the conditions a proctologist treats include hemorrhoids (enlarged blood vessels around the anus) and rectal cancer.

Proctologists complete a residency in general surgery plus a one- or two-year training period in colon and rectal surgery.

Psychiatry

A psychiatrist is a medical doctor—with the authority to write prescriptions and make medical decisions—who deals with mental disorders. Psychologists, on the other hand, do not have to have a medical degree and cannot prescribe drugs. Many psychiatrists do psychoanalysis as part of their therapeutic or diagnostic method and all psychiatrists have intensive training in psychology.

There are four chief branches of psychiatry: (1) descriptive psychiatry, which is based on the observation of external factors that may be the cause of mental illness; (2) dynamic psychiatry, which is the study of the processes, origins, and mechanisms of emotional states; (3) forensic psychiatry, which deals with the legal aspects of mental illness; and (4) orthomolecular psychiatry, which is the study of the molecular bases of mental illnesses. Areas such as psychopharmacology (the effect of drugs on mental behavior) and psychophysiology (the study of the physiology of mental illness) are offshoots of the last type of psychiatry mentioned.

Psychiatrists go through the usual medical sequence: medical school, internship, and residency. The psychiatrist may spend over five years in specialized training in psychiatry and neurology.

Pulmonary medicine

This field deals with the study, diagnosis, and treatment of diseases and disorders of the lungs and their related passages. Among the diseases included are:

- Lung cancer
- Tuberculosis
- Pneumonia, an inflammation of the lungs
- Bronchitis, an inflammation of the bronchi (passageways from windpipe into lungs)
- Tracheitis, an inflammation of the trachea (windpipe)
- Black lung, lungs clogged with coal dust
- Pleurisy, an inflammation of the lining of the lungs and the chest cavity
- Emphysema, destruction of lung tissue causing air to become trapped within the lungs, often accompanied by severe breathing problems.

These specialists also perform bronchoscopy (viewing the trachea and bronchial passages directly through flexible tubes) and specialize in managing ventilators or respirators, artificial breathing machines.

The pulmonary specialist trains in internal medicine, followed by two years of special training in pulmonary diseases and disorders.

Radiology/radiotherapy/ nuclear medicine

A radiologist is a medical doctor who uses X rays to diagnose diseases and other disorders. A radiologist is primarily concerned with the administration and interpretation of X rays. Many perform sophisticated procedures, such as arteriography of peripheral arteries and arteries of the brain. Some choose to subspecialize in areas such as neuroradiology ("neuro" means nerves).

Radiologists have training in physics and instrumentation as well as in biochemistry and the effects of radiation on human tissue. A radiologist will have completed a three- or four-year residency in diagnostic radiology plus a one-year internship in a medical field other than radiology.

A radiation therapist is primarily concerned with the application of radiation in the treatment of cancer. A radiation therapist will have completed a one-year internship, either rotating or in internal medicine, followed by a three-year residency in the specialty.

Nuclear medicine is the field in which radioactive substances, called isotopes, are used to diagnose and treat diseases, such as an overactive thyroid. Specialists in this field are trained in the use of scans as opposed to X rays for diagnosis. A nuclear medicine specialist completes a two-year training period in either internal medicine, pathology, or radiology plus a two-year residency in nuclear medicine.

Rheumatology

Rheumatology is the field of medicine concerned with the study, diagnosis, and medical treatment of diseases and disorders of bones, joints, and muscles. These disorders are often characterized by inflammation or degeneration and include such conditions as arthritis, gout, lupus erythematosus, and other diseases of the connective tissues.

A rheumatologist has completed an internship and residency in internal medicine followed by two or more years of training and experience in rheumatology.

Sports medicine

This is one of the newest fields in medicine and has come into its own largely as a result of two factors: the training and rehabilitation needs of both amateur and professional athletes, and the tremendous growth in fitness and sports-related activities among members of the public. Doctors from a variety of fields now list themselves as sports medicine practitioners. Exercise physiology has become an integral part of medical and sports training programs, and what was once a collection of lore on how to get the most out of your body in a game has become a field of medical research and practice.

Sports medicine has made great contributions to the general public welfare, by producing hard evidence of the benefits of healthful exercise. As a consequence, information about subjects such as nutrition, kinesiology (the study of movements), and biomechanics (study of lever systems and their effect on performance) has come to be available to the average weekend athlete. Training need no longer be haphazard; by using the information developed by sports medicine practitioners, you can train for strength, power, endurance, and speed without incurring injuries. Each goal calls for a different kind of training method. Sports medicine and exercise physiology have made a science out of athletic training.

In one sense, with the advent of sports medicine as a medical field, athletics serves the same function for ordinary people that auto racing serves for the development of new ways to make the family car better: high performance calls for research and ingenuity in converting research into practical applications. Sports medicine converts the lessons learned on the playing field into insights into the medical problems of ordinary people who want to play a little golf, do a little swimming, tone up, and trim down.

You'll find sports medicine practitioners in the training rooms of pro ball clubs, and you'll also find them on the running track. Many of them have trained as orthopedists since that specialty field is concerned with the mechanics of muscular and skeletal function. Therefore, if you need the services of a sports medicine practitioner, you may want to contact an orthopedist for a recommendation.

Surgery

Surgery is the branch of medicine that uses surgical operations to treat disease, injury, or deformity. Surgeons go into the human body by way of incisions through the skin and muscles to alter, correct, or remove and/or replace the offending organ or tissue. There seems to be a surgical specialty for almost every region of the body. Among the usual subspecialties in surgery are the following:

- General surgery (including surgery of the abdomen and breasts)
- Thoracic surgery (of the chest)
- Heart surgery (often included in thoracic surgery)
- Oral surgery (of the mouth) usually performed by dentists with a sub-

specialty in oral surgery except in the case of an ear, nose, and throat specialist

- Neurosurgery (of the nervous system, particularly the brain and the spinal cord)
- Plastic or cosmetic surgery (to correct damage caused by injury or for reasons of appearance)
- Orthopedic surgery (of the bones, joints, ligaments, tendons)
- Eye surgery (for repair or treatment of eye problems)
- Foot surgery (usually performed by a podiatrist or orthopedist).

Surgeons work closely with internists, pathologists, radiologists, anesthesiologists, and other related specialists. In a very real sense, everything that physicians know about diagnosing and treating illnesses is relevant in an operating room.

Surgeons have the usual four years of medical school followed by a general surgery internship and a varying time period in a general surgery residency. In addition, surgeons must also complete additional training in their specific field of surgery.

Urology

Urology deals with diseases and disorders of the urinary tract, the kidneys, the prostate gland, and the male sex organs. The urologist's skills include knowledge of diagnostic procedures and surgical techniques, as well as the ability to treat infections and inflammations of the urinary tract and the male reproductive system.

After completing medical school, the urologist has two years of training in general surgery, followed by a three-year training period in urology and urologic surgery and an 18-month period of practice. Specialty board exams are then required.

What you need to know about medical tests

The basis of medical care is a complete medical history and physical examination. Common health problems are primarily detected and diagnosed by means of the history and physical examination. Nevertheless, your doctor will also use a variety of diagnostic aids and tests to rule out a disease, to confirm a diagnosis, or to detect a disorder that is not apparent. Modern technology now enables medical professionals to inspect the structure of a cell, to see the inside of an organ, or to examine a detailed cross-sectional picture of an internal structure. Used properly, these tests provide vital information to aid your doctor in both the diagnosis of illness and the selection of appropriate treatment.

To help you understand what procedures are available and how they are carried out, this section is a guide to some of the more common medical tests.

Common tests

Blood tests

The complete blood count, the most common of the blood tests, and blood chemistry screening tests are usually based on blood samples drawn by venipuncture (puncture of a vein by a hypodermic needle). While some blood tests may be done from a finger prick, most tests require more blood for the sample and it will be necessary to take blood from a vein. The procedure is quick and relatively painless. The doctor who orders the tests will most often submit all the test orders together, so that multiple venipunctures are not needed.

Although some patients fear that a great volume of blood is being drawn in venipuncture, the usual laboratory tests do not ordinarily require more than 10 to 20 ml (two to four teaspoons). Remember that the total amount of blood circulating in the body of the average person is at least six quarts at any given time and is constantly being replenished. Therefore, fears about unusual blood loss from the usual testing are groundless.

Complete blood count (CBC)

A complete blood count determines the number and types of blood cells in the blood. The CBC includes:

- Hematocrit, a measure of how much of the blood is made up of red blood cells alone
- Hemoglobin test, to measure the amount of hemoglobin (the blood substance that carries oxygen to the body tissues) present in a given volume of red blood cells
- White blood cell count, to find

out how many white blood cells are in the blood

- Differential count, to learn how many of each type of white blood cell are present in the blood
- Platelet count, to determine the number of platelets (the blood elements that aid in clotting the blood) that are present (usually the platelet count is expressed in terms of "adequate," "increased," or "decreased;" if a full count is needed, it must be ordered separately).

Blood chemistry panels

Besides the complete blood count, there are other blood tests that taken together constitute what is known as a blood chemistry panel. These tests, which analyze many components and chemicals in the blood, can be done from a single sample of blood within minutes using an automated blood chemistry machine.

Blood chemistries are performed routinely as screening tests for detection of certain disorders, such as diabetes or kidney disease. They are also used as particular diagnostic tests when specific diseases are suspected, such as hepatitis. Blood chemistry profiles are frequently used to determine the overall function of an organ, especially the liver (the usual profiles contain three or four indicators of liver function). These tests may not pinpoint a specific disease of the liver, but instead provide a general indication of whether or not the liver is functioning normally, leading the physician to perform more specific diagnostic tests. Many illnesses affect more than one organ; furthermore, failure in one organ may cause problems in another. It is here that blood chemistry profiles have great utility; they give information about the function of several organs (particularly the liver and kidneys) at once, using one sample.

The following list contains some of the more common blood chemistry tests with a brief description about the purpose of each:

- Blood glucose (sugar)—to measure blood glucose levels, especially in suspected or diagnosed diabetes mellitus (in many cases, if the blood sugar is high enough on a screening panel, the diagnosis of diabetes mellitus can be made from this alone)
- Blood urea nitrogen (BUN)—to assess kidney function
- Creatinine — to assess kidney function
- Electrolytes — to check body fluid and salt balance (salts include sodium, potassium, and chloride)
- Uric acid—to aid in diagnosing gout
- Cholesterol or triglycerides—to measure fat levels in blood
- Bilirubin — to assess liver function; to evaluate jaundice; to help diagnose hemolytic anemia
- Albumin — to measure protein (albumin) in blood in order to assess general nutritional status as well as a general idea of liver function (albumin is produced by the liver).

Urinalysis

A routine urine analysis is a microscopic examination and a chemical analysis of the urine. Under the microscope, red or white blood cells in the urine can be seen, indicating bleeding and/or an infection somewhere along the urinary tract. Other microscopic elements such as "casts" (formations of protein with and without cellular elements that usually indicate disease in the kidney) and crystals (uric acid or calcium, for example) may also be seen. A chemical analysis can determine the presence of sugar, protein, or other substances that may indicate kidney or bladder diseases as well as other disorders unrelated to the urinary tract such as diabetes and starvation. There is no risk to this test.

The patient is given a clean container and told to urinate directly into it. When a urine culture is indicated, a "midstream" specimen is usually requested, that is, a specimen obtained after proper cleansing of the urinary opening and after the initial spurt of urine is passed. If you are to collect the specimen at home, you should also be provided with a clean container with a cap. If not, you should use a clean glass or plastic container. A container that has held food, perfume, chemicals, or cosmetics should not be used. Such containers are difficult to empty and may still contain traces of the original contents, thus invalidating the test results.

Chest X ray

The most common standard X-ray examination is the chest X ray. This is an X ray usually used to check for signs of lung diseases and abnormalities. In addition, in a standard chest X ray, the heart, parts of the aorta, the ribs, the upper backbones, the shoulders, the upper arm bones, and the collar bones are seen along with the lungs. Often, diseases other than those that affect the lungs, such as osteoporosis (thin, brittle bones) and congestive heart failure (enlarged heart with the characteristic pattern of fluid in the lungs and lung vessels), may be diagnosed and followed with chest X rays.

The patient undresses from the waist up. The usual chest X ray is taken in two positions: sideways and with the patient standing with his or her front side resting against an X-ray cassette (where the film is) and with the X-ray machine at his or her back. Correct positioning and inactivity are critical in obtaining good X-ray pictures. The actual time of exposure to radiation is quite short. The test is painless but, as with any X-ray procedure (if the test is overused), it may carry a risk of long-term effects of radiation exposure. Routine X rays should be avoided by pregnant women; however, if necessary, a lead shield may be used to protect the fetus (unborn baby).

Electrocardiogram

An electrocardiogram (ECG) is a visual record of the heart's electrical impulses that control the rate and rhythm of beating and reflect many alterations of the heart muscle. This test, along with the history and physical examination, is used to diagnose numerous heart disorders, including previous and new myocardial infarction (heart attack), some congenital (present at birth) abnormalities of the heart, pericarditis (inflammation of the lining sac of the heart), and abnormal thickness of the muscle (such as is seen in long-term high blood pressure), among many others. There is no risk to this test, and it is totally painless.

Electrodes (small metal disks) sensitive to the heart's impulses are taped onto the body at various points on the chest, arms, and legs. The electrode cables are connected to the electrocardiograph, a machine that produces a visual record of the impulses. A normal heart produces an ECG tracing consisting of regularly occurring wave patterns whereas an arrhythmic heart (beating in other than a normal rhythm) or one with some other condition will produce alterations in the cadence and/or appearance of the wave patterns.

Stool blood test

This test is used to detect tiny quantities of occult (hidden) blood in the stool (feces or solid waste material) that are not visible to the eye and that may signal bowel disease or bleeding somewhere along the digestive tract.

The test is usually done by the patient at home and mailed to a laboratory. The patient places a small sample of stool on specially coated paper that will reveal any blood when treated with a special developer. The test may have to be done several times, since the bleeding may be intermittent, that is, it may start and stop rather than be constant. The patient will be instructed to eat a diet that is free of red meat for at least three days before taking the stool specimen (since the blood from meat, including cooked meat, may cause a false positive result on the test) and to take no aspirin-containing medications (aspirin may cause bleeding from the stomach).

This test is painless and has no risk. It is an excellent method of screening for colon cancer.

Throat culture

This common procedure is used to determine the type of microorganisms causing infection in the throat. The most common reason for its use is to differentiate streptococcal (beta hemolytic group A) infection from viral sore throat.

The test involves obtaining a sample of bacteria by rolling a cotton-tipped applicator around the swollen area. The test is painless, but may cause gagging. There is no risk.

The cell samples are placed in a culture medium (a special mixture of chemicals and nutrients designed to support growth of bacteria), so that growth of microorganisms can be detected and measured. Special procedures are used to identify the specific bacteria. This procedure usually takes from 24 to 48 hours for definitive results.

Special diagnostic tests

Allergy tests

Tests to determine the existence of various allergies are as numerous and complex as the substances (called allergens) that cause the allergic responses. One of the most common allergy tests is the skin test. This procedure can be either a scratch skin test or an intracutaneous skin test. In the scratch test, suspected allergens are applied in small amounts to individual, tiny scratches on the skin, often several at a time and in a prescribed order. In the intracutaneous skin test small quantities of the suspected allergens are injected into or under the skin. After a short period of time—about one half hour—the doctor notes which substances have caused a reaction. In both of these tests, a swollen reddish bump at the site of the application is a positive reaction to that allergen. The skin scratches and injections can be uncomfortable while the procedures are being performed. In addition, there is a risk to the skin tests in that an extremely sensitive individual may react strongly to an applied or injected allergen.

Although skin tests are relatively safe and reliable, there is also a blood test to help diagnose allergens. The test, called radioallergosorbent technique (RAST), measures specific (allergic-group) antibodies in the blood. Antibodies are substances formed by the immune system in response to foreign invaders, such as an allergen. The test can be used for those people who should not have skin tests: people with extremely sensitive skin, very young children, and those individuals suspected to be extremely sensitive to an injected allergen. However, the RAST may not be as sensitive as skin tests and is more expensive.

In the case of food allergies, diagnosis is often difficult. One method of identifying allergens is to have samples of suspected allergy-causing foods eaten in small quantities, at times when there is nothing in the digestive system. Symptoms, if any, are noted. Adequate time is required between food samples so that each sample can clear the system before the next food is given. Someone with a history of severe reactions should not be tested in this fashion. Skin testing can be done, but may not be accurate.

Biopsy

A biopsy is the removal of a small sample of tissue for examination under a microscope. This procedure is done to establish a precise diagnosis of abnormalities, including cancer. The tissue may be removed by cutting, by aspirating (suctioning) with a needle, or by other methods, depending on the part of the body from which the tissue sample is removed. For example, endoscopic biopsy is removal of tissue by instruments attached to or passed through an endoscope (a device — usually a flexible lighted tube — used for direct visualization of the interior of a hollow organ) into a hollow organ, such as the colon.

The procedure varies with the type of biopsy to be performed. Some require hospitalization — especially if surgery is required to conduct a biopsy on internal organs. Other procedures, such as removal and/or biopsy of small skin growths or needle aspiration (suctioning) of a breast lump, can be done in a doctor's office or an outpatient clinic. Although many biopsies are done with some type of anesthesia, there may be some discomfort if a biopsy involves some sort of cutting or invasive (entering the body) technique. Additionally, depending on the surgical or invasive procedures involved, there is some risk, which varies with the procedure being performed. The risks of outpatient biopsies are usually minimal; but complications, such as excessive bleeding, can occur.

Contrast examinations

Contrast media, popularly known as "dyes," are materials introduced into the body that alter radiopacity (the capacity to be "seen" by X ray or fluoroscope) of one part of the body in comparison with surrounding parts. The contrast materials are opaque, that is, they are able to be seen on the X ray or fluoroscope, and are essential to visualize certain internal body areas, such as the stomach and intestines. When the contrast medium is introduced into the body, the radiologist performing the test often uses fluoroscopy (the projection of moving X rays onto a special screen) to observe the working of the internal body organs and then takes still X-ray films of the area being examined. Common contrast examinations include the upper gastrointestinal tract examination (upper GI series), lower gastrointestinal series (barium enema), intravenous pyelogram (IVP or kidney X ray), the gallbladder series, and angiogram (visualization of blood vessels).

Upper GI series

The upper GI series is a contrast medium/X-ray examination of the esophagus, stomach, and first part of the small intestine (duodenum). This X ray is used to detect ulcers, cancers, and other abnormalities. The contrast medium used is barium sulfate, and it is introduced by having the patient drink it after fasting overnight. It is necessary that the patient's stomach be empty to accommodate the barium meal and also to avoid having food particles confuse the results. The radiologist observes the filling of the stomach on the fluoroscope as the patient drinks. The time required for the exam is about 30 minutes. In some instances, such as suspected regional enteritis or an obstruction, the doctor will order what is known as "small bowel follow-through," a series of X rays following the barium throughout the small intestine. In this procedure, many films are taken at specified time intervals. This X ray may take hours. Patients can expect very light-colored stools after the test because of the presence of the barium sulfate. As with any X-ray examination, there may be a risk of effects from radiation exposure, but modern equipment and techniques have minimized this.

Lower GI series

The lower GI series, or barium enema, is a contrast medium/X-ray examination of the large intestine (colon) that is useful in detecting tumors, polyps, and other problems in the colon. For this examination, the colon must be cleared of all fecal matter. This is usually accomplished by a liquid diet for 24 to 48 hours, accompanied by laxatives and enemas. Nothing is then allowed by mouth until the examination is completed. The time for the examination itself is usually about 30 minutes. The patient is given an enema consisting of a barium solution (that makes the colon opaque) introduced into the large intestine through a tube inserted into the anus and must retain the enema until all the films are made. When looking for polyps or when a detailed view of the lining of the colon is required, air is put into the colon to form a double contrast with the barium. This technique is referred to as an "air contrast barium enema" and is rapidly becoming more common than the plain lower GI.

At the time of the examination, the radiologist fluoroscopically observes the colon filling with the liquid suspension of barium sulfate. Before, during, and after emptying of the solution, films are made of the barium-coated colon. Afterward the patient is usually given a cleansing enema and occasionally a mild laxative to rid the colon of barium.

There is the usual risk from radiation exposure and, rarely, an obstruction of the colon by impacted (hardened) barium or a perforation of the colon because of the enema may occur.

Intravenous pyelogram (IVP)

This test is used to determine the size and functioning of as well as the presence of obstructions in the kidneys and the urinary tract. In men, an enlarged prostate gland may also be noted. The test is done by injecting contrast material — into a vein in the arm — which then is eliminated through the kidneys and urinary tract. X-ray films are made at given time intervals to observe the rate of excretion, the concentration of the contrast medium inside the kidneys, and the outlines of the ureters (tubes from kidneys to bladder) and the bladder. Since fecal matter and gas in the intestinal tract obscure the observation of urinary tract structures, the lower bowel needs to be cleared for this examination. There is the usual risk of the effects of radiation exposure. Patients with diabetes mellitus, known kidney disease, or a history of previous reactions to X-ray contrast materials may be at risk of kidney damage or serious allergic-type reactions. These patients should inform their physicians and the radiologist of these facts, since adequate precautions can be taken to minimize the chance of complication.

Gallbladder series

This series, called the oral cholecystogram is performed to test gallbladder function and to detect gallstones.

Contrast medium (a dye in tablet form) is given to the patient after the evening meal the day before the X ray. Usually nothing is given by mouth until the examination is completed. If the gallbladder does not show up (concentrate the contrast), the next day the dose of contrast is repeated and another film is taken now 48 hours after the first dose. If the gallbladder is still not visible, this indicates a diseased gallbladder (assuming that the gastrointestinal tract and liver are processing the contrast normally). In some X-ray departments, after the films of the contrast-filled gallbladder have been made, the patient is given a fatty meal to stimulate the gallbladder to empty and then another film is made to judge this function. The time required for the examination is about one hour, excluding the time for the fatty meal. The oral cholecystogram will correctly diagnose gallbladder disease (including both poor function and or stones) about 96 percent of the time.

For this examination, as with pyelography (kidney X ray), it is helpful to clear the intestinal tract of fecal matter and gas to allow for adequate viewing of the gallbladder. This is done with a special diet 24 hours prior to the examination and administration of enemas. Avoiding creams, butters, and other fatty foods (fats stimulate the gallbladder, which must be at rest in order to concentrate the dye well) is also required. There may be some side effects such as nausea, vomiting, or diarrhea. There is the usual risk from exposure to radiation, along with the risk (although uncommon) of allergic-type reaction to the contrast. Patients with diabetes and known kidney disease may be at risk of kidney damage and should inform their doctor of these facts so that precautions can be taken.

Cardiac catheterization

Cardiac catheterization, often referred to as the "angiogram," is required before most heart surgery and for diagnosis of some heart diseases. In this procedure the cardiologist introduces a tube (called a catheter) into the heart. This is usually done through a puncture in an artery in the groin or arm. Through this tube, an opaque contrast is injected so that moving pictures of the heart can be clearly seen. Through the catheterization, the cardiologist and the cardiovascular surgeon obtain crucial information such as the location of defects in the various walls and valves of the heart, the location and degree of narrowing of the cornary arteries (the arteries that supply the heart muscle itself with blood), and even the different pressures in the chambers giving an idea as to the overall functional situation of the heart. Nowadays, this procedure is commonly performed, and carries a very low risk potential in the hands of experienced physicians. After the procedure, there is occasional bleeding at the catheter introduction site along with some mild discomfort there. During contrast injection, many patients complain of a "hot flash" or nausea. There is the usual risk of radiation exposure in this test. Also, patients with previous history of reaction to contrast materials, diabetes, or kidney disease may be at risk from the contrast. Adequate precautions can be taken to prevent complications when the physician performing the procedure is informed of these problems prior to the test.

It is important to note that there are other (uncommon) complications that can occur with cardiac catheterization. Detailed explanations of the risks should be obtained from the doctor.

Electroencephalogram

An electroencephalogram (EEG) is a visual record of the electrical impulses discharged by the brain cells. The EEG is used to diagnose and interpret possible abnormalities in the brain. The test is painless and carries no risk.

Electrodes (small metal disks) are placed at specified points on the surface of the head (in special circumstances, disks may be inserted through the nose into the throat, which may be annoying but not painful or dangerous) and then attached to the electroencephalograph machine, which produces a visual tracing of the brain's electrical waves. When, for instance, the brain has been damaged or the patient has epilepsy, the waves produced by the electrical discharges form patterns characteristic of that disorder. Tracings are taken when the patient is awake but calm; when he or she has been asked to hyperventilate (breathe rapidly) and has been stimulated with a flashing light which may evoke changes characteristic of epileptic grand mal seizures; and when the patient is asleep. An EEG usually takes about one hour to complete. Careful pretest preparation of the patient is essential for accurate results. On the day of the test, no coffee, tea, cola drinks, or other stimulants are permitted. Alcohol, which as a depressant would affect the accuracy of the EEG, must also be avoided. The physician ordering the test must be informed of any medications the patient is taking as these can have profound effects on the EEG. After shampooing, no hair preparations should be used until after the tracing is made. Since part of the tracing may be made while you are asleep, it is helpful if no naps are taken on the day of the test.

Endoscopy

Endoscopy is a method of directly viewing the inside of hollow organs by inserting an endoscope (lighted tube) into the organ. Five common endoscopic examinations are described below, in order from the most frequently performed to the least frequently done.

Proctosigmoidoscopy

This is an examination of the rectum and colon for detection of cancers and other ailments of the lower 12 inches of the large intestine. In addition to cancer, the examination can reveal muscle tone, swollen veins (hemorrhoids), infected areas, anal fistulas (abnormal passages in the anus), rectal polyps (growths protruding from rectal wall), abnormal narrowing of the intestine, tumors, and foreign bodies, among other problems.

The examination is frequently recommended as part of any complete checkup. It is a must for anyone with rectal bleeding and/or a change in bowel habits. The examination usually takes place on a tilting-top table with the patient in the knee-chest position or lying in a head-down position. After a manual examination (insertion of the physician's finger into the anus), the doctor inserts a lubricated anuscope to examine closely the anus (the opening from the rectum to the outside). Then the sigmoidoscope (a lighted hollow rigid tube also known as a proctoscope) is inserted through the anal canal into the large intestine.

Patients are advised to prepare for this examination by eating a light diet for 24 to 48 hours before the test and by emptying the lower intestinal tract with one or two enemas. If a barium X ray of the colon is to follow the sigmoidoscopic examination (which it commonly does), a more detailed preparation involving laxatives and a number of enemas is undertaken.

There are few risks to a routine screening. Perforation of the colon is possible, but quite rare. There may be some discomfort or cramping during the examination, but there should be no actual pain.

Gastroscopy

Gastroscopy is an examination of the interior of the esophagus, stomach, and duodenum (the first part of the small intestine). The test is performed to detect and examine ulcers or tumors and to determine the cause of gastrointestinal bleeding or any other known or suspected abnormalities. The response of an ulcer to treatment can also be followed endoscopically rather than by X ray. Often during this procedure tissue samples (biopsies) are collected or stomach contents suctioned out for examination.

In the procedure, the throat is first anesthesized by a spray and/or gargle. The patient is then given a sedative to induce relaxation. A flexible lighted tube (the gastroscope) is then passed down the throat through the esophagus into the stomach and duodenum. The patient can have no solid food for the evening meal the night before the test is done. Water may be taken in the evening, but not on the day of or within eight hours prior to the test. Smoking is prohibited on the day of the test until the examination is completed, since smoking stimulates the stomach's secretion of gastric juices. Any other stimulation, such as alcohol, caffeine, or colas should also be avoided. There is little risk to this test (very rarely, there may be a risk of the gastroscope injuring or perforating an organ or of the patient vomiting and inhaling the contents of the stomach). The patient may experience a temporary sore throat afterward.

Colonoscopy

This procedure is similar to proctosigmoidoscopy except that the entire colon (large intestine) is examined, and the instrument is a long, flexible tube. Usually, colonoscopy is performed to detect and/or remove polyps (small growths), to biopsy tumors or suspicious areas, to look for sites of occult (hidden) or obvious bleeding, and to inspect the entire colon for inflammatory bowel disease. In this test the patient is asked to stay on a liquid diet for about 48 hours before the procedure. Laxatives and enemas are also given to cleanse the colon thoroughly. During the test mild sedatives are given to aid in relaxation. Some discomfort and cramping are common, but actual pain should not occur. The risks are mainly perforation and bleeding from the site of the biopsy or growth removal. However, both are uncommon.

Cystoscopy

Cystoscopy is the direct viewing of the interior of the urinary bladder, the urethra (the passageway from the bladder to the outside of the body), and part of the prostate gland in men. A flexible, lighted tube, called a cystoscope, is passed through the urethra into the bladder. The inside of the bladder and urethra are examined for cancer, polyps (growths), and other abnormalities. The procedure includes collecting tissue samples (biopsy), if indicated, for later examination. An overgrown prostate gland can also be "shaved down" through the cystoscope. This is referred to as a transurethral resection of the prostate and is considered a surgical procedure.

The male patient is usually given a sedative before the test and a spinal or general anesthetic during the procedure. Women frequently only need local anesthesia and often have the procedure done as outpatients. Men, however, generally enter the hospital for the procedure. There is little risk to the diagnostic cystoscopy, although there may be a slight chance of damage to the lining of the urethra, of perforation of the bladder, and of temporary retention of urine after the test.

Bronchoscopy

Bronchoscopy is the direct viewing of the trachea (windpipe), larynx (voice box), and bronchi, the breathing tubes through which air travels from the trachea into the lungs. This examination can be performed to pinpoint the cause of an unexplained persistent cough, wheeze, or pneumonia. It is also used to investigate an undiagnosed abnormality on a chest X ray or to diagnose a lung tumor. As with other forms of endoscopy, bronchoscopy may also be used to take a tissue sample or remove a small obstruction, such as a foreign body.

A lighted tube, either flexible or rigid and varying in diameter, is threaded from the mouth or nose through the trachea into the bronchi. Some bronchoscopes are small enough in diameter to offer a view of even the smallest structures in the bronchial tree. A sedative and topical anesthetic are used; the anesthetic may be in a spray form for the mouth and nose and in a lubricating jelly to protect and anesthesize the tissues of the nose and throat. The patient fasts for at least eight hours prior to the test. Patients with a history of heart disease or those over age 50 are frequently monitored with an electrocardiograph. There is a minor risk of possible damage to the teeth, throat, or bronchial structures, but damage to the respiratory tract is very rare. Bleeding from biopsy sites and areas of growth removal also occurs, but uncommonly. This procedure is almost always done in a hospital setting, but actual admission to the hospital is unnecessary in most cases.

Lumbar puncture

The lumbar puncture, also called spinal tap, is a procedure used to withdraw a small amount of cerebrospinal fluid from an area (the subarachnoid space) surrounding the spinal cord. The cerebrospinal fluid is then examined microscopically and analyzed chemically to detect conditions that may exist in the brain and spinal cord (both of which comprise the central nervous system). The conditions include bleeding, infections, and other abnormalities of the brain and spinal cord. Often the appearance of the fluid, which is normally crystal clear, will provide a preliminary diagnosis of a problem; if, for example, the fluid is cloudy, an infection may be indicated.

The patient usually lies on his or her side with knees drawn up sufficiently to bow the back. After a local anesthetic is administered, the subarachnoid space (where the cerebrospinal fluid circulates) is entered with a special needle inserted through the skin and soft tissues and between two of the lower lumbar vertebrae (backbones). The pressure of the cerebrospinal fluid in the central nervous system is measured with a manometer (an instrument for measuring the pressure of liquids and gases). The fluid is then allowed to drip into a series of small, sterile test tubes.

Although patients are sometimes apprehensive about the lumbar puncture procedure, it is not usually painful. Headache after the tap is not uncommon. It is not possible, however, to predict who will develop one. It seems that maintaining a lying-flat position for an hour or so after the tap decreases the incidence of headache. Furthermore, if a headache should develop, lying flat seems to ease the pain.

There is a slight risk of nerve damage from the needle, but this is extremely rare. The site of the puncture is below the end of the spinal cord, so the cord itself cannot be injured in any way. In conditions in which pressure in the central nervous system is elevated, such as with a brain tumor or other mass, or if there is swelling of the brain because of disease or injury, a lumbar puncture may lead to a "dropping" of the brain downward. This is a serious complication, but fortunately a rare one. New procedures, such as computerized tomography (CAT scan) have minimized this problem by providing a noninvasive means of ruling out a large mass or swelling before performing a spinal tap. Also, as with any procedure that invades the body, there is a risk of infection, but the incidence of infections following lumbar punctures is quite low.

Pulmonary function tests

Pulmonary function testing (PFT) is a procedure to assess the physical functioning of the lungs, especially lung capacity. The results of this group of tests often reveal the existence of various diseases of the lungs, including asthma and emphysema. Diseases that cause restriction of lung movement can also be diagnosed and differentiated from those that cause airways obstruction, such as asthma. Pulmonary function tests are also used as a baseline to monitor the course of a disease and the effects of therapy.

The routine PFT is done with a spirometer; long tubes resembling vacuum-cleaner hoses are connected to a device that measures (in graphic form) the volume of air breathed in and out against time. The patient breathes into the spirometer according to instructions given during the test. The amount of air inhaled and exhaled as well as the rate of inhalation and exhalation are measured, and sometimes specific exhaled gases are also measured. Some pulmonary function tests also require a blood sample from an artery to determine if the arterial blood (freshly oxygenated in the lungs) has adequate oxygen and a normal concentration of carbon dioxide.

The test is painless and without risk, with the possible exceptions of discomfort during and complications after an arterial puncture for the blood sample.

Cardiac stress test

The stress test, also often called the treadmill test, is done basically to determine the reaction of the heart and circulatory system to physical exercise. Devices other than a treadmill, such as a bicycle, can also be used, depending on the situation. A stress test can be done for many reasons: to determine if the cause of chest pain is the heart; to detect the presence of coronary artery disease; and to follow the progress of a patient in cardiac rehabilitation, among others.

For this test, the patient is told to sleep well the night before the test and to eat lightly more than three hours before the test. At the lab the patient will put on exercise clothes and running shoes. The patient is questioned about recent medical history and exercise habits. An individual in good health who has not exercised for a long time may have a treadmill negative for coronary disease, but the test will indicate poor cardiovascular conditioning.

For the test, electrodes for continuous electrocardiogram are attached so that the tester (usually a cardiologist) can monitor the heart rate and the electrocardiographic response of the heart to graded exercise. A blood pressure cuff is also attached to an arm.

The patient is then started on the treadmill at a low work load. The work load (speed and incline of the treadmill) is then increased, usually at three-minute intervals until the patient either (1) attains about 90 percent of the predicted maximum heart rate for his or her age (obtained from standardized tables); (2) develops symptoms or electrocardiographic changes consistent with heart disease; or (3) cannot continue the test for any reason (for example, leg cramps or shortness of breath). The time it takes to reach the target heart rate is related to the degree of cardiovascular fitness, but not necessarily related to the presence or absence of heart disease. That is, an individual who attains his or her peak heart rate at only six minutes is less fit ("cardiovascular-wise") than someone who can exercise 12 minutes on the treadmill. Both, however, may or may not have changes or symptoms indicating heart disease. At the individual's maximum performance level, the closer he or she comes to the predicted maximum heart rate, the more meaningful the test. In other words, if one's age-predicted maximum is 180 beats per minute and the patient must stop at 130 beats because of a leg cramp, fatigue, or other non-cardiovascular reason, this test is considered "submaximal." In this case, the negative ECG (meaning there is no heart disease) carries less diagnostic importance than a negative ECG at a heart rate of 180 beats.

Stress tests may cause discomfort because of fatigue, tired muscles, and so forth. The main risk is of precipitating a cardiac event, such as arrhythmia (abnormal heart rhythm) or a coronary. In centers with well-trained and well-equipped staff, and with carefully chosen patients, these risks are minimized.

Tomography

Tomography is a type of X-ray examination in which the shadows in front of and behind the part of the body being studied are blurred out on the X-ray picture. Successive exposures are made at different depths within the structure of the body part under study and from different angles. The effect is the same as that achieved when a microscope is adjusted back and forth and up and down while looking at a piece of tissue: it is possible to get a picture of a structure at different levels, each one pinpointed and sharply focused.

Nowadays these multiple images can be fed into a computer that has been programmed to coordinate such data, and a cross-sectional "map" of the body part under study can be constructed in picture form. The expansion of computer capabilities has led to a high degree of sophistication in tomography, resulting in what is called "Computerized Axial Tomography" (also known as the CAT scan). As the name implies, the computer produces a tomographic picture of a body part with exposures taken around the axial or longitudinal line of the body (which is a line from the head to the toes that runs exactly through the center of the body).

The most widely known use of the CAT scan has been in the detection and description of brain disorders. However, in recent years this scanning technique has been extended to other parts of the body, so, for example, cross-sectional images of organs in the abdomen, such as the liver and pancreas, can now be produced. These scans are quite sensitive and have greatly aided the effort for early detection of tumors. One of the breakthroughs that has made this possible is the development of scanners that can complete their scan in five seconds or less. The brain scan does not require such fast scanning, since the head can be easily immobilized. The abdominal area, on the other hand, is in constant movement, because of the action of the stomach, the intestines, and the diaphragm. Consequently, the scan must be made fast enough to provide a clear image in the same way that a fast shutter speed on an ordinary camera can "stop" the motion of the subject. The test is painless, but there is a risk of radiation exposure. Also, intravenous X-ray contrast solution is used to enhance the picture. Persons with a sensitivity to the dye, kidney disease, or diabetes may be at risk of kidney damage or serious allergic-type reactions when contrast solution is used. These individuals should tell their physician of these facts so that adequate precautions can be taken to minimize the chance of complication. This type of testing is expensive and therefore not done routinely.

Computerized Tomography is known by a variety of names, depending on the method and the sequence of scanning: Computerized Axial Tomography (CAT), Computerized Transverse Axial Tomography (CTAT), Computer-Assisted Transaxial Tomography (CATT).

Ultrasonography

Ultrasonography, often called ultrasound, is a method of visualizing the deep structures of the body by recording the reflection off those structures of high-frequency sound waves. The procedure is painless and uses no radiation. Ultrasound, the sound range used in diagnostic procedures, is a vibration beyond the range of human hearing. Ultrasound diagnosis is based on interactions between the sound waves and biological structures in the human body.

The instrument used in ultrasonography is called a transducer. The transducer, placed over the area to be examined, directs ultrasonic waves at the tissue. The sounds returning from the internal structure are processed by machines that produce a multidimensional, detailed visualization of the structure. Formerly, only still pictures could be obtained. Now, however, moving pictures in "real time" are routinely done, as in pregnancy, when the baby's movements and beating heart can actually be seen.

The development of sonography as an alternate way of visualizing body structures reflects not only current technological advances, but also present-day concern about the potential dangers of over-reliance on X rays. Sonography offers an alternative to X rays in the examination of soft tissues in those cases in which X rays might be ineffective or potentially harmful. Another advantage is that sonography does not require invasive procedures (for example, injections, catheterization, incisions) or the use of contrast media such as opaque dyes. There is no known risk for sonography, although the long-term effects of sound waves have not been determined.

Tests for women

Amniocentesis

Amniocentesis is the surgical penetration through the abdomen of the pregnant uterus and the amniotic sac surrounding the unborn baby in order to withdraw some amniotic fluid to be tested. The analysis of amniotic fluid is useful in determining the condition and health of the fetus (unborn baby), since the amniotic fluid contains cells that normally are discarded by the baby. Examination of these cells for chromosomal and chemical makeup can detect numerous genetic defects and hereditary disorders. Testing certain chemicals in the fluid itself is done to determine fetal lung maturity and to detect certain fetal abnormalities, such as spina bifida. The fetal cells will also indicate the sex of the baby. Identifying the sex of the baby before birth may be important when a sex-linked hereditary disorder (such as hemophilia, a blood-clotting disease occurring almost exclusively in males) is suspected. However, amniocentesis is never performed simply to satisfy curiosity about the sex of a baby. In fact, the test is not routine; it is performed most often in pregnant women over the age of 35 or with a family history of certain hereditary disorders. The incidence of chromosome abnormalities of the fetus increases rapidly after a woman reaches the age of 35. As each year passes, the chances of chromosome abnormalities increase.

The sample of amniotic fluid is obtained by inserting a hollow needle through the mother's abdomen into the uterus and amniotic sac and drawing out fluid with a syringe attached to the needle. The procedure should be relatively painless since a local anesthetic is used around the injection site. The test is usually done around the sixteenth to eighteenth week of pregnancy (before this time the test results are inconclusive), but final results are often not available for about three to four weeks. Therefore, the waiting period can be the most difficult part of the test. However, studies have shown that approximately 95 percent of amniocentesis results are normal.

There is some risk to this test, which is why it is not routinely used. There is a risk of miscarriage as well as a chance of striking the placenta or baby. However, much of the risk is minimized, or even eliminated, by the use of ultrasonography to reveal the position of both the fetus and placenta before the needle is inserted. In addition, as with any technique that invades the body, there is a chance of infection. A patient experiencing any pain, fever, or discharge from the puncture site or from the vagina should notify her doctor.

Mammography

Mammography is a simple, painless examination of the breasts by means of a special X-ray machine that is specially designed to be used for soft tissue. This procedure is especially valuable for the detection of early breast cancers before they can be manually felt by the woman or her doctor. Mammography can also differentiate between malignant (cancerous) and nonmalignant (noncancerous) lumps and can provide information about fibrocystic breast disease.

Many medical experts recommend that a baseline mammogram (of the normal breasts) be made when a woman is around the age of 40. This can later be used for comparison purposes if subsequent mammograms reveal changes in the breasts. After the first mammogram, it is recommended that the test be repeated every one to five years, depending on individual risk factors such as a family history of breast cancer. Some doctors suggest a mammogram every year for women past the age of 50 regardless of risk factors. However, a mammogram should not replace a monthly breast self-examination nor regular breast examinations by a doctor; rather, the mammogram should be done in conjunction with these manual examinations.

Other related techniques for breast examination are xerography and thermography. Xerography is a form of mammography that records the image using a photo-electric process rather than standard X-ray film. Thermography is a diagnostic technique that, unlike mammography and xerography, uses no X rays and thus can be repeated as often as desired. Thermography records any variations in the temperature of various parts of the breast.

The basic premise of thermography is that rapidly growing cancer cells give off more heat than does normal tissue. Thermography, however, is not as accurate as mammography and should only be used to augment information obtained from a physical examination and a mammogram.

There is some question about the risk of radiation exposure in mammography, especially for those women who receive a yearly mammogram. The radiation dosage has been reduced in modern testing, and many physicians feel that because of this the benefits of early detection outweighs any risks. However, most doctors are conservative about the use of mammography, and a woman should discuss the benefits and risks of this test procedure with her doctor who knows her medical history. It is important to remember, too, that mammography should not be used on a pregnant woman; the radiation may be harmful to the unborn baby.

Pap test

The Pap test (abbreviation of Papanicolaou, the scientist who developed the test) is a standard part of the gynecological examination for women. It is used to detect early cell changes that might indicate cancer or other abnormalities of the cervix, the neck of the uterus.

The Pap test involves scraping a smear of cells from the surface of the external area where the cervix opens into the vagina. The scraping is done with a small plastic spatula and the scrapings are spread to dry on a glass slide. The test is painless, and there is no risk.

The test results are categorized into five groups: Class I—no abnormal cells; Class II–atypical cells, usually caused by inflammation or infection; Class III—cells suspected to be cancerous; and Classes IV and V–cancer cells present. In some laboratories, a modification of this classification system is used so that the report simply states that the smear is negative, doubtful, unsatisfactory, or positive.

A woman should have her first Pap test at about 18 years of age, and then every one to two years. Women over age 40 should have an annual test. Any woman with a history of cervical or uterine cancer or of abnormal Pap tests should have the test done every six months.

Pelvic examination

The pelvic examination is a physical and visual inspection of the female reproductive tract. It is done to assess the condition of and to detect disorders in the reproductive organs, including the vagina, cervix, uterus, and ovaries. A pelvic examination can also reveal pregnancy.

The patient lies on an examination table and places her heels in metal holders resembling the stirrups on a horse's saddle. The doctor inserts into the vagina a speculum, a special instrument that expands the vagina to permit visual examination of the vagina and cervix. After removing the speculum the doctor will also insert two fingers into the vagina while simultaneously pressing lightly on the patient's abdomen. This procedure enables the doctor to feel the uterus and ovaries and detect any abnormalities in these organs. Sometimes the doctor also inserts a finger into the rectum while pressing on the abdomen; this, too, enables the doctor to feel the uterus and ovaries.

A pelvic examination takes only a few minutes, is painless, and has no risk.

What you need to know about prescription drugs

Because of the variety of drugs now available, both over the pharmacy counter and also by prescription from our physicians, a wide range of illnesses and disorders can be controlled, relieved, or even cured. We can control hypertension, eliminate the irritating effects of allergies and hay fever, relieve cold discomfort, cure a variety of stomach and intestinal disorders, control stress and insomnia, and end bacterial and fungal infections—all by taking a medication.

Along with the benefits of modern drug therapy, however, comes responsibility. There is a great deal that the informed patient ought to know about the medicine he or she is taking: how to take it; how often to take it; what its possible side effects can be; and how it might react with other medications, foods, or alcohol. In short, there's a wealth of information that can help you in buying, using, understanding, and taking the drugs and medications that you need for your continuing good health.

The process of buying and taking a drug starts when your doctor writes out a prescription. The choice of drug is determined by many facts you have already told your doctor, including information about drugs that you have taken at various times in your life, any allergic reactions you might have suffered, any chronic conditions for which you are still taking medication, any special side effects that you have experienced with certain drugs or classes of drugs, and any chronic health problems you have. Based on this information, the doctor makes a decision as to what he or she thinks is the right drug for your particular condition. The doctor's part of the process is now complete; your part is just beginning.

You need to know many facts before you take your first pill or swallow your first tablespoon of medicine. You need to know how to administer the medicine. You need to understand the dosage schedule: how often you're to take the drug, how much each time, whether to schedule medication at night as well as in the daytime. You need to know something about common side effects in order to distinguish between those that are truly "minor side effects" and those that are signs that a serious drug reaction may be taking place. You need to know whether or not you should continue the medicine after your symptoms have completely disappeared, or whether you should stop the medication when you no longer show symptoms. You need to know if the drug might interact negatively with other drugs you are taking (even nonprescription drugs, such as cold pills, aspirin, or vitamins), with alcohol, with caffeine, with other foods, and, if you are a woman on the birth control pill, with your own brand of oral contraceptive. You need to know the possible consequences of overdosage or underdosage. In short, you need to know answers to many questions in order to assume responsibility for taking your prescription drugs.

As you read on, you will learn how some common types of drugs work to relieve certain conditions or symptoms. You will learn how to read a prescription correctly and how to buy, store, and use drugs. You will learn how to administer the most common forms of medication either to yourself or to someone else. You will learn how to save money, in many cases, by substituting a less expensive generic drug for a more expensive trade name or brand name medication. Finally, you will learn to identify some common side effects of the most widely-used prescription drugs and to recognize symptoms that will help you decide when your drug response is not a cause for concern and when it calls for prompt medical attention.

As with other sections of the book, this section is not a substitute for informed advice from your doctor and pharmacist. You should keep these two persons informed at all times of your condition and of any reactions you are experiencing, as well as of other medication you take on a regular basis. You should also consult your doctor or pharmacist about the latest information about your medications; although every effort has been made to assure that the information here is up-to-date, new developments occur rapidly in drug research. What this section can do, however, is help you to work better with both pharmacist and doctor or other health care professionals in becoming a wise, well-informed, and aware patient who receives the maximum benefits from his or her medication and treatment.

How drugs work

Prescription drugs may fall into any one of a number of different categories, depending on their use and the kind of condition they are commonly prescribed for. For example, one category of drugs is prescribed for the cardiovascular (circulatory) system, another for the eyes, another for the ears, another for the respiratory system, and so on. This section describes the various classes of drugs, their therapeutic effects, and how they work to correct your condition or illness.

Cardiovascular drugs

Anti-anginals

The type of chest pain known as angina pectoris (or simply angina) is caused by an insufficient supply of blood, and consequently of oxygen, to the heart. Anti-anginal drugs cause a drop in blood pressure and allow an increased amount of oxygen to enter certain parts of the heart. A frequently prescribed anti-anginal is nitroglycerin.

Anti-arrhythmics

The condition called arrhythmia is characterized by lack of a smooth, steady rhythm in the heartbeat. Anti-arrhythmics are the drugs prescribed to remedy this condition by regulating the heartbeat. The most common anti-arrhythmics are Inderal, Norpace, Pronestyl, and quinidine sulfate. Another drug, Dilantin (or phenytoin) can become an anti-arrhythmic drug when injected intravenously; it is normally used as an anticonvulsant in treating epilepsy.

Antihypertensives

High blood pressure, or hypertension, is a condition in which the pressure of the blood against the walls of the blood vessels is higher than normal (that is, does not fall within normal ranges for a person's age and sex). High blood pressure, fortunately, can be controlled which in turn can control other diseases or conditions linked to hypertension. This is a vital class of drugs, for antihypertensives, by counteracting and reducing high blood pressure, can help to prolong a hypertensive's life and improve the general state of his or her health.

Antihypertensive drugs can work in a variety of different ways. Some antihypertensives block the nerve impulses that cause the arteries to constrict. Some actually slow the heart rate and reduce the force of its contractions. Others may lower the amounts of a hormone that causes the blood pressure to increase. Often, antihypertensive therapy is built around diuretics, drugs that reduce body fluids (see next category).

Examples of common antihypertensive drugs include Aldomet, Aldoril, Apresoline, Catapres, Dyazide, Diupres, Hydropres, Minipress, reserpine, Salutensin, and Ser-Ap-Es.

Diuretics

Diuretics, or "water pills," are widely used in the treatment of hypertension since they lower blood pressure by encouraging the loss of water and salt through increased urination (excessive salt in the body can increase blood pressure). Often, antihypertensive drugs are used along with diuretics. There are many types of diuretics, each with its own specific action, so that diuretic therapy can be individualized to suit a patient's needs.

Thiazide diuretics are among the most popular "water pills" that are available today. They rarely become toxic, usually have minimal side effects, and can be taken once or twice a day. Thiazide diuretics are effective all day, unlike other types of diuretics, which have a shorter period of effectiveness. Also, patients do not develop a tolerance for their antihypertensive effect, so the therapy can be continued over a longer period of time. However, a major drawback is their tendency to deplete potassium stores in the body—a problem that can be corrected with a potassium supplement (K-Lor or Slow-K) or with potassium-rich foods and drinks, such as bananas, apricots, and orange juice, or with the use of potassium-containing salt substitutes. Diuril is an example of a mild thiazide diuretic.

Loop diuretics are more potent than the thiazides. They promote more water loss but also deplete more potassium. Lasix is a loop diuretic.

In recent years, manufacturers have developed potassium-sparing diuretics that remove the excess water without depleting the body's potassium stores. These potassium-sparing diuretics (Aldactone, for example) help in the treatment of heart failure, high blood pressure, and low potassium levels in the body. Also, in such medications as Aldactazide and Dyazide, potassium-sparing diuretics and thiazide diuretics are combined to enhance the antihypertensive effect and reduce the loss of potassium.

The most common diuretics are Aldactazide, Aldactone, Diuril, Dyazide, Enduron, Esidrix, hydrochlorothiazide, HydroDiuril, Hygroton, Lasix, Regroton, and Zaroxolyn.

Digitalis

Drugs that are derivatives of digitalis, such as digoxin or Lanoxin, affect the heart rate. However, they are not considered in the strict sense to be antiarrhythmics. Digitalis slows the heart rate but at the same time increases the force of the heart's contractions. It is often used to regulate an erratic heart rhythm or to strengthen heart output in cases of heart failure.

Anticoagulants

Anticoagulants are drugs that prevent blood clotting. There are two categories of anticoagulants: heparin anticoagulants, which must be given by injection (usually reserved for patients hospitalized with a heart attack, stroke, pulmonary embolism, or thrombophlebitis), and oral anticoagulants, generally derivatives of the drug warfarin. These anticoagulants are used to treat strokes, heart attacks, and abnormal blood clotting, as well as to prevent the movement of a blood clot in a critical position in the body.

The use of warfarin after a heart attack remains controversial; some physicians believe that anticoagulants are not useful after the first month or two following a heart attack.

There are some special precautions that patients on warfarin must observe. They must avoid taking many other drugs, including aspirin, because their interaction with warfarin could cause internal bleeding. Patients on warfarin are advised to have blood samples checked regularly by their doctors.

Antilipidemics

Antilipidemics are drugs that are used to treat arteriosclerosis, or hardening of the arteries, by reducing the cholesterol and trigylcerides (fats) that form plaques on the arterial walls. Atromid-S is one of the most common of these drugs. Many physicians, however, question the value of the antilipidemics; a low-fat diet and a good exercise program with emphasis on cardiovascular fitness and general weight reduction may be quite as beneficial in the long run.

Vasodilators

Vasodilating drugs are drugs that cause the blood vessels to enlarge. Vasodilators are used in the treatment of stroke and disorders characterized by poor circulation. Hydergine (used to treat the symptoms of senility) and Pavabid (used in post-stroke therapy) are two examples of vasodilators. Neither drug, however, has been proven effective, both are expensive, and the use of both is still controversial in medical circles.

Beta blockers

Beta blocking drugs are medications that "block" the heart's response to stimulation, thus slowing the heart rate and reducing high blood pressure. Propranolol (Inderal), metoprolol (Lopressor), nadolol (Corgard), pindolol (Visken), atenolol (Tenormin), and timolol (Blocadren) are all examples of beta blockers, used chiefly in the treatment of angina, high blood pressure, and cardiac arrhythmias (heartbeat irregularities), as well as after a heart attack.

Gastrointestinal drugs

Antinauseants

Antinauseants are exactly what the name implies: drugs that are used to reduce the urge to vomit. Antihistamines are used to prevent nausea and vomiting especially when these symptoms are caused by motion sickness (plane, train, car, or water travel).

Non-antihistamine antinauseants are also used—chiefly, phenothiazine derivatives, such as Compazine. It usually alleviates acute nausea and vomiting within a short time—from a few minutes to an hour.

Anticholinergics

Anticholinergic drugs, such as Librax and Pro-Banthine, slow the action of the bowel by relaxing the intestinal muscles and relieving muscle spasms and cramps. Thus they have an antispasmodic action. They also work to lower the amount of stomach acid present.

Antidiarrheals

Antidiarrheals work to slow the action of the bowel and reduce the frequency of bowel movements. Common antidiarrheals include narcotics, such as paregoric, and anticholinergics, such as atropine. Lomotil, a popular antidiarrheal, is a combination of a narcotic and an anticholinergic.

Anti-ulcer medications

Anti-ulcer drugs relieve the symptoms and promote healing of an ulcer. Tagamet, an antisecretory drug, suppresses the production of excess stomach acid. Carafate, another anti-ulcer medication, works by forming a chemical barrier over an ulcer to protect the ulcer from stomach acid. Both of these drugs promote healing of the ulcer while providing relief of pain.

Respiratory drugs

Antitussives

Antitussives are drugs that control coughs and thus are popularly known as cough medicine. The narcotic codeine is an antitussive; dextromethorphan is a non-narcotic antitussive. Cough medicines do not coat the throat. Instead, most cough drops and syrups must be absorbed into the blood and circulate through the brain before they can act to control a cough. They should be taken with a glass of water in order to speed this absorption process.

Expectorants

Expectorants are used to change a "nonproductive" cough to a "productive" one—that is, a cough that brings up phlegm into the throat. Expectorants supposedly increase the amount of mucus produced; however, their effectiveness has yet to be proved. Drinking water or using a vaporizer/humidifier is equally effective with most coughs. Two popular expectorants are Ambenyl and Phenergan Expectorant.

Decongestants

The decongestants are agents that constrict the blood vessels in the nose and sinuses and thus open up air passages. These agents can be taken orally or in the form of nose drops or nose sprays. The oral decongestants are slow-acting and they can increase the blood pressure; however, they have the advantage of not interfering with the production of mucus or the movement of the cilia (tiny hair-like processes of the respiratory tract). Nose drops and sprays provide immediate relief and do not increase blood pressure as much as the oral form, but they do slow the movement of the cilia. It should be remembered that persons who use decongestants regularly develop a tolerance for them rather quickly. It is recommended that they be used for only a few days at a time.

Bronchodilators

Bronchodilators are drugs that relax airways in the lungs. They are often prescribed in combination with smooth muscle relaxants, or agents that relax the smooth muscle tissues of the body—in this case, the smooth muscle tissues of the lungs. Bronchodilators include aminophylline, theophylline, Elixophyllin, Slo-Phyllin, and Brethine. Quibron is a smooth muscle relaxant that is used to treat asthma and pulmonary emphysema.

Allergy medications

The allergy medications most often used are antihistamines, which, as the name suggests, counteract the effects of histamine, a chemical released in the body that causes swelling and itching. Severe allergy attacks are best treated with injectable epinephrine, or adrenaline, which is fast and potent for severe allergic symptoms. For mild or chronic respiratory allergies (for example, hay fever or pollen allergies), slower-acting, less potent antihistamines like Benadryl can be used.

Central nervous system drugs

Sedatives and hypnotics

The drugs that are commonly used in the treatment of anxiety and/or insomnia work to reduce selectively central nervous system activity. Anxiety-reducing drugs include Atarax, barbiturates, Equanil, Valium, Tranxene, Sinequan, Serax, Miltown, and Librium. Common sleep-inducing drugs are Dalmane, Butisol Sodium, and Seconal. The actions of all the drugs listed above are similar, but those that are used to induce sleep (the hypnotics) are the more powerful of the two.

Tranquilizers/antipsychotic agents

Drugs known variously as tranquilizers or antipsychotic agents calm the activity of certain areas of the brain but allow the rest to function normally; in other words, they act as a screening device to allow the transmission of some nerve impulses and to restrict others. The most common tranquilizers include the phenothiazines: Mellaril, Stelazine, Thorazine, and Haldol, a butyrophenone with an action similar to Thorazine.

Antidepressants, such as Elavil or the monoamine oxidase inhibitors, are also used with psychotic patients to help combat severe depression. The antidepressants must be used with great caution, since they often produce dangerous side effects and can interact with other drugs in harmful ways. The monoamine oxidase inhibitors must be used with particular care because they can interact with certain cheeses and other foods and beverages to increase blood pressure to dangerously high levels.

Anorectics

Anorectic drugs, or appetite suppressants, reduce appetite by quieting the part of the brain that causes hunger. As side effects, however, they may cause or increase sleeplessness, raise the blood pressure, and accelerate the heartbeat. Generally, they lose their effectiveness after a two- to three-week period. Once widely used as "diet pills," the anorectics (largely amphetamines) have fallen into disfavor because of these side effects.

While most people are stimulated into activity by amphetamines, hyperkinetic (hyperactive) children are calmed by them. Both amphetamines and the adrenergic Ritalin slow down the normal pace of hyperactive youngsters for inexplicable reasons—probably because they selectively stimulate parts of the brain that ordinarily provide control of activity.

Anticonvulsants

Such drugs as Dilantin, Tegretol, Depakane, and phenobarbital are effective in controlling most of the symptoms, including convulsions, of epilepsy by selectively reducing excess stimulation in the brain.

Antiparkinson agents

Such drugs as Artane or Cogentin anticholinergics or levodopa are used to correct the chemical imbalance in the brain that causes Parkinson's disease. They also provide symptomatic relief for the tremors, characteristic stoop, and inability to walk well that are specific to Parkinson's disease. These drugs are also used, in other cases, to counterbalance the side effects of other drugs that are known to cause tremors.

Analgesics

Analgesics are drugs used to relieve pain, which is not a disease but a symptom or warning signal of a disease or other abnormal condition.

Analgesics can be either narcotic or non-narcotic. The narcotics are derived from the opium poppy and act on the brain to cause deep analgesia (absence of pain) and often drowsiness. Narcotics can relieve coughing spasms and are thus used in many cough syrups. Narcotics relieve pain within a short time span and also give the patient a feeling of well-being, but, unfortunately, are highly addictive. Attempts to produce synthetic narcotic derivatives which are non-addictive have so far failed.

The most common non-narcotic pain relievers are the salicylates (aspirin is the best-known example). The aspirin substitute acetaminophen, used in Tylenol, is often used instead of aspirin and is effective against headache and other minor pains. However, it cannot relieve arthritis-induced inflammation and is toxic to the liver in overdose. (Aspirin, too, can be fatal in overdose.)

Many analgesics contain codeine or another narcotic as well as analgesics such as aspirin or acetaminophen—for example, such drugs as Empirin with Codeine, Tylenol with Codeine, or Fiorinal with Codeine. While these analgesics are not as strong as the pure narcotics, they are often as effective and are potentially less addictive.

Anti-inflammatory drugs

Inflammation is the body's response to injury and causes pain, fever, itching, and redness as accompaniments to inflammatory swelling. Aspirin is among the most effective anti-inflammatory drugs, but there are other nonsteroid anti-inflammatories: Butazolidin, Dolobid, Feldene, Indocin, Motrin, Naprosyn, and Tolectin. Steroids are also used to relieve inflammation (see section on hormones).

Gout, an inflammatory disease resulting from excessive uric acid that causes swelling and pain in the toes and joints, is also treated effectively by other agents: Benemid uricosuric to stimulate the excretion of the uric acid in urine, colchicine antigout remedy (to prevent swelling), and Zyloprim (to decrease the body's production of uric acid). Colchicine is effective in relieving the pain of a gout attack, while Benemid and Zyloprim guard against gout attacks.

The analgesics called skeletal muscle relaxants, including Equagesic, Norgesic, and Parafon Forte, can relieve the pain of sore, tense, or inflamed muscles. Skeletal muscle relaxants such as these often are prescribed in combination with an anti-inflammatory drug such as aspirin.

Local anesthetics

Local anesthetics are also pain-relieving drugs which can be applied directly to a painful area to relieve localized pain, such as a toothache, earache, or hemorrhoidal pain. They are not effective, however, for major or generalized pain. Some of the local anesthetics, such as lidocaine, are often prescribed in the treatment of heart disease (given intravenously or by intramuscular injection), since they can restore the heartbeat to normal. One side effect of the local anesthetics is an allergic reaction—many people are allergic to these drugs.

Topical drugs

Topical drugs, applied directly to or on the affected area are used chiefly in the treatment of common skin problems, such as infections and inflammations. (Antibiotics in cream or ointment form can treat skin infections while steroid preparations treat inflammations.)

Another common skin problem, acne, can be treated with over-the-counter preparations but sometimes is serious enough to require prescription medicines —usually such antibiotics as the tetracyclines, erythromycin, or clindamycin, taken orally or applied topically. Sometimes keratolytics, or agents that soften the skin causing the outer cells to slough off, are also used. Retin-A, a skin irritant and derivative of Vitamin A in topical form, can also be used in the treatment of acne. Isotretinoin, which is also related to Vitamin A, is available in oral form as Accutane. It is used to treat severe cystic acne resistant to other forms of treatment.

Drugs for the ears

A physician treating an ear infection will usually prescribe two types of medication—an antibiotic and a steroid. A common treatment, for example, would be Cortisporin otic suspension. The antibiotic attacks the infecting bacteria while the steroid will reduce inflammation and/or pain. Local anesthetics such as benzocaine or lidocaine may also be used for pain.

If the problem is the result of impacted earwax, the earwax is usually removed or dissolved with Auralgan eardrops.

Drugs for the eyes

Almost all the drugs used to treat common eye infections and problems can be used in treating other areas of the body as well.

Antibiotics will usually cure common eye infections. Steroids (usually in the form of eyedrops or eye ointments) can treat eye inflammations, provided they are not used for too long a period of time. Pharmacists are particularly careful in refilling prescriptions for eyedrops containing steroids and often refuse a refill until the attending physician is consulted.

Glaucoma, an eye disorder caused by increased pressure within the eyeball because of fluid buildup, can be treated nonsurgically through the use of three eyedrops: epinephrine, pilocarpine, and timolol. Epinephrine is an adrenergic agent (which increases blood sugar, accelerates the heartbeat, and dilates the pupils of the eyes) while pilocarpine is a cholinergic drug, or a medication that stimulates the body's parasympathetic nerve endings (which assist in the control of the heart, lungs, bowels, and eyes). Timolol is a beta blocker that may reduce the fluid production in the eye.

Hormones

Hormones are substances that are produced and secreted by glands in order to stimulate certain bodily functions. Hormones in drug form imitate or "mimic" the effects of naturally-produced hormones in the body. The hormones that are commercially available include thyroid drugs, diabetic drugs, steroids, and sex hormones.

Thyroid drugs

The thyroid hormone was among the first synthetically-produced and marketed hormones. The first thyroid preparations were obtained by drying the thyroid glands of animals and pulverizing them into tablets; these preparations are still used for patients with reduced levels of thyroid production. However, a synthetic thyroid hormone called Synthroid is also available today.

Two other drugs, propylthiouracil and radioactive-iodine, are used to slow down thyroid hormone production in hyperthyroid patients (persons with excessive amounts of the hormone).

Antidiabetics

Diabetes is a condition in which the body is unable to produce and/or utilize insulin, a hormone secreted by the pancreas that regulates the level of sugar in the blood and also controls carbohydrate and fat metabolism. Glucagon is a substance that stimulates the liver to release stored glucose, or sugar; both insulin and glucagon are crucial in maintaining the proper blood sugar levels in the body.

Treating diabetes may involve adjusting the patient's diet and also administering insulin. Glucagon is usually given by injection only in emergencies—for example in the case of insulin shock when it is necessary to raise the patient's blood sugar level quickly.

A group of oral antidiabetic drugs, Diabinese, Orinase, and Tolinase, act on small groups of cells within the pancreas and stimulate the pancreas to produce more insulin. These oral antidiabetic drugs are normally used only by those diabetic patients whose pancreases still produce some amount of insulin. The oral antidiabetics cannot be used by "insulin-dependent" diabetics (juvenile-onset diabetics) whose condition can be controlled only by insulin injections.

Steroids

Steroids in their natural form are secreted by the adrenal glands, the glands lying above the kidneys. The process is simple: the pituitary gland secretes ACTH, or adrenocorticotropic hormone, which in turn stimulates the adrenal glands to produce steroids.

The main function of the steroids is to fight inflammation. ACTH is often injected directly in order to combat inflammatory diseases.

Such oral steroid preparations as Medrol and prednisone are often prescribed for inflammatory diseases such as arthritis or for minor inflammations, including poison ivy rashes or other rashes, hay fever, and insect bites. Topical steroid preparations or creams such as Kenalog and Lidex may also be applied directly to the skin for local irritations and inflammations.

Sex hormones

The sex hormones are produced chiefly by the sex glands themselves, although the adrenal glands also secrete small amounts of these substances. Estrogens are the female hormones that are responsible for the development of secondary female sex characteristics (breast development, maintenance of the uterus lining, and enlargement of the hips during puberty). Progesterone, another female hormone, prepares the body for pregnancy.

Estrogen's corresponding male hormone is called testosterone, or androgen, and is responsible for male secondary sex characteristics such as beards, enlarged muscles, and deeper voice. Testosterone is responsible for the retention of protein in the body, leading to increased muscle size. Because of this effect, athletes, especially professional bodybuilders, often take drugs called anabolic steroids, which are similar in effect to testosterone, but these drugs can adversely affect the heart, kidneys, and nervous system.

Most of the commercially available oral contraceptives contain a combination of estrogen and progesterone, although some (especially the so-called "mini-pills") contain only progesterone. The estrogen in the pills prevents the production and release of the egg. The progesterone content also aids in preventing ovulation, alters the uterus lining, and thickens the cervical mucus secretions, all of which prevents conception. Oral contraceptives are prescription-only drugs and because of their side effects should be taken only under medical supervision.

Premarin estrogen hormone is used to treat some of the unpleasant symptoms of menopause, such as hot flashes and drying of the vaginal secretions. Provera progesterone hormone is often prescribed for menstural problems and abnormal uterine bleeding.

Anti-infectives

Antibiotics

Antibiotics are a specific kind of antibacterial drug (drugs used to combat bacterial infections). Antibiotics can either be derived from molds or synthetically produced; as drugs, they are capable of destroying or prohibiting the growth of bacteria and fungi.

Although antibiotics are very effective in treating bacteria infections, they are not effective in fighting viral infections such as the common cold virus. Their use in cold therapy is not recommended.

The common antibiotics include aminoglycosides, cephalosporins, erythromycins, penicillins (including ampicillin and amoxicillin), and the tetracyclines.

Antibiotics must be taken properly with great care to follow the physician's specific instructions. An antibiotic must be taken regularly for the prescribed period of time. If the patient does not take the antibiotic regularly for the prescribed period, the infection may not be eliminated and microorganisms that are resistant to the antibiotic may appear.

Chemotherapeutics

The chemotherapeutics are another group of drugs that are used to treat infections; this group includes synthetically produced drugs like the sulfonamides (Gantrisin) and the nitrofurantoins (Macrodantin).

The antineoplastics are other chemotherapeutic agents used specifically in the treatment of cancer. Although they are highly toxic and cause serious side effects, the benefits in certain cancer patients outweigh the risks.

Antivirals

Antivirals are drugs used to combat virus infections. For example, an antiviral called Zovirax reduces the reproduction of the herpes virus in the initial stages and generally speeds up the healing of the herpes blisters. However, this antiviral does not "cure" herpes; rather, it lessens the severity of the disease.

Vaccines

Vaccines contain weakened or dead disease-causing microorganisms that stimulate the body's defense system to produce a natural immunity or resistance to a specific disease (polio, measles, diphtheria, for example). A vaccine is most commonly used as a preventive against a specific disease, although some are used to alleviate or treat infectious diseases.

Antifungals and other anti-infectives

Fungal infections are treated with antifungal drugs, such as Mycostatin and other drugs that destroy fungi and prevent their growth. Anthelmintics are used to treat worm infestations. Pediculocides treat lice infestations and scabicides cure scabies.

Vitamins and minerals

Vitamins and minerals are not drugs at all, but are chemical substances which help maintain normal body functions. Fortunately, most vitamins and minerals are readily available in a normal diet; true vitamin deficiencies are actually quite rare except for persons with severely restricted diets. Patients whose diet is restricted for weight loss programs or for the treatment of certain disorders or illnesses and some pregnant and breast-feeding women may benefit from vitamin and mineral supplements, as may some persons engaged in strenuous athletics. However, even these patients should consult a doctor to see if there is a true vitamin or mineral deficiency.

How to read and understand your prescription

Part of the process of becoming an educated participating patient is to understand as much as possible about the medications you are taking. This process starts in the doctor's office. Make sure that you understand what medication is prescribed for you, how often and how it should be taken, and for how long. Ask specifically if you should continue the medication once the symptoms subside. Some drugs, such as antibiotics, should be taken for a certain minimum period of time, even though all the symptoms have disappeared. Other drugs should be discontinued when the symptoms subside. Make sure, too, that you understand your dosage schedule, any precautions you need to take to prevent or reduce possible side effects, and how (if at all) you should alter your normal eating or drinking habits while you are on the medication. You should also learn what side effects are to be expected that are within the "normal" range and which ones are signals that you need to consult your doctor again. Be sure that you know and understand all of these facts before you leave your doctor's office.

A more detailed step by step review will be helpful.

Step 1: Read your prescription

You cannot be sure that your prescription has been filled correctly unless you can read it, so your first step is to read the prescription. There is nothing mysterious or secret about a prescription; the "indecipherable" notations are simply abbreviations of Latin and/or Greek words and phrases (actually, holdovers from a time when doctors wrote in Latin). The chart below will help you understand the abbreviations—for example, "gtts" is an abbreviation for Latin *guttae*, or "drops," "ut dict" is from *ut dictum* meaning "as directed" and "bid" stands for the Latin *bis in die*, or "twice daily."

Once you have familiarized yourself with this simple table, you will be able to check your actual prescription with the label on the drug container to make sure that the two coincide. The chart lists the most commonly used symbols and abbreviations that doctors use in writing prescriptions. Read it; then check your skills by reading the sample prescription reproduced in this book.

Common abbreviations and symbols used in writing prescriptions

Abbreviation	Meaning	Derivation and notes
A_2	both ears	*auris* (Latin)
aa	of each	*ana* (Greek)
ac	before meals	*anti cibum* (Latin)
AD	right ear	*auris dextra* (Latin)
AL	left ear	*auris laeva* (Latin)
AM	morning	*ante meridiem* (Latin)
AS	left ear	*auris sinistra* (Latin)
bid	twice a day	*bis in die* (Latin)
$\bar{c}$	with	*cum* (Latin)
cap	capsule	—
cc or cm^3	cubic centimeter	30 cc equal one ounce
disp	dispense	—
dtd#	give this number	*dentur tales doses* (Latin)
ea	each	—
ext	for external use	—
gtts	drops	*guttae* (Latin)
gutta	drop	*gutta* (Latin)
h	hour	*hora* (Latin)
HS	bedtime	*hora somni* (Latin)
M ft	make	*misce fiat* (Latin)
mitt#	give this number	*mitte* (Latin)
ml	milliliter	30 ml equal one ounce
O	pint	*octarius* (Latin)
O_2	both eyes	*oculus* (Latin)
OD	right eye	*oculus dexter* (Latin)
OJ	orange juice	—
OL	left eye	*oculus laevus* (Latin)
OS	left eye	*oculus sinister* (Latin)
OU	each eye	*oculus uterque* (Latin)
pc	after meals	*post cibum* (Latin)
PM	evening	*post meridiem* (Latin)
po	by mouth	*per os* (Latin)
prn	as needed	*pro re nata* (Latin)
$\bar{q}$	every	*quaqua* (Latin)
qd	once a day	*quaqua die* (Latin)
qid	four times a day	*quater in die* (Latin)
qod	every other day	—
$\bar{s}$	without	*sine* (Latin)
Sig	label as follows	*signetur* (Latin)
sl	under the tongue	*sub lingua* (Latin)
SOB	shortness of breath	—

Common abbreviations and symbols used in writing prescriptions

Abbreviation	*Meaning*	*Derivation and notes*
sol	solution	—
ss	half unit	*semis* (Latin)
stat	at once, first dose	*statim* (Latin)
susp	suspension	—
tab	tablet	—
tid	three times a day	*ter in die* (Latin)
top	apply topically	—
ung or ungt	ointment	*unguentum* (Latin)
UT	under the tongue	—
ut dict	as directed	*ut dictum* (Latin)
x	times	—

Step 2: Try reading a sample prescription

The sample prescription reproduced here is for Darvon Compound-65 (appearing on the prescription as Darvon cpd-65). The prescription tells the pharmacist to give you 24 capsules (#24). It also directs you to take one capsule (cap i) every four hours (q4h) as needed (prn) for pain. In the space for refills the prescription indicates that you should receive up to five refills (5x) and that the label on the drug container states the name of the drug (LABEL-yes). It also gives your name and address, perhaps your age, the date of the prescription, and the name of the physician. Many physicians' prescription blanks will also give their office address and telephone number in case the pharmacist needs to call for clarification on anything.

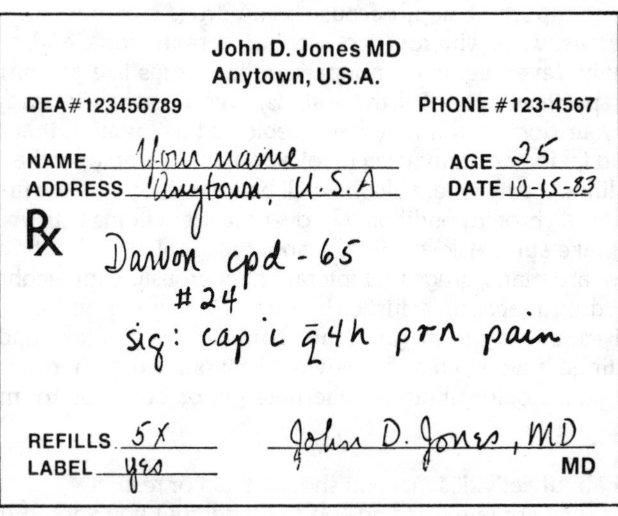

John D. Jones MD
Anytown, U.S.A.

DEA#123456789 PHONE #123-4567

NAME Your name AGE 25
ADDRESS Anytown, U.S.A DATE 10-15-83

℞ Darvon cpd-65
#24
sig: cap i q̄4h prn pain

REFILLS 5X
LABEL yes

John D. Jones, MD
MD

Step 3: Talk with your pharmacist

Once you have read the prescription, you may feel that you understand the instructions. But you may not understand them clearly enough. Using the sample Darvon prescription as an example, the prescription states that you can take one capsule every four hours as needed. What does "as needed" mean? Surely you shouldn't take a capsule each hour even if you feel you need one. How many capsules is your maximum for the day—four, five, six? You need to know your per day limit on this prescription.

As another example, suppose your prescription states that you should "take one tablet four times a day." Does that mean one tablet every six hours around the clock (which means getting up at night to take a tablet) or one tablet in the early morning, one at noon, one in the late afternoon or early evening, and one at bedtime? For other medications, it might mean one tablet every hour for the first four hours after arising in the morning. If you are confused about these instructions, be sure to ask the pharmacist while you are there in the pharmacy. He or she can always call the physician for clarification if necessary.

Step 4: Check with your pharmacist about how to take this medication

For some medications, it makes a difference as to whether you take the drug before a meal, after a meal, or along with it. *When* you take the drug can make an important difference; often the drug's effectiveness depends upon following exactly the directions for its use. Your pharmacist can help you understand directions such as "as directed," "as needed," and "take with fluid." For example, with some drugs you may take water, while with others you should take milk or fruit juice. Some diuretics, for example, should be taken with orange, other citrus, or tomato juice to decrease potassium loss, since these foods have natural potassium. And be sure to check on the maximum number of doses per day if your prescription simply says "as needed."

Step 5: Ask about any foods, beverages, or other drugs that you should avoid

This is a very important step, because some drugs may interact in negative, even dangerous, ways with tobacco, alcohol, certain foods, and/or drugs you habitually take (even common nonprescription drugs like aspirin). Ask your pharmacist specifically about all these items, even if you have already discussed them with your doctor. You may have neglected to mention that you will be traveling and taking an antinausea medication, for example, or that you will be going to a dinner party where alcohol will be served, or that you take a certain medication for a chronic condition. Go over the list of items with your pharmacist just to make sure. Ask specifically about alcohol and about avoiding any foods. There are many drugs that interact dangerously with alcohol, so don't become a "drug reaction" statistic. If you are a woman and are taking oral contraceptives, be sure to mention the contraceptive you take and ask if you should continue it along with the new medication. If the pharmacist says no, check with your doctor about an alternate pill or birth control method that is safe.

Step 6: Ask about activities that you should avoid or restrict

Some drugs now contain warnings on the label that you should not drive or operate equipment/machinery because the drug causes drowsiness and slowed reactions. Even if your medication does not carry such a warning, ask anyway. Drowsiness is a common side effect and, in a driver, can be lethal. Also ask if you need to restrict travel or exposure to sun. Some drugs, especially in combination with other drugs, cause *photosensitivity* (sensitivity to light—that is, to sun) and you may end up with an uncomfortable rash and other side effects.

Step 7: Make sure you know how long to continue the medication
The length of time you need to take a medication varies with your condition and also with the drug itself. In some cases, it is advisable to stop the drug as soon as your symptoms disappear in order to minimize side effects or, in some cases, to avoid building up a tolerance to the drug. In other cases, you should continue taking the drug for a specified length of time regardless of whether or not you are free from symptoms. In some special cases, such as kidney infection, the treatment is long-range and you'll need to take the medication for several weeks or months.

Step 8: Be certain you are familiar with possible side effects
This is probably the most important step of all. Your doctor will probably have already mentioned possible side effects to you, but check again with your pharmacist. What are the most common side effects of this drug? Write down the list if you have trouble remembering. Which can you expect and which are rare? Which side effects are "just side effects" and nothing to be concerned about and which are serious? For example, the drug Butazolidin may cause a blood disorder and one of the first symptoms of that disorder is a sore throat. Thus your pharmacist will urge you to check with your doctor if you develop a sore throat in the course of your medication. (This topic is discussed in more detail in the section on managing side effects.)

Step 9: Learn how to store your medication
Finally, before you leave the drugstore or pharmacy, ask the pharmacist how to store the medication. This is important because many drugs can lose potency and therefore become ineffective if they are not stored correctly.

Most prescription drugs can be safely stored at room temperature, out of direct sunlight. (Even if your pills or tablets are in dark or colored bottles, keep them out of direct sunlight.)

There are some drugs that require refrigerator storage. However, "refrigerate" does not mean to store the drug in the freezer. Some medications, especially sugar-coated tablets, will crack if frozen and thawed; also some liquid medications will separate into layers and can't be remixed.

There are also some drugs that cannot be stored in the refrigerator at all—for example, a cough suppressant Tussionex, which thickens and ceases to pour when cold. Contrary to popular belief, nitroglycerin does not become more stable when refrigerated. In fact, it should not be refrigerated at all.

The bathroom medicine cabinet is not a good place to keep your medication, since the temperature and humidity changes in the bathroom can have adverse effects on the stability of many prescription drugs. Also, if there are small children in the house, a bathroom cabinet is an easily accessible place for them to reach and overdose on the drugs, which they may assume are candy or gum.

Remember to keep your medications away from children at all times. When you are finished with the prescription, flush the unused portion down the toilet or pour it in the sink. Discard capsules or tablets you no longer use. What is a small overdose to an adult can be fatal to a small child.

You will notice that prescription drugs have expiration dates on the container. This is a date established by the manufacturer to indicate a time beyond which the drug is no longer effective. In most cases the time is five years after the drug is made (not after it is purchased) and is based on the time by which 5 percent of the drug will have been lost or converted.

The expiration date on certain antibiotics, such as tetracycline, is very important, because after that date, the antibiotic becomes toxic. After the expiration date, tetracycline actually converts into another chemical that can damage the kidneys. Other antibiotics, such as penicillin, do not become toxic but completely lose their effectiveness and become worthless as medication.

Definitions of ideal storage temperatures

Cold	**Any temperature under 46°F (8°C)**
Refrigerator	**Any cold place where the temperature is between 36°-46°F (2°-8°C)**
Cool	**Any temperature between 46°-59°F (8°-15°C)**
Room temperature	**Temperature usually between 59°-86°F (15°-30°C)**
Excessive heat	**Any temperature above 104°F (40°C)**

Buying drugs: spending and saving money

Prescription drugs can be expensive. Therefore, you might want to ask your pharmacist about substituting a generic drug for your prescription medication, particularly if your drug therapy is a long-term affair.

A "generic" drug is one that is not protected by trademark registration. The generic name of a drug is like a shortened form of its chemical name so that any manufacturer can use this generic name when the drug is marketed (for example, many manufacturers make the drug called tetracycline).

Usually a manufacturer will use both a trade name and a generic name for a drug. A trade name is registered and reserved for the manufacturer who holds that trademark. Thus, to follow our example above, only Lederle Laboratories can call their tetracycline Achromycin, and only Upjohn can use the name Panmycin for the same drug. (If you're confused about what the trade name looks like, it is usually capitalized in print and will include the register symbol ® after it.)

It is not necessarily true that trade name drugs are made by large manufacturers and generic drugs by small ones. Often a manufacturer will market large quantities of a certain drug under a trade name and then sell the base chemical to several other companies, some of which will sell the drug generically while others will sell it under their own trade name.

The major difference in trade name and generic drugs is in cost. Generic drugs are usually priced lower than trademarked equivalents because they are less widely advertised. You should be aware, however, that not all drugs are available generically. Furthermore, not every generic drug is significantly cheaper than nor equivalent to the trademarked drug. You should seek your pharmacist's advice on these matters, since some trademarked drugs are superior to their generic equivalent, yet others are not significantly different either in quality or in price. Remember, however, that although the Food and Drug Administration reports that there is no evidence of "serious differences" between generic and trade name drugs, private research has demonstrated differences in quality between certain brands.

If you do find an acceptable, safe generic equivalent for your drug, your cost savings can be significant. One hundred capsules of Darvon Compound-65 analgesic may cost $12 to $15 while the generic equivalent can be bought for about $8. Pavabid vasodilator can cost $17 per 100 capsules, but the generic drug may be as low as $9 per 100.

In most states, it is now legal for consumers to inquire about and to request pharmacists to fill prescriptions with the cheapest generic brand. If this subsitution is not legal in your state, you might ask your doctor to prescribe drugs by their generic name so that the pharmacist will fill the prescription in this form. This is especially helpful if the medication is one that you take on a long-term or regular basis.

Your pharmacist can also help you save money by recommending the use of over-the-counter drugs (OTC drugs). These are, of course, drugs that can be purchased without a prescription and consequently can be sold anywhere. There are no legal requirements and no limitations on who can buy them.

In general, OTC drugs are safer to use than prescription drugs since they are less active or potent than those that require a doctor's signature. Often, a pharmacist—or even the doctor—can recommend an OTC drug that is less costly and potent, but as effective as a prescription medication. For example, aspirin, which is cheap and widely available, is a highly effective anti-inflammatory drug that can be used in the treatment of arthritis and other inflammatory diseases.

Finally, if you are on a medication for a long period of time or if you are very sensitive to drugs and suspect that you might react badly to one, you might wish to save money by purchasing larger or smaller quantities of the medication. In the first instance, patients with chronic conditions such as heart disease, high blood pressure, or diabetes may want to purchase medication in quantity. Generally, the price per dose decreases with the amount purchased. For example, a drug that costs 6¢ per tablet when bought in amounts of 25 or 30 tablets decreases to 4 to 5¢ per tablet when bought in bottles of 100 or more. Many doctors will prescribe one to six months' supply of drugs that you take regularly.

On the other hand, if you have a history of drug reactions or allergies and are concerned about the side effects of a certain drug, you might ask the pharmacist to fill one half or one quarter of the prescription to see if the drug "agrees" with you. You may have to pay more per dose when you buy in small amounts, but you will then have a chance to test the drug on yourself. Make sure that the pharmacist realizes that you took only half the prescription (or a third, or whatever) so that you can get the rest if you want it. For many drugs, however, you must get another prescription once any part of the first has been filled.

How to administer medication

If you want to receive full benefit from your medication, you must learn to administer it correctly. Otherwise, you waste your money and time and slow your own or your family member's recovery. Furthermore, improper administration of a drug may be dangerous, because some drugs become toxic when improperly used. It is important to learn how to use each type of medication, properly.

Liquids

Medication in liquid form can be used externally on the skin, placed into the eye, ear, nose or throat, or taken internally by mouth. So before you use any liquid medication, read the label carefully to see if there are specific directions as to how to take or apply the medicine.

Some liquid medications will contain specific directions such as shaking the container before measuring the dose. This is an important instruction. Some liquids contain particles that will settle to the bottom of the container so that it must be shaken each time you use it to assure the right amount of the active ingredient. If you don't shake before you pour, the drug becomes more concentrated as the amount of liquid decreases. Eventually, you get more active ingredients with each dose and perhaps even a toxic amount with the last few doses.

When you open a bottle of liquid medication, point it away from you, since some liquids may build up pressure inside the bottle. The liquid could spurt out and stain clothing or household items if the opening is pointed toward you.

If the liquid medication is intended to be applied directly to the skin, your pharmacist will probably have already given you instructions on application. If not, use a cotton pad or small gauze square and pour a small amount of the liquid onto the cotton or gauze. Don't use too large a piece of material or too much of the liquid will be absorbed and wasted. Don't pour the medicine into your cupped hand—it is too easy for spills to occur. If there is only a small area involved, a cotton-tipped applicator is recommended. Do *not* dip cotton-tipped applicators or pieces of gauze or cotton directly into the bottle; this might contaminate the rest of the medicine.

If your liquid medication is to be swallowed, measure it accurately. Your doctor means by "one teaspoonful" a 5 ml medical teaspoon. An ordinary kitchen teaspoon can contain anywhere from 2 to 10 ml of liquid. Ask your pharmacist for a medical teaspoon or use a measuring spoon for best results.

Capsules and tablets

Capsules and tablets are among the easiest types of medication to take properly. However, some people find them hard to swallow. If that's your case, try rinsing your mouth with water before you try to swallow the tablet/capsule. Place it on the back of your tongue, take a drink of water, and then swallow. If you find that a very large tablet or capsule "sticks" in your throat, empty the contents of the capsule or crush the tablet and mix the particles with applesauce, soup, yogurt, or even a syrup. However, be sure to check with your pharmacist first and also check the tables below since some tablets and capsules must be swallowed whole.

If you continually have trouble swallowing a tablet/capsule and don't want to mix the preparation with food each time you take it, ask your doctor if the medication is available as a liquid preparation or chewable tablet.

Examples of drugs that must be swallowed whole

Aminodur Dura-Tabs	Donnatal Extentabs	Naldecon
Choledyl	Drixoral	Tagamet
Dimetapp Extentabs	E-Mycin	Tenuate Dospan
Disophrol Chronotabs	Equanil Wyseals	Tepanil Ten-tabs
	Isordil Tembids	

Examples of drugs that should be used quickly (within 12 hours) if crushed or opened

Combid Spansules	Haldol	Stelazine
Compazine	Mellaril	Thorazine
Elavil	Phenergan	Tofranil
Etrafon	Sinequan	Triavil

Sublingual tablets

Sublingual tablets are those that must be placed under the tongue; the prime example is nitroglycerin. To take this type of tablet properly, place the tablet under your tongue, close your mouth, holding the saliva under the tongue also as long as possible without swallowing. If you have a bitter taste in your mouth after five minutes, this indicates that the drug has not been completely absorbed, so wait five more minutes before drinking water. The water may wash the medication into the stomach before it has been thoroughly absorbed if you drink water too soon. This is an instance where it is important to follow your instructions to the letter.

Eyedrops and eye ointments

Before you administer eyedrops or eye ointments, wash your hands thoroughly. Then lie or sit down and tilt your head back. Use your thumb and forefinger to pull the lower eyelid down to form a sort of "pouch" and drop the drops or squeeze the ointment into the eye.

If you are applying eyedrops, place your second finger alongside your nose and press gently to close off a duct that drains fluid away from the eye. If you do not close this duct, the drops will drain away too soon. Hold the dropper close to the eye but don't touch it. Do not place the drops directly on the eyeball or you will blink and lose the medication. Close your eye and keep it closed for a few minutes. Do not wash or wipe the dropper before replacing it into the bottle and make sure you close the bottle tightly to keep out moisture.

If you are applying an eye ointment, pull down the lower eyelid and make the pouch as described above. Then squeeze a one-quarter to one-half inch line of ointment into the pouch and close your eye. Roll your eye a few times to spread the ointment evenly.

Always make sure that the drops or ointment are explicitly intended for use in the eye and that you are observing the expiration date on the label. If the eye product changes color or becomes contaminated with foreign particles—bits of dust or eye makeup, for example—discard it and get a fresh refill.

Eardrops

Eardrops must fill the ear canal to be effective. Tilt your head to one side and turn the affected ear upward. Grasp the earlobe and pull it upward and back to straighten the ear canal before you drop the drops inside. Be sure to put the prescribed number of drops (usually "one dropperful") into the ear. Be careful not to touch the ear canal with the dropper to avoid contamination.

Keep your ear tilted upward for five to ten seconds and keep holding the earlobe. Then insert a small piece of clean cotton into the ear to keep the drops in. Replace the dropper in the bottle and seal tightly to keep out moisture.

If you wish, you may warm the bottle of eardrops by rolling the bottle back and forth between your hands to bring the solution to your body temperature. Do *not* heat the eardrops in a pan of boiling water; extremely hot eardrops can cause pain and even damage the ear. The water may also destroy the medication if it is too hot.

Nose drops and sprays

Before using this type of medication, blow your nose if you can. Then fill the dropper, tilt your head back and place the prescribed number of drops in the nose. Do not touch the dropper to the nasal membranes to avoid contamination. Keep your head tilted back for five to ten seconds and sniff gently two or three times.

Nasal sprays should not be used with the head tilted back. Insert the sprayer into the nose without touching the nasal membranes. Sniff and squeeze the sprayer at the same time. Do not release the sprayer until you have removed it from your nose to prevent nasal mucus and bacteria from being pulled into the container. After you have finished spraying, sniff gently two or three times.

Unless you have different instructions from your doctor, do not use nose drops or sprays for more than a few days at a time. Never use the same container for more than a week. Bacteria from your nose can easily enter the container and cause contamination. If you need long-term medication, buy refills or new prescriptions frequently and never exchange them with anyone else in your family.

Rectal suppositories

These suppositories can be used either as laxatives or for symptomatic relief of hemorrhoids. They all are inserted the same way. In order to be inserted properly, they must be firm, so if melting occurs in hot weather, chill the suppository in its wrappings in the refrigerator or in a cold glass of water. Then remove the aluminum wrappings and insert.

To insert the suppository, lie on your left side (if you are right-handed) and push the suppository into the rectum as far as possible. The pointed end is pushed in first. If insertion is difficult or painful, coat the suppository with a thin layer of petroleum jelly or mineral oil. If you feel like defecating after insertion, lie still until the urge has passed.

Some hemorrhoidal suppositories should be stored in the refrigerator; be sure to ask your pharmacist about the preferred method of storage.

Vaginal ointments and creams

Most vaginal ointments and creams prescribed by your doctor will come with instructions for use and an applicator. However, most of these products are used in the same way. Attach the special applicator to the top of the tube. Squeeze the tube from the bottom until the applicator is completely full of cream or ointment. Then lie on your back with your knees drawn up. Holding the applicator horizontally and pointed slightly downward, insert it into the vagina as far as it will comfortably go. When it is fully inserted, press the plunger down to empty the cream into the vagina. Withdraw the plunger and wash it in warm, soapy water. Rinse it thoroughly and allow it to air-dry completely. Return the plunger to the package only when it is thoroughly dry.

Although these general instructions apply to many vaginal creams and ointments, always read the directions carefully. There may be important differences in your medication. Check with your physician if you have any problems with applying the medication.

Vaginal tablets and suppositories

Most packages of vaginal tablets and/or suppositories will include complete instructions, but the following procedure is fairly standard for this type of medication.

Remove any foil wrappings from the medication. Place the tablet or suppository in the applicator. Lie on your back with your knees drawn up. Hold the applicator horizontally and tilted slightly downward. You should depress the plunger when the applicator is fully inserted so that the tablet or suppository is released into the vagina. The muscles of the vagina will hold the tablet or suppository in place. As with the cream or ointment, withdraw the plunger, wash it in warm, soapy water, rinse and allow to air-dry. Return it to its package only when it is completely dry.

Unless you have other instructions from your physician, you should not douche for two to three weeks before or after you use vaginal tablets or suppositories. However, check with your physician about specific instructions since each case will be slightly different.

Throat lozenges and discs

Although throat lozenges and discs are slightly different (lozenges are crystallized sugar whereas the discs are not), both release medications in the mouth that can soothe a sore throat, treat laryngitis, and reduce coughing.

Do not try to chew either a lozenge or a disc but allow it to dissolve in your mouth. Once it is dissolved, do not swallow or drink fluids for a short time to allow the medication to run down the back of your throat.

Throat sprays

When you are administering a throat spray, open your mouth wide and spray the medication as far back into the throat as possible. Try not to swallow. Hold the spray in your mouth as long as possible. Avoid drinking any fluids for several minutes.

Although the sprays are not meant to be swallowed in large quantities, swallowing the spray is not harmful. If you find that the spray upsets your stomach, simply spit it out after you have held it in your mouth for a few minutes.

Topical ointments and creams

Before you apply a topical ointment or cream—that is, a cream or ointment designed only for external use, such as on a cut, rash, or insect bite—moisten the skin or dab the area with a clean, wet cloth. Blot the skin dry and apply the cream or ointment. Apply it as thinly as possible. Many of the topical preparations, especially the steroid creams, are expensive. Furthermore, there is no special advantage to a thick layer; in fact, some steroid-containing creams and ointments can cause toxic side effects if the application is too heavy.

Once the cream or ointment has been applied, gently massage it into the area until it has disappeared. The ointment will make the skin feel slightly greasy, but the cream will not. If you have a choice between a cream and an ointment, ask for the cream; it is usually greaseless and will not stain clothing. Creams are also best for the scalp or other hairy areas. However, if you have very dry skin, an ointment is preferable since it will keep the skin soft for a longer period.

In some cases, your doctor will advise putting a wrap on the skin after a cream or ointment has been applied to hold the medication close to the skin and to keep the skin moist. This will help the drug to be absorbed and will hasten healing. For this, you can use a layer of transparent plastic film such as that used for wrapping food. Use the wrap only for the length of time specified and then remove it. A wrap that is kept on too long may cause too much of the drug to be absorbed, possibly resulting in negative side effects.

Never use wraps of this kind without your doctor's approval and do not use them on "weeping" lesions.

Powders

Powders are among the simplest medications to apply. They can be applied to any part of the body for which they are prescribed. They are especially good for tender or sensitive areas because they can be applied without touching the area.

Sprinkle the powder evenly over dry skin; any excess will blow or shake off. If you are using a foot powder, sprinkle some of it in your shoes and socks or stockings. Be sure to avoid inhaling any powder; it can cause respiratory problems if inhaled in any quantity.

Aerosol sprays

Topical preparations are often packaged as pressurized aerosol sprays—usually more costly than the same product in cream or ointment form. They are best used on sensitive or hairy areas of the body where creams and ointments may be difficult to apply.

Before you use a medication in aerosol spray form, shake the can. Hold the container upright four to six inches from the area being sprayed. Press the nozzle lightly, then release.

Do not use aerosol sprays in the area of the face and eyes. If the spray is intended for a part of the face (as with a spray for a skin rash), apply the spray to your hand and rub it on the area. Aerosol sprays can be very damaging to the eyes and mucous membranes such as those of the nose or mouth.

Do not be surprised if the aerosol spray feels cold to the skin; this is a normal sensation. Ask if another form of the product is available if this sensation bothers you.

How to manage side effects

Drugs obviously have many beneficial effects; they relieve unpleasant or dangerous symptoms, eliminate pain, and in many cases, attack the underlying cause of a disorder, such as a bacterial infection or a virus. However, from time to time, drugs can have undesirable effects called "side effects" or "adverse reactions." Some of these are simply annoyances, such as dry mouth or minor itching. Some are more serious, though not dangerous: slight dizziness, fluid retention, drowsiness. Finally, some are dangerous: severe diarrhea, erratic heartbeat and palpitations, throbbing headaches, kidney problems. Such adverse reactions are serious and are even capable in extreme cases of causing death. Remember that although all adverse reactions are side effects, not all side effects are adverse reactions. Most "side effects" are simply very minor annoyances that disappear spontaneously as your body becomes used to the drug; "adverse reactions," on the other hand, are more serious and may outweigh the benefits of the drug.

It is useful to distinguish between predictable, common side effects and those that are unusual or unexpected. Your doctor or pharmacist will probably warn you to anticipate the former ("you may experience drowsiness or a dry mouth with this capsule"). The latter, more severe reaction is almost always unexpected and should be reported to your doctor immediately. Often it is a completely individual response to the drug and means that you have an unusual sensitivity to the drug.

If you know that a particular side effect is common with a certain drug, you can relax a little because you know it is temporary and no cause for alarm. You can also plan your schedule to accommodate the reaction. For example, if you are on a program of antihistamine therapy for hay fever, you may become drowsy when you take your medication. You can ask your doctor if you can take your capsule at intervals during the day when you do not need to drive or operate equipment; you may also be able to schedule medication for "non-peak" times in your working day when you can nap or relax if necessary. In addition, you may find ways to minimize some side effects: if your doctor approves, you can take the medication with meals or change the dosage to eliminate the bothersome side effects. Always consult your doctor before making any of these changes, however.

On the other hand, sometimes a side effect is completely unexpected and potentially dangerous. You take a dose of your medication and experience sudden rapid or irregular heartbeat, difficulty in breathing, severe diarrhea or stomach cramps, or a feeling of faintness as if you are going to "black out." In these cases, take whatever emergency measures you need to stabilize your condition; then call your doctor immediately. Do not assume it is "just a side effect." Check it out to be safe.

Furthermore, don't assume that because the drug you are taking is a common or mild one that you will be free from side effects. Individual body chemistries react differently to different drugs. Some people have allergic reactions to common tranquilizers such as Valium, to painkillers such as Darvon and its derivatives, or to steroids and steroid preparations. If a problem presents itself or recurs, check with your physician before you take another dose of your medication.

Types of side effects

There are basically two types of side effects: those that are obvious to the patient and those that can be detected only with laboratory tests.

Obvious side effects

This discussion considers side effects categorized by the parts of the body that are affected by the side effects. It will help you identify some common types of side effects, but for additional information about your particular medication, be sure to consult your doctor.

Ear. Few drugs cause loss of hearing or even hearing problems. More common side effects that involve the ear include dizziness and tinnitus, or a sensation of ringing, thumping, or "hollowness" in the ear. If these sensations persist for more than three days, be sure to consult your doctor. Call your doctor immediately if you have any symptoms of hearing loss.

Eye. Blurred vision is one of the more common drug side effects. Some drugs, such as digitalis, may cause the patient to see a sort of "halo" around a lighted object (a lamp, television screen, or traffic light). Other drugs may cause "night blindness." Among the most serious side effects involving the eye is blindness which has been known to be an adverse reaction of quinine, a drug used to treat malaria. Librax (a sedative) may make it difficult to judge distances accurately and also may make the eyes very sensitive to sunlight.

While blurred vision, sensitivity to light, and difficulty in judging distances are all minor reactions, the quinine and digitalis reactions described above are signs of a toxic drug reaction. In any case, however, a disturbance in vision should be taken seriously and reported to a physician.

Gastrointestinal system. Gastrointestinal (digestive) symptoms are among the most common of all drug reactions. The symptoms include dry mouth, mouth sores, difficulty in swallowing, heartburn, nausea, vomiting, diarrhea, constipation, loss of appetite, stomach cramps, bloating and gas, and rectal itching.

Examples of drugs that may cause ulcers

Aristocort	**Clinoril**	**Medrol**
Butazolidin	**Indocin**	**prednisone**

Diarrhea is a common side effect of many drugs. Drugs often cause localized reactions in intestinal tissue that produce a temporary diarrhea. Usually, this lasts only a day or so—often less than 24 hours. But some antibiotics can cause a severe diarrhea, leading to ulcerated areas in the intestines and gastrointestinal bleeding. Be sure to consult your physician if diarrhea develops while you are taking an antibiotic.

If the diarrhea is proved to be a "normal" side effect, it should disappear within three days. During this time do not take any diarrhea remedy that might interfere or interact with your medication. Drink plenty of liquids to replace lost fluid and call your physician if the diarrhea persists for more than three days.

Examples of drugs that may cause diarrhea

Actifed
Aldactazide
Aldactone
Aldomet
Aldoril
Ambenyl
Apresoline
Atromid-S
Benadryl
Butazolidin
Clinoril
Coumadin
Dalmane
Dimetane
Dimetapp Extentabs
Diuril
Dyazide
Enduron
erythromycin
Flagyl
Haldol
Inderal
Indocin
Keflex
K-Lyte
Lanoxin
meprobamate
Minipress
Minocin
Motrin
Norpace
oral antidiabetics
Ornade
Pavabid
penicillins
Pronestyl
reserpine
sulfa drugs
Tagamet
Talwin
tetracycline
Thorazine
Tofranil
Zyloprim

The opposite reaction, constipation, is also a common drug reaction. Drugs such as Librax and Thorazine can slow down the action of the bowel, resulting in constipation that can last from a few days to a week. Some drugs absorb moisture in the bowel; and others, for example, Aldomet antihypertensive, act on the nervous system which then decreases nerve impulses in the intestine. If you suspect constipation is caused by a drug, do not take laxatives; instead, try increasing fluid intake (at least eight glasses of water a day) and eating some high-fiber foods such as vegetables and fruits. If the constipation continues more than three days, call your doctor.

Examples of drugs that may cause constipation

Actifed
Aldomet
Aldoril
Ambenyl
Benadryl
Bentyl
Catapres
Clinoril
Combid Spansules
Compazine
Dalmane
Dilantin
Dimetane
Dyazide
Flagyl
Haldol
Inderal
Librax
Librium
Mellaril
Minipress
Pavabid
Percodan
Sinequan
Stelazine
Talwin
Thorazine
Tussionex
Valium

Circulatory system. Certain drugs speed up or slow the heartbeat. If the drug slows the heartbeat too much, you may feel drowsy, tired, and sometimes dizzy. If, on the other hand, the drug accelerates the heartbeat, you may have palpitations that you may experience as thumping or fluttering sensations in the chest. You may feel that your heart is "skipping beats," and you may also have headaches. Usually, these symptoms are only temporary and are not serious; however, you should contact your doctor if they persist or are severe.

Some drugs that affect the circulatory system may also cause fluid retention or edema. When edema forms, fluid from the blood will collect outside the blood vessels. Ordinarily, edema is not serious and is only temporary. You may experience swollen ankles, feet, or fingers; a weight gain of a pound or two; and a mild headache. But if you are gaining weight steadily or have gained more than two or three pounds in a week, check with your doctor.

Drugs may also increase or decrease blood pressure. If your blood pressure decreases too much, you may feel drowsy and tired; you may also experience dizziness and a feeling of faintness when you get up from a reclining or kneeling position. If your blood pressure increases, you may be dizzy, have a headache and/or blurred vision, or hear a ringing or buzzing in your ears. Be sure to contact your doctor if you experience any of these symptoms.

*Examples of drugs that may cause fluid retention**

Apresoline	**Librax**	**oral contraceptives**
Aristocort	**Librium**	**prednisone**
Butazolidin	**Medrol**	**Premarin**
Clinoril	**Mellaril**	**Stelazine**
Combid Spansules	**Motrin**	**sulfa drugs**
Compazine	**Nalfon**	**Tolectin**
Elavil	**Naprosyn**	**Triavil**
	Norpace	

****Indicated by a weight gain of two or more pounds a week.***

Respiratory system. The most common side effects in the respiratory system include stuffy nose, dry throat, shortness of breath, and slowed breathing. The stuffy nose and dry throat usually disappear within a few days. You can use nose drops or spray (consult your doctor first), throat lozenges, or a warm salt water gargle, or you can suck on ice cubes to relieve these symptoms.

Shortness of breath is a common side effect of many drugs, for example, Inderal anti-arrhythmic. It sometimes lasts for several days to a week. Consult your doctor if this occurs.

Barbiturates or sleep-promoting drugs sometimes slow respiration. Slowed breathing is not serious, but you should inform your doctor if it continues.

Nervous system. Drugs that work on the nervous system can affect you in two ways: you will either become drowsy and lethargic or stimulated and overactive. If the drug causes drowsiness, you may feel sleepy, lethargic, dizzy, and lacking in coordination. If the drug causes stimulation, you may become nervous and jittery or have insomnia or tremors. Either set of symptoms may be accompanied by headaches or tingling in the fingers and toes. If the symptoms persist, call your doctor.

Examples of drugs that may cause dizziness

Actifed	Dalmane	Norpace
Aldactazide	Dimetane	oral antidiabetics
Aldactone	Dimetapp Extentabs	oral contraceptives
Aldomet	Diuril	Ornade
Ambenyl	Enduron	Pavabid
Aristocort	Flagyl	reserpine
Ativan	Keflex	Tagamet
Atromid-S	Lomotil	Talwin
Benadryl	Medrol	Tofranil
Benemid	meprobamate	Triavil
Bentyl	Minipress	Tussionex
Clinoril	Nitro-Bid	Vasodilan
	Nitrostat	

Skin. Common skin reactions include rash, swelling, itching, and sweating. Itching, swelling, and rash often indicate a drug allergy that may be dangerous if you continue the drug. Consult your doctor immediately if you develop these symptoms.

Some drugs increase sweating while others decrease it. If the weather is very hot and your medication decreases sweat output, your body may have a harder time adjusting to the high temperatures.

If you have a mild skin reaction that is not an allergic reaction to the drug, ask your pharmacist for a soothing cream, ointment or powder.

Examples of drugs that may cause a mild rash

Actifed	Compazine	Norpace
Aldactazide	Dimetane	Ornade
Aldactone	Dimetapp Extentabs	Pronestyl
Aldoril	Diuril	reserpine
Ambenyl	Dyazide	Stelazine
Ativan	Elavil	Tagamet
Atromid-S	Enduron	Thorazine
Benadryl	Haldol	Tofranil
Benemid	Indocin	Triavil
Butazolidin	Librax	Tussionex
Catapres	Librium	Valium
Clinoril	Lomotil	Zyloprim
Combid Spansules	Minipress	

Another type of skin reaction is photosensitivity (a more extreme form is phototoxicity or sun poisoning). This means unusual sensitivity to the sun. Tetracycline can cause such a reaction. After taking such a drug, you may receive a severe sunburn after only ten to 15 minutes of exposure. It is not necessary to stay inside all the time; just make sure you are fully covered with clothing if you are outside for a long period of time. Stay out of the sun for prolonged periods if possible. Continue taking these precautions for two or three days after you have finished your medication therapy with these drugs.

Examples of drugs that may cause photosensitivity

Benadryl	Haldol	sulfa drugs
Compazine	hydrochlorothiazide	tetracycline
Diuril	oral antidiabetics	Thorazine
Enduron	Phenergan	Tofranil

Side effects detected by laboratory tests

As was mentioned before, some side effects are very difficult to detect and can be confirmed only with laboratory testing. If you suspect any of these effects, consult your doctor immediately.

Kidneys. Some drugs reduce the kidneys' ability to remove chemicals and other substances from the blood. If drug therapy continues over a period of time, these substances accumulate in body tissues. This accumulation, if it continues, causes vague symptoms such as swelling, fluid retention, nausea, headache, weakness, and a general fatigue. Pain and other obvious symptoms are usually absent.

Liver. Drug-induced liver damage may result in fat accumulation in the liver. Often such damage occurs because the drug either increases or decreases the liver's ability to metabolize other drugs, foods, and alcohol. Liver damage may be rather advanced before it produces any symptoms. Therefore, periodic tests of liver function are made during many kinds of drug therapy.

Blood. Many drugs affect the blood and the circulatory system without producing noticeable symptoms. If a drug lowers blood sugar levels, for example, you may not know it for an hour to several hours. The symptoms of lowered blood sugar can include tiredness, muscular weakness, palpitations, and ringing or buzzing in the ears. Similarly, low levels of blood potassium produce dry mouth, thirst, and muscle cramps or weakness.

Some drugs, also, can decrease the number of red blood cells, causing a mild anemia and feelings of tiredness, weakness, dizziness, and hunger. Other drugs will decrease the number of white blood cells and thus increase your susceptibility to infection and minor illnesses. If a sore throat or fever begins while you are taking a drug, call your doctor; you may have an infection and too few white blood cells to combat it.

*Examples of drugs that may cause blood diseases**

Aldactazide	Lasix	sulfa drugs
Apresoline	Mellaril	Tagamet
Butazolidin	Minocin	Thorazine
Dyazide	oral contraceptives	Tofranil
Elavil	Orinase	Tolinase
Hygroton	Regroton	Zyloprim
	Stelazine	

***Indicated by a sore throat that doesn't go away in one or two days.**

Managing possible side effects

Consult your physician and also the lists and charts in this book to discover whether your side effects are minor (expected, common, and usually not serious) or whether they suggest that something is wrong in your drug therapy. In the latter case, you may need to adjust your dosage (with your doctor's guidance) or you may need to switch to another drug that does not produce these side effects. Perhaps you should not be taking this drug, or class of drugs, at all.

If, however, your doctor assures you that your side effects are minor and temporary, here are some ways to manage common but irritating side effects:

- Blurred vision: Avoid operating machinery or driving; avoid bright lights and heavy reading tasks
- Decreased sweating: Curtail exercise; avoid work in the sun; try to stay in shady, cool places
- Diarrhea: Drink plenty of fluids and water, including potassium-rich citrus juices and commercial mineral and electrolyte mixtures; if diarrhea persists beyond three days, call the doctor
- Dizziness: Avoid operating machinery or driving; lie or sit down and be careful on stairs
- Drowsiness: Avoid operating machinery or driving; schedule frequent rest periods
- Dry mouth or throat: Suck ice chips or chew gum
- Dry nose and throat: Use a humidifier or vaporizer; boil water on the stove
- Fluid retention: Follow a low-salt diet; avoid adding salt to foods; avoid sodium-heavy cola drinks
- Headache: Remain quiet and rest; take aspirin or aspirin substitutes with your doctor's permission
- Insomnia: Take the last dose of the drug earlier in the day instead of at bedtime (with doctor's permission); drink a warm glass of milk at bedtime; ask your doctor about light exercise or walking in the evenings
- Itching: Take frequent (not hot) showers or baths
- Nasal congestion: Use nose drops or spray if permitted; use a vaporizer or humidifier
- Palpitations (mild): Rest, avoid tension; avoid coffee, tea, cola drinks, and alcohol; stop smoking
- Upset stomach: Take medication with milk or food if your doctor permits.

The medical guide to diseases, disorders, syndromes, and medical terms

This section of the medical guide, arranged in alphabetical order for easy and fast reference, covers diseases, disorders, conditions, syndromes, symptoms, diagnostic procedures, treatments, and medical terms. Each entry is presented in clear, easy-to-understand language with practical advice about when to treat a problem at home, when to consult a doctor, and when to administer emergency first aid or to seek immediate emergency care. Since this section can be used as a reference manual, each entry is designed to be self-contained; for example, terms that may not be a part of everyday vocabulary are defined where they occur, even if they have been defined elsewhere. On the other hand, if another entry or section of the book naturally expands or complements a topic, there is a cross reference for you to find the additional information.

In those entries that discuss a disease or disorder, the description of the problem, the cause (if known), the symptoms, the treatment, the prognosis, and the risk factors are discussed. In addition, preventive action is outlined, if appropriate or possible. In those entries that define a term or discuss a procedure, the explanation often includes examples to illustrate the concept or idea. In short, each entry attempts to be as inclusive as possible without being technical and hard to understand.

A

Acne

Acne is a condition of the skin that ranges in appearance from small raised bumps to pustules, large cysts and pimples on the skin surface. Acne is so common that more than 80 percent of the population can claim having had some form of it at some time.

Although there are several theories about what causes acne, authorities generally believe that acne is a by-product of hormonal changes in the body during puberty —that period of life when a child develops the secondary sex characteristics (such as facial and body hair, deepened voice, and increased muscle mass in boys and breast development and menstruation in girls) of an adult. At this time, hormone production increases, particularly the male hormone testosterone, and stimulates the sebaceous (oil) glands that lie within the skin.

Most excess oil produced by these glands leaves the skin through a series of tubes called hair follicles that contain small hairs. Sometimes, oil clogs these tubes and creates comedones or blocked hair follicles. Comedones are what form the initial lumps in acne.

If comedones are open to the surface of the skin, they are called blackheads. They contain oil (sebum) from the glands, bacteria, and any skin tissue that accumulates near the surface. Comedones that are closed at the surface are called whiteheads. Plugged follicles can rupture internally, resulting in a discharge of their contents into the surrounding tissues. This process sets up an intense inflammatory response that sets the stage for the development of acne.

The role of bacteria in acne is unclear. Bacteria may act by causing chemical reactions in the sebaceous fluid, leading to the release of very irritating compounds called "fatty acids." These in turn may cause inflammation that increases susceptibility to infection.

Authorities vary about emphasizing diet as a cause of acne. Diet alone does not cure acne, nor does acne stem from an allergic reaction to a specific food. However, some cases of acne improve after eliminating certain foods, particularly chocolates and fats. In addition, emotional stress seems to increase acne in certain cases.

Acne causes raised swellings most frequently on the face, neck, back,

Blackhead
Hair follicle
Sebaceous gland

When excess material produced by the sebaceous glands clogs the hair follicle tube, a blackhead results. A blackhead is open on the surface of the skin, but nevertheless blocks the normal release of material from the sebaceous gland to the skin's surface.

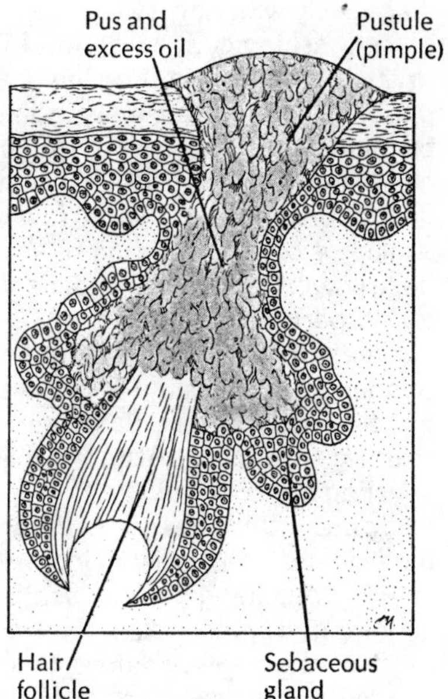

When a blocked hair follicle is not open on the surface of the skin, it may eventually rupture internally, discharging its contents into the surrounding tissues. This results in an inflammatory response that sets the stage for the development of acne.

chest, and shoulders. Severe acne may have pus-filled sacs that break open and discharge fluid. Soreness, pain, or itching may accompany the bumps. These symptoms could be acne, or they could indicate other skin reactions to such substances as cosmetics, medications, and grooming or cleaning products.

Since puberty plays a role in the onset of acne, the condition usually appears during teenage years. Nevertheless, it can extend to age 25 and over, particularly in women. Although acne is not life-threatening, it can be problematic. If untreated, comedones can leave permanent scars which can result in embarrassment and emotional stress.

Acne has no prevention or cure, but there are several treatments. The simplest home remedy is to wash the affected areas thoroughly at least twice a day with warm water and mild soap. Washing gently will not dry or irritate sensitive skin. Regular shampooing also helps acne, especially if the hair is oily. Use of makeup should be limited. In addition, skin may heal with exposure to the sun. However, sunlamps or ultraviolet lamps should be used very cautiously under a doctor's supervision.

One form of treatment not recommended is picking or squeezing pimples, since more inflammation or scarring may result. Also, the risk of infection is increased.

Some over-the-counter acne medications, particularly lotions or creams containing benzoyl peroxide, can help troubled skin. However, most of these preparations tend to dry the skin if manufacturer's directions are not followed carefully.

For persistent acne, a doctor may prescribe a preparation that can be applied on the skin or oral antibiotics such as tetracycline or erythromycin. These antibiotics act to suppress bacteria that may cause the aforementioned chain of events.

Another drug, tretinoin (Vitamin A acid), has reduced acne in more than 50 percent of the people who have tried it. This drug can be taken independently or in combination with an antibiotic—all under a doctor's supervision. A newer drug, isotretinoin, is related to tretinoin and is used to treat severe cystic acne. It is usually not prescribed, however, unless all other acne treatments have failed. These drugs work by temporarily suppressing the activity of the sebaceous glands.

See also Boils.

ACTH

ACTH (adrenocorticotropic hormone), also known as corticotropin, is a hormone (a chemical "messenger" that acts upon a body process) produced by the pituitary, a pea-sized gland that is attached by a stalk to the base of the brain. ACTH is also manufactured synthetically or extracted from the pituitary glands of cattle and sheep and used as a drug. ACTH travels through the bloodstream to affect the adrenal glands, two small but very important organs located over each kidney. It stimulates the cortex, the outer layer of the adrenal glands, to produce various hormones known as steroids. These include the corticosteroids (the most important of which is cortisol), androgens, which are male sex hormones (also produced in far smaller quantity by the adrenal gland in the female), and mineralocorticoids. The first of these, cortisol, has numerous functions. It is important in protein formation and breakdown, blood sugar control, reduction of inflammation, and is necessary for the body to mount an effective response against severe stress, be it a disease or multiple injuries with resultant shock. Androgens also have many functions, mainly the development and maintenance of male sex characteristics, reproductive capability, and musculature. They are also important in bone marrow function and protein biochemistry. Mineralocorticoids are steroid hormones involved in maintaining salt and water balance in the body.

The drug forms of ACTH and the corticosteroids are used to treat a disease in the same way the natural hormones would or as substitute or supplement hormones for people who have lost the ability to manufacture their own. The primary difference is that ACTH acts less directly and more generally. It stimulates the adrenal glands to enlarge and produce more steroids that then perform their various functions throughout the body. Corticosteroid drugs, on the other hand, can be administered to the part of the body that needs them most. Thus, a dab of hydrocortisone cream will eliminate a rash and a hydrocortisone injection will diminish the swelling of a painful knee joint virtually without affecting any other part of the body. Sometimes, however, corticosteroids are considered for generalized use throughout the body. In those instances, corticosteroids have an advantage over ACTH in that they can be taken by mouth and may be given in doses that far exceed what the body's adrenal glands can produce. ACTH must be injected because it would otherwise be destroyed by digestive enzymes, which do not affect the corticosteroids. Regardless of why they are used or how they are administered, all are powerful drugs that must be used with great care.

See also Addison's disease, Adrenal glands, and Corticosteroids.

Acupuncture

Acupuncture is a method of relieving pain and treating disease by inserting fine needles through the skin. Having originated in China thousands of years ago, acupuncture is still widely used throughout the Orient. It has also been used recently in Russia, France, England, and Germany and in the 1970s gained some popularity in the United States as a means of relieving chronic pain. However, most physicians in the United States do not employ it nor recommend it as a very effective treatment. Others reserve it as a last resort when other methods fail or use it in combination with other therapies.

Practitioners of acupuncture follow ancient charts of the body showing 12 meridians, or lines, along which the "life force" is said to flow. These lines do not correspond to known nerve pathways. By inserting fine needles at specifically marked points (often far distant from the source of pain) along the meridians, the practitioner attempts to relieve pain or to improve the condition of a particular organ or area of the body. As many as ten or 20 needles may be inserted at one time and left in place for 20 or 30 minutes or more. Because they are so fine, the needles do not produce much pain themselves. Each has a tiny brass knob on one end to serve as a handle and to permit the practitioner to spin the needle rapidly between two fingers and thus stimulate sensation.

Acupuncture has long been used in China to treat a wide variety of ailments including arthritis, asthma, headaches, stomach trouble, and even mental illness. In the United States it is most often used to relieve arthritis symptoms, prolonged backaches, and other chronic pains.

It is widely recognized that some people have their pain relieved, at least temporarily, following acupuncture. But no one knows why this happens. One theory, greatly simplified, holds that nerve impulses that are generated by the acupuncture needles and carried on large nerve fibers block off the pain impulses that are carried on small nerve fibers, at the point where they enter the spinal cord. A newer theory states that the nerve impulses from the needles stimulate the production of natural painkilling chemicals by the body.

Addison's disease

Addison's disease is a gradually worsening condition occurring when the adrenal cortex, the outer layer of the adrenal glands, fails to produce enough hormones to meet the needs of the body. The adrenal glands, situated just above each kidney, produce many different hormones—chemicals which travel through the bloodstream and have specific effects on cells in another part of the body.

Formerly, the cause of this disease in 70 to 90 percent of the cases was tuberculosis or a fungal infection. However, in recent years, the disease is most commonly referred to as idiopathic, or "of unknown cause." The predominant theory is that most cases of Addison's disease are due to autoimmune destruction of the adrenal cortex; that is, the body produces antibodies against its own tissues, leading to their ultimate breakdown. Other known causes include partial destruction of the adrenal cortex by cancer, surgery, or degeneration of the tissue, or by deposits of amyloid, an abnormal body substance. A similar condition known as secondary adrenal insufficiency is caused by failure of the pituitary (a small gland attached to the base of the brain) to produce enough of the hormone known as ACTH, which stimulates the adrenal cortex to produce its hormones.

Early symptoms of Addison's disease are weakness, fatigue, and a tendency to become faint when arising suddenly from a bed or chair. Increased pigmentation of the skin, producing a "tan" all over the body on exposed and unexposed areas alike with even darker pigmentation on creases and bony pressure points, occurs in most cases. (The increase in pigmentation is caused by overactivity of the pituitary gland as it tries to stimulate the failing adrenal cortex by producing more ACTH thereby also increasing production of a related substance that actually causes the pigmentation.) In certain places the tan may be broken by completely white patches, known as vitiligo. Black freckles appear on the forehead, face, shoulders, and neck. There may be bluish-white discoloration around the nipples and the mucous membranes of the lips, mouth, vagina, and rectum.

Later symptoms include weight loss, dehydration (loss of fluid in body tissues), low blood pressure, and sometimes loss of appetite, nausea, vomiting, diarrhea, dizziness, and inability to keep warm.

The most alarming symptoms are those of a life-threatening condition known as an adrenal crisis, which requires immediate attention and hospitalization. Signs of this are extreme weakness; severe pains in the lower back, abdomen, or legs; collapse of the circulatory system; and a shutdown of the kidneys. Such a crisis may be brought on by severe stress such as infection, injury, surgery, or by loss of salt through perspiration during hot weather.

One laboratory sign of Addison's disease is a high level of ACTH but a low level of cortisol (an adrenal hormone) in the blood. This indicates that the pituitary gland is working overtime to stimulate the adrenal cortex with ACTH to produce cortisol, but the cortex is failing to produce.

The basic treatment for Addison's disease is to provide steroid hormones, principally cortisone, to replace those not being produced by the adrenal cortex. An additional steroid drug may be added to the cortisone as part of the continuing treatment. It enables the body to retain salt, which helps the body retain water in tissues and blood. In doing so, it prevents the loss of salt and fluid with resulting low blood pressure (caused by too little water in the blood resulting in low blood volume) of severe Addison's disease.

The outlook for patients on hormone treatment is excellent. Good medical supervision and intelligent patient cooperation can prevent emergencies caused by a sudden withdrawal or neglect of treatment or by an increased need for hormones because of infection, injury, surgery, pregnancy, or other stress on the body. It is important to avoid infection, to treat infection that develops as soon as possible, and at all times to carry a card or wear a bracelet describing the condition and the need for cortisone. It is also critical to take the medication reliably and to be in touch with a physician who can increase or decrease the dosage as the need arises. With proper care, a person with Addison's disease can lead a normal life.

Prevention of Addison's disease, except by eliminating certain known causes such as tuberculosis, will probably have to wait until more is known about the mysterious failures of the adrenal cortex.

See also ACTH, Adrenal glands, and Pituitary gland.

Adenoids

Adenoids are masses of protective (lymphoid) tissue located in the lining of the nasopharynx, the cavity above the throat and behind the nose. Like the tonsils located below them, the adenoids (technically known as the nasopharyngeal tonsil) are lymph glands containing a fluid (lymph) rich in white blood cells that help localize and destroy harmful bacteria and viruses. They thus provide an important defense against diseases of the respiratory (breathing) system.

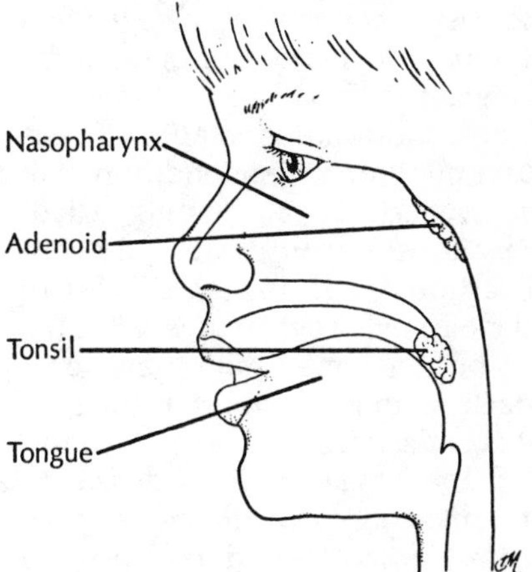

An adenoid is a mass of lymphoid tissue, located above the throat and behind the nose, whose function is to trap and destroy harmful bacteria and viruses.

It is normal for adenoids to become enlarged during throat infections, just as the tonsils do, and then diminish in size after the infection passes. Sometimes, however, as a result of continuing infection or allergies the adenoids remain enlarged.

The resulting obstruction of the nasal passage may cause mouth breathing, the characteristic "nasal" voice, and continuing drainage down the throat of pus-filled mucus. It may also cause a blockage of the two eustachian tubes, which connect the throat to the inner ears, resulting in retention of fluid in the middle ear, impaired hearing, earache, and sometimes serious recurring ear infections.

Treatment of infected adenoids is with antibiotics, taken by mouth. Surgery may be recommended when the infected or enlarged adenoids themselves are the source of the disease (usually the tonsils beneath are infected as well and are removed in the same operation). This would be the case when there is recurrent or continuing infection of the adenoids that cannot be eliminated with antibiotics, when the adenoids cause repeated ear infections, or when there is cancer or an abscess (a mass of pus in a cavity surrounded by decaying tissue). When chronically infected adenoids may increase susceptibility to a condition like rheumatic fever or nephritis (a kidney disease), your doctor may consider surgical removal of the adenoids. However, surgery should not be performed during an acute attack of tonsillitis, because it may worsen the infection.

Surgery may not be the answer to prevent snoring, mouth breathing, or "nasal" voice caused by enlarged adenoids, since the enlargement usually diminishes after childhood.

See also Tonsillitis.

Adrenal glands

The adrenal glands are two tiny, vital glands that lie on the upper part of each kidney and produce more than 30 different hormones (hormones are chemical substances which are created by cells in one part of the body and carried by body fluids to another part, where they act as messengers to help regulate a body process). All but two of these hormones are produced in the cortex, the outer layer of the adrenal glands, and are known as steroids. The remaining hormones, known as adrenaline and noradrenaline, are manufactured in the adrenal medulla, the inner portion of the adrenal glands.

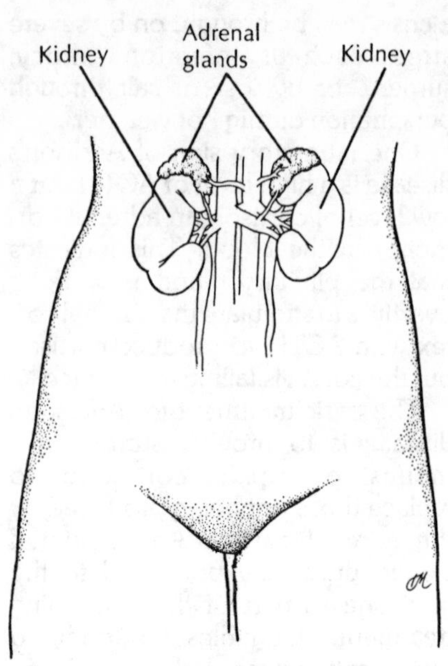

The adrenal glands are two small glands that are located on the upper part of each kidney and that produce more than 30 different hormones to help regulate body processes.

Adrenaline and noradrenaline help to prepare your body for immediate action when you are in danger or excited. Messages from your brain cause a part of your brain known as the hypothalamus to stimulate your pituitary gland, located just beneath. The pituitary gland releases a hormone known as ACTH, which travels through the bloodstream to your adrenal glands and causes the adrenal cortex to pour corticosteroids into your blood, which further cause an increase in the production and release of adrenaline and noradrenaline. There are also more direct chemical responses stimulating the adrenal medulla. One of these is through the neurotransmitter (a chemical involved in activating the nerves to perform a function) called acetylcholine. This chemical acts as a direct stimulus to the adrenal medulla, causing an increased production and release of adrenaline and noradrenaline. These two hormones speed up your heart and lungs, release sugar into your bloodstream to give you more energy, increase blood flow to your muscles, sharpen your senses, and release chemicals to initiate clotting of your blood if you are injured. Your body is thus better able to fight, run, or otherwise handle an emergency. Pain, injuries, starvation, extreme emotion, and insufficient air supply can also cause this general protective reaction.

The steroid hormones produced in the outer layer of the adrenal glands affect all organs and tissues throughout the body; they are essential to life. One group of these hormones, known as mineralocorticoids, controls the distribution of body fluids and the sodium and potassium mineral salts dissolved within them. If production of these hormones is decreased, the tissues and blood are depleted of salt and water. The blood volume decreases, so blood pressure falls. In an extreme case only the rapid injection of salt water into the bloodstream can prevent death from shock caused by collapse of the blood-circulation system.

A second group of hormones produced in the outer layer are known as glucocorticoids. They help regulate the body's reserves of and use of sugars and proteins, among other complex metabolic processes. They assist chemical processes throughout the body, and they also act to control inflammation. (Cortisol, one of these hormones, is known for this effect. For example, when given as a drug such as hydrocortisone or prednisone, it reduces the swollen joints of arthritis and can eliminate skin rashes.) Finally, these hormones also participate in the body's reaction to stress.

A third class of hormones produced by the outer layer of the adrenal glands in both men and women are the sex hormones. These hormones, the best known of which are testosterone (also produced in the male testes) and estrogen (also produced in the female ovaries), cause masculine and feminine characteristics, respectively. Abnormal production of testosterone in women and children results in beard growth, enlarged muscle development, and changes in sex organs. One cause of this condition is a tumor (growth) on the adrenal cortex. If it is removed, the patient returns to normal.

A deficient functioning of the outer layer of the adrenal glands produces Addison's disease. It can result in fatigue, low blood pressure, poor digestion, and even death. However, those with this condition can usually be restored to a normal life by regular doses of replacement hormones.

See also ACTH, Addison's disease, and Corticosteroids.

Adrenocorticotropic hormone

See ACTH.

Agoraphobia

Agoraphobia is the abnormal fear of being in open places. This greatly restricts the life of the person with the fear, who in extreme cases will not leave home—except perhaps if accompanied by a close friend or relative. The first sign of the condition may be a panic attack when out in public, with feelings of anxiety, restlessness, breathlessness, rapid or irregular heartbeat, and approaching doom. Thereafter, the person may stay at home to prevent another panic attack.

Agoraphobia is by far the most common of all phobias, accounting for 60 percent of cases. It is also the most persistent and the hardest to cure. Phobias are unreasonable or exaggerated fears of a specific object or situation. As long as it is avoided, the sufferer is relatively free of anxiety. Phobias are thought to be the mind's way of providing a substitute for feelings or desires the person refuses to face. The choice of the symbol, whether open places (agoraphobia), closed places (claustrophobia) or whatever, may occur by chance. Thus, a person may be in an open, public place when overcome by a panic created by the real fear the mind is trying to avoid. Ever after, the person automatically associates open, public places with the panic and avoids them. Another theory is that some phobias at least may be caused by physical or chemical disorders of the body.

The standard treatment of a phobia, usually by a psychiatrist or psychologist, is to talk with the patient, try to discover the real fear behind the substitute fear, and help the patient face it and deal with the problem behind it. If the cause of the agoraphobia is fear in getting along with other people, group therapy may be the best treatment (in group therapy, people with the same problem—sometimes members of the same family—get together and talk about it under the leadership of a trained therapist). If nothing else works, the therapist may instead be able to persuade the patient to face and overcome the substitute fear. Thus the person with agoraphobia would become determined to conquer it and would do so by going out into open, public places time and again until the fear is gone. At first this might be with a friend and later completely alone. To ease the anxiety during this period, the therapist may prescribe tranquilizers and teach the patient methods of relaxation and self-hypnosis. Recently, many other medications, particularly antidepressants, have been shown to lessen the symptoms of phobias.

All phobias including agoraphobia, it would seem, are best prevented by a continuing effort to understand and acknowledge one's own true feelings. When problems arise, you should try to solve them rather than refusing to admit to yourself that they exist. Such refusal could lead to the substitute fear—the phobia—that hides your real problem.

See also Phobia.

AIDS—acquired immune deficiency syndrome

Acquired immune deficiency syndrome (AIDS) is a condition in which the body's immunity, its natural defense system against disease, is somehow severely jeopardized thus enabling organisms that are normally fought off by the body quite effectively to become deadly.

The cause of the new disease, discovered in 1979, is unknown. What is known is that male homosexuals, drug addicts who inject drugs, and hemophiliacs who receive blood transfusions for their disorder are all high risk groups. Homosexual practices (for example, rectal intercourse), use of nonsterile needles within a group, possible environmental factors, and multiple transfusions of pooled blood factors have all been respectively mentioned as possible means of transmission of an agent causing the syndrome. Of early known victims, 75 percent were male homosexuals, 12 percent intravenous drug abusers, 0.5 percent hemophiliacs—but 6 percent were Haitian immigrants who were neither homosexuals nor drug abusers. More recently, AIDS is affecting more of the general population especially the sex partners and children of its victims. Many investigators think that AIDS can be transmitted by prolonged intimate contact, but this has not been proved.

Symptoms include low-grade fever, swollen lymph glands, weight loss, fatigue, night sweats, longstanding diarrhea, and a general sick feeling. Up to one third of the victims develop a previously rare cancer known as Kaposi's sarcoma, which can appear as purplish bumps on the skin. Many come down with a severe form of pneumonia. The main problem, however, is the inability of the body to fight many diseases that come along, including various cancers, skin infections, fungus growths, and tuberculosis.

Individuals with AIDS almost uniformly have reduced numbers of lymphocytes. These are specialized white blood cells that are critical in combating infectious diseases, particularly those caused by tuberculosis, fungi, and viruses. Lymphocytes may also be instrumental in destroying malignancies in their early stages. There are two types of lymphocytes actively engaged in coping with infection: the T-cell and the B-cell. The T-cell is mainly concerned with direct cytotoxicity, that is, by a series of complex processes, it directly kills invaders. The B-cell, on the other hand, is concerned with the production of infection-fighting antibodies when stimulated. In AIDS the T-cells are greatly reduced; in fact, it is the "helper" T-cell (a further subdivision) that is most profoundly decreased. So far, this has been a constant finding in almost all AIDS victims and will possibly serve as a link toward the discovery of a treatment.

Treatment to counter the effects of AIDS may involve the use of antibiotics, surgery to remove skin cancer, chemotherapy, and drugs to raise the body's resistance to diseases. No cure for the disease itself has been yet found. In addition, no specific means of preventing AIDS is known.

See also Immunity.

Albumin

Albumin is the name given to a protein found in nearly every body tissue and in body fluids. Serum albumin, produced in the liver, makes up some 55 percent of the proteins in the blood plasma (the fluid content of the blood). Albumin combines chemically with many substances carried by the blood, including various acids and drugs, helping them to be transported to sites throughout the body. Together with other blood proteins, albumin also acts in a significant way to regulate the distribution of water in the body. In an emergency when the body is in shock, a condition when blood volume is very low and circulation is failing, albumin solution may be injected to restore the volume of fluid. This acts to improve circulation and the pumping action of the heart. The solution may also be used to prevent shock in an injured person.

Albumin when found in the urine in excess amounts, a condition known as albuminuria, can be an important sign of kidney disease. It indicates that the kidneys, in processing the blood, are allowing an important part of it to pass out of the body. However, fever, intense exercise, extreme dehydration (loss of water from body tissue), and other shocks to the system can create harmless albuminuria in a healthy person.

Alcoholism

Alcoholism is a disorder in which a person repeatedly drinks excessive amounts of alcoholic beverages, with resulting harm to health, relations with other people, and work performance. The person becomes physically dependent upon alcohol as well as psychologically dependent. There is a genuine craving for alcohol, and unpleasant symptoms such as delirium tremens (a syndrome of fever, hallucinations, tremors, and a tremendous stress response) are seen. Withdrawal seizures or convulsions are also common. These and other withdrawal symptoms may follow an attempt to stop drinking "cold turkey."

Various causes of alcoholism have been suggested. These include a shy, lonely, immature, or dependent personality; depression; and self-hate. Some societies and groups within those societies encourage overuse of alcohol as recreation and as an escape from life's problems. It has been suggested but not proved that a tendency to alcoholism may be inherited or is the result of a chemical defect in one's makeup. Whatever the cause, alcoholism is a self-damaging disease and an ineffective way to deal with life. An estimated one American in ten suffers from alcoholism at some time in life.

The fact that a person is an alcoholic (one who suffers from alcoholism) is not always obvious. Alcoholics often do not recognize their own alcoholism and commonly hide symptoms from spouses, family, friends, and employers. Signs of alcoholism include:

- Frequent drunkenness
- Tolerance to alcohol (a great deal of liquor is required before the person shows signs of intoxication; however, this is not true in all cases, especially where alcohol has damaged the liver)
- Physical dependence, resulting in withdrawal symptoms a day or more after drinking is stopped; symptoms may range from tremors and physical pain to seizures and visions of bugs or strange creatures
- Continued drinking even when it is harming the person's health and personal life
- Poor job performance
- Depression

Other signs may include an odor of liquor on the breath in the morning; "sneaked" drinks; suspicious work absences (due to sleeping off hangovers); and frequent falls, accidents, and cigarette burns on hands and body (caused by drunken carelessness). Several years of alcoholism can cause permanent damage to the liver, brain, heart, and nervous system. Heavy drinking by a pregnant woman (six drinks a day, perhaps fewer) can result in mental retardation, low birth weight, and birth defects in her baby.

In the worst cases, in which the alcoholic has been drinking as much as a gallon of beer or a pint of whiskey a day for several months, sudden withdrawal of alcohol may even result in death because of convulsions and/or delirium tremens.

Treatment of severe alcoholism involves two stages: immediate and long-term. Both require a physician's attention.

The first step is to stop the drinking while treating the symptoms of withdrawal. Sometimes, with the patient's consent, a drug known as disulfiram is taken daily by mouth; it causes vomiting if the patient drinks anything alcoholic. It stops the person from drinking, but the patient may refuse to continue it because of its unpleasant results. In a crisis situation, withdrawal is best done in a hospital alcoholic unit. Under a doctor's care, psychologic support and reassurance may be enough to comfort the patient during the withdrawal stage. But frequently other measures are needed. The patient may be undernourished from drinking so much and eating so little and may need replacement doses of vitamins, particularly thiamine (Vitamin B_1). Fluids containing glucose (a sugar) and salt water may be added to the blood, which has been robbed of water and glucose by the effects of overuse of alcohol. Tranquilizing drugs may be given to help ease withdrawal symptoms, which may continue for days.

Long-term treatment may include psychiatric help to treat the problem that caused the alcoholism in the first place, such as depression or mental illness. For many alcoholics the solution is to join an organization known as Alcoholics Anonymous (AA). Members help each other overcome their drinking problems and vow to stay away from alcohol completely. In helping each other, they develop badly needed confidence and positive feelings about themselves. No other approach has been nearly as successful.

Alcoholism is a significant social and medical problem that cannot be easily stopped. However, it may be diminished if people:

- learn the full extent of its dangers;
- find more healthful ways to deal with life's problems and disappointments—by facing, rather than avoiding, them;
- learn to recognize the symptoms of alcoholism; and
- seek help for problem drinking from their physicians and/or a group like Alcoholics Anonymous.

Allergy

An allergy is an extraordinary reaction or sensitivity to a particular environmental substance by the immune system, the body's natural defense system against disease.

Although it can be present almost immediately after exposure to the irritant, an allergy usually develops over time, while the immune system forms protective substances called antibodies as a reaction to an invasion by a foreign substance. Under normal conditions, such antibodies work to protect the body from further attack. In the case of an allergy, however, the antibodies and other specialized cells involved in this protective function trigger an unusual sensitivity to the foreign substance (called an allergen). The antibodies then stimulate the special cells to produce histamine, a powerful chemical released from the cells that causes the small blood vessels to enlarge, the smooth muscles (such as those in the air passages or the digestive tract) to constrict, and hives to develop.

No one knows why allergies develop, but it is known that an allergy can appear, disappear, or reappear at any time and at any age. Allergic reactions rarely occur during the first encounter with the troublesome allergen because the body needs time to accumulate the antibodies. Also, a family history of allergies seems to be related to an individual's sensitivity to certain allergens. People who show a tendency to develop allergies are referred to as "atopic." This state of atopy frequently runs in families.

An allergic reaction can be so mild that it is barely noticeable or so severe that a person's life is threatened. Common symptoms of allergy are watery eyes, runny nose, itching or inflamed skin, or a swollen mouth or throat. Some allergic reactions may be accompanied by headaches, sinus stuffiness, a reduced sense of taste or smell, or difficult breathing.

An extremely severe allergic reaction, called anaphylactic shock, is characterized by breathing difficulties (caused by swelling of the throat and larynx and narrowing of the bronchial tubes), itching skin, hives, and collapse of the blood vessels, as well as by vomiting, diarrhea, and cramps. This advanced condition can be fatal if not promptly treated.

There are four categories of allergens: inhalants, contactants, ingestants, and injectants.

Inhalant allergens are breathed in, and include such substances as dust, pollen, feathers, and animal dander (small scales from the animal's skin). Hay fever is an inhalant allergy in which the mucous membranes react to various inhaled substances, usually the pollens associated with the changing seasons. Year-round hay fever may be a reaction to pet dander, feathers, mold, or dust. Hay fever symptoms include itching of the nose, eyes, and roof of the mouth; sneezing; headache; and watery eyes.

Contactant allergens are those that are touched and include such substances as poison ivy, cosmetics, detergents, fabrics, and dyes. Contact dermatitis is an example of an allergic-type reaction resulting from exposure to a contactant. Skin becomes inflamed, burning, and itching where it has come in contact with soaps, detergents, household cleaners, drugs, or chemicals found in food or cosmetics. Poison ivy and poison oak rashes are other examples of contactant allergic reactions.

Ingestant allergens are swallowed or eaten. A variety of foods and medications can act as ingestant allergens to persons overly sensitive to them. A food allergy usually occurs in children and is a reaction to an ingestant allergen, often milk, eggs, shellfish and other fish, peanuts, chocolate, strawberries, and citrus fruits. Symptoms of food allergies include abdominal cramps, nausea, vomiting, and diarrhea. Hives, rash, headache, nasal congestion, even anaphylactic shock can also accompany a food allergy.

Injectant allergens are substances that penetrate the skin, such as insect venom or drugs that are injected. For example, people who have severe allergic reactions to insect bites or stings are suffering from a reaction to an injectant allergen. Shortness of breath; strong, rapid heartbeat; coughing; wheezing; and lightheadedness are common symptoms. The bite area swells and becomes tender or numb, and, in extreme cases, anaphylactic shock may occur.

In any allergy case, identifying the offending allergen may be painful, time-consuming, and expensive, but it is necessary to avoid future allergic reactions. A medical history, a record of any recent changes in daily habits, and both skin scratch tests (in which small amounts of the suspected allergens are applied to tiny scratches in the skin) and intracutaneous skin tests (in which allergens are injected under the skin) are used to help detect the troublesome foreign substance. A blood test called RAST (radioallergosorbent technique) is often taken to measure the amount of antibodies in the blood that have been manufactured in response to an invading substance.

Once the allergen is pinpointed, half the battle is won. Obviously, avoiding the troublesome allergen is a good start toward relieving an allergy problem. However, if the allergen cannot be avoided or removed, two treatments may be recommended: medication or immunotherapy. Three types of medication have commonly been prescribed: antihistamine drugs, which combat the effect of the histamines in the body; corticosteroids, which reduce inflammation and swelling; and bronchodilators, which ease breathing by opening bronchial tubes.

Allergy immunotherapy, or treatment by "desensitization shots," consists of the injection into the body of first small, then increasingly larger, quantities of the allergen. This allows the body to build up a form of resistance or immunity to the offending substance. Immunotherapy works best in controlling allergies to pollen, (especially hay fever), insect venom, and dust.

A little common sense goes a long way in controlling allergies. Obviously, the offending allergen needs to be avoided, removed, or replaced. Natural fibers in the home can be replaced with synthetics; air conditioners or air filters can be installed for hay fever sufferers; those susceptible to insect bites can wear protective clothes and avoid bright clothing and perfumes, both of which attract insects; babies born into allergy-prone families should be breastfed as long as possible to delay exposure to cow's milk, eggs, and citrus fruits.

Allergies cannot really be prevented, but much can be done to help to control or diminish their effects on the overly sensitive body.

See also Anaphylactic shock, Antibody/antigen, Asthma, Contact dermatitis, Hay fever, Hives, Immunity, and Insect bite and sting.

Alzheimer's disease

Alzheimer's disease is a disorder in which there is a steady deterioration of brain function resulting in continuing loss of memory, of recognition of friends and family, of personality, and of mental powers. Beginning as early as age 40 but most prevalent in the aged, it accounts for about half of all serious mental impairment in persons over age 65.

This disease has been studied extensively. As in any senile (characteristic of old age) condition, there is atrophy (shrinkage or wasting) of the cerebral cortex, which is the outer layer of the brain mostly concerned with intellectual and social functioning. In Alzheimer's disease, however, there are more specific abnormalities such as tangles or whorls of fibers within the nerve cells and senile plaques, deposits of a material, probably amyloid (a semisolid protein complex seen in many degenerative diseases). These abnormal changes are scattered throughout the cortex of an Alzheimer's victim and serve to distinguish the disease from other forms of senility. It is important to note that brain biopsies (tissue samples taken from the brain) are not performed on individuals without very specific reasons and without intention of specific treatment. Therefore, these changes are only seen after death except in very unusual circumstances.

Theories abound as to the possible causes of Alzheimer's disease. Slow viruses (viruses acquired early in life that have taken many years to do their damage) have been considered as have been environmental factors and damage from previous disease(s). Recently, in some patients, a diminished amount of the enzyme choline-acetyltransferase — necessary to manufacture the critically important neurotransmitter acetylcholine (a chemical that promotes the passage of nerve signals in numerous brain functions) — has been found, and theories about replacement of the enzyme and/or neurotransmitter are being formulated. High levels of aluminum have also been found in the brains of Alzheimer's patients, and drugs that combine with the aluminum and draw it out of the tissues (a process called chelation therapy) have been tried—in order to slow the deterioration — with mixed results. Heredity seems to play some part, since a family member of an Alzheimer's victim is more likely than others to develop the condition. It is generally agreed that hardening of the arteries is not a cause. The disease does not appear to be contagious, nor is it caused by emotional upsets and stress.

Symptoms vary considerably from one person to another and may occur days or months apart. They begin with small memory lapses, almost always first involving loss of recall for recent events. This can happen to anyone, but in Alzheimer's disease they grow more serious in time. A man may forget his son's name or lose his way home from the office. A person may forget to turn off the oven, misplace articles, recheck to see if a task was done, or repeat questions already answered. Eventually the gaps in memory, and failure to recognize friends and family members, interfere with normal work and social life. The individual starts having trouble with figures when working on bills, with understanding what is being read, with organizing the day's work. As the disease progresses, the victim of Alzheimer's disease becomes confused, frustrated, and irritable. Although at first the person seems physically unaffected by the disease, as the condition advances the patient becomes restless, always moving about, and must be watched so that he or she does not wander away or into danger. Endless repetition of meaningless actions, such as the opening and closing of drawers, is another characteristic of the disease. Some victims of the condition may become extremely agitated with little or no provocation.

The course of the disease, which eventually can result in damage to the body and nervous system (apart from the brain) and in loss of control over bladder and bowels, may range from one to 20 years. It may cut life expectancy by as much as one-half by contributing to death from another cause such as pneumonia or heart or kidney failure.

Other conditions can cause many of the symptoms of Alzheimer's disease, and many of these conditions are treatable. So it is very important for the patient to undergo a general medical examination with tests and extensive neurological and psychological studies. These involve computerized axial tomography (CAT scan—three-dimensional X-ray pictures), electroencephalography (EEG—a study of brain waves), blood tests, and often a sampling of spinal fluid. These procedures can rule out or identify possible causes such as a series of "little strokes," brain tumors or infections, pernicious anemia (curable with Vitamin B_{12}), overmedication with barbiturates or bromides, alcoholism, drug side effects, abnormal thyroid, or a blockage of cerebrospinal fluid in the head (hydrocephalus). Psychological depression is also an important—and treatable—cause of senile symptoms in the elderly and others, with symptoms of apathy, slowness of thought, inattention, and poor concentration. Death of a spouse or a shock such as moving to a nursing home could cause such symptoms temporarily.

Medical science does not now know how to prevent or treat Alzheimer's disease. However, it is important to find a physician who is able to help the patient and family handle the many problems that are bound to arise. At times, tranquilizers can lessen agitation, anxiety, and undesirable behavior. Medication may also help improve sleeping patterns and treat depression caused by the disease.

It is important that the patient continue the daily routine, exercise as usual, and keep in touch with friends. Memory aids such as lists of daily chores, reminders about safety, and a large calendar can help in day-to-day living. As care of the patient becomes more difficult, it may be best for the patient and family alike to move the patient to a health facility where a professional staff can provide round-the-clock care. Families can find support and receive latest information about the disease from the self-help Alzheimer's Disease and Related Disorders Association, 360 North Michigan Avenue, Chicago, IL 60601.

Amblyopia

Amblyopia is the name for diminished vision in one or both eyes, usually without any obvious defect. (Amblyopia is not the same as nearsightedness, farsightedness, or astigmatism which can be corrected with eyeglasses or contact lenses.)

There are two main types of amblyopia, depending upon the cause: "lazy eye" amblyopia and toxic amblyopia.

"Lazy eye" amblyopia occurs frequently in young children whose eyes, because they are not parallel, do not line up images correctly (a condition known as strabismus). In order to prevent double vision (in which you see two images of everything instead of one), the brain suppresses the sight of one eye; the other eye does all the work. Thus the popular term "lazy eye" is used for the eye that is not working. The eye, like any other organ, will not develop properly if not used; therefore, the structures of the suppressed eye may atrophy (waste away) or fail to develop.

Unfortunately, there are usually no obvious symptoms of "lazy eye." By the time the condition is recognized, the eye may be permanently damaged. The child usually appears to see as well as the next boy or girl. On the other hand, sometimes the condition that causes the amblyopia may be very noticeable. The eyes may turn either inward or outward or one may be looking up while the other is looking down.

To fully restore sight in the lazy eye, treatment must begin before the child is four to six years of age. If the eyes are out of focus because some of the muscles of the eye are weaker than others, the condition may be corrected by special glasses or contact lenses, by eye exercises, by eyedrops in or a patch on the normal eye that diminishes the ability of the normal eye to focus thereby forcing the lazy eye to work, or occasionally by surgery. Follow-up by the doctor is needed until the child is at least ten years of age.

Prevention of "lazy eye" amblyopia can begin soon after birth. If the eyes of a baby in the first weeks of life are continually out of alignment or still out of alignment from time to time at six months of age, the condition should be investigated. Otherwise, there may be a possibility of amblyopia. A simple eye test given in the doctor's office or even at home or nursery school should be able to show that one eye is not working and that treatment is needed. It should not be delayed. The child will not "grow out" of either strabismus or amblyopia.

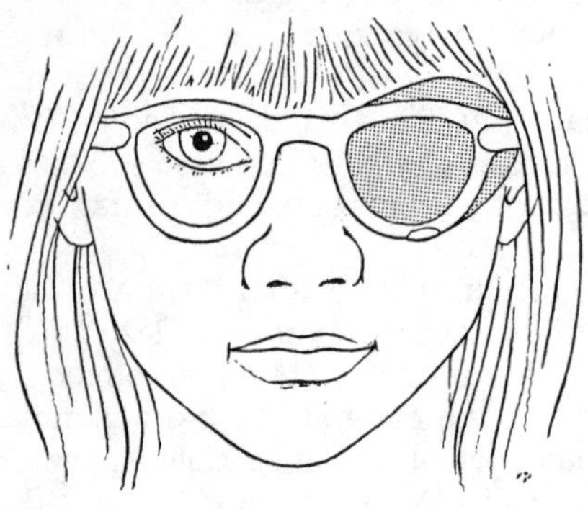

"Lazy eye" amblyopia may be corrected by patching or hindering the vision in the good eye, thus forcing the lazy eye to work.

Toxic amblyopia, usually occurring in both eyes, can result from excessive drinking of alcoholic beverages over a long period of time (and may be due mainly to the poor nutrition of heavy drinkers, who get most of their calories from alcohol and so do not eat enough nourishing food). It is also found, rarely, in heavy cigarette smokers and in people exposed to various chemicals, including lead, methanol (wood alcohol), digitalis, chloramphenicol, and arsenic. The toxic substance causes swelling and irritation of the optic nerve around the site where it enters the eyeball, and if the irritation continues, it can cause lasting damage to the nerve and even total blindness.

Symptoms include pain on moving the eyeball and an increasing area of poor eyesight in or near the center of one's field of vision.

Treatment is to stop exposure to the poison, if it can be discovered. In lead poisoning, the patient is given medicine that combines with the lead and draws it out of body tissues. The treatment is known as chelation therapy.

If the cause is removed at once, vision may improve—unless there is permanent damage to the optic nerve.

See also Strabismus.

Amenorrhea

Amenorrhea is defined as the absence of menstruation. There are two categories of this disorder. Primary amenorrhea is the failure to begin menstruating by the age of 16; secondary amenorrhea, the more common of the two conditions, is the absence of three or more periods in a row in a woman who has been menstruating for some time. Primary amenorrhea is specifically defined at the age of 16 and can go on indefinitely; secondary amenorrhea is usually a temporary condition, since the periods generally resume when the underlying cause for the interruption has been corrected.

Primary amenorrhea may be caused by endocrine gland disorders (such as hyper- or hypothyroidism); genetic abnormalities; damaged or missing ovaries, uterus, or vagina; or an excessively thick hymen (the membrane that covers the vaginal opening in young girls), which prevents the menstrual blood from flowing out.

Secondary amenorrhea is caused, most commonly, by pregnancy. It can also be triggered by strenuous sports training; poor nutrition; drastic weight gain; jet lag; certain medications, including birth control pills; serious surgery or disease; emotional shock; or the loss of a certain percentage of body fat, different for each individual (often seen in women afflicted with anorexia nervosa).

The symptoms that commonly accompany primary amenorrhea indicate abnormal or inhibited physical development; the young girl may fail to develop breasts or body hair, indicating that a genetic disorder may be present that is preventing her from attaining sexual maturity. These girls are also usually short.

Secondary amenorrhea has no symptoms other than the absence of menstrual periods.

Diagnosis of both categories will probably include a pregnancy test to rule out that possibility as its cause, as well as tests to determine genetic or hormonal disorders and X rays to check the condition of the reproductive organs.

Primary amenorrhea may be treated with an extensive hormone therapy program to stimulate physical development or, if the cause is a thick hymen, with surgery to open the hymen. Some cases of primary amenorrhea, however, are untreatable.

Secondary amenorrhea may be treated with a hormone that will trigger ovulation and reestablish the menstrual cycle. However, quite often this condition will reverse itself without treatment, especially if the cause is merely an interruption in the patient's normal routine, an emotional upset, or, of course, pregnancy.

Maintaining good nutrition habits and a normal weight and avoiding overexerting sports can probably be beneficial in preventing secondary amenorrhea; no specific precautions can be taken, however, to prevent primary amenorrhea.

See also Anorexia nervosa.

Amino acids

Amino acids are the main building blocks of proteins and are found in all living cells. There are 20 or more different kinds of amino acids, each of which contains carbon, hydrogen, oxygen, nitrogen, and in some cases sulfur. Each protein molecule is made up of thousands of amino acid molecules, linked to each other in chains.

In the body, food proteins in the small intestine are broken down to their amino acids, which are transported through the bloodstream to form, repair, and maintain body protein. Sometimes they are also used as fuel. In the cells, enzymes (substances, often proteins, which stimulate body processes) break down some amino acids into simpler compounds, use some for structure, and form others into chains of new proteins.

Nutritionists divide amino acids into two groups:

- nonessential amino acids, which can be manufactured by the body if we don't eat enough of them, and
- essential amino acids, which must be included in our diets if we are to remain healthy.

Rich sources of amino acids include meat, fish, fowl, egg white, milk, cheese, and various peas and beans. The proteins from animal sources are much more complete—that is, they contain more essential amino acids in the right proportions—than those from plant sources. Thus the person who avoids meat and dairy products should take care to include substantial amounts of two or more plant proteins in each day's meals.

Amnesia

Amnesia is the loss of memory and the inability to form new memories. It can be either temporary or permanent. The cause may range from brain damage to a psychological reason.

A certain type of amnesia (called retrograde) usually follows any severe head injury that produces unconsciousness. The patient is not able to recall what happened immediately before the accident causing the injury, the accident itself, nor some of the events of the recovery period. In most cases, this type of amnesia is not significant because no other memory is affected, and no treatment is needed.

An inability to record new memory along with a defect in memory of the past and usually accompanied by "confabulation" (storytelling of fabricated events) is known as Korsakoff's syndrome. It may be caused by head injury, stroke, encephalitis (inflammation of the lining of the brain), deficiency of Vitamin B, cancer of the brain, or poor blood supply to memory tissue or pathways in the brain. However, heavy drinking of alcohol, with resultant brain damage, is commonly the cause.

Although there may be little or no loss of memory or skills that were acquired before the disease begins, the person with Korsakoff's syndrome cannot effectively learn new skills or remember recent events. To hide this loss, from self as well as others, the patient may describe imaginary or confused experiences to take the place of the missing experiences. Sometimes the stories are so convincing the patient appears normal.

Treatment of Korsakoff's syndrome is limited to treating the condition that caused it. Permanent brain damage, however, may make it incurable. Frequently, however, especially if it is caused by a brain concussion (a swelling in the head that puts pressure on the brain), it will disappear of its own accord.

Amnesia of psychological cause is less common but more dramatic and newsworthy than other amnesias. A person disappears from home, job, and family, travels to a new place, assumes a new name, perhaps a new job, all without being aware that anything has changed. After days or weeks, the person "awakes," becomes his or her old self and wonders what happened. There is no memory of the period of amnesia.

Anxiety is the cause of this type of amnesia. The person is faced with an intolerable situation of high emotional stress or pain. To protect itself, the mind forgets the anxieties and everything related, including the person's identity.

Treatment may not be necessary, since most affected persons recover without help. However, if the problem that caused the amnesia still remains, it must be faced and solved. Family therapy and change of work or activities may help. Hypnosis may be used to bring back the memory of the "lost days" and unlock the ideas and feelings that caused the original flight from home and self.

Anaphylactic shock

Anaphylactic shock, most correctly known as anaphylaxis, is a violent allergic reaction characterized by itching skin, hives, breathing trouble, collapse of the blood circulation system, and sometimes vomiting, diarrhea, and cramps in the abdomen. It can occur in a person who is extremely sensitive to a substance on first exposure and certainly can reoccur if the person then is exposed to the substance again. The result is an explosive overreaction of the body's defense system to the foreign matter.

Often, the reaction is set off by an insect sting, such as that of a bee or wasp; by animal serum used in a vaccine; by desensitizing injections; or by one of various drugs. The allergen (the actual substance that sets off the reaction) is usually a protein, called an antigen. When it first enters the body, certain body cells treat it like an invading microorganism and create antibodies, which are protective substances that fight infection—in part by stimulating body defensive processes such as inflammation and vomiting. On later exposures, the antibodies are ready for the "invader" and stimulate release of certain chemicals including that known as histamine, which causes smooth muscles such as those in the digestive and breathing systems to contract, resulting in symptoms in those areas such as cramps and wheezing respectively. Histamine also causes the small blood vessels to enlarge and lose plasma (blood fluid) to surrounding tissues. This results in a drop in blood pressure that may lead to shock, or collapse of the blood circulation system.

Symptoms develop rapidly. Within one to 15 minutes, the exposed person becomes uneasy, upset, and red in the face. Rapid heartbeat, prickly and itching skin, throbbing in the ears, sneezing, coughing, and breathing difficulty are also likely. Vomiting, incontinence (involuntary release of urine and bowel contents), and even convulsions may occur. In another one or two minutes, shock may result, in which blood vessels collapse, the pulse becomes weak and rapid, and the person becomes cold, clammy, and faint. Without immediate medical aid, death may result.

Medical aid should be obtained as fast as possible; call an emergency squad. Keep the patient's airway open. With the patient lying down, keep legs elevated. Immediate treatment with the drug known as epinephrine is critical. It counteracts the action of the histamines released in the blood that are causing the symptoms of anaphylactic shock. If a drug injection has caused the reaction, a tourniquet should be applied above the site of the injection and more epinephrine should be injected into the site. Antihistamine drugs should also be given. In extreme cases, especially when shock has occurred or there is great breathing difficulty, intravenous (IV) solutions of salt water are given to restore blood volume and raise blood pressure. Anyone with a severe reaction should be hospitalized for at least 24 hours, to guard against a relapse.

A preventive measure against possible anaphylactic shock is routine allergy skin testing before the use of substances about which there is a question of sensitivity or substances, such as animal serums in vaccines, that are commonly known to cause anaphylactic shock. In addition, anyone who has had an anaphylactic reaction to a stinging insect should carry a kit containing a filled syringe of epinephrine and also an epinephrine-filled nasal sprayer, for prompt self-treatment when stung again. Desensitization injections of the insect venom to allow the body to build up a resistance to the venom should also be considered, if your doctor feels that such injections will not trigger an anaphylactic reaction.

Somewhat similar to anaphylaxis are anaphylactoid reactions, which can occur on the first injection of certain drugs, including contrast media (used when taking X-ray pictures), histamine, and morphine. These are not allergic reactions in the pure sense, but are serious nevertheless.

See also Allergy and Insect bite and sting.

Anemia

Anemia is a general term referring to a shortage of red blood cells or a reduction of their hemoglobin content. Hemoglobin is the pigment (colored agent) in the blood that carries oxygen in the blood cells. Therefore, a shortage of red blood cells or hemoglobin means that the blood will be unable to carry adequate oxygen to all parts of the body.

There are many types of anemia, such as iron deficiency anemia, folic acid deficiency anemia, pernicious anemia (Vitamin B_{12} deficiency), aplastic anemia, and various hemolytic anemias (in which red blood cells are broken up) including sickle cell anemia. Each type has its own cause and therefore its own methods of treatment, but all types of anemia are the result of an excessive loss or destruction of red blood cells or an inadequate production of red blood cells and hemoglobin.

Anemia can be caused by vitamin deficiencies or the body's inability to absorb certain vitamins, the destruction of red blood cells, inherited abnormalities in the blood, or the bone marrow's failure to manufacture red blood cells. Such diverse conditions as bleeding ulcers, drug allergies, cancer, and exposure to radioactivity, among many more, can lead to anemia.

People with poor diets or histories of alcoholism are more likely to develop one of the anemias caused by vitamin deficiencies. Women are particularly susceptible to iron deficiency anemia (a shortage of the mineral iron, which is necessary to produce hemoglobin) because of regular loss of blood during menstruation as well as depletion of iron during pregnancy by the unborn baby. A tendency toward anemia can also be inherited, in the form of sickle cell anemia, for instance.

Anemia can range from a severe case which may lead to extreme exhaustion or even death, to a mild condition which may be recognized only by a persistent tiredness.

The symptoms of anemia are fatigue, shortness of breath, pounding and increased heartbeat, headaches, loss of appetite, dizziness, ringing in the ears, and weakness or faintness. Burning of the tongue, and/or a change in its appearance, may also be a clue. A physical sign of anemia may be paleness in the creases of the palms, under the fingernails, and in the lining of the eye. Very severe cases may be signaled by swollen ankles and other signs of heart failure, and shock.

Diagnosis includes a physical exam as well as tests of the blood and often the bone marrow to detect shortages of red blood cells or hemoglobin.

Each type of anemia has different causes and therefore different treatments. Iron deficiency anemia is caused by a shortage of the mineral iron, which is necessary to produce hemoglobin. This shortage can be caused by a variety of conditions: a drastic blood loss, such as from an accident, or a chronic blood loss, such as from a bleeding ulcer or excessive menstrual flow; hookworm; a diet lacking in dark green vegetables and organ meats, which are good sources of iron; and pregnancy. This type of anemia can be treated with iron supplements (ferrous sulfate or ferrous gluconate tablets).

Folic acid deficiency is caused by insufficient folic acid in the diet, also necessary for hemoglobin production. This deficiency may be caused or aggravated by malnourishment and alcoholism. Some disorders of the small intestine, such as inflammatory bowel disease, may also cause it. It is treated with folic acid and sometimes additional vitamin supplements.

Pernicious anemia is caused by the body's inability to absorb Vitamin B_{12}, necessary for the production of red blood cells in the bone marrow. A substance called the intrinsic factor, which helps to absorb Vitamin B_{12}, is lacking in the stomach of someone suffering from this condition. Pernicious anemia is treated with Vitamin B_{12} injections directly into the bloodstream, bypassing the stomach completely. Inability to absorb Vitamin B_{12} can be caused by some parasites, inflammatory bowel disease, and other diseases of the small intestine.

Aplastic anemia is caused by the bone marrow's inability to produce blood cells. This deficiency affects the production of white and red blood cells, as well as the platelets (the blood cells that work to coagulate or clot the blood). The bone marrow's ability can be inhibited by cancer or exposure to radioactivity, hazardous chemicals, or some drugs. This variety of anemia is treated with blood transfusions and bone marrow transplants. It is a serious condition.

Hemolytic anemias are caused by the destruction of red blood cells. These anemias can be either acquired (developed over time) or congenital (present at birth).

Acquired hemolytic anemias can be caused by mismatched blood transfusions, a drug allergy, cancer, or a serious infection. Treatment of the source is necessary to treat the resulting anemia; blood transfusions can treat the condition temporarily.

Congenital hemolytic anemias are caused by an inherited abnormality in the red blood cells. The most common type is sickle cell anemia, a disorder that strikes mostly black people, in which the red blood cells, sickle-shaped instead of disclike, cannot carry enough oxygen throughout the body. These cells are also very fragile and break easily (or hemolyze). This disease is characterized by crisis period bouts of severe joint or abdominal pain and can lead to complications such as kidney disease, gallstones, and heart failure. Sickle cell anemia is treated with painkillers, oxygen, and transfusions. Avoiding situations in which oxygen may be scarce, such as high altitudes, is advisable.

There are no specific methods to prevent anemias other than a balanced diet to prevent anemia caused by vitamin and mineral deficiencies.

See also Sickle cell anemia.

Anesthesia

Anesthesia is an absence of sensation or feeling, with or without unconsciousness. Doctors use the term to describe complete loss of sensation in a body part even if it is the result of disease or injury or coldness. Most often, however, it refers to loss of feeling brought about by a drug known as an anesthetic, used to prevent pain during surgery or other painful procedures.

General anesthetics, most often used for major surgery, put the patient to sleep and eliminate pain throughout the body. They may be inhaled, through the nose or the mouth usually by means of a slender tube that goes into a nostril or the mouth and down the windpipe. This method permits both better control of the process by the anesthesiologist (a physician specially trained to relieve pain) or an anesthetist (a nurse trained in anesthesia) and the maintenance of an open airway. The doctor or nurse must keep constant watch over the anesthetized patient's resultant slowed heartbeat, breathing, and other vital functions to make sure that anesthesia is not slowing the body down to the danger point. In fact, during most general anesthesia, the patient is being artificially ventilated—that is, the patient's breathing is controlled by the use of a bag or breathing machine.

Before the operation, an injection may be given to relax the patient and reduce the amount of general anesthesia that is necessary. This is known as a basal anesthetic. An injection of a short-term general anesthetic may also be used alone, for brief operations. General anesthesia can also be given intravenously (into a vein, fed through a line from a bottle) or by an injection.

Where possible, physicians prefer to use anesthetics that do not put the patient to sleep. There is less danger of complications and in some cases such as childbirth the patient may be asked to perform certain tasks during the procedure. (Another reason general anesthesia is avoided when possible in childbirth is that it reduces the heartbeat and breathing of mother and baby alike. This weakens the strength of the mother's uterine contractions, so that birth may be more difficult. It can also result in less oxygen traveling to the baby's brain — severe lack of oxygen can cause temporary or permanent brain damage.) Descriptions of these various types of anesthetics follow.

Local anesthetics, such as the drug a dentist injects into the gums to "freeze" a tooth or a surgeon injects for a minor operation, prevent pain only in the area where they are applied. Certain sunburn lotions contain such a local anesthetic; rubbed on the skin, they take away the burning sensation temporarily.

Spinal anesthesia, often used in surgery of the abdomen and legs, is accomplished by injecting a local anesthetic into the sac surrounding the spinal cord. This stops the flow of pain messages carried by nerves from the lower part of the body.

Saddle block anesthesia is a form of spinal anesthesia produced by injecting anesthetic near the lower end of the spinal cord. It is so called because it blocks off sensation from the parts of the body that rest on the saddle in riding a horse.

Regional anesthesia prevents pain in a region of the body that is injected with a local anesthetic. The anesthetic may be injected into the area surrounding a region to be operated on. Or it may be injected close to the nerves leading from the region, in which case it is called a nerve block, block anesthesia, or conduction anesthesia.

Anesthesia used during childbirth includes pudendal block, paracervical, spinal, epidural, and caudal anesthesia.

In pudendal block, local anesthetic is injected through the wall of the vagina or through the skin of the buttock to reach the pudendal nerve. Blocking off this nerve eliminates pain and feeling from the lower part of the vagina, the rear portion of the vulva (the external genitals), and the surrounding outside skin. It is often used when delivery is going well and the mother wants to push. Sometimes this type of anesthesia is used following a paracervical block, in which a local anesthetic is injected around the mouth of the womb.

Various types of spinal anesthesia are used in childbirth. In one popular method, with the patient sitting up, a heavy solution containing local anesthetic is injected between the fourth and fifth vertebrae of the lower back into the fluid-filled sac surrounding the spinal cord. The heavy solution mixes with the spinal fluid and settles downward, blocking off pain messages from below the waist for about an hour.

Epidural anesthetic has a similar effect and is injected at the same place, but instead of being introduced into the spinal fluid in a single shot it can be fed for hours through a fine plastic tube that rests its tip against the tough dural membrane covering the spinal cord (hence the term epidural; "epi" means "upon"). The nerves are blocked where they enter the spinal cord to produce a numbing effect. An advantage of this is the fact that the dural membrane is not punctured, thus reducing the chances of complications, such as headache and infection.

Caudal anesthesia is the same as epidural except that the tube is introduced at the very tip of the spine, the "caudal" or "tail" area.

Because both the epidural and the caudal anesthesia can slow labor if given too soon, they are not given until the woman is in active labor.

There are various anesthetic methods that do not involve drugs, such as acupuncture, hypnotism, and electricity, but they are not widely used in the United States. Acupuncture, which originated in China thousands of years ago, involves inserting into the skin one or several fine needles, which are left in for 20 to 30 minutes for each treatment. Usually the method is used in an attempt to cure the disease or lessen long-lasting pain rather than to eliminate pain during surgery. Hypnotism has occasionally been used successfully to block from the mind the pain of surgery or childbirth, but as with acupuncture it is hard to predict or guarantee the results of a given procedure. Victims of chronic pain can sometimes relieve it with electricity—by using a device known as a transcutaneous nerve stimulator. The small battery-powered device is worn beneath the clothes and attached each day to the skin area where pain occurs. Upon feeling pain, the wearer presses a button to block the pain with an electrical current.

See also Acupuncture.

Aneurysm

An aneurysm is a bulge in a blood vessel, usually an artery, due to a weakness in the vessel wall particularly in the elastic, muscular layer of the artery wall. An artery has three layers: the intima, which is the smooth inner layer; the media, composed of the elastic and muscular fibers; and the adventitia, the tough outer layer. A true aneurysm involves all three layers, whereas a "false" aneurysm is a disruption and/or clot in one or two of the layers causing a bulge in the vessel. A dissecting aneurysm occurs when blood enters the layers of the media, causing it to become separated from the other layers, thereby creating an extra channel through which blood flows and is diverted from the organs. This dangerous condition can develop rapidly, in hours or days. Once between the media layers, the blood keeps creating a new channel that may finally extend the full length of the artery.

The main danger of most untreated aneurysms is that they may rupture or dissect causing death from loss of blood. If death does not occur, blood loss may so decrease blood flow to the heart that the heart cannot work properly.

There are various causes of aneurysms. Those occurring in the arteries of the brain are often due to a genetic (inherited) defect—a weakness in or lack of elastic tissue in the media. If they rupture, a stroke can result.

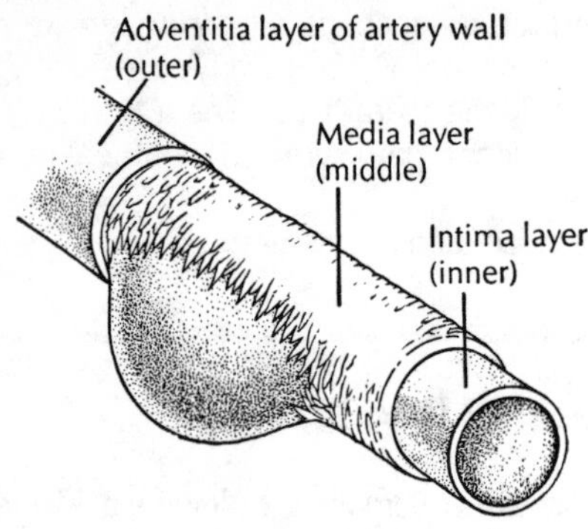

An aneurysm is a bulge in an artery because of a weakness in the vessel wall. A true aneurysm involves all three layers of the vessel wall, whereas a "false" aneurysm, shown here, is a disruption in one or two of the layers causing a bulge in the vessel.

Aneurysms in the small arteries may be caused by blood infections that weaken the vessel wall. Penetrating wounds occasionally can cause aneurysms. The sexually transmitted disease syphilis may also be a cause of aneurysms. Syphilis can cause an inflammation of the microscopic arteries that feed a large one (this is called vasculitis). When this occurs, these small arteries are lost, thereby causing a loss of nourishment to and a dying off and scarring of parts of the large arterial wall. This process leads to weakness of the wall and consequent formation of an aneurysm.

Dissecting aneurysms usually occur in the aorta (the main blood vessel leading away from the heart through the chest and abdomen), with atherosclerosis (hardening and scarring of the arteries) the most common cause, especially in the elderly. However, when dissecting aneurysms occur in the young, the cause is usually an inherited condition that results in damage to the media.

Symptoms of dissecting aneurysms of the aorta, if in the chest, include sudden, severe pain in the area of the aneurysm, often resembling a heart attack. There may be pain under the breastbone, in the back of the neck, difficulty in swallowing, shortness of breath, hoarseness, or a heavy cough. An aneurysm in a neck artery may create a pulsating swishing sound that the patient can detect.

Evidence of an aneurysm can be a tender, pulsating mass in the abdomen, or a painful, tender mass at the back of the knee (the latter can lead to blood clots that can travel downward and may result in gangrene—death of tissue—in the toes). Symptoms of dissection or rupture in the abdomen can include sudden, severe central or low abdominal pain radiating to the back, a loss of blood flow to the legs, and shock—collapse of circulation with fainting, pale and clammy skin, and rapid weak pulse. Death can result quickly.

X-ray and ultrasound pictures are taken of affected areas and used to locate aneurysms and determine their extent. The most reliable test is called an arteriogram or angiogram. In this test an X-ray dye is injected directly into the aorta providing an excellent visual picture on an X ray.

Treatment of most aneurysms, especially dissecting aneurysms, should begin as soon as possible. Patients with dissecting aneurysms belong in an intensive care unit. Drugs are given to lower high blood pressure (which worsens a dissecting aneurysm) and thus to reduce the chances of rupture. Occasionally, under lessened pressure, a dissecting aneurysm heals itself. Long-term medication which keeps blood pressure low is standard treatment for those who cannot be operated on. Surgery, however, is by far the most satisfactory solution where it is possible. The damaged portion of the blood vessel is removed and replaced with a synthetic or natural vessel. Patients with ruptured aortic and, in most cases, dissecting aneurysms need emergency surgery. Rapid replacement of blood is necessary, as is intensive monitoring. Surgery for aneurysm is usually long and difficult. However, with newer methods of diagnosis, many more people are being spared the risks of surgery by correction of the aneurysm before it becomes a problem.

Angina pectoris

Angina pectoris, usually referred to simply as angina, is a warning signal in the form of chest pain, commonly dull and pressure-like, indicating that the heart muscle is getting insufficient blood and therefore insufficient oxygen. Angina occurs when the heart is using oxygen beyond what its blood supply can provide and is a sign that the body needs to slow down to permit the heart to catch up.

An angina attack is not a heart attack. Its pain is usually not as severe or as long-lasting as that experienced during a heart attack, and it does not destroy the heart muscle, as does a heart attack. However, those who suffer from this condition are probably more prone to heart attack than are those who do not.

Angina can be caused by any number of factors that prevent the heart muscle from getting enough blood from the circulatory system. By far the most common cause of angina is coronary artery narrowing due to atherosclerosis. The coronary arteries supply the heart muscle itself with blood. When an increased demand is placed upon the heart by the body, for instance, by exercise, the heart must work harder to supply blood (and thereby oxygen) to keep the muscles and organs nourished. This increased work effort causes the heart muscle itself to require more blood. When narrowing of the coronary artery is present, the areas of heart muscle supplied by that part of the coronary artery cannot get enough blood in time to keep up with the demand. When this occurs, the muscle reacts by causing pain — angina pain. Exercise, emotional stress, or even cold weather can trigger an attack.

Overeating and smoking can also trigger and aggravate angina: overeating by drawing much needed blood to a full stomach to aid in digestion, and smoking by causing the coronary arteries to contract thus reducing the oxygen-carrying capacity of the arteries.

Several so-called "risk factors" are associated with the development of coronary artery disease and angina. Family history of heart attack, smoking, high cholesterol levels, and high blood pressure are among the best-known. There is much controversy in medicine regarding the degree of impact these factors have. It is not yet clearly established whether alteration of one or more of these will definitely prevent or delay the onset of heart disease. However, there is much evidence favoring reduction of any and all of these factors. Furthermore, common sense would dictate that one attempt to do this.

The major symptom of angina is a dull pressure or a sensation of squeezing or burning in the center of the chest behind the breastbone.

This dull pain in the chest is often compared to that accompanying indigestion. Angina pain can also be felt in the uppermost part of the abdomen and along the neck, and numbness may extend down the arm and wrist to the little finger. The bodily location and severity of the pain vary among angina patients, but the same symptoms usually reoccur for the same patient with each incident.

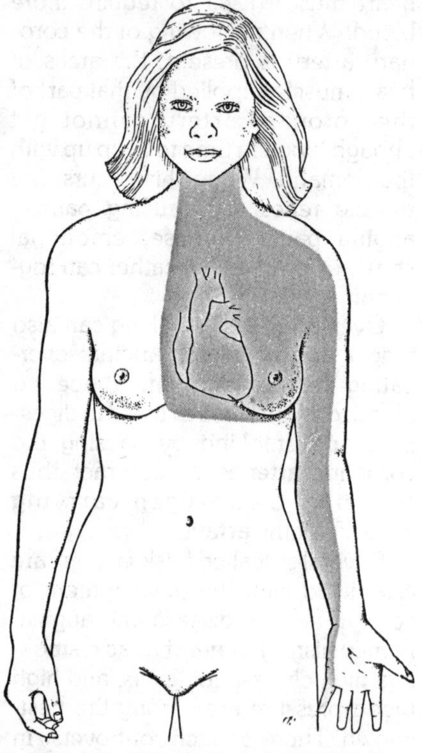

Although anginal pain is most often felt in the chest, it can also be felt below the breastbone near the uppermost part of the abdomen and along the neck. Pain and numbness may also extend down the arm and wrist to the little finger.

This pain usually occurs during or after physical exertion or emotional stress, lasts only three to five minutes, and is relieved by resting or relaxing. If the pain does not go away within five minutes or if the pain increases in severity, the condition causing it may not be angina. It may be another disorder unrelated to the heart or it may be a heart attack.

Angina is diagnosed by first eliminating the possibility that the pain is originating from some other disorder, such as gallbladder disease, rib injury, muscle spasm, or pleurisy (an inflammation of the membrane that covers the lung). The doctor will take a complete medical history, physical exam, and probably an exercise or stress test using an ECG (electrocardiograph) which measures the heart's electrical impulses during exercise. This test can indicate abnormalities in the arteries that are preventing sufficient blood to flow to the heart. Also, radioactive isotopes or X-ray opaque fluids can be injected into the bloodstream to monitor the flow of blood through the heart. The most definitive test for the diagnosis of coronary artery disease is the cardiac catheterization or angiogram. In this test, a radiopaque (able to be seen on X rays) dye is injected through a tube (catheter) placed directly into the heart through an artery in the leg or arm. Once the dye is injected, X-ray films are taken, and the areas of obstruction to the dye within the coronary arteries can be clearly seen. During this procedure, other important information, such as the overall condition of the heart muscle, can also be obtained.

Angina is often treated by recommending changes in the patient's lifestyle, to reduce the strain on the heart, and by administering medication, to modify the supply-demand relationship of the heart muscle and its blood supply.

A change in lifestyle will be necessary for patients who smoke, overeat, or overexert themselves. Certain types of exercise may be too stressful, but regular exercise is necessary to improve collateral circulation (the natural development of a system of small blood vessels that detour obstructions in the arteries and supply blood directly to the heart).

The medication most often used to treat angina attacks is nitroglycerin, which may act by expanding blood vessels to increase blood flow and/or by altering the distribution and volume of blood in the heart. Nitroglycerin is taken in the form of a tablet that is dissolved under the tongue. Pain should stop within three or four minutes; if it does not, the pain may not be due to simple angina. Nitroglycerin can also be prescribed as an ointment. This is used for the prevention of attacks, not for the treatment of an acute episode.

Surgery to bypass the obstructions in the arteries is performed only when angina cannot be controlled with medication or when its pain is becoming increasingly severe. There has been much controversy surrounding bypass surgery, mainly centering around the question of whether this procedure can increase life expectancy in those with coronary artery disease and angina. At present, there is no question that the surgery relieves pain and allows for greater exercise tolerance in the majority of patients who undergo it for severe angina. In certain patterns of disease such as obstruction of the "left-main" coronary artery, the operation definitely prolongs life expectancy. In other patterns such as "triple vessel disease" where branches of all three coronaries (except for the left-main) are involved, the surgery most likely allows a longer life. In still other patterns, the question is unsettled. Whether or not the surgery will prevent a heart attack is also an unsettled issue.

Incidents of angina pain can be prevented with several drugs: nitrates and calcium antagonists (drugs such as nifedipine and verapamil that act by blocking the constricting actions of calcium on arterial muscle), which have a longer lasting effect than plain nitroglycerin and may be taken on a regular basis; and beta blockers, which also effectively prevent angina, since they decrease the work of the heart, thereby lessening its oxygen needs and making it less likely that angina will occur. (One additional note: beta blockers should be used with caution if at all by asthma patients, as these drugs may cause spasms in the breathing tubes and subsequent breathing difficulties.)

See also Atherosclerosis, Bypass surgery, and Heart attack.

Ankylosing spondylitis

Ankylosing spondylitis is a form of arthritis, mainly affecting the sacroiliac joints, the spine, and nearby structures, in which joints become inflamed and eventually stiff and immovable. The elastic cartilage discs between the vertebrae (bones of the backbone) turn to dense tissue as does adjacent connective tissue, and bony connections between the vertebrae (ankylosis) are formed. The vertebrae may become fused together, creating a straight "poker spine" frequently with a curve in the upper spine.

The cause of ankylosing spondylitis is unknown, but there appears to be an inherited tendency toward the disease. The disease affects men ten times as often as women, and many are born with a certain trait, called HLA-B27, in their blood. Persons carrying this trait are much more likely to develop the disease than those without it.

Ankylosing spondylitis is mostly a disease of young men, occurring most commonly between the ages of 15 and 40. The disease may progress slowly for ten to 20 years and then stop or slow down of its own accord.

Chronic low back pain and stiffness in a young man is a chief sign of the disease; hip pain is also quite common as is an inflammation of the eye known as anterior uveitis. Symptoms begin gradually, usually as low backaches. There may be morning stiffness and pain extending down the leg along the sciatic nerve commonly alternating from one side to the other. The back pain and stiffness eventually affect the upper spine and sometimes the neck. In up to a third of the cases, large joints such as those of the hips and shoulders are affected. Knees and other smaller joints are affected less often, with symptoms matching those of rheumatoid arthritis. The heart is affected in up to 3 percent of cases (after many years of disease), and inflammation of the lining of the eye occurs in around 25 percent of the cases. As the disease progresses, it is harder for the patient to flex the back and expand the chest; neck movements may be limited. X-ray pictures of the back-related joints—especially those between the upper portion of the hipbone and the sacrum (the bony structure at the base of the spine)—reveal changes typical of ankylosing spondylitis. A sign of advanced disease is "bamboo spine," seen on the X ray, showing bony bands around the discs, cementing the vertebrae to each other.

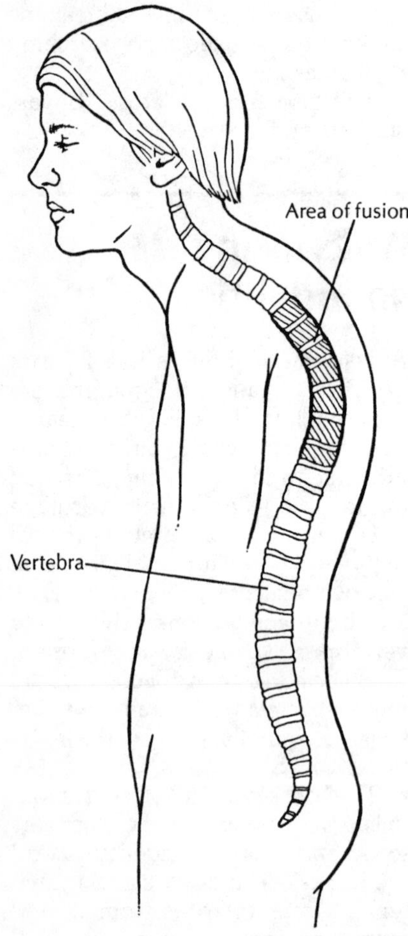

Ankylosing spondylitis is a form of arthritis in which the vertebrae (backbones) may become fused together often with a curve in the upper spine.

Although there is no cure for ankylosing spondylitis, certain measures can lessen the effects of the disease. These include breathing exercises and exercises to maintain posture, to help with curvature of the upper spine, and to keep the back as flexible as possible. To prevent curvature of the upper spine, sleeping on the back on a firm mattress with a small or no pillow is advised. Locking the fingers behind the head and pushing the elbows back as far as possible is a good way to straighten the upper back and stretch the chest muscles. Painkillers and anti-inflammatory drugs may be given. Surgery is rarely needed, nor is a back brace. Plenty of rest is recommended.

Anorexia nervosa

Anorexia nervosa is an eating disorder that strikes mostly young women who suppress the urge to eat and continue to lose weight to the point of malnutrition and starvation. It can be fatal, because an anorexic can literally starve herself to death while she continues to think of herself as fat.

Anorexics continue to starve themselves because they mistakenly believe that they are fat and need to diet. The result is not only an unattractively skinny appearance, but also an end to menstrual periods (which very frequently cease when a certain percentage of body fat is lost), and, most importantly, the destruction of healthy muscle and organ tissue, which the body, when starved, uses as energy sources instead of food.

Ninety-five percent of all anorexics are female; most are teenagers from upper or upper-middle class homes. About one in 200 women of this age and social class is estimated to have anorexia nervosa.

Anorexia seems to be a psychological disorder as well, as it often develops in young women with deep-seated problems, although the classic anorexic may not seem to be a "troubled" teenager. The young girl who has always been "perfect," obedient, and who has tried to fulfill all the wishes of her parents, teachers,

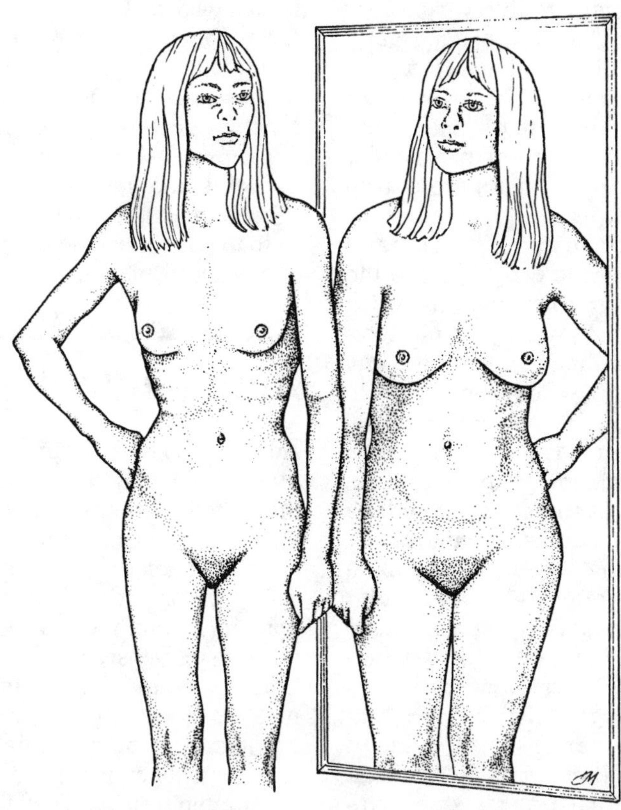

A person with anorexia nervosa has a distorted body image that makes her think she is fat even as she views her extremely thin body in a mirror.

and friends may become anorexic due to a subconscious need to have total control over at least one area of her life.

Impending adulthood and all that it entails may scare the anorexic into dieting away all that reminds her of her developing maturity: her larger breasts, curved hips, and fuller thighs. The lack of menstrual periods, too, is a reminder of the happier days of childhood.

Our culture's obsession with thinness as the ideal in beauty can also trigger the desire in an adolescent girl to diet down to her "perfect" weight; often a casual remark that a girl is slightly overweight has led to a case of anorexia in a susceptible person.

In addition, people with jobs or hobbies that require strict weight control, such as athletes, ballerinas, and fashion models, may find that simply watching their weight has become an obsession with dieting. In fact, the few males who develop this disorder often do so in an attempt to qualify for an athletic team.

The major symptom of anorexia nervosa is drastic weight loss to the point of extreme underweight, which can be accompanied by overly vigorous exercise that burns off the few calories that are consumed. Anorexics cannot be convinced to eat with threats or reasoning; they have a distorted body image that tells them they are fat even as they view their extremely thin bodies in a mirror.

Despite the refusal to eat more than tiny amounts of particular foods, the anorexic may be obsessed with the idea of food. She may prepare elaborate meals for others or go on eating binges followed by vomiting, which can be self-induced (bulimia), and excessive use of laxatives. Menstrual periods stop completely, and a growth of fine, downy hair appears all over the body.

Positive diagnosis of anorexia nervosa will require the doctor first to rule out that the extreme weight loss has been caused by a serious illness such as cancer, infectious disease, disorders of the digestive organs, or inadequate absorption of vitamins and minerals. Anorexia can usually be positively diagnosed when the patient displays the classic symptoms before the age of 25 and has lost 25 percent of her original body weight.

Anorexia is sometimes treated with hospitalization and forced feeding; but usually, anorexics can be treated on an out-patient basis by a doctor, psychiatrist, or specialist in eating disorders, whose job is to convince the anorexic that she must eat and gain weight, but that she will not be allowed to become fat. Her distorted body image as well as her eating habits must be changed in order for her to conquer this disorder. Most importantly, the underlying psychological problems must be exposed and resolved. Often, this means psychological therapy for both the anorexic and her family.

See also Bulimia.

Antibody/antigen

An antibody is a substance produced by the body to fight a specific invading foreign agent. The invading agent, known as an antigen, may be a virus, bacterium, a poison produced by bacteria, or a foreign protein. Each antibody is designed to work only against a particular antigen and no other. There is one for measles, another for mumps, and so on. The antibody molecule combines with the antigen molecule by matching combining sites. They fit together like the pieces of a jigsaw puzzle.

Antibodies are produced by the

B-lymphocytes (a type of white blood cell) that are manufactured and developed in the bone marrow. Lymphocytes circulate in the blood and are stored in great quantities in the spleen, lymph glands, tonsils, adenoids, and elsewhere. In a normal healthy person, enough antibodies are produced quickly by the lymphocytes — usually in hours or days — to overwhelm and defeat the invading antigens of disease. After the invaders are destroyed, antibodies to that specific disease remain in the system to produce immunity, a natural resistance that protects against future infection from that particular antigen.

Antibodies are not always beneficial. For example, when tissue from another body, such as a transplanted heart, is introduced, antibodies are produced to destroy the "invader." Transplants usually are made possible only by means of drugs and occasionally radiation that act against the body's immune response. Also, when you have a blood transfusion, it must be of a matching type; otherwise your body will manufacture antibodies to destroy it.

Apgar score

The Apgar score is a general evaluation of a baby's condition, made one and five minutes after birth, to determine immediately if the newborn needs emergency care. The score, devised by the late Virginia Apgar, M.D., is now used throughout the world and is based on the letters of her last name.

One minute and five minutes after birth, a delivery room nurse, anesthesiologist, or pediatrician rates the baby on five indicators, using a scale of 0 to 2:

A (Appearance): the baby gets a top score of 2 if the skin is completely pink, 1 if it is pink but hands and feet are bluish, and 0 if the entire body is blue (indicating lack of oxygen).

P (Pulse): a score of 2 is given for a pulse, or heart rate, above 100; 1 for less than 100; 0 for no pulse.

G (Grimace, or reflex irritability): to score a 2, the baby must cry vigorously when slapped lightly on the soles of the feet; a grimace or slight cry scores as a 1; no response gets a 0.

A (Activity): active motions score a 2; some movement of arms and legs is a 1; but a limp and motionless infant scores 0.

R (Respiration; breathing): strong efforts to breathe together with vigorous crying score a 2; slow, irregular breathing, 1; no breathing, 0.

Most babies score between 7 and 10 when tested one minute after birth. They are breathing well, crying, pinkish in color, active, and need no emergency measures.

Those babies who score from 4 to 6 usually need help immediately. The throat is suctioned to remove thick mucus, small blood clots, or bits of swallowed membrane (from the amniotic sac that enclosed the baby before birth). Oxygen is sometimes given to assist breathing and restore color.

The baby with the Apgar score below 4 is limp, pale or bluish, perhaps without heartbeat, and is in grave danger. The throat is suctioned and the baby is placed on a mechanical respirator which pumps air in and out of the lungs until the baby can breathe on his or her own.

A second Apgar score is taken five minutes after birth and recorded on the baby's chart beside the first score. The second score is a good measure of the baby's adaptation to the world outside the womb.

Apnea

Apnea is an interruption in breathing that occurs in some very premature babies and also during the sleep of some adults. The usual cause in infants is immaturity of the brain centers that regulate breathing. In adults, most often the cause is obstruction of the upper airway; the second most common cause is malfunction of the breathing control centers of the brain.

Apnea in a tiny baby appears frightening. From time to time, the infant suddenly stops breathing completely and turns blue. If the baby is stimulated in some way, as by a flick of the finger on the bottom of the foot, he or she will usually start breathing normally at once. Seldom is it necessary to use first-aid measures or a mechanical respirator to restart breathing. Even without stimulation, the baby will usually start to breathe again on its own. But the condition is dangerous, so such babies in hospital newborn intensive care units are guarded by equipment (called an apnea alarm) that detects any stoppage of breathing and sounds an alarm. A nurse then rushes to the baby's side and stimulates it to resume breathing. The condition usually disappears in a few weeks after the baby's breathing control centers mature.

Apnea during the sleep of certain adults, particularly fat people, has just recently been recognized. A typical sleep pattern is loud snoring, followed by silence (when the breathing stops), and then a loud choke or gasp as the sleeper partially wakes, clears the air passage, and resumes breathing. This may occur many times within an hour for a number of hours during the night. In some sleep-apnea patients such as those with severe emphysema, during the apnea, carbon dioxide in the blood builds up, occasionally to a dangerous level. The reason for the closure of the airway is not fully known, but obesity is thought to play a part in many cases. Apnea also occurs in some adults of normal weight, perhaps because of inborn defects in the upper airway. Victims of sleep apnea are likely to be drowsy during the day and irritable, from lack of sleep, with decreased memory and attention span.

Treatment includes weight reduction for fat patients. In extreme cases of airway obstruction, the only solution is for a surgeon to create a tracheostomy—a hole in the windpipe and neck, below the upper airway, through which the patient breathes. Drugs are sometimes given to help correct sleep apnea, and stimulation of the diaphragm (the muscle, separating the chest and abdomen, that is instrumental in breathing) with an electronic pacemaker—like a heart pacemaker—has been tried with some success.

Appendicitis

Appendicitis is an inflammation of the appendix that results from a bacterial infection.

The appendix is a small worm-like portion of intestinal tissue located at the juncture of the small and large intestines. Although it may have had a function at some point in human development, the appendix serves no purpose now.

Nevertheless, despite its uselessness, the appendix can cause problems when it becomes inflamed. Inflammation occurs when the hollow tubular structure clogs with masses of waste matter, intestinal worms, or other material that can prevent normal drainage. The blockage provides a fertile environment for bacteria to grow and multiply, thereby causing infection and inflammation.

In the beginning, appendicitis may produce a dull or sharp pain in the navel area of the abdomen. Any movement, coughing, or sneezing can intensify the pain. Patients in early stages may also feel nauseous and be unable to eat. Constipation usually accompanies appendicitis; nonetheless about 10 percent of the patients may have diarrhea instead. Adults may run a mild fever (up to 102°F), but children generally experience higher fevers. Occasionally, pulse rates accelerate to about 100 beats per minute.

Within hours, the pain becomes continuous and moves to the lower right side of the abdomen over the appendix. Because the location of the appendix may vary depending upon the individual, pain may emanate from the back, side or pelvis, or even the opposite side of the abdomen. The entire appendix area becomes extremely tender as abdominal muscles tighten.

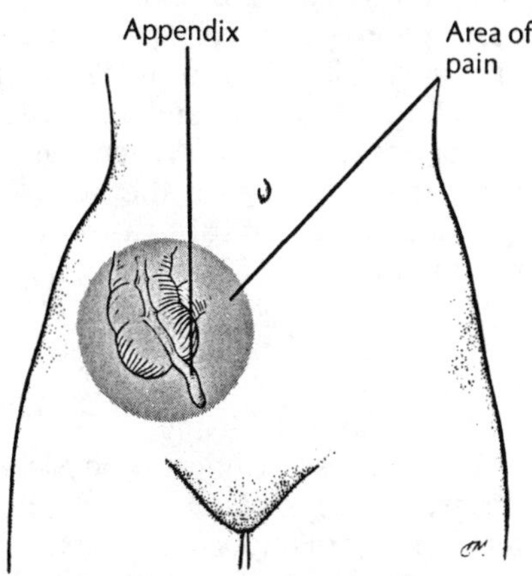

In appendicitis, the lower right side of the abdomen becomes painful and tender.

If fever rises and pain grows more intense, chances of rupture become greater. Rupture results when the appendix becomes so swollen and filled with pus from bacteria that it bursts, spreading infection to surrounding organs. Infection spreads so quickly that gangrene of the appendix (death of tissue) may occur within hours after the first symptoms. One serious complication of rupture is peritonitis, an inflammation of the lining of the abdominal cavity.

Any fever with nausea and abdominal pain should be reported to a physician. More severe pain is an immediate medical emergency that must be diagnosed to prevent potentially fatal complications. Appendicitis can affect anyone but the disease is more prevalent among people between ten and 30 years of age.

When confirming appendicitis, the doctor checks for tenderness over the appendix. A blood test determines whether or not there is a high white blood cell count (with an infection, the body produces extra white blood cells to help fight the disease). Morever, the doctor may perform additional tests to rule out other diseases sometimes mistaken for appendicitis, such as gallbladder attack, kidney stones, or kidney infection. In women a twisted ovarian cyst (growth on the female sex organ) or a ruptured ectopic (tubal) pregnancy may produce symptoms similar to those of appendicitis.

Although appendicitis cannot be prevented, prompt diagnosis can lead to effective treatment. Patients who suspect appendicitis should not eat or drink food or water, or take drugs to relieve pain until a doctor is consulted. Eating or drinking any substance, including laxatives, may cause the appendix to rupture by stimulating activity in the intestine.

A mild case of appendicitis may subside by itself, but some people may have recurrent attacks. The most common cure for acute appendicitis is surgery to remove the inflamed organ and to avoid complications. To insure against further infection, antibiotics may be prescribed in addition to surgery.

Arrhythmia

See Heartbeat irregularities.

Arteriosclerosis

See Atherosclerosis.

Arthritis

Arthritis is an inflammation of the joints, the junctures where the ends of two bones meet.

Inflammation develops in one of two ways. With *osteoarthritis,* there is gradual wearing away of cartilage in the joints. Healthy cartilage is the elastic tissue that cushions the joints and prevents the bones from touching. When this cartilage deteriorates, the bones rub together causing pain and swelling. Although osteoarthritis can result from direct injury to the joint, it commonly occurs in most adults over the age of 55 because of long-term wear and tear on the joints.

Rheumatoid arthritis, on the other hand, can attack at any age. This form of arthritis affects all the connective tissues in the body. The precise cause of rheumatoid arthritis is unknown. Some researchers believe that a virus may trigger the disease, causing an autoimmune response whereby the body develops a sensitivity or allergy to its own tissues. However, evidence for this theory is inconclusive as yet. What is confirmed is the progression of the condition. First, the synovium, which is a thin membrane lining and lubricating the joint, becomes inflamed. The inflammation eventually destroys the cartilage. As scar tissue gradually replaces the damaged cartilage, the joint becomes misshapen and rigid.

Arthritis is not an inherited disease. Nonetheless, people who have arthritis in their family are more prone to develop the disease. Women have a greater tendency to develop arthritis than men, although the reason for this is unclear. In addition, excess body weight may promote osteoarthritis because of increased load on the joints. Constant joint abuse from strains of sports or employment may encourage arthritis, but inactivity can also cause the problem.

Symptoms of arthritis include swelling, tenderness, pain, stiffness, or redness in one or more joints. For many patients, pain is greater in the morning, and it subsides as the day advances. Damp weather and emotional stress do not cause arthritis, but they can make symptoms worse.

With rheumatoid arthritis, these symptoms may be accompanied by more generalized feelings of fatigue and fever. Often, this form of arthritis goes into periods of remission when symptoms disappear. When symptoms return, however, they can be more severe. If left untreated, rheumatoid arthritis may damage heart, lungs, nerves, and eyes, whereas complications of osteoarthritis can cause permanent damage and stiffness of the joints.

To diagnose arthritis, a physician observes the symptoms and administers a standard physical examination. X rays and laboratory tests may be recommended for confirmation of joint swelling.

The most effective treatment program for arthritis consists of drug therapy, exercise, and rest. Treatment should begin early after diagnosis to prevent permanent damage.

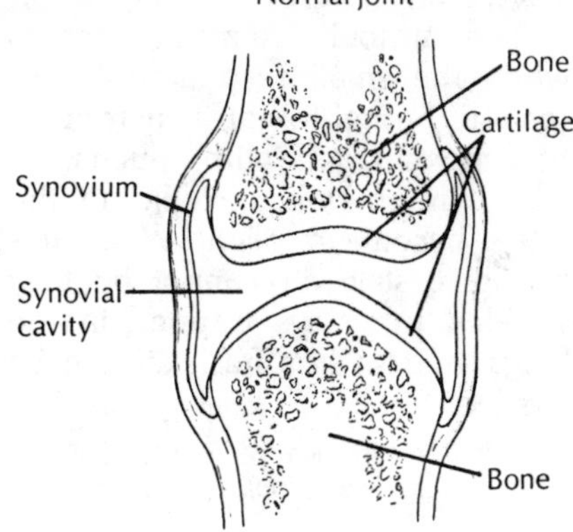

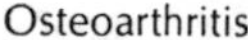

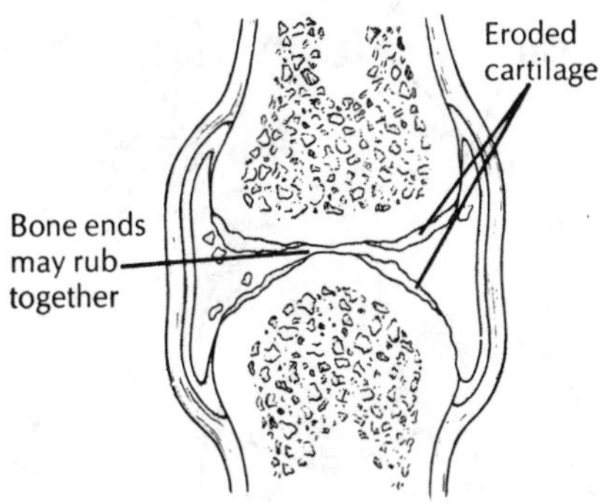

In osteoarthritis, the cushioning cartilage at the ends of bones wears away or erodes, possibly causing the bones to rub together which results in swelling and pain.

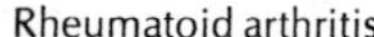

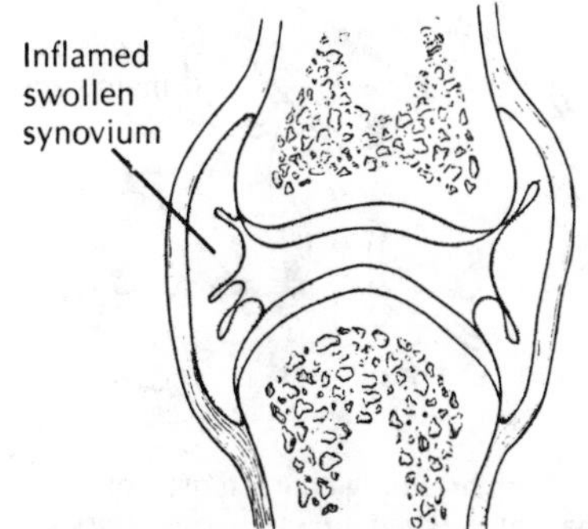

Rheumatoid arthritis is characterized by a swollen and inflamed synovium, the membrane that lines the joint and produces lubricating fluid.

Of the drugs administered for arthritis, aspirin is the most common. Doctors prescribe two to three tablets several times a day to relieve pain and reduce inflammation. To prevent stomach irritation, they suggest taking aspirin after meals or in a coated tablet form.

Often nonaspirin pain relievers and nonsteroid anti-inflammatory drugs (for example, ibuprofen, naproxen, tolmetin, or sulindac) may be prescribed. Corticosteroids also relieve inflammation, but they can cause adverse side effects. Sometimes, a doctor needs to try several different drugs before finding an effective one that produces no side effects.

Moderate daily exercise, such as swimming, walking, or perhaps physical therapy, is critical to maintaining mobility in arthritic joints. A supervised exercise program interspersed with rest periods helps to reduce joint inflammation. To lessen pain while increasing movement, moist heat often helps. In addition, maintaining correct posture and body weight eliminates extra burden on sore joints.

Some severe cases of rheumatoid arthritis may require surgery to remove inflamed synovial tissue. With either form of arthritis, artificial joints may be implanted to replace those damaged beyond repair.

Artificial insemination

Artificial insemination is the introduction of a man's semen (the fluid containing the sperm) into a woman's vagina or uterus by artificial means, usually by a special syringe, in the hope of accomplishing a pregnancy. The semen may be from the woman's husband or from an unknown donor.

Artificial insemination from the husband is sometimes done when the husband has a low sperm count—that is, when there are not enough sperm per unit of fluid to cause pregnancy. To obtain enough sperm, several collections may be made over days or weeks, frozen, and used in one insertion. Artificial insemination may also be used when one or the other partner cannot perform the sexual act in a normal manner, for example because of a physical condition or an emotional problem.

Artificial insemination from a donor can also be an alternative to adoption when the husband cannot father a child, whether because of low sperm count, absence of sperm, poor quality and lack of motion in sperm, or because of inability to perform sexual intercourse. It may also be considered when the husband carries an inborn defect that he does not want to pass on to his child. The woman's physician arranges for the sperm to be obtained from an unknown donor and inserts it at or before the time of her ovulation. The sperm may be fresh or obtained from a "sperm bank," which collects sperm in advance, freezes it, and stores it for this purpose. This procedure should never be done without the husband's permission; in fact, in most states it is illegal without a legal agreement signed by both husband and wife.

Asthma

Asthma is a respiratory disease characterized by unpredictable periods of acute breathlessness and wheezing. Asthma attacks can last from less than an hour to a week or more and can strike frequently or only every few years. Attacks may be mild or severe and can occur sporadically, at any time, even during sleep.

The difficult breathing occurs when the small respiratory tubes (called bronchioles) constrict or become clogged with mucus, or when the membranes lining the tubes become swollen. When this happens, stale air cannot be fully exhaled but stays trapped in the lungs, and so less fresh air can be inhaled.

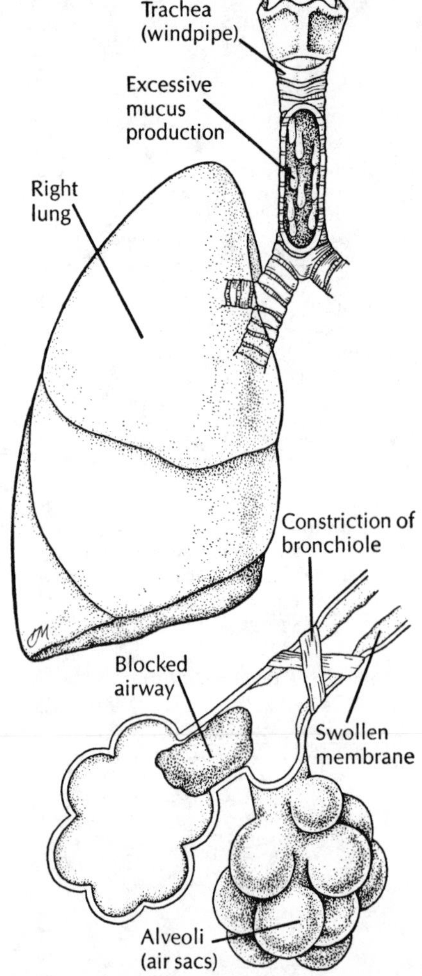

The difficult breathing characteristic of asthma occurs when the small respiratory tubes (bronchioles) constrict or become clogged with mucus, or when the membranes lining the tubes become swollen. Stale air is trapped in the air sacs and less fresh air can be inhaled.

Asthma attacks can result from the bronchial system's oversensitivity to a variety of outside substances or environmental conditions. About one half of all attacks are triggered by allergies to such substances as dust, smoke, pollen, feathers, pet hair, insects, mold spores, and a variety of foods and medications. Attacks not related to allergies can be set off by environmental conditions such as ear, nose, or throat infections, strenuous exercise, breathing cold air, or even emotional stress. Heredity may play a part in the tendency to develop asthma; children with one or both asthmatic parents have a 50 percent chance of developing the condition.

Asthma is rarely fatal, but it can be a very serious condition, especially in young children. Nevertheless, attacks often become less frequent and less severe as children grow up.

Common symptoms of an asthma attack include tightness in the chest, difficult breathing, coughing, and the characteristic wheezing that is caused by the effort to push the flow of air through the narrowed bronchioles. As the attack progresses, muscles surrounding the bronchioles constrict further, breathing becomes even more difficult, and mucus collects.

Diagnostic procedures may include a complete medical history, physical examination, chest X ray, and allergy and skin scratch tests.

Asthma cannot be cured, but it can be controlled with a variety of drugs. An epinephrine (adrenaline) injection or an adrenaline aerosol may be administered during an acute attack in order to enlarge the bronchioles; however, these drugs may overstimulate the heart and so cannot be used for long periods of time (they, therefore, are usually used only in an emergency). Adrenaline-like drugs, taken orally, can be administered for longer periods because they lack this stimulating effect on the heart since they affect only the muscles of the airways. However, these drugs are usually recommended to be taken for only a few days after an attack, because constant use may result in the body's building a tolerance to the drugs, thus making the next attack more difficult to treat.

For long-term therapy, the drug theophylline can be used to keep the bronchioles constantly cleared. Its prescribed dosage, however, must be closely supervised because its rate of absorption into the body can vary widely among patients; some persons eliminate the drug so quickly it is almost ineffective while in others the drug accumulates in the body at times to toxic levels. Also, nausea, vomiting, and agitation are common side effects.

Corticosteroids can control asthma, but patients may become dependent on them and they may have such undesirable side effects as weight gain, ulcers, high blood pressure—even a stunting of growth and development in children.

Cromolyn, the only known drug that actually prevents attacks, acts to inhibit the release of histamines, the chemicals manufactured by the body during an allergy reaction. Cromolyn, however, cannot relieve an attack already in progress and is usually only for mild cases.

Regardless of which drug is prescribed, all asthmatic patients should drink plenty of water to keep the bronchial tubes moistened and to replace fluids which may be depleted by the use of drugs.

If an allergy is causing the attacks, the troublesome foreign substance (called an allergen) must be removed. If this cannot be accomplished, allergy shots to reduce the patient's sensitivity to the allergen may be beneficial. The use of antihistamines may also bring some relief.

Several precautions can be taken to reduce the possibility of an asthma condition developing. Since the tendency to develop asthma is inherited, babies of asthmatic parents should be fed breast milk or soy protein formula, since these are less likely than cow's milk to cause allergic reactions. Smoke and pet hair, as well as rugs, drapes, and overstuffed furniture, which tend to attract dust, can be removed from the home. Moderate exercise is a good preventive method, although strenuous exercise may cause an attack.

One additional note: asthmatics who also suffer from angina or heart problems should take beta blocker drugs only with extreme caution, as these drugs may cause spasms in the airways.

See also Allergy.

Astigmatism

Astigmatism is a type of distorted vision caused by a defect in the curvature of the eye. This prevents all the rays of light entering the eye from being properly focused on the retina at the back of the eye. Some rays are misplaced, causing the image to be partially out of focus.

Most people with astigmatism can see clearly those objects directly in front of them. However, their peripheral vision is imperfect. They may have vertical astigmatism, in which the scene above and below their direct gaze is imperfect. They may have horizontal astigmatism in which the right and left sides of their field of vision are warped; for example, a straight horizontal line may appear curved to the right and to the left. The astigmatism may also be diagonal.

Fortunately, the defect in the curvature of the eye is usually uniform and can be easily corrected by eyeglasses or contact lenses. The fault is usually in the shape of the cornea, the clear "window" in front of the iris and pupil, which may be slightly flattened vertically or horizontally. The eyeglass or contact lenses do not bend rays entering the band of clear vision but are curved to adjust the angle of rays entering from either side or top and bottom, depending upon the prescription.

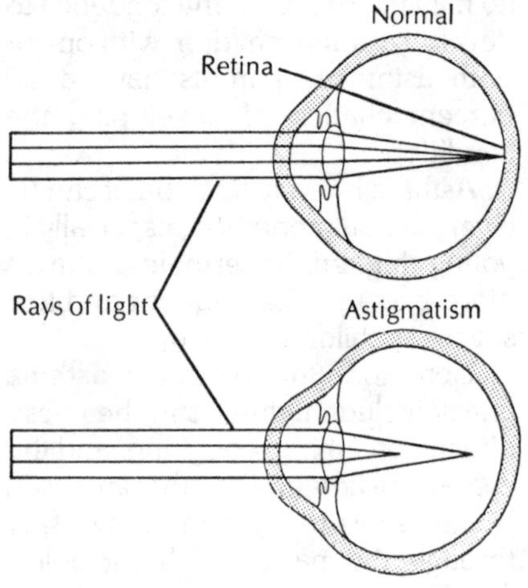

Astigmatism is a form of distorted vision in which rays of light entering the eye are not properly focused on the retina at the back of the eye because of a defect in the curvature of the eye. This can be corrected by the proper eyeglasses or contact lenses.

Although most people with astigmatism were born with a tendency toward the condition, a few cases are caused by eye disease or injury. These may be more difficult to correct. Regardless of the cause, astigmatism—as with any vision problem — should be corrected as early as possible. A child, in particular, with an uncorrected vision problem may develop permanently defective vision.

See also Amblyopia and Myopia.

Ataxia

Ataxia is a condition characterized by muscular incoordination, producing irregular and inaccurate movements of the body. The result may be a clumsy manner of walking with feet wide apart, a lack of balance, tremors of the arms, or slurring of speech.

Ataxia may be caused by anything that affects the motor control centers of the brain, or the nerve pathways leading from them. Drunkenness can produce a temporary staggering ataxia. Permanent ataxia is caused by damage to the central nervous system (the brain, spinal cord, and spinal nerves).

Locomotor ataxia may be a late result of untreated syphilis. Its symptoms include sharp, stabbing pains, usually in the legs; an unsteady walk; and a feeling of walking on foam rubber. There may be an increased sensitivity of the skin, sometimes with burning, prickling, creeping, or crawling sensations.

Ataxia occurs in one case in ten of cerebral palsy, which is a group of movement disorders caused by damage to the brain or nerve pathways before or around the time of birth. Weakness, unsteadiness, clumsy walking, and difficulty with fine or rapid movements are typical. Physical and occupational therapy help patients handle daily life despite their condition.

Ataxia may also be caused by any one of a group of hereditary spinocerebellar diseases that attack the central nervous system. They cause degeneration of the spinal cord and cerebellum (the lower part of the brain, which controls muscle movements) and also frequently damage the brainstem and various nerves. Inherited disorders of body chemistry and body chemicals are believed to be involved, but little is known about them. Only one, Refsum's syndrome, can be treated—by reducing the excessive level of a body chemical known as phytanic acid.

Symptoms of the hereditary ataxias include unsteadiness in walking or tremor of the arms, muscle weakness, wasting away of muscle, and various other disorders depending upon the disease. For example, Friedreich's ataxia, the commonest, causes curvature of the spine (scoliosis) and damages heart tissue.

All of these diseases continue throughout life and none can be treated effectively.

See also Cerebral palsy.

Atherosclerosis

Atherosclerosis is a slow, progressive disease of the arteries in which various fatty deposits partially clog or, eventually, totally block the blood flow. It is often called "hardening of the arteries."

This blockage of various arteries, depending on their location in the body, can result in serious complications when the arteries involved lead to vital organs: heart attack can result when an artery to the heart is totally blocked, and angina pectoris (chest pain) can be caused by partial clogging of an artery; stroke occurs when an artery to the brain is blocked; kidney disease can develop from obstructions in the arteries leading to the kidneys; blindness or diseases of the extremities can result from blockages of the arteries supplying these areas of the body.

Atherosclerosis occurs when the normally smooth, firm linings of the arteries have become roughened, thickened, and clogged with deposits of fat, fibrin (a clotting substance), calcium, and cellular debris. This condition develops over time, in a step-by-step procedure. Fats (called lipids), necessary for the production of certain hormones and tissues, are constantly present in the bloodstream. When the level of these fats is greatly increased, however, fatty streaks form along the artery walls. These streaks, harmless in themselves, can cause small nodules of fatty deposits (cholesterol) to jut out from the normally smooth linings of the artery walls. Fibrous scar tissue grows under these nodules and further attracts calcium deposits; accumulated calcium develops into a hard, chalky film called plaque that cannot be removed. This permanent coating inside the arteries hampers their ability to expand and contract properly and slows the blood flow through the now narrowed channels. Clots may now easily form, totally preventing the blood from traveling through the artery.

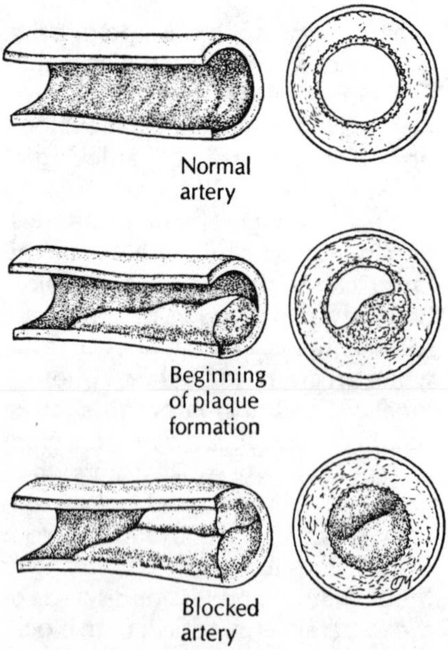

The exact cause of this process has not been pinpointed, but the initial increase of the blood's fat content may be triggered by diets high in saturated fats (fats that are usually solid at room temperature, including all animal fats such as those found in butter and meats). Also, the body's inability to absorb these fats from the bloodstream may lead to their increased buildup in the arteries.

Hypertension (high blood pressure) can increase the risk of atherosclerosis because it puts constant strain on the arteries, thus speeding up the clogging and hardening process. Smoking narrows the arteries, thus restricting blood flow and inviting atherosclerosis to set in.

Atherosclerosis alone has no visible symptoms. In fact, the disease often remains undetected until the arteries are totally blocked and strain or damage to the affected organs produces symptoms. For example, if an artery supplying the heart is afflicted with atherosclerosis, chest pain may be felt; if atherosclerosis affects a cerebral (head) artery, the patient may experience dizziness, blurred vision, and faintness.

Diagnosis of atherosclerosis involves several methods: an exercise tolerance or stress test using an ECG (electrocardiograph), which measures the electrical impulses generated by the heart and which will indicate damaged heart tissue or blocked arteries; ultrasound, which records blockage in the arteries, abnormalities of the heart chambers and valves, and the movement of blood through the heart; and radioactive isotopes or X-ray opaque fluid, which, when injected into the bloodstream, can be traced through the circulatory system to indicate

Normal artery

Beginning of plaque formation

Blocked artery

Atherosclerosis occurs when the normally smooth, firm linings of the arteries become roughened and thickened with deposits of fat, calcium, and cellular debris. Developing into a hard film called plaque, this deposit eventually may build up and block the artery.

obstructions or areas insufficiently supplied with blood.

Treatment of this disorder aims at reducing the strain on the heart and preventing further artery damage. Changes in lifestyle and eating habits along with the administration of medication can accomplish this. Currently there are no available medications that will actually dissolve the deposits that have clogged the arteries. Delicate surgical procedures, however, may be performed to remove those deposits that are blocking arteries to vital organs. These procedures, called endarterectomies, are performed on relatively large vessels such as those entering the brain, heart, kidneys, and legs. Surgery cannot remove deposits in small blood vessels of these organs.

Lifestyle changes include cutting out smoking; reducing cholesterol intake; perhaps losing weight (obesity puts a strain on the heart); and maintaining a moderate, but not overly strenuous, exercise program (exercise helps develop the collateral circulation, a system of small blood vessels that can bypass the partially blocked arteries and directly supply organs with blood).

Anticoagulants may be prescribed to thin the blood and prevent clotting. If atherosclerosis has led to angina, several other drugs may help to suppress chest pain by expanding the arteries and increasing blood flow; they are nitroglycerin, nitrates, and calcium antagonists. If high blood pressure contributes to the problem, two other types of drugs may be prescribed: diuretics, which lower the resistance in the blood vessels, and beta blockers, which reduce both the heart rate and the amount of blood pumped from the heart with each beat. (Note: asthma sufferers should use beta blockers only with extreme caution, as these drugs can cause spasms in the respiratory passages and lead to breathing difficulties.)

When medication is not sufficient and the individual suffers from severe and recurrent chest pain, surgery may be performed to bypass the major obstructions in the arteries, by creating a detour around the blockage in the artery.

See also Angina, Bypass surgery, Heart attack, Hypertension, and Stroke.

Athlete's foot

Athlete's foot (whose medical name is *tinea pedis*) is ringworm of the foot. A fungus infection of the skin between the toes and also of the skin on the soles of the feet, it causes itching, burning, and stinging sensations. The skin between the toes reddens, cracks open, and crumbles. In extreme long-lasting cases, the toenails may become infected, discolored, and overgrown. The fungus may spread to the underside of the foot, beneath the arch, producing groups of itching blisters and peeling of the skin (a related disorder, *tinea rubrum* causes a scaling and thickening of skin around the edges of the soles).

It is important to rule out other causes of similar symptoms. For example, hot, tight shoes may produce sweaty feet in warm weather; the moisture and friction may cause softening and peeling of the skin on the soles. Dyes, adhesive cements, and other substances inside the shoes may cause irritation, as may powders and nail polishes. Eczema, psoriasis, and scabies are other sources of symptoms.

If sweaty feet are the cause, athlete's foot ointments should not be used. Instead, you should ask your doctor for suggestions about controlling the excessive sweating; there are ointments and solutions that can help this condition. Changing shoes may eliminate the problem if the feet are sensitive to chemicals inside the shoes.

Most people can treat their athlete's foot condition at home using one of several good salves, powders, or liquids obtainable without prescription from the drugstore. These include compound undecylenic acid ointment, tolnaftate, and miconazole. Clotrimazole is another good medicine, but it requires a prescription from a physician. Directions usually call for application morning and night, to continue until one week after all symptoms have vanished. As long as loose skin remains, the feet should be soaked before the ointment is applied, and the loose skin removed carefully.

Severe cases of athlete's foot call for treatment by a physician. To relieve symptoms, the doctor may prescribe soaking the feet three times a day in a solution of aluminum sulfate and calcium acetate (often called Burow's solution) with an antiseptic solution added if a secondary infection is present. In extreme cases the antifungal drug griseofulvin may be prescribed, to be taken by mouth.

Athlete's foot can recur despite any treatment, especially during the hot summer months. The organisms that cause athlete's foot thrive in a hot, moist setting. However, there are several things you can do to help prevent the disease. You can keep your feet clean, dry between your toes after bathing, and change socks frequently. Use dusting and drying powders to keep the feet dry. Separate your toes with small wads of cotton when you are sleeping. Wear wooden or rubber clogs in motel and community showers and sandals, open-toed shoes, or no shoes at all during hot weather.

Autism

Autism is a form of mental illness (psychosis) in children. The word autism comes from "auto," the Greek word for "self," and literally means "self-ism." The autistic child is wrapped up in his or her own unrealistic inner thoughts, unable to communicate or relate to other people.

Although the cause of autism remains a mystery, several reasons for the disorder have been suggested. In some cases, an inborn mental defect may play a part, since many of these children from birth do not smile and do not accept affectionate cuddling. In other instances, severe mental or physical trauma during childhood may contribute to the disorder. The sex of the child may also be a factor; males are four times as likely as females to be autistic.

Autism is a collection of symptoms, of unknown cause, beginning in the first 30 months of life. The autistic child is very withdrawn, unaffectionate, and uninterested in people including parents, brothers, and sisters. The child seems to behave as if he or she is alone in the world. Accompanying this attitude is a speech and language disorder: the child may learn to speak late or not at all, and if speech develops it is odd and limited. One common practice is echolalia (repeating or "echoing" the last phrase or word of everything the other person says). Other marks of autism are a total resistance to change (even something so minor as rearrangement of furniture) and the repetition of meaningless acts such as rocking, arm-flapping, or head-banging. Finally, mental development is often uneven. Usually the child does best in non-language subjects and may learn best with methods that emphasize memorization and drill. There are no particular signs of nervous system defects, although half of all autistic children experience seizures before reaching their teens.

In diagnosing autism, the doctor must distinguish it from childhood schizophrenia, a mental illness that usually strikes later than does autism but that may also cause a child to be silent and withdrawn. The doctor must also make certain that deafness or severely impaired hearing is not present. The child is given intelligence tests, to help determine the potential for training and education, and tests of the nervous system. A tranquilizer drug may be prescribed if needed for emergency use to quiet screaming or violent outbursts.

An autistic child may have to be cared for in an institution or a specialized school. But day care programs for autistic children are available in some cities, and the trend is to train parents to care for their children at home (information about available programs may be obtained from The National Society for Autistic Children).

The method of treatment used by professionals today, and taught to parents, is known as behavior therapy. The main goals are to limit self-destructive or meaningless actions, to promote language development, and to make the child more social. In behavior therapy, the professional—or parent—works hard to develop a close relationship with the child, so that the child will want to imitate the adult. The adult also uses direct action such as rewards and praise to promote speech, playing with other children, self-care skills (such as dressing and washing), and helpfulness. With such methods, some autistic children of average or near-average intelligence are able to develop into normal adults.

Unfortunately, because the cause of autism is unknown, there is no recognized method of prevention.

Autoimmune diseases

Autoimmune diseases are disorders in which the body's immune (defense) system reacts against some of its own tissue and produces antibodies (protective substances) to destroy it.

Ailments believed to be autoimmune diseases include Hashimoto's thyroiditis and Grave's disease, disorders of the thyroid; systemic lupus erythematosus, which attacks connective tissue; myasthenia gravis, a muscular disease; and autoimmune hemolytic anemia, in which red blood cells are destroyed before the end of their normal 120-day life span.

Diseases that *probably* are autoimmune disorders include the joint disease rheumatoid arthritis; pernicious anemia, a blood disorder; Addison's disease, which attacks the adrenal glands; and some forms of diabetes mellitus, which is a breakdown of the body's ability to handle starches and sugars.

Possible autoimmune diseases are chronic active hepatitis, a liver disorder; some forms of vasculitis, an inflammation of blood vessel walls; and many other diseases that produce inflammation, degeneration, or wasting away of body tissue.

An autoimmune disease can begin in several ways:

- Some body substance that ordinarily never enters the bloodstream may do so because of injury. For example, a disease known as sympathetic opthalmia occurs when tissue from the inside an injured eye is released into the bloodstream. The tissue is recognized as "out of place" or "foreign" by the body's immune system and antibodies attack it—causing irritation in both the injured eye and in the noninjured eye. The reaction may be severe enough to cause blindness.

- Body substances may be altered by chemicals, sunlight, or a virus so that they become "foreign" to the body's immune system. The substance is then attacked by antibodies. This occurs in contact dermatitis, when, for example, metal in a bracelet causes chemical changes in the skin on one's wrist. The body reacts against the "different" skin and attacks it, causing a rash.
- Finally, infection of the body may cause the body to react with an immune response so strong that the body reacts against some of its own normal tissues.

There seems to be an inherited tendency to autoimmune diseases. Women are affected more often than men.

See also Antibody/antigen and Immunity.

B

Backache

A backache is generally a gripping pain near the inward curve of the back above the base of the spine. It is one of the most common physical ailments, affecting about 80 percent of the population at some time in their lives.

Pain results from a variety of causes. Strains are especially common when overworked or underexercised back muscles perform beyond their normal capacity. Muscles will then contract or go into spasm and become a tight mass of tissue. Meanwhile, the body transmits a sharp pain signal as nearby muscles tighten in an effort to protect strained muscles and prevent further damage. Strain of back muscles can be due to sports, a sudden jerking motion such as a car braking, or reflex actions like sneezing.

Overweight is a leading cofactor of backache, since excess pounds increase stress on back muscles. Similarly, pregnancy can produce back pain because of the weight or position of the unborn child. For some women, menstruation results in back discomfort.

Many people develop back pain as they age and joint tissues deteriorate or shift. Psychological tension, stress, or anxiety about everyday problems can also lead to backache. In addition, back pain can result from diseases of the kidneys, heart, lungs, intestinal tract, or reproductive organs.

Occasionally, backache stems from a congenital (present from birth) malformation. In this case, pain usually results from unusual stresses the deformity imposes on surrounding muscular structures rather than from the abnormality itself. For example, having one leg shorter than another forces the neighboring muscles out of alignment and may cause back pain.

Backaches can appear abruptly after physical activity or develop slowly. The pain may feel like a sharp jab or a dull ache. Sometimes, pain becomes so piercing that a person who is bending over may not be able to straighten up. Severe back pain may also be accompanied by pain or numbness radiating down the leg(s). Most muscular back pains disappear within a week or two of their onset, while some will last one to two months, but pain may recur unless preventive measures are taken.

Sufferers of prolonged back pain (more than two to three weeks) should consult a physician to check for underlying disorders such as kidney or lung problems that may be causing the backache. Once other medical causes have been ruled out, an orthopedic physician specializing in bone and muscle conditions may be able to determine the cause of the discomfort.

During the examination, the physician asks questions about the type of pain and its location, general health, previous illnesses, and physical activity routines. The patient walks, sits, stands, and performs exercises while being observed. If an X ray is recommended, it may or may not reveal adverse changes in the bones of the spine since not all problems can be revealed on film.

If there are no physical causes for the backache, physicians usually recommend an exercise program to strengthen weak muscles. Losing weight can also relieve unnecessary pressure on the back.

For immediate symptoms, hot pads at the site of the pain will reduce soreness. Over-the-counter preparations in the form of a rub containing menthol salicylate (oil of wintergreen) or similar ingredients may produce a soothing heat sensation when applied to the pain site. Physicians may also prescribe muscle relaxant drugs.

When backache is the result of some deformity, surgery may be necessary to correct the problem. Sometimes, braces, corsets, or shoe lifts improve the condition. Specific exercises strengthen participating muscles and counter stress caused by the malformation.

Almost all types of musculoskeletal backache respond well to complete bed rest that allows muscles to relax and inflammation to subside. Here, time is the best healer, especially in extreme situations.

To prevent back pain, stress to the spine should be avoided. Good posture when awake and asleep relieves tension on the spinal column. Properly-fitted shoes encourage good posture, as does a semi-firm bed. Contrary to popular belief, a hard mattress distorts alignment of the spine and causes back problems as much as a soft mattress does. A semi-rigid mattress is recommended because it conforms to the arch of the back and maintains spine alignment.

Good posture is also important when performing daily activities. Kneeling, rather then bending from the waist, when lifting objects keeps the weight of the object on the legs, leaving the back straight. Avoid sitting for long periods of time at a desk looking down or watching television with the chin on the chest.

Bacteria

Bacteria are one-celled microscopic organisms. Some exist as chains or clumps of single cells. Some of the many different kinds of bacteria cause disease in humans and animals, but many others are beneficial. Bacteria dispose of organic waste, enrich the soil, and ferment wine and beer. They help make vinegar, cheese, and yogurt. In human beings certain beneficial bacteria live in the intestine where they help digestion.

Bacteria are different from viruses in that they are able to multiply on their own outside a living cell whereas viruses can grow and multiply only in living cells. Bacteria are different from two other causes of infection — protozoa (one-celled animals) and fungi (plant-like organisms) — in two ways: they have a primitive nucleus (center where their genetic material is kept) rather than a well-defined one with an enclosing membrane and chromosomes; and they reproduce simply by splitting in two, as opposed to reproducing by means of a complex process (mitosis) in which their genetic material is duplicated prior to splitting.

There are two main types of bacteria, classified by shape:

- Rod-shaped bacteria are known as *bacilli.* They often have one or many waving projections known as flagella, which propel them about. Some form small thick-walled cells known as "spores," which can survive for long periods even after the "parent" bacteria have been killed by freezing, disinfectants, or other harsh forces. When conditions are favorable, the spores come to life and generate new bacteria. Typhoid fever is caused by a bacillus bacterium.
- Round or egg-shaped bacteria are known as *cocci.* They occur singly (micrococcus), in chains (streptococcus, the cause of strep sore throat), in pairs (diplococcus), in irregular bunches (staphylococcus — the cause of many infections), and in cube-shaped packets (sarcina). Cocci do not form spores nor do they usually move about.

Bacteria also exist as comma-shaped organisms called vibrios (the organism responsible for cholera) and as spirals such as the spirochete of syphilis.

Another way to classify bacteria is by whether or not they can live in the open air. Those who can are called *aerobic.* Those who cannot are called *anaerobic.* Some can live either with or without air and are called *facultative.* Tetanus (lockjaw) is an example of a disease caused by an anaerobic bacterium that is common in the soil. It poses no danger to humans unless it enters the body through a wound, particularly a puncture wound such as that made by a dirty, rusty nail. The air then cannot get to the tetanus organisms to destroy them and so they multiply within the body unless the infected person is vaccinated against tetanus.

Disease bacteria enter the body in many different ways. Those that cause pneumonia and sore throat are carried in droplets that an infected person sneezes or coughs into the air; the bacteria are then inhaled and deposited on the mucous membranes of the throat or lungs by a healthy person where they multiply and eventually cause disease unless checked by the body's immune system. The bacteria of intestinal diseases like cholera and typhoid can be transmitted by foods that have been handled by an infected person or by water tainted by body wastes from an infected individual. Another important route for infection is any break in the skin, which is why it is important to clean any cut in the skin as soon as possible.

Once inside the body, disease bacteria do their damage in two main ways: by direct destruction of tissue or by producing toxins, or poisons, that poison remote parts of the body. Certain white blood cells known as lymphocytes produce substances called antitoxins, which neutralize the toxins of the bacteria, and antibodies, which are tailored to cause the destruction and removal of the invading bacteria (once created, the antibodies to a specific disease can persist in the body or be reproduced when needed creating continuous immunity to the invading disease organism — sometimes for life). Still other white blood cells known as phagocytes entrap and destroy the bacteria. The phagocytes literally eat and digest the bacteria.

Baldness

Baldness (the technical term is alopecia) is partial or complete loss of hair on the head. This may be caused by an inherited tendency and/or by aging, fever, infection, certain drugs, radiation, injury, or disease.

Male-pattern baldness is the most common form. There seems to be an inherited tendency toward it, and androgen, a male hormone, contributes to it. However, the exact way it occurs is not known. Hair loss is gradual, occurring at the forehead, on either side of the front (sometimes leaving a center tuft known as a "widow's peak"), and on the top of the head. It can begin as early as age 15 or 16, in which case it may indicate that considerable baldness is likely later (however, male-pattern baldness does not usually advance at a steady or predictable rate). Female-pattern baldness is fairly common in women of menopausal age and usually involves only the thinning of the hair in the area around the crown. It is also believed to be due to hormonal causes as is male-pattern baldness.

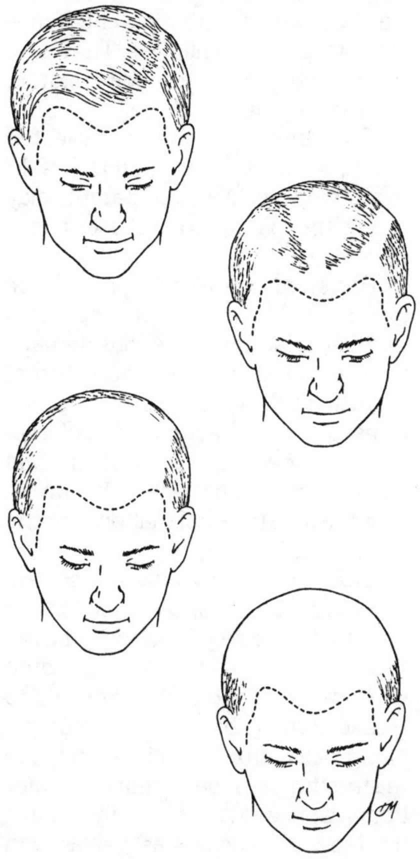

Hair loss in male pattern baldness is gradual, beginning at the forehead on either side of the front and continuing to the top of the head.

Temporary baldness sometimes occurs up to three or four months following a severe illness, especially one with fever such as scarlet fever. It can result from lowered activity of the pituitary or thyroid glands, from early syphilis, pregnancy, birth-control pills, "crash" dieting or malnutrition, certain medications, or too much Vitamin A. When the cause is no longer present, the missing hair usually returns.

Spotty baldness (alopecia areata) may affect areas of the head and beard. The cause is unknown, but it often clears up after a few months if there are just a few spots and if it first occurs in adulthood. However, it may reoccur. The outlook is less favorable for spotty baldness that begins in childhood or if hair loss is widespread.

Occasionally, all body hair is lost. When this happens, and there is no readily apparent cause such as fever or severe illness, the hair is not likely to return.

Permanent baldness results when the scalp is scarred by burns, other injury, or disease. Diseases which can cause scarring baldness include severe bacterial infections, tuberculosis ulcers, severe ringworm of the scalp, lupus erythematosus, and certain slow-growing tumors.

There is no satisfactory medical treatment at this time to cure or prevent baldness. However, hair transplants can be effective. Scalp plugs containing active follicles (hair cells) to be transplanted are taken from the back of the head, which is not affected by male-pattern baldness. The transplanted follicles continue to grow hair just as before, despite the new location.

Battered child syndrome

The battered child syndrome is a group of symptoms indicating that a child has been injured, usually repeatedly, by a parent, guardian, or other family member. The injury may be either physical, emotional, or sexual and is known as *child abuse.* Closely related is *child neglect,* in which the parent or guardian fails to provide for the nutritional, emotional, physical, or health needs of the child — even though resources such as food, shelter, clothing, and health care are available.

The principal cause of child abuse is a failure of self-control by the parent or guardian. There are four main reasons for this:

Inadequate parent. Many parents who abuse their children did not receive much love from their own parents and may themselves have been abused. They did not learn how to give affection and thus find it hard to develop a good relationship with their own children. They do not have a very high opinion of themselves. Easily frustrated, they lose their tempers and resort to harsh punishment methods that they learned as children. In addition, some abusing parents are simply mentally disturbed.

"Difficult" or "different" child. Some children are so overactive, irritable, or demanding that they drive a parent to unacceptable behavior. The parent strikes out and injures the child. Another reason may be that the child may not be able to perform as well as brothers or sisters, or as well as the parent expected, in school or elsewhere. The parent may lash out to punish the child for this "failure" or "defiance," either with blows or hurtful words.

"Lonely family." Some parents without close friends or relatives nearby, to help out and talk to, become overburdened with the constant demands of rearing children — especially small children. They lose their tempers and hurt their children, without meaning to do so.

Emergency. Some unexpected event, such as when a child breaks something or defies the parent, may cause the parent to strike out in a blind rage:

Physical symptoms of abuse include old and new bruises; scars from cuts and burns; serious damage to the eyes, mouth, or internal organs; and evidence in X-ray pictures of bone fractures in different stages of healing. The test of child abuse comes when parents cannot give reasonable explanations for the child's injuries.

Signs of emotional abuse are more difficult to spot. In babies, it may be failure to put on weight even though no illness is present. Children who are "too good," too anxious to please adults, but who do not get along well with other children and are mistrustful may be victims of emotional abuse. At school, they have trouble with teachers as well as with other children. Threats, ridicule, and unreasonable punishment by nonphysical means are some of the ways parents abuse their children emotionally.

Sexual abuse is fairly common, often by a parent or an older brother or sister. Of all kinds of abuse, it may be the hardest to detect. There are usually no physical symptoms, although venereal disease in a child is grounds for suspicion. The child may willingly consent to sexual activity or may be too embarrassed to reveal the facts to anyone outside the family. The most typical sexual abuse occurs when a father establishes a sexual relationship with his daughter often with the knowledge of the mother. The mother may be afraid to complain or may simply accept the situation. As in other forms of child abuse, sexually abused children often grow up to abuse their children just as they were abused.

Child neglect can be as harmful as child abuse. An extreme example is when a live newborn baby is found in a garbage can. Parents who did not want a child in the first place may not give it the love and attention it needs to do well. Babies who have been neglected emotionally may appear uninterested in people and even retarded.

Parents who neglect their children may be incompetent because of drug or alcohol abuse or medical problems, because of a depressed state of mind, or because of a whole set of problems they just cannot seem to handle.

When physicians suspect child abuse, they are required by law in most states to report it to a government social service agency or welfare department. However, punishment of the parents is not the goal of the law. Jailing a parent might injure the child even more than the original abuse, if the parent is capable of being a good father or mother in the future. Removing the child from the family may be necessary to protect the youngster from future injury, but in most cases this is not done or the removal is only temporary. The child may simply stay in the hospital a few days while the case is studied and parents are interviewed. In many communities, a team made up of a social worker, pediatrician, psychiatrist, and other specialists talk to the child and parents and develop a long-term treatment plan. This often involves periodic visits by a social worker to the home and psychological help for one or both parents. Practical help such as day care for small children and household help by a trained homemaker can ease the burdens on an overworked mother. Trained nonprofessional "parent aides" can provide good support as can "Parents Anonymous" chapters —made up of parents who formerly abused their children.

Those most likely to abuse their children are young parents with their first child, unmarried adolescent mothers rebelling against their parents, parents who were abused as children, and parents of ill or premature babies who are separated from them shortly after birth. Such parents need special attention and support in order to get their families off to a good start.

Even before the first child is born, planning is useful. The father should realize the need for his encouragement of the mother and help with the baby and chores. Perhaps relatives and friends or others can be lined up to help with emergencies or babysitting. If the baby is born ill or prematurely and must stay in the hospital intensive care unit after the mother comes home, parents should visit the baby at least every day and stay as close as possible so that the baby will not be a stranger when he or she comes home. Many mothers of young children find it helpful to get together once a week or so while their children play to share ideas and support each other.

Parents who are afraid they may abuse their children should talk to other parents about how they handle their problems with children and to their family doctor who may be able to provide the name of a specialist in family problems. In some communities, a parent can call a parental stress "hot line."

Bell's palsy

Bell's palsy is a sudden paralysis (loss of function or movement), total or partial, of one side of the face. It is believed to be due to inflammation of the nerve that controls the facial muscles. The inflammation, often of unknown cause but suspected to be the result of viral infection, causes the nerve to swell and to be compressed inside its bony passage in the skull. This reduces its blood supply and ability to function.

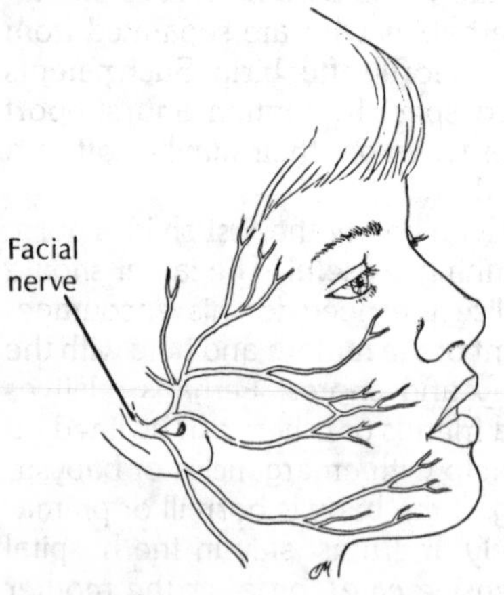

Bell's palsy, a paralysis of one side of the face, is thought to be due to inflammation of the facial nerve and its branches that control the facial muscles.

The disease can occur in someone of any age, but is most common from age 20 to 50. The first sign may be an aching pain behind or below the ear. Paralysis may develop in a few hours or more slowly, causing the entire side of the face to be flat and without expression (this is different from the facial paralysis caused by stroke or brain tumor, where the weakness is mostly below the forehead). The mouth droops on the weak side, with saliva drooling from the corner. Taste may be affected. The eyebrow cannot be raised. In most cases, the eye cannot be shut. When the patient tries to close the eye, it rolls upward (which happens in a normal person, but the movement is not seen). False tears may come from the affected eye.

In diagnosing the case, the doctor must determine if the paralysis might be caused by other diseases affecting the facial nerve, including ear infections or skull fracture. The facial nerve can also be affected by many other conditions, cancers among them. However, other nerves are usually involved, and other signs and symptoms are frequently present. Head X rays may be taken during this investigation.

Primary treatment is aimed at reducing the inflammation of the nerve before any permanent damage is done to it. A cortisone hormone known as prednisone is given by mouth for this purpose. However, in many if not most uncomplicated cases, treatment with medication is unnecessary. After two weeks, if there has been no improvement in the ability of the muscles to move, the muscles of the weak side of the face may be stimulated electrically to maintain their condition.

The affected eye should be covered with an eyepatch, especially out of doors, and protected from dirt and wind. A facial sling is used to keep the mouth shut. Moist heat (not too hot) on the weak side of the face can reduce pain. Brief periods of upward facial massage help maintain muscle tone. So do facial exercises the patient can perform before a mirror. The patient needs help while eating, privacy to prevent embarrassment, and soft, easy-to-eat food (no hot food or drinks).

Fortunately, most Bell's palsy patients recover in one to eight weeks. Elderly patients may take much longer—up to two years. Complete recovery usually follows within several months if the paralysis is partial.

Beriberi

Beriberi is a disease that results when the body does not get enough thiamine (Vitamin B_1). It has been most common in those parts of the world where people's diets have been limited almost entirely to polished (white) rice. Milling removes the brown rice husks, which are rich in thiamine. Other causes include:

- Increased need for thiamine, such as with fever, pregnancy, breast-feeding, or an overactive thyroid gland (which severely increases energy requirements and causes the body to increase the rate at which it burns nutrients)
- Failure of the body to absorb enough thiamine, such as may occur with long-lasting diarrhea
- Poor use of the vitamin by the body, for example, in severe liver disease.

A combination of these factors occurs in alcoholism, because of less food intake, poor vitamin absorption, increased need for thiamine, and poor use of it by the body.

Because thiamine is necessary for the proper use by the body of fats, starches, and sugars, and for the normal functioning of nervous tissue and of enzymes (which stimulate body processes), symptoms of beriberi usually occur in the digestive and nervous systems. In severe cases, heart muscle is damaged. Early symptoms include fatigue, irritation, poor memory, loss of appetite, constipation, discomfort in the abdomen, and difficulty in arising from the squatting position. There may be burning of the feet, prickling of the soles, or tenderness and cramps in the calves. Certain muscle reflexes are lost. Mental confusion, paralysis of speech and eye muscles, coma, and death can occur in untreated beriberi affecting the brain. Heart damage from beriberi produces heart failure with buildup of body fluids, seen as swelling in the abdomen and/or legs, and difficulty in breathing.

Babies who are breast-fed by mothers deficient in thiamine may develop heart failure, paralysis of speech, and lose certain muscle reflexes.

Treatment for beriberi consists of daily doses of thiamine, at first by injection into a muscle or vein and later by mouth. Improvement usually begins in one or two days.

Eating a well-balanced diet of fruits, vegetables, meat, and whole grains is the best way to prevent B-vitamin deficiency diseases like beriberi. Beriberi itself is rare in the United States because flours are enriched with added thiamine.

Beta-adrenergic blockers

Beta-adrenergic blockers, often known simply as "beta blockers," are drugs that, along with other drugs known as "alpha blockers," fight the action of adrenaline and noradrenaline in the body. Adrenaline and noradrenaline hormones, produced by the adrenal glands, have major effects on blood vessels, the heart, the smaller air passages of the lungs, and the nervous system. These are known as "alpha" and "beta" effects. The beta effects include stimulation of the body in various ways such as dilating (enlarging) blood vessels and increasing heart rate and strength of heart contractions, among others. Beta-blocking drugs, such as propranolol, metoprolol, atenolol, pindolol, timolol, and nadolol, work to block the beta effects in many conditions where a stimulant effect is undesirable. Thus, they are useful for heart diseases, such as angina pectoris (chest pains caused by lack of blood flow to the heart muscle), and many arrhythmias (irregular heartbeat), because their blocking action reduces stimulation to the heart and therefore decreases the work of the heart. They can also be used to counteract the adrenaline-like effects of too much thyroid hormone produced by an overactive thyroid gland. This condition alone can cause a rapid heartbeat and heart "flutter." Beta blockers are used in the treatment of high blood pressure; for example, propranolol interferes with renin, a hormone produced by the kidney that plays a role in contracting blood vessels and raising blood pressure. In addition, because of its ability to block the dilation of blood vessels, propranolol has been used to prevent (but not treat acute attacks) migraine headaches, which may result from the enlargement of blood vessels of the scalp as well as from blood vessel changes inside the brain and neck.

Other possible uses of the beta blockers may be calming victims of schizophrenia (a mental disease), decreasing tremors, aiding in withdrawal from alcohol, and reducing the number of second heart attacks. (Note: beta blockers, especially propanolol, pindolol, nadolol, and timolol, should be used with caution or not at all by persons with asthma or other respiratory diseases because of the drugs' effects on the lung's air passages.)

Bile

Bile is a fluid produced by the liver and discharged into the small intestine, where it helps in the digestion of food, particularly fats. Yellow-green or golden in color and bitter to the taste, bile is made up of water, salts, bile acids, cholesterol (a fatlike substance), and lecithin (a fatty acid).

Bile acts like a detergent to break down fat in the intestine into tiny globules that can be dissolved and suspended in water so that they can pass through the walls of the small intestine's cells into the bloodstream (to provide fuel for the body). The bile "detergent" (known as bile salts) is also absorbed through the walls of the intestine but is returned to the liver to reform new bile. The color of bile is due to pigments known as bilirubin and biliverdin. Bilirubin is a yellow pigment derived from decomposed red blood cells. Biliverdin is a green pigment derived from conversion of bilirubin by a chemical reaction. These pigments are also responsible for some of the coloration of body wastes, in which the pigments are passed out of the body.

Bile is continually produced in the liver and passes through ducts to be stored in the gallbladder, a hollow organ located just beneath the liver, until mealtime when it is emptied into the duodenum, the entrance to the small intestine just below the stomach. Digestive disturbances result if the flow of bile is stopped or reduced, either because of a liver disorder or because a duct has been blocked by inflammation or a gallstone (a solid chunk of deposited material, usually calcium, cholesterol, bilirubin, or combinations thereof, formed in the gallbladder). Any of these conditions can also cause jaundice, in which the pigments bilirubin and, to a lesser extent, biliverdin, accumulate in the blood. Jaundice is a symptom of trouble, not a disease in itself, and shows up as a yellow staining of the skin, eyes, and body fluids.

See also Gallstones and Jaundice.

Birth control

Birth control, also called contraception, is the voluntary prevention of pregnancy. A variety of methods are available for preventing pregnancy. Couples who use no contraceptive have a 90 percent chance of achieving pregnancy over a 12-month period.

Natural family planning. Natural family planning is based on calculating when a women ovulates—that is, releases the egg from the ovary each month — and is most fertile. The couple then abstains from intercourse during the fertile period.

The male's sperm can live in the female's body for about two days before fertilizing an egg. The egg can live for about 24 hours after ovulation. A day or two is added to this fertile period for safety's sake because it is so difficult to determine just when ovulation occurs. All told, a couple needs to abstain from intercourse eight to nine days a month to prevent pregnancy.

There are three methods a woman can use to determine when she ovulates. The temperature method is one of the most reliable. Each morning upon awakening and before getting out of bed, you take your temperature with a special basal temperature thermometer (which only measures temperatures between 96 and 100 degrees Fahrenheit) and record it on graph paper. At the end of a menstrual cycle, you will note that your temperature dropped suddenly on one day followed by a rapid climb for the next three days. The sudden drop in temperature indicates that you are about to ovulate. After ovulation your temperature rises quickly for three days and does not return to pre-ovulation levels until the beginning of the menstrual period. The safe days to have intercourse are from four days after the sudden drop in temperature until three or four days after the end of your period. It is important to become familiar with your cycle by recording your temperature levels for several months before relying on this method of birth control.

The mucus method may also help determine when you ovulate. Each morning you examine the mucus from the vagina and cervix. Cervical mucus undergoes changes as hormone levels vary during the course of the cycle. To determine these changes, you can blot the vaginal area each morning with a facial tissue and then test the mucus between your thumb and forefinger. You are watching for the following changes. After your period you will have several days with no mucus. This is followed by several days of a yellow or white thick, sticky discharge. There will then be one or two days when the mucus becomes transparent and very *slippery* with the consistency of raw egg whites. The mucus will form a string between the thumb and forefinger. This is when ovulation occurs. After ovulation the mucus again becomes thick and sticky or there may be no mucus at all. The fertile period begins with the yellow/white thick, sticky discharge and continues until about three days after the phase when the mucus is slippery with the consistency of egg whites. You should avoid intercourse during this time. In other words, the safe period is from three days after the slippery mucus stage to about three days after the end of the menstrual period.

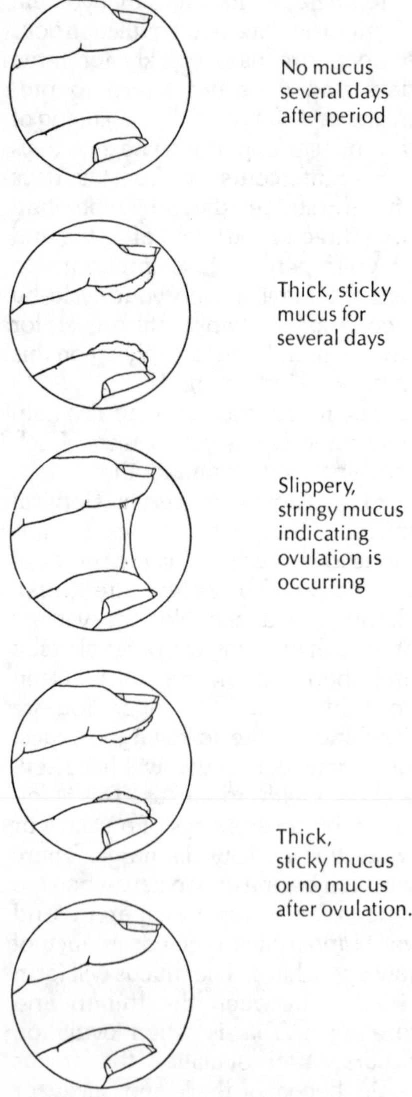

Mucus from the cervix (neck of uterus) undergoes changes as hormone levels vary during the menstrual cycle. Testing the mucus between thumb and forefinger indicates the changes shown here.

The calendar method is also an option. You keep a record of your menstrual cycles for one year or more. You and your doctor then use the record to work out the probable day of ovulation, based on the fact that the average woman menstruates 14 days after she ovulates. However, any individual woman may vary from the average, so this is not precise.

Natural family planning is entirely natural and does not require the use of mechanical aids or drugs. The effectiveness rate for this kind of birth control is up to about 75 to 80 percent, depending on the care with which the techniques are followed. However, even in women with regular cycles, illness, fatigue, stress, or even a vacation can delay ovulation and throw off all careful calculations.

Spermicides. The spermicide is a chemical foam, cream, suppository, or jelly applied to the woman's vagina to kill sperm. Used alone, a spermicide is about 75 to 85 percent effective when used correctly. Some disadvantages of a spermicide are that it must be applied before each separate act of intercourse, it has chemical odors, and it may irritate the vagina. A chief advantage is that spermicides are readily available at every drugstore without a prescription.

Diaphragm. The diaphragm is a molded rubber cap that the woman places inside the vagina to cover the cervix, the opening of the lower end of the uterus that projects into the vagina. The cap blocks the sperm, preventing them from entering the uterus. Diaphragms come in different sizes and must be fitted by a physician. Used alone, the diaphragm may occasionally fail, because it may not be inserted correctly or may shift slightly during intercourse. Used with spermicides, however, diaphragms are quite effective, with only about a 3 to 5 percent chance of pregnancy.

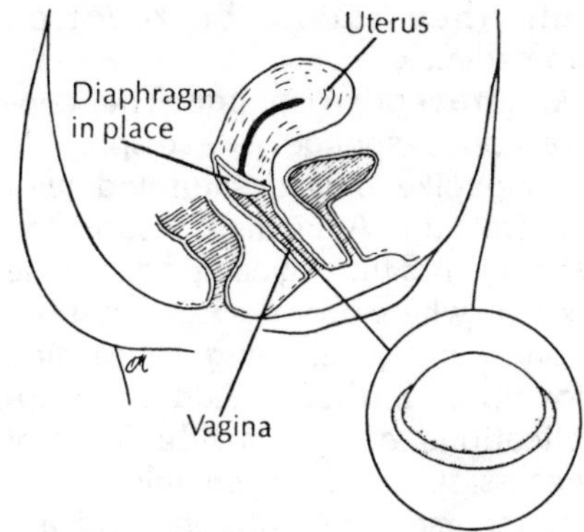

The diaphragm is a molded rubber cap that a woman places inside the vagina to cover the cervix, the opening of the lower end of the uterus. The diaphragm blocks the sperm, preventing them from entering the uterus.

Condom. The condom or "rubber," is a thin rubber or synthetic sheath that the man fits over his penis just before intercourse. A condom used alone is about 70 to 90 percent effective, depending on the care with which it is used. Several problems may occur with the use of the condom. For example, tiny holes or tears may develop in the sheath causing leakage of sperm. Also, when the penis withdraws from the vagina as intercourse is completed, the condom sometimes breaks or unrolls partially inside the vagina—releasing its contents. However, a condom used regularly with a spermicide is approximately 95 percent effective in preventing pregnancy. Condoms have the great advantage of being readily available in any drugstore without a prescription. They also have the theoretical advantage of preventing the spread of venereal disease.

IUD. The intrauterine device (IUD) is a small plastic device inserted into the woman's uterus by a physician. They are available in a variety of shapes. The IUD has a string attached to it that hangs into the cervix, so the woman or her partner can check to be sure the IUD is still in place. The IUD apparently prevents pregnancy by causing changes in the uterine lining that disrupt the normal environment of an egg. For the woman who can use an IUD, the advantages are great, as she does not have to worry about contraception each day. The effectiveness rate is high, with only about a 5 percent chance of pregnancy.

However, severe menstrual cramps and increased menstrual bleeding may follow the insertion of an IUD. Sometimes these side effects lessen after a month or two. In other cases, severe cramps and prolonged bleeding continue, and the physician may advise removal of the IUD. The IUD is also thought to increase the probability of pelvic infections and ectopic (outside the uterus) pregnancies.

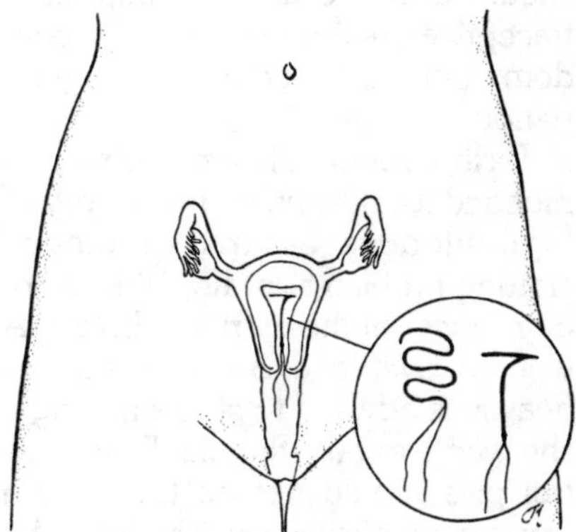

The IUD, available in several shapes, is a small plastic device inserted into a woman's uterus by a doctor. It is thought that the IUD prevents pregnancy by causing changes in the lining of the uterus that disrupt the normal environment of the egg.

Oral contraceptives. Oral contraceptives, or birth control pills, are the most effective reversible method of contraception. A woman taking the pill has less than a 1 percent chance of getting pregnant.

The pill — which is available by prescription only — uses synthetic female hormones, estrogen and progestin, to override the natural hormonal regulation that results in the release of an egg. The pill signals the pituitary gland, which directs hormonal activity in the body, not to release the hormones that would normally stimulate the ovary to release an egg.

Each day you take one pill, at about the same time of day, removing it from a container that has the required number of pills for one cycle —usually 21. From one to three days after you take the last pill for that cycle, your menstrual period begins. Menstrual periods may be lighter in flow, and cramps are reduced or absent.

If you forget to take one pill or more, menstrual bleeding may begin. In that case, you should continue taking the pills daily, but you should also use an additional contraceptive method, such as a condom, until after your next regular period.

Birth control pills are not recommended for women with a history of high blood pressure, of blood-clotting problems, of hepatitis, or of any cancer of the uterus or breast. A woman over age 35 who smokes heavily is advised to stop smoking if she wants to take the pill. Birth control pills should not be taken by a woman who suspects she may be pregnant. In addition, women with diabetes, epilepsy, heart disease, and thyroid disease may be advised not to take the birth control pill, depending on the nature and severity of the disease.

It is important for a woman on the birth control pill to report to her doctor if any of the following symptoms occur: severe headache, blurred vision, severe chest pain, sudden shortness of breath, and pain and swelling of the legs. Since these symptoms may indicate complications caused by the birth control pill, they should be reported immediately.

Contraceptive sponge. The contraceptive sponge is a disposable sponge-like device saturated with spermicide. A woman inserts the sponge into the vagina up against the cervix where the device works by continuously releasing spermicide for up to 24 hours. Additional applications of spermicide are not necessary, even for multiple acts of intercourse. There are other advantages as well: the sponge is available as an over-the-counter contraceptive that does not need a prescription; unlike a diaphragm, the sponge does not have to be fitted; and the sponge can be inserted ahead of time, which allows greater spontaneity in sexual relations. The sponge has been found to be about 85 percent effective.

Because the contraceptive sponge is a relatively new product, some doctors think that more needs to be known about side effects. So far there have been a few cases of a local irritation or an allergic reaction; however, these have been mild and infrequent. There is also concern that the sponge could become a breeding ground for infection, especially if used improperly. You should consult your doctor about the sponge and its proper use before trying this method of birth control.

Sterilization. A woman may be sterilized by an operation that blocks the fallopian tubes that carry eggs from the ovaries to the uterus. A man may be sterilized by a procedure called a vasectomy, in which the vas deferens, ducts that carry the sperm from the testes to the penis, are cut. These procedures may be reversed, but only by complicated surgery that is not always successful. Therefore, physicians recommend sterilization only when the couple has decided without reservation that no further pregnancies are desired.

See also Conception and Ovulation.

Bleeding

See Emergency first aid section at the end of this book.

Blepharitis

Blepharitis is an inflammation of the edges of the eyelids, with redness and thickening. Scales and crusts or shallow ulcers (eroded areas) may also appear. The disease is common, especially in children, and often affects both eyes and upper and lower eyelids.

Bacterial (*Staphylococcus aureus*) infection of eyelash follicles and oil glands causes blepharitis with ulcers. The non-ulcerous variety may be the result of an allergic reaction, or it may be linked with seborrheic dermatitis, an inflammatory scaling of the scalp, eyebrows, and sometimes ears. Occasionally the non-ulcerous form is caused by lice on brows and lashes, which irritate lid margins.

Symptoms of blepharitis include itching, burning, "red-rimmed" eyes; swelling of the lids; loss of eyelashes; and irritation of the underside of the lid, as if dirt or sand were underneath. The eyes may tear and be sensitive to light. In blepharitis with ulcers, tough dry crusts form that leave a bleeding surface when removed. Greasy, easily removed scales appear on the edges of the lids in the non-ulcerous variety.

Blepharitis caused by a bacterial infection can be treated with an antibiotic ointment, such as erythromycin or bacitracin specially formulated for use around the eyes. The salve is applied three times a day to the eyelash margins with a cotton-tipped swab, after the margins have been softened with warm compresses for ten minutes and the crusts removed. Sulfacetamide-corticosteroid drops are often used to combat irritation or other types of bacterial infection and may replace the second application of ointment.

If an allergy is the cause, a cosmetic may be at fault and should be removed. If there is scaling on the eyebrows and scalp — that is, seborrheic dermatitis — the doctor is likely to recommend a special shampoo such as a sulfur or tar shampoo to control the dandruff and to prescribe a cortisone lotion or cream to be rubbed into hairy areas. Absolute cleanliness of hair, scalp, eyebrows, and eyelid margins is necessary during treatment.

If the blepharitis is caused by lice, nits (lice eggs) are carefully removed with tweezers and steps taken to keep the patient free of lice.

Both of the principal varieties are difficult to cure and often recur. Blepharitis without ulcers causes no permanent damage. However, ulcerous blepharitis, if it recurs often enough, can cause scarring of eyelids, loss of lashes, and even ulcers of the cornea (the transparent covering across the front of the eyeball).

Complete cleanliness may help prevent the disease. If it is treated promptly when it occurs, permanent damage can probably be prevented.

Blood

Blood is the fluid that travels in blood vessels throughout the body transporting oxygen and other nutrients to the tissues and waste products away from the tissues. It consists of plasma, a faint yellow liquid comprised of protein and water. Within the plasma are three formed elements — red blood cells, white blood cells, and platelets — that are visible only under a microscope. These elements are manufactured by the soft tissue, called bone marrow, in the center of bones.

Red blood cells carry oxygen from the lungs to various body tissues. Oxygen travels attached to hemoglobin, a pigmented substance in red blood cells that contains iron. When the amount of hemoglobin or the total number of red blood cells falls below a specified amount, anemia develops. Normally, there are about 27 million red blood cells in one teaspoon of blood.

The job of the white blood cells is to protect the body from invading organisms. Whenever the body becomes wounded or infected, white blood cells attack and kill disease-causing agents in the affected area. In addition, certain white blood cells produce antibodies. These substances counteract harmful agents by destroying or inactivating them so they are powerless. Because the body produces more white blood cells in response to infection, any change in their number signals disease. From 25,000 to 50,000 white blood cells exist in one teaspoon of blood.

Platelets are small colorless disks numbering between 750,000 to 1,750,000 in a single teaspoon of blood. They work to help the blood clot should bleeding develop.

See also Lymphocytes and Platelets.

Blood vessels

Blood vessels comprise the network of passageways transporting blood throughout the body. The blood within this network carries nutrients to and waste products from body cells.

This complex system consists of various types of blood vessels that are defined according to their size, function, and physical properties. Arteries can be large and elastic, medium-sized and muscular, or small, called arterioles. Their job is to receive blood from the heart and move it out to body tissues.

In the tissues, smaller subdivided arteries, called capillaries, exchange nutrients for waste products. Then, veins carry the "used" blood back to the heart to be recirculated through the lungs and then back through the heart and arteries to the rest of the body. The entire network is the basis of the circulatory system that keeps the body nourished.

Boils

A boil, or furuncle, is a contagious bacterial infection and irritation of the skin and its underlying structures. It is a painful swelling in the skin that is easily detected by touch. When a group of boils interconnect below the surface of the skin, a carbuncle forms.

Boils develop when staphylococci bacteria enter the skin through a hair follicle and multiply in its warm, moist environment. Bacteria continue to grow while producing substances that invade surrounding cells. In the body's defense, white blood cells (whose job is to attack and kill invading organisms) travel to the infected hair follicle and enclose the bacteria. As more white blood cells gather, they eventually consume the bacteria and eliminate the infection. This counterattack by the white blood cells is what produces the pustule in the center of the boil as the white blood cells build. When the pustule ruptures, pus and dead skin cells

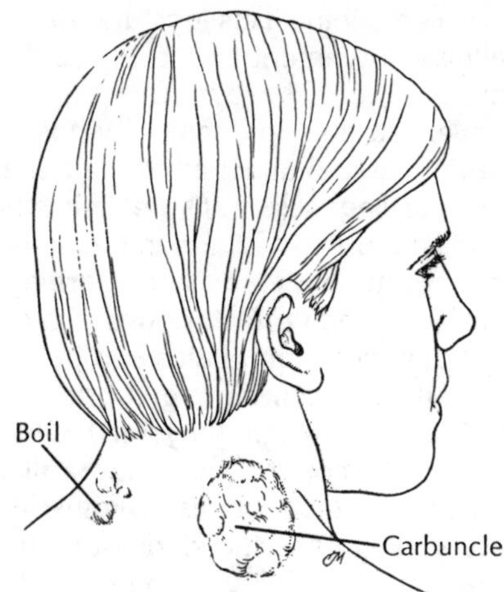

A boil is a contagious bacterial infection and irritation of the skin and its underlying structures. When a group of boils interconnect below the surface of the skin, a carbuncle forms.

killed by the bacteria drain out, and the boil heals.

Staphylococci germs are often found in the nose and throat where washing cannot reach them. They spread to a hair follicle from there or another site on the body, by contact with another person, or by contact with an infected article such as a washcloth or towel. In most cases, however, other people coming in contact with the bacteria do not get boils.

People with diseases such as anemia (deficiency of red blood cells), diabetes, or localized infections that weaken their natural defenses against bacteria seem more susceptible to boils. Others who are physically run down may also have greater difficulty fighting the infection. Often, those who work with greasy or oily substances are more likely to develop boils because these materials trap bacteria against the skin. Poor bathing habits, especially in summer months when sweaty skin provides the moist climate conducive to bacteria growth, also invite infection.

Boils can develop anywhere on the skin. They appear most frequently on the neck, face, and back, and they can erupt in several places at once. Although boils vary in size, they characteristically form white or yellow pustules. As the infection progresses, the pustule becomes red and hot. Excess fluid in the boil produces pressure on the nerves underneath that can result in considerable pain. When boils contain little pus, they are called *blind boils*. In this instance, the inflammation recedes slowly without rupturing, but sometimes it leaves a scar.

If boils are large or extensive, the person may also experience fever and general weakened feeling. Sometimes, the infection gets into the bloodstream and spreads throughout the body. The same bacteria that cause the boil may also produce a toxin (poison) that causes blood clots, usually in the small blood vessels around the boil.

Any treatment plan for boils and carbuncles emphasizes that they should *never* be squeezed, particularly if they are on the face. Squeezing may force the infection deeper into the skin and possibly into the bloodstream. Only a physician should lance a boil to encourage drainage. Afterwards, the doctor may prescribe an oral antibiotic such as penicillin or erythromycin to fight further infection.

Many boils will rupture and heal on their own. However, holding a soft cloth soaked with warm water against the boil for 15 to 20 minutes at least four times a day will speed the process. These warm compresses increase blood flow to the area and encourage pustule formation. Since bacteria from the boil is contagious, the cloth should be disinfected in boiling water or in the hot cycle of a washing machine.

When a boil bursts, the infected area should be washed thoroughly and covered with an antibiotic cream and sterile gauze. If the boil does not heal within a few days, or if the boil is located on or near the face, a physician should be consulted.

To prevent new eruptions, the skin needs to be kept cool and dry. Sometimes, physicians advise washing the entire body with an antiseptic (germ-fighting) soap twice a day. If boils frequently recur, underclothing and bed linen should be changed every day.

See also Acne.

Bones

Bones are hardened masses of living tissue that have several functions. They collect calcium for the entire body, storing 99 percent of this mineral that is required to keep all bones firm and strong. In addition, bones produce large numbers of red and white blood cells within their softer tissue center called marrow.

There are 206 bones in the body. Together they form the skeleton or framework for the body. The total structure maintains the body's shape and protects internal organs from injury. For example, bones in the skull shield the brain while bones comprising the rib cage encircle the lungs and heart.

The place where two bones meet is called a joint. This juncture usually allows movement of the bones that are involved. However, movement is governed by ligaments (bands of fibrous tissue) attached to the bones and cartilage (elastic tissue) lining the ends of bones. Ligaments connect one bone with another. Cartilage cushions and protects bones with the aid of various joint fluids and bursae (small sacs containing lubricating fluid located within the joints). Other bands of connective tissue called tendons attach bones to muscles. Muscles are specific kinds of tissues that have the ability to contract. This contraction and pull on the tendon are what actually create movement of the bones. In order to move any part of the skeletal structure, coordination of ligaments, tendons, and muscles is necessary.

Brain

The brain is the control center for the entire body. The brain sends out to and receives stimulation from all body parts. Specifically, nerve cells from the brain transmit messages throughout the nervous system, the network of specialized tissue responsible for mental processes, sensations, actions, and emotions. More than ten billion interwoven brain cells

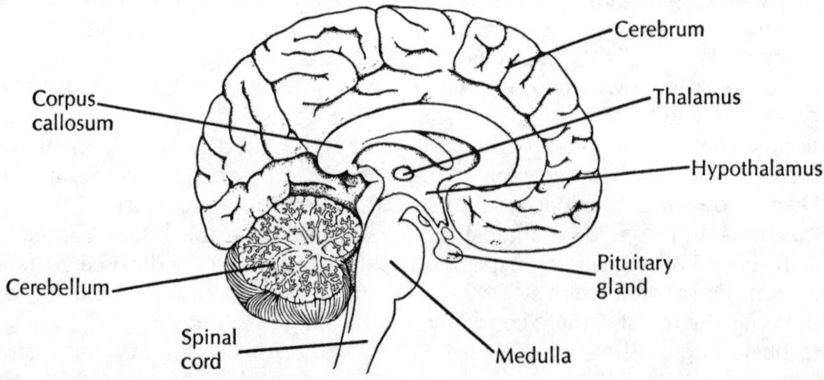

The brain is the control center for the entire body.

regulate mechanisms during sleep and wakefulness.

Different areas of the brain control different body functions. The entire brain lies within the protective bony structure called the skull. At the back of the skull is the cerebellum. This part of the brain determines coordination of movements, balance, and posture.

Deep inside the brain is the thalamus, the center for pain, touch, temperature, and consciousness. In addition, the thalamus is the relay station for incoming impulses from the body, conveying these impulses to other parts of the brain.

Beneath the thalamus is the hypothalamus, which governs involuntary or automatic body operations such as heartbeat, blood pressure, and blood circulation. The master gland, or pituitary gland, of the endocrine system is attached to the hypothalamus by a thin stalk. Because the pituitary gland controls most of the hormones in the body, the hypothalamus is considered a major influence upon primary drives governed by hormones, such as sexual desire, hunger, and thirst.

Covering the inner parts of the brain is the cerebrum, which consists of two cerebral hemispheres. In these hemispheres are the nerve centers that regulate voluntary thought and action. Connecting the left and right cerebral hemispheres are bands of fibers called the corpus callosum. Because nerve fibers from the two cerebral hemispheres cross one another at the base of the brain (medulla) before progressing down the spinal cord, each hemisphere generally controls functions in the opposite side of the body.

The brain is the most complex part of the body. Although research has identified many of its capabilities for memory, reasoning, and creative thought processes, many functions of the brain remain a mystery.

Breast disease

See Fibrocystic breast disease.

Bright's disease

See Glomerulonephritis.

Bronchiectasis

Bronchiectasis is a lung condition in which some of the small and medium-sized bronchi (air tubes) have lost their elasticity and have expanded and filled with fluid. Most often, bronchiectasis follows pneumonia, whooping cough, tuberculosis, or other lung disease or is the result of an obstruction. (Fortunately, the use of antibiotics has reduced the number of cases.) Other causes include the hereditary disease cystic fibrosis, with its thick secretions of mucus; a rare inherited condition in which the little air sacs at the end of the bronchi are not developed completely; and a condition in which the cilia do not work properly (the cilia are hair-like projections that line the bronchial walls and wave mucus, pus, and dirt upward).

Bronchiectasis is a chronic condition that persists for life. The individual almost always has some symptoms that will at times worsen if an acute infection occurs. The most typical symptom is a chronic cough, producing a thick white or green sputum (discharge). In older cases the sputum may be foul-smelling and abundant and settle into three layers if placed in a cup: a thick film of pus on the bottom, green or brownish fluid in the middle, and froth on top. It may also contain blood. The individual generally coughs up large amounts of sputum after changing position, for example, after rising from bed. The doctor, listening to the chest with a stethoscope, can hear abnormal sounds inside the lungs as the patient breathes. An X ray, made with the use of dye injected into the bloodstream or directly into the bronchi, will show up the characteristic appearance of the disease. Chronic bronchitis (continued inflammation of the mucous membrane in the bronchi) must be ruled out as a cause, along with tuberculosis, certain fungus infections, cancer or other tumor, and objects that the patient may have inhaled that are lodged in the bronchi.

Treatment of an active case of bronchiectasis includes fighting the infection with antibiotics such as penicillin or tetracycline and eliminating the fluid with postural drainage. In this procedure, the patient lies face down in bed with pillows elevating the hips as a therapist strikes the back over the chest area with cupped hands to loosen mucus. The treatment, which can be taught to a family member, requires two to four 10-minute sessions a day. Inhaling warm mists may also help to loosen sticky fluids in the lungs. The patient should avoid anything that can irritate the lungs, such as smoke (especially cigarette smoke), fumes, and dust.

Most attacks of bronchiectasis can be handled well with the above methods. However, in a few cases in which the infection is progressing despite antibiotics and is confined to a small part of the lung, it may be best to remove the portion of the lung that contains the bronchiectasis with surgery.

You can prevent repeated attacks by being immunized against flu and pneumonia, avoiding anyone with a cold or cough, and stopping smoking. Prompt treatment with antibiotics can help to control new infections.

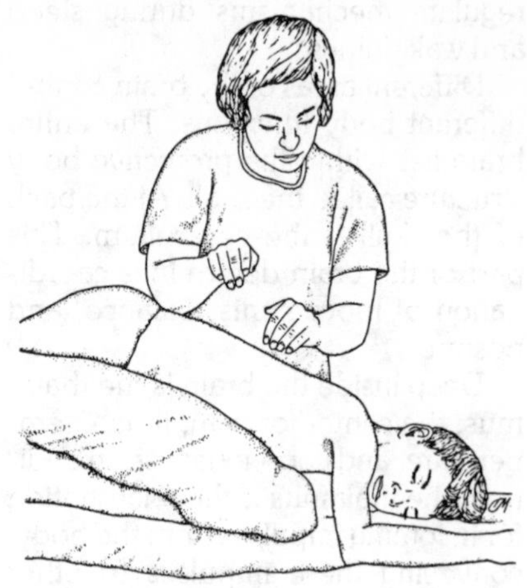

Postural drainage, a way of eliminating fluid from the respiratory system, is one method of treatment for bronchiectasis. In this procedure, the patient lies head down in bed with pillows elevating the hips as a therapist strikes the back over the chest area with cupped hands to loosen mucus.

Bronchitis

Bronchitis is a respiratory disease characterized by an inflammation and swelling of the main breathing tubes (called the bronchi) that connect the windpipe and lungs. When these tubes develop inflammation in their inner linings or mucous membranes, the mucous glands located in the membranes will expand and release more mucus. The bronchi, already narrowed by the swelling, become further clogged with the excess mucus. This mucus must then be coughed up in order to keep the breathing tubes free for normal air flow into the lungs.

When the excess mucus is produced and coughed up, the patient has what is known as a productive cough. A short period of productive coughing is called acute bronchitis; when the coughing lingers for six months, or when it occurs for three months a year and for two years in a row, it is called chronic bronchitis. In either case, the coughing stops only when the source of inflammation has been removed or overcome and the inner linings of the bronchi have returned to normal.

Bronchitis alone can be fatal, but more likely it will lead to another condition that proves to be fatal. For example, in some severe long-standing cases, bronchitis-damaged lungs can deprive the heart of adequate oxygen, resulting in death from heart failure. Also, bronchitis can be very serious when combined with other respiratory diseases. Such is the case for people who suffer from a category of respiratory conditions called chronic obstructive pulmonary disease (COPD). Bronchitis, emphysema, and several other diseases are included in this category, and patients may suffer from two or three of the COPD conditions, or one may lead to another.

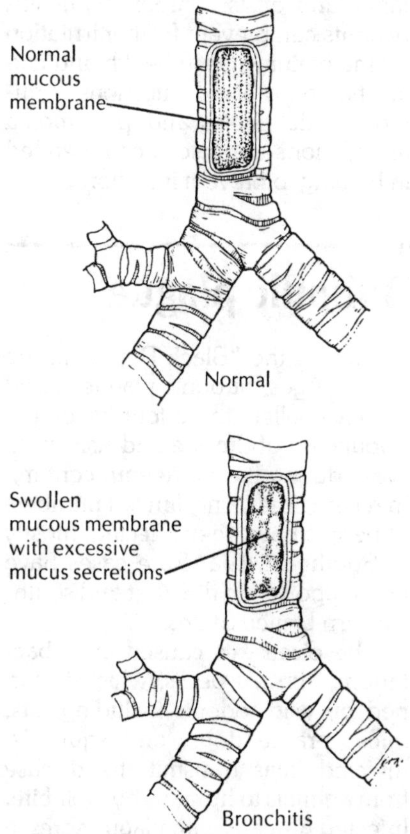

Bronchitis is an inflammation of the mucous membranes (inner linings) of the bronchial tubes. As the membranes swell, they secrete more mucus, resulting in clogged bronchial tubes and a reduced air flow into the lungs.

Bronchitis occurs when the bronchial tubes are infected or irritated. A cold, flu, or strep throat may lead to acute bronchitis, or even chronic bronchitis, if these infections occur often enough. However, chronic bronchitis is more commonly triggered by the constant irritation of environmental substances such as cigarette smoke, air pollutants, or occupational dusts.

Cigarette smoking is the predominant cause of chronic bronchitis. Seventy-five percent of all those who suffer from bronchitis are cigarette smokers. When tobacco smoke reaches the bronchial linings, it stops the action of the cilia, the hair-like projections whose job it is to sweep mucus out of the lungs, mucus that normally carries with it dust and bacteria. Once the cilia are stilled by smoke, these irritating particles remain trapped in the stagnant mucus, aggravating the delicate bronchial tubes and eventually creating a breeding ground for infection.

Some degree of bronchitis occurs in about 90 percent of all smokers who live in polluted environments or who are exposed to occupational dusts. Babies and young children with chronic bronchitis usually overcome the condition, but are more likely to contract it later in life. People who are undernourished, inadequately housed, or often fatigued are more likely to contract bronchitis. Also, this disorder tends to occur within certain families, but the reason is not yet known.

Bronchitis can be recognized by its major symptom, the persistent cough that brings up the lung's excess mucus. Acute bronchitis may be accompanied by hoarseness, chest discomfort, slight fever, wheezing, and shortness of breath. In children, the productive cough may establish itself after several short-term infections and chronic bronchitis will set in. In adults, the beginnings of chronic bronchitis can be recognized by regular coughing and clearing of the throat the first thing each morning; the coughing will become more persistent and the mucus more plentiful as the disease progresses, and these symptoms may be accompanied by wheezing, shortness of breath, chest infections, and heavy panting after exercise.

As the years pass, chronic bronchitis may cause the bronchial tubes to become severely obstructed and the breathing irreversibly impaired. The heart will pump harder to get its needed oxygen and sometimes become enlarged. Nails, lips, and skin may even develop a blue tinge from lack of oxygen.

To diagnose bronchitis, the doctor will take a medical history, physical examination of the chest with a stethoscope, and perhaps a chest X ray. Special machines can measure the amount of air flowing in and out of the lungs, and others can measure how well oxygen is being transported from the lungs to the bloodstream.

Bronchitis is treated by removing the troublesome outside irritants, clearing the lungs of mucus, and trying to prevent infections. A chronic bronchitis patient will need to quit smoking and to avoid constant exposure to pollutants or hazardous dusts. Humidity plays a large part in treating bronchitis; patients should drink plenty of water and hot liquids, breathe warmed and humidified air from a vaporizer or humidifier, or even inhale steam from hot water or hot liquids, like chicken soup, a popular home remedy. Humid air and steam will act to loosen trapped mucus in the lungs.

A drug that relaxes the air passages, called a bronchodilator, may be prescribed, to be used along with the humidity treatments. Also, mucus may be more easily loosened and the bronchial tubes drained when the head is lower than the chest, so lying on a bed with the head hanging off the edge may bring some relief.

Bronchitis can best be prevented by avoiding the irritants that cause it, namely cigarette smoke, air pollutants, and dusts. Chronic bronchitis patients can prevent further irritation by maintaining good health and eating habits to avoid infections. Antibiotics, flu shots, and pneumonia inoculations are also recommended in helping to prevent infection.

Bubonic plague

Known as the "Black Death" in the Middle Ages, bubonic plague is said to have killed three-fourths of the population of Europe and Asia in 20 years during the fourteenth century. In recent times, only limited numbers of people have been infected, mostly in Southeast Asia. Rare cases have been reported in the west and southwestern United States.

The disease is caused by a bacterium, *Yersinia pestis,* which is carried by wild rodents including rats, mice, prairie dogs, and squirrels. Infected fleas transmit the disease from animals to humans by their bite. Infected humans with plague sores in their lungs can pass the bacteria to other people when they cough. The result of this direct infection of the lungs is known as *primary pneumonic plague.*

In bubonic plague transmitted by flea bite, chills and high fever occur after an incubation period—the time between exposure to the disease and the development of symptoms—that is usually two to five days (although it can vary from a few hours to 12 days). However, the chief symptom is the development of enlarged, painful lymph glands (called buboes) that fill with pus and may later rupture. The patient is often restless, delirious, and uncoordinated. Without treatment, 60 percent of victims die, as the plague bacteria rapidly spread to affect all organs of the body, usually in three to five days.

Primary pneumonic plague kills even more quickly. Two or three days after being infected, the victim experiences high fever, chills, rapid heartbeat, and headache. A cough develops, with blood specks in the mucus discharge that eventually turns red and foamy. Breathing is rapid and irregular as pneumonia develops. Untreated persons usually die within 48 hours.

Immediate treatment as soon as plague is suspected can reduce the death rate to below 5 percent. Streptomycin or tetracycline antibiotic is given around the clock every six hours for seven to 10 days. Patients with primary pneumonic plague need to be isolated and watched closely. Anyone who is in contact with a plague victim should also be closely watched for the development of fever, cough, and painful lymph glands. Preventive antibiotics, to prevent the onset of the infection, should generally be given to those exposed to plague victims.

To prevent plague, travelers to the parts of Southeast Asia and India, where bubonic plague is present, should be immunized with killed plague vaccine. Insect repellants help prevent bites from infected fleas, and rodent control can reduce the source.

Bulimia

Bulimia is abnormal and excessive eating, usually caused by emotional factors. Victims of the disorder overeat far beyond the needs of their bodies. In extreme cases, they resemble alcoholics, employing food instead of drink as an escape from the problems of life. When distressed, they may even go on food binges and eat themselves into a stupor. Sometimes they may feel guilty after overeating and induce themselves to vomit.

To a bulimia victim, food provides a way to relieve stress. Some think that excessive eating is an unconscious attempt to recapture the feelings of security experienced in childhood when food was received from the mother. Psychiatrists have speculated that overeating may also represent a hunger for affection that was denied in early childhood when the child's attention was focused on the mouth and eating. It may be a substitute for affection, attention, or sexual relations that the person is not now receiving. It may be an outlet for hostile feelings, since food is being destroyed by the acts of biting and chewing. Finally, the person may unconsciously seek to become more important and safer by becoming larger—through weight gain.

Bulimia is sometimes found among mental patients, especially those who have regressed to babyish behavior. Excessive eating may also result from hyperthyroidism (overactivity of the thyroid gland), whose victims burn up great quantities of calories without adding weight. In a very small percentage of cases, bulimia may be caused by damage to the appetite control center of the brain.

Attempts to cure bulimia have not been very successful and have frequently caused the patient to become even more distressed. However, it is generally agreed that a logical first step is to help the patient discover the emotional causes of his or her disorder. This may require individual or family counseling by a psychiatrist or clinical psychologist, who also tries to help the patient gain confidence, become more sociable and self-reliant. New satisfactions are sought to replace the satisfactions formerly found in overeating. A program of diet and exercise may follow.

See also Anorexia nervosa.

Bunion

A bunion is a swelling on the foot usually at the joint of the big toe. Often, a bony protuberance is found at the joint of the big toe, which gives the bunion its bulging appearance.

Bunions are most often caused by poorly fitting footwear, but they can also be the result of inherited deformities in bone structure. In a normal foot, the two main bones of the big toe must align to fit together. However, some people have loose bone joints in the foot that allow their big toe to point outward toward the other foot. This inherited condition causes problems when footwear encloses the foot. Shoes force the big toe inward and the big toe joint outward so that the joint rubs against the inner surface of the footwear. Friction from such rubbing produces a bunion. The same action results when pointed-toed or tight shoes put pressure on the joint—whether or not the genetic tendency exists.

A bunion is characterized by swelling at the big toe joint that may be accompanied by pain and tenderness. Bunion formations can be acute or chronic. Acute bunions are a type of bursitis, which is an inflammation of the bursae. A bursa is a fluid-filled sac that cushions the juncture where two bones meet. With an acute bunion, the bursa covering the big toe joint becomes inflamed from friction at the joint, often producing considerable pain. Chronic, or long-term, bunions develop an inflexible bony protrusion that results from continued pressure at the joint.

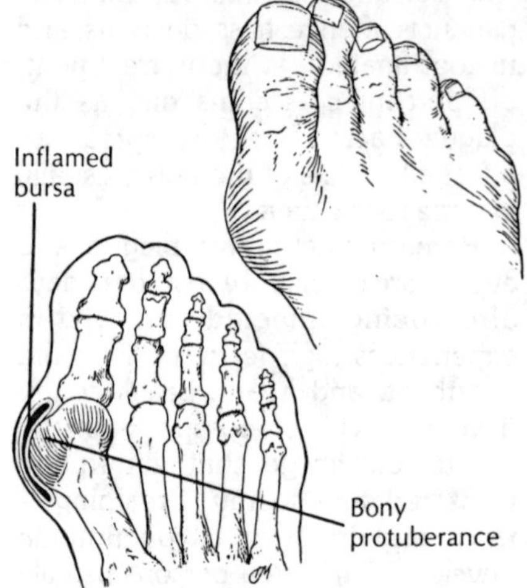

A bunion is a swelling at the joint of the big toe, often accompanied by a bony protuberance and an inflamed bursa—the fluid-filled sac that acts as a cushion in the joint. A bunion is most often caused by friction or pressure on the joint.

Complications can develop if the bunion grows and increases pressure on the big toe. This pressure may force the other toes to overlap, encouraging corns (mounds of dead skin found on toes) or other problems that could result from friction on the skin of the distorted toes.

A physician diagnoses a bunion by general physical examination. To verify bone problems, X rays may be necessary.

Surgery is the only permanent cure for bunions. It can entail simple removal of the excess bone or more complex realignment of the bones, muscles, and tendons that led to formation of the bunion. Sometimes a doctor can remove a bony protrusion in the office with local anesthetic. Pain is minimal, and the incision is probably only about an inch long. With this treatment, the patient has full use of the foot in about six weeks.

For more extensive surgery, the patient goes to a hospital and requires longer recuperation time. Usually, an orthopedic surgeon performs this type of surgery.

Nonsurgical devices can relieve the pain and discomfort of bunions. Padding can be used to shift the weight of the foot in the shoe, lessening friction. Protective shields can also prevent contact between the bunion and the inside of the shoe.

Wearing properly fitting footwear is the best prevention of bunions. Even a child's first shoes should have a sturdy sole and be wide enough to accommodate all toes without cramping, since early childhood is when most foot problems begin.

When buying shoes, the width and length of each foot needs to be measured separately. If one foot is larger than the other, shoe size should correspond to the size of the larger foot. A one-inch gap between the big toe and the tip of the shoe allows enough moving space. Even more room is needed with pointed-toed shoes. Shoes should be comfortable from the first wearing—without requiring a breaking-in period.

Women who wear stylish high-heeled or pointed-toed shoes may be damaging their feet. Heels about one inch in height are actually best for feet. However, if higher heels are chosen, open-toed styles cause fewer problems. Similarly, narrow-toed shoes are less damaging with low heels.

Nothing is better for feet than walking barefoot on unlittered sand or grass. Sandals or thongs are the next best kind of footwear to avoid the cramping effects of shoes. For some people, wooden clogs provide the same relief.

Burns

See Emergency first aid section at the end of this book.

Bursitis

Bursitis is an inflammation of the bursae, the sacs or pouches located at the ends of the bones in the joints. Bursae contain lubricating fluid and normally eliminate friction in the area and maintain smooth muscle movement over the bones.

In some forms of bursitis, calcium deposits from the bones cause swelling that may render the surrounding area immobile. This swelling produces inflammation of the bursae. Continual stress on a particular joint or a combination of calcium build-up and stress can also create the problem.

The inflammation can result from either sudden extreme pressure or from continuous strain. Some occupations and sports that require constant use of certain joints contribute to acute or chronic bursitis. For example, "typist's shoulder" and "baseball pitcher's elbow" are forms of chronic bursitis. Acute bursitis can develop suddenly and may be triggered by a chill or draft.

Inflamed bursae produce tenderness and swelling near the affected joint. Pain from bursitis can be very disabling. At times, it is so severe that movement becomes impossible. Any joint in the body can be the site of bursitis, but shoulders, knees, and elbows are most commonly affected.

To diagnose bursitis, your physician may suggest an X ray to determine if there are calcium deposits in the bursae. For bursitis that is stress-related, however, X rays only show bursae that are swollen.

Acute bursitis may heal with time if the joint is immobilized. Patients may consider using a sling, crutches, or complete bed rest to relieve pressure on the affected area.

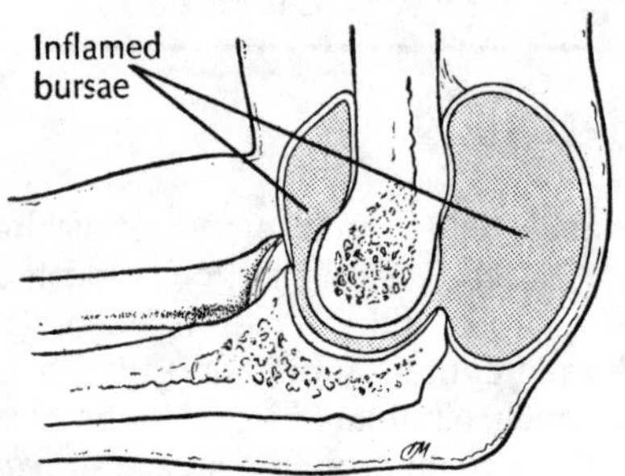

The elbow is a common site of bursitis, an inflammation of the bursae, the fluid-filled sacs located in the joints. Bursae normally eliminate friction in the joints and maintain smooth muscle movement over the bones.

Applying moist heat directly to the inflamed joint frequently reduces the discomfort of bursitis, although some patients find cold compresses more effective. Aspirin and other over-the-counter pain relievers may also alleviate pain. In some cases, anti-inflammatory corticosteroid drugs may be injected directly into the inflamed area, but these drugs should be used judiciously since they have been known to cause adverse side effects.

For severe cases of bursitis, a doctor may recommend surgery by an orthopedic surgeon to remove calcium deposits or free the area from chronic inflammation by removing part of the bursa.

Bypass surgery

Bypass surgery is a term that usually refers to either (1) coronary bypass surgery or (2) intestinal or gastric bypass surgery. Both will be discussed.

Coronary bypass surgery is performed on one or more of the three great blood vessels, the coronary arteries, that lie on the outer surface of the heart and supply heart muscle with the oxygen and nutrients it needs. In coronary artery disease, a section or sections of the arteries gradually become obstructed with a buildup of cholesterol, calcium, and scar tissue. The purpose of the operation is to bypass the blood around the obstruction using a section of blood vessel (usually a vein taken from the leg) that is sewn into the artery in front of and behind the blockage. This permits free blood flow again. Without it, heart muscle below the obstruction is starved for blood and oxygen, especially during exercise. This creates the chest pains known as "angina." If one or more of the coronary arteries become completely obstructed, the result may be a heart attack, in which a portion of heart muscle becomes so starved for blood that it dies.

Usually if there is one obstruction in the coronary arteries, there are others (there may be two in the same artery). A "double bypass" operation means that two obstructions are bypassed, a "triple bypass" means that three are, and so forth. Three or more bypasses are common.

Bypass surgery is usually considered when a person suffers frequent chest pains from angina. However, not all persons with angina need bypass surgery. Advances are being made in medication to control angina. Furthermore, some angina is caused by spasms (sudden, violent contractions) of the coronary arteries, which bypass surgery may not prevent or help. In the future, obstructions in the coronary arteries may be eliminated by methods that do not require cutting open the chest, perhaps by a cutting or crushing instrument that is threaded to the site of the obstruction through the blood vessel. Even without outside help, and given enough time, the heart creates its own partial bypass, by developing blood vessels that detour the blood around the obstruction; this is known as "collateral circulation."

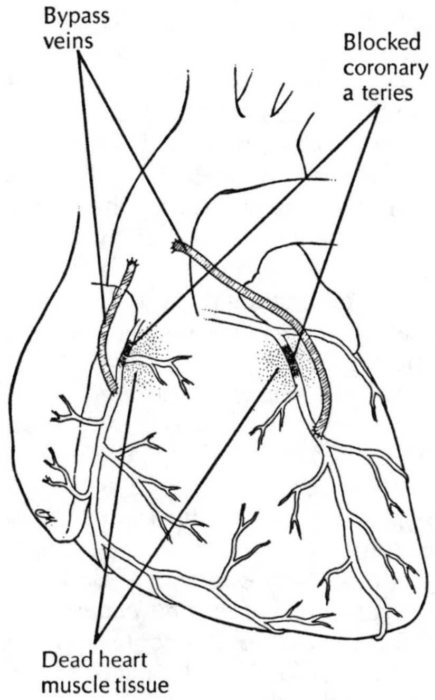

In coronary artery disease, a section of the coronary arteries gradually becomes obstructed with a buildup of cholesterol, calcium, and scar tissue. The coronary bypass operation bypasses the blood around the obstruction in the coronary arteries using a section of blood vessel—usually a vein taken from the leg—that is sewn into the artery in front of and behind the blockage. This permits free blood flow again.

If you have severe chest pains often and they cannot be controlled by medication, your doctor may decide to order that X-ray motion pictures of your heart be taken. Through a thin woven plastic catheter (tube) entering at the arm or leg and passing through large blood vessels to your heart, X-ray contrast medium is injected so that it flows into the coronary arteries, outlining them on the X-ray screen. The pictures show exactly where the blood vessels are narrowed or blocked. Thus the doctor can determine whether bypasses are needed and where. The most urgent reason to operate is the obstruction, of 50 to 70 percent or more, of the left main coronary artery, which supplies two-thirds of the blood to the heart muscle by means of its two lower branches.

The bypass surgery operation takes about four hours or more depending on the number of bypasses. An assisting surgeon cuts several incisions in one leg to obtain a long section of a large vein for use as bypass tubing. Next, the surgeon makes an incision down the middle of the chest, divides the breastbone with an electric saw, and separates the two sides of the rib cage enough to expose the beating heart. The heartbeat is then stopped using either electric shock, ice water, or certain drugs. A heart-lung machine, connected to large vessels carrying blood from and to the heart, takes over the job of adding oxygen, removing carbon dioxide, and pumping the blood through the body.

The surgeon cuts through the pericardial sac (a bag of tissue around the heart) to expose the coronary arteries outlined on the heart surface. On either side of each coronary artery blockage, the surgeon cuts open the artery and sews in either end of bypass tube—a piece of vein taken from the leg. Thereafter, blood will flow freely around the obstructed portion to nourish the heart muscle and thereby protect the patient against chest pains and heart attacks. Usually the patient can walk about three or four days following the operation, and return home in little more than a week.

For such a major operation, the death rate is very low—less than 1 percent in some hospitals. In 80 percent of cases, angina pains are eliminated and the patient can return to a normal life. Life expectancy may improve but it cannot be guaranteed in all cases. There has been much controversy surrounding bypass surgery, mainly centering around the question of whether this procedure can increase life expectancy in those with coronary artery disease and angina. At present, there is no question that the surgery relieves pain and allows for greater exercise tolerance in the majority of patients who undergo it for severe angina. In certain patterns of disease such as obstruction of the "left-main" coronary artery, the operation definitely prolongs life expectancy. In other patterns such as "triple vessel disease" where branches of all three coronaries (except for the left-main) are involved, the surgery most likely allows a longer life. In still other patterns, the question is unsettled. Whether or not the surgery will prevent a heart attack is also an unsettled issue.

Intestinal bypass surgery and *gastric bypass surgery* are means of treating massive obesity (excessive fat). Because of their potential dangers, such methods should be limited to persons who are at least 100 pounds over their ideal weight and who have failed to lose weight by various other means such as diet and exercise. These persons are at serious risk for diabetes, high blood pressure, heart disease, arthritis, and other major disorders.

Various types of operations have been tried in the past two decades to detour digesting food around a long section of the small intestine, thus limiting the area of intestine that can absorb fats and carbohydrates from the food. The most recent intestinal bypass is the jejunoileal (named for the upper portion of small intestine, the jejunum, and the lower part, the ileum) in which all but 18 inches of the 240 inches of the small intestine are bypassed (the unused portion remains in the body and drains into the colon). The method is very effective in reducing weight—from 80 to 150 pounds in most patients—but frequently produces persistent diarrhea, severe liver disease, imbalances in body salts, kidney stones, urinary stones, mental disturbances, and joint inflammations. The mortality rate caused by the above complications may be as high as 5 percent. Because of this high complication rate, many physicians believe that the intestinal bypass method should no longer be used. This surgery is seldom performed today since safer methods have been developed.

Replacements for the intestinal bypass, said to have far fewer complications, are the *gastric bypass* and *gastric stapling* operations. Both are designed to reduce the capacity of the stomach so that only a small amount of food can be eaten at one time. In the gastric bypass operation, the lower part of the stomach is cut off, and the remaining top part is connected to the upper portion of the small intestine. In the gastric stapling operation, stomach capacity is reduced by stapling off most of the fundus, the uppermost portion of the stomach.

The long-term results and side effects of gastric bypass and gastric stapling, when known, will probably determine whether these operations will replace the older methods.

Other forms of bypass surgery are

used in various parts of the body either to route blood around an obstruction or to increase blood supply to an area. For example, a blocked artery in the leg may be bypassed to increase the blood supply to the foot, and a blocked artery in the neck may be bypassed to increase the blood supply to the brain.

See also Atherosclerosis, Agina pectoris, Heart attack, and Obesity.

C

Calluses

Calluses are thickened areas of the skin. They develop most often on the balls and heels of the feet and on the hands.

Skin buildup is the result of excessive friction or pressure against the surface of the skin. As pressure mounts, dead skin cells accumulate, and the skin thickens. Improperly fitting shoes or tightly held pencils can create the problem. Since calluses often follow blisters on the same site, they are considered to be the body's way of shielding the area against further injury.

People with flat feet have greater incidence of calluses. The reason for this is that because of the abnormal shape of the foot, the small bones in the front portion of the foot are forced downward against the skin of the sole with great pressure while walking. This creates pressure points, thus leading to callus formation. In addition, those who wear high heels promote growth of calluses by increasing pressure on the balls of their feet.

Calluses vary in size and shape depending upon where they grow and how much skin is affected. Sometimes, calluses grow so thick and irregular in shape that the skin becomes inflexible and cracks.

When pressure is relieved, calluses usually produce no pain. However, continued irritation, especially against split skin, can cause enough discomfort to interfere with physical activities, such as walking or sports.

Immediate treatment involves removal of the pressure that caused the callus in the first place. Extremely persistent or painful calluses should be examined by a doctor. In rare instances, surgery may be necessary to alleviate intense pressure. In milder cases, calluses can often be eased by padding the exposed area to reduce further friction.

There are over-the-counter remedies that soften the callused tissue, making it easier to remove. Salicylic acid plasters, which are sold in medicated sheets, can be placed over the callus after bathing and secured with tape. The pad should be removed just before the next bath so that the softened skin can be gently removed with a pumice stone or other rough surface.

Home remedies should not be used by people who have diabetes, atherosclerosis, or other circulatory disorders because risk of infection is greater with these diseases. These individuals should consult their doctor before attempting any form of treatment.

Cancer

Cancer is the term used to describe a broad group of diseases which have certain common characteristics. Most cells in the body grow and reproduce in an orderly manner, as dictated by the body's genetic information. A cancer cell does not follow the same genetic direction that normal body cells do.

Cancer cells grow at an uncontrolled rate, taking over, causing the death of, or replacing normal cells as they grow inside the body. As cancer progresses, cells are often sent through the circulatory system to start growth at other parts of the body. When this occurs, it is called *metastasis.*

The term *tumor* means, literally, "a growth." A tumor may be either malignant (cancerous) or benign (noncancerous). A benign tumor commonly grows within a self-produced capsule and does not invade surrounding tissue (although it can cause trouble by pressing on the surrounding tissue), nor does it spread itself throughout the body. Malignant tissues may grow out of control and quite commonly spread.

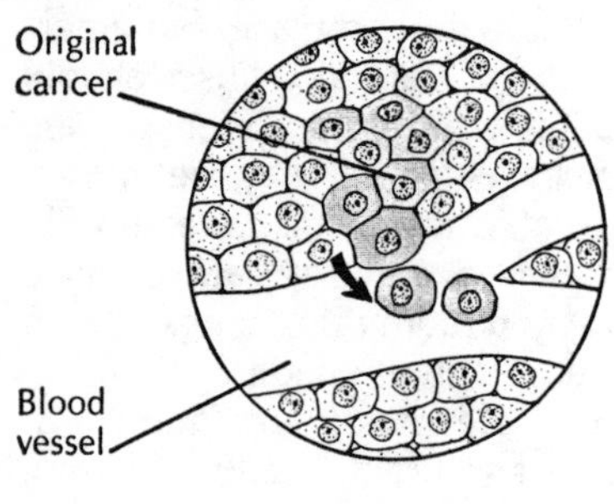

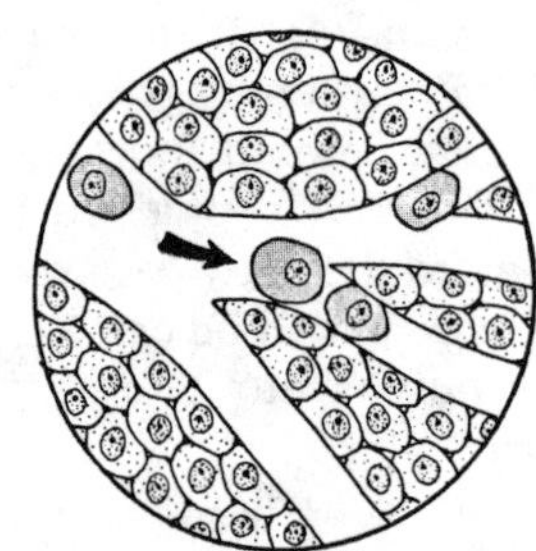

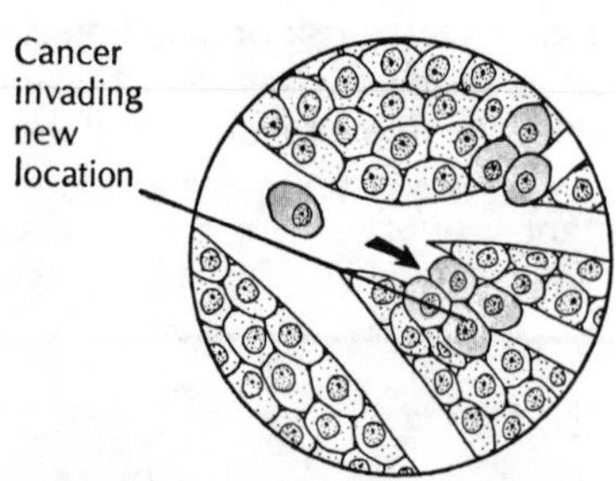

The spread of cancer from its original site to other locations in the body is called metastasis. As cancer progresses, cells are often sent through the circulatory and/or lymphatic system to start growth at other parts of the body.

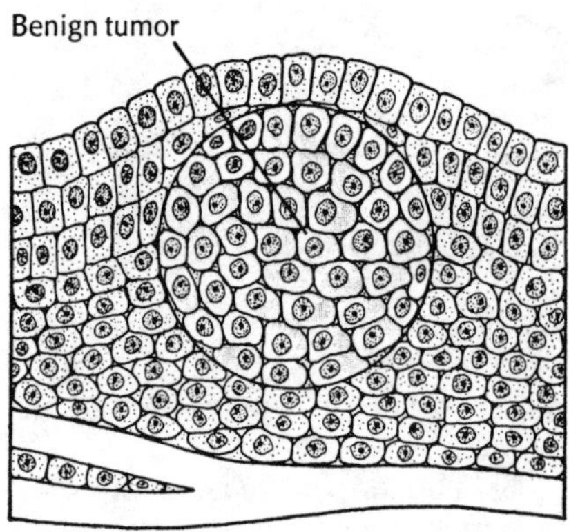

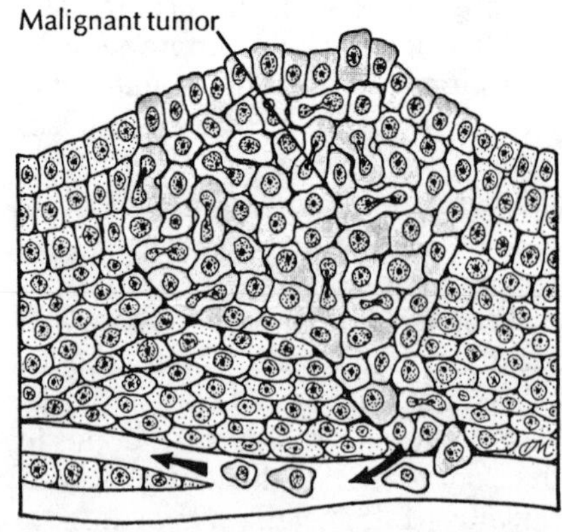

A tumor may be either benign (noncancerous) or malignant (cancerous). A benign tumor commonly grows within a self-produced capsule and does not invade surrounding tissue nor spread itself throughout the body (metastasize). A malignant (cancerous) tumor may grow out of control and does metastasize.

There are over 200 types of cancer that have been identified by pathologists, the physicians who study the body's tissues. In spite of the large numbers, there are three basic categories of cancer: carcinoma (cancer of the cells, known as epithelium cells, that line organs and serve many purposes including production of mucus and protection), sarcoma (cancer of the bony, fat, and muscle tissues), and fluid cancers (leukemia is one example of a fluid cancer). Some cancers may fall into more than one category.

Often a patient is the first to suspect cancer. This is why it is important to learn cancer's seven warning signals:

1. Change in bowel and/or bladder habits
2. A sore that does not heal
3. Unusual bleeding or discharge
4. Thickening or lump in the breast or elsewhere
5. Indigestion or difficulty in swallowing
6. Obvious change in wart or mole
7. A nagging cough or hoarseness.

Since the chances of cure are greatest for the cancer discovered at an early stage, you should learn to perform the important self-examinations. If you are a woman, you (or a mate) should learn to perform the breast self-examination to detect suspicious lumps as early as possible. If you are a man, many physicians recommend testicle self-examination for testicular cancer.

If you suspect you may have cancer, *do not delay* in seeing a physician. Following a physical examination, if the doctor suspects possible abnormal growth, he or she may order a series of tests, including X-ray examinations (for example, tomograms or CAT scans which are X rays utilizing an in-depth technique), nuclear medicine scans (liver-spleen scan, thyroid scan), ultrasound examination, cytology tests (examination of body cells such as is done in a Pap smear), and a group of laboratory evaluations. The doctor may also order a biopsy (microscopic examination of a tissue sample) to determine the cell type of the suspected growth and whether it is benign or malignant.

Your physician may also refer you to a specialist in the area of your suspected cancer. This may be an oncologist (cancer specialist), cancer surgeon, radiation therapist, hematologist (specialist in blood diseases), or a number of other specialty physicians. These physicians are specially trained to deal with diagnosis and treatment of your cancer.

There are many ways of treating cancer. Many treatment programs (called protocols) have been developed that have been most effective in certain types of disease. Cancer therapy often includes surgery to remove the cancer, to clear obstructions of vital passageways caused by the cancer, or to cut nerve paths sending pain messages to your brain; chemotherapy (use of powerful drugs to kill cancer cells); radiation therapy (use of radioactive materials in the form of energy beams or radioactive implants to destroy cancer cells); or a number of other newly developed techniques. Often, combinations of the above therapies are used.

Most methods of treatment have side effects. Surgery sometimes can be disfiguring; however, specialists can often repair the damage at or near the time of surgery. Radiation therapy and chemotherapy can also cause side effects such as skin soreness, loss of hair, or digestive upsets. The alternative to such treatments, of course, is often much worse.

Sometimes, in desperation, a patient or the family will seek unor-

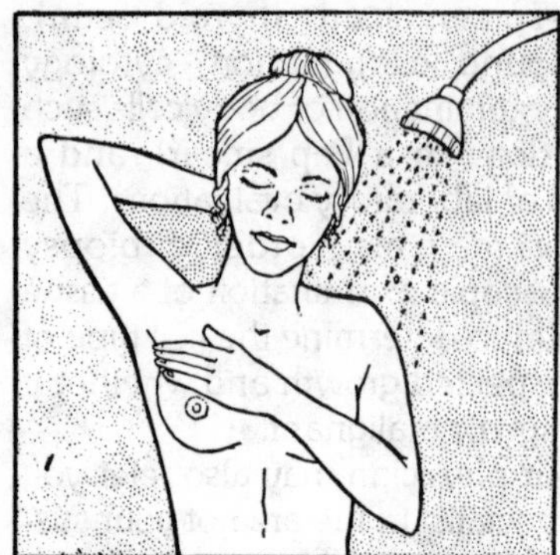

In the shower, keep one hand overhead and examine each breast with opposite hand. Wet, soapy skin may make it easier to feel lumps.

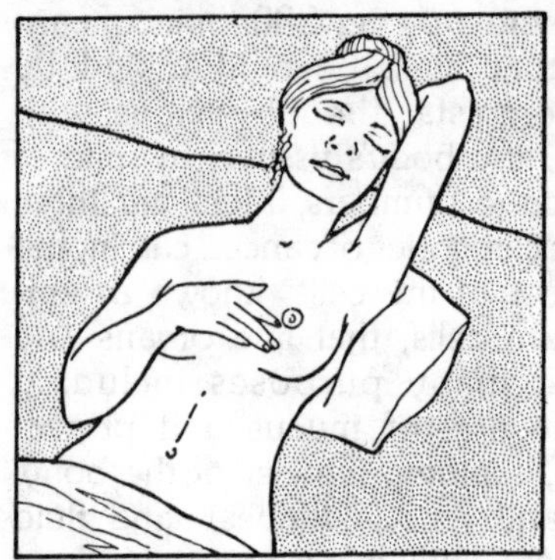

Lying in bed, place a pillow under one shoulder to elevate and flatten breast. Examine each breast, with the opposite hand, first with arm under head and again with arm at side.

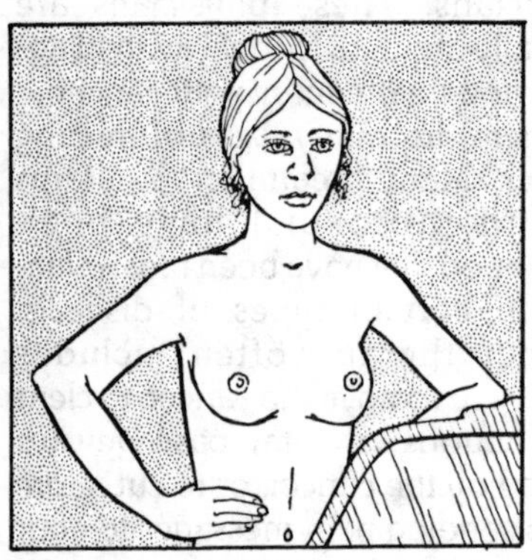

In front of a mirror, stand with hands resting on hips. Examine breasts for swelling, dimpling, bulges, and changes in skin.

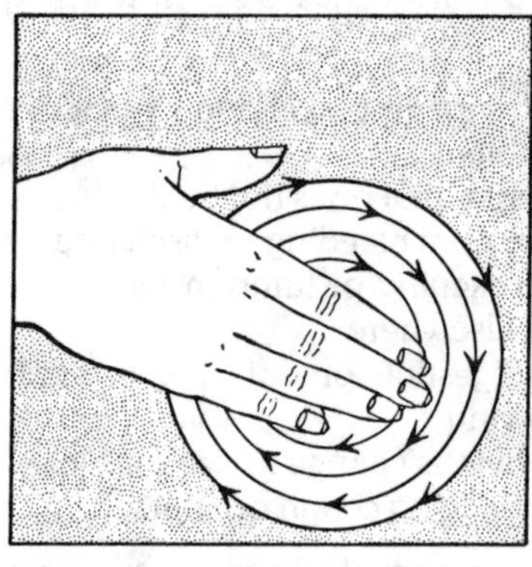

Make rotary motions—with flat pads, not tips, of fingers, in concentric circles inward toward nipple. Feel for knots, lumps, or indentations. Be sure to include the armpit area.

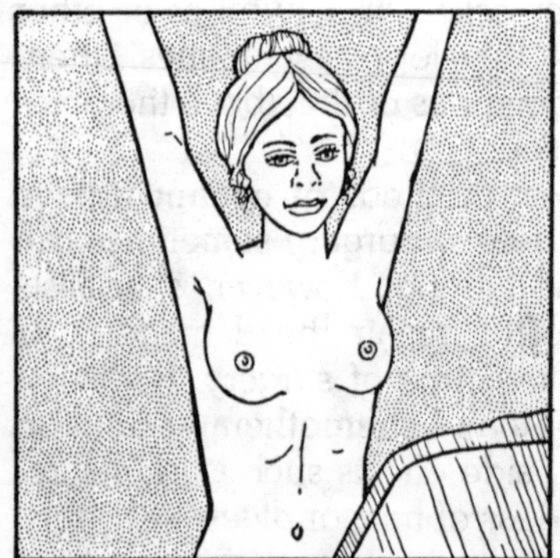

In front of mirror, examine breasts for changes with arms extended overhead. This position highlights bulges and indentations which may indicate a lump.

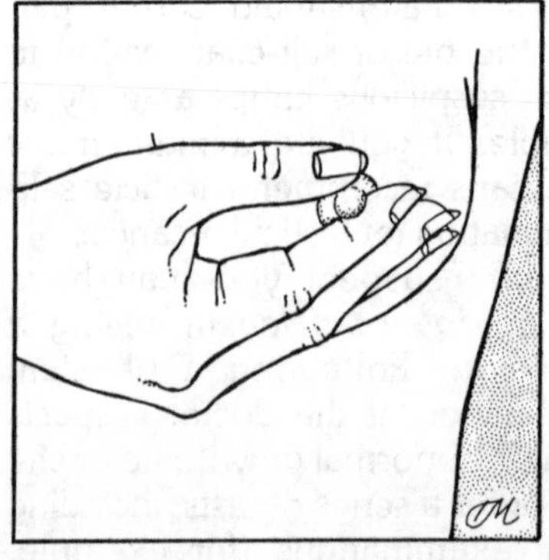

Squeeze nipples gently to inspect for any discharge. Report any suspicious findings to your doctor.

thodox methods of treatment. The medical community is actively researching all known methods of treating cancer and carefully evaluating those that look most promising. Many treatments are slow, and often have severe side effects. Many quack cures, however, offer — but do not deliver — rapid cure with fewer side effects. The harm done by quack practitioners is that they prevent a patient from seeking *effective* treatment until it is too late for *any* treatment to be of use. The best advice is to trust a physician to treat cancer and not waste time, money, and hope on an unproven, unlicensed quack cure.

There are many places to get cancer treatment. Most cancers can be effectively treated at a well-equipped and staffed community hospital. There are, however, a number of large cancer centers throughout the country where specialized protocols are available. Often diagnosis and/or treatment is initiated at a special center and then continued in the community by an oncologist and/or family physician. If you need information or referrals, cancer hotlines or the American Cancer Society are valuable resources. In the event you wish a second opinion about your case, either resource, or your physician, should assist you in getting another opinion.

Who develops cancer? This is a question that is very difficult, if not impossible, to answer. There are, however, certain risk factors that increase the possibility that you may develop cancer in your lifetime. Among these are age—as a rule, the older you are, the higher your risk of getting cancer; in some cases family history, for example, if your mother or sister had breast cancer, your risk of developing breast cancer is increased; and environmental and other factors.

The rapid increase in cancer rates during this century has been blamed, to a large part, on the environment. Polluted air and water, food additives and colorings, changes in diet from "natural" to "processed" foods all have been implicated as possible causes. Cigarette smoking has been relatively conclusively implicated as a cause of lung and other related cancers. If you wish to reduce your risk of getting cancer, it is best to control the factors that you can control — obviously one person alone cannot clean the environment. However, you can stop smoking.

If you do develop cancer, there are a number of prognostic factors (factors that predict length of survival) that are important. Most important are the stage and the type of the disease. The earlier the stage of the disease, that is, the sooner it is diagnosed, the better the prognosis will be. The type of tumor also makes a major difference, since different tumors respond differently to treatment. Furthermore, within a specific organ there are different cell types of cancer that can occur. For example, all lung cancers are not the same type of cell. Often these types are important in determining both response to therapy and prognosis. Your age and overall physical condition are also important in determining your ability to win the fight over cancer.

Cancer should no longer be considered the dreaded scourge that it was thought to be 20 years ago. It is not always fatal and is in many instances curable. The keys to living today should be to avoid cancer-causing materials (for example, cigarettes), to consult your physician regularly (and discuss possible risk factors), and to perform regularly the self-examination procedures that your doctor suggests. Early detection is of extreme importance and you are the best source of early detection.

Candida albicans

Candida albicans is a fungus that is normally present on the skin and on membranes of the mouth, throat, intestines, and vagina. It becomes an infecting agent only when there is some change in the body environment that allows it to multiply and to invade normal tissue. The most common cause may be the use of antibiotics that destroy beneficial as well as harmful microscopic organisms in the body and permit *Candida* to multiply in their place. The resulting infection is known as candidiasis, candidosis, or moniliasis. In the mouth, it becomes thrush; on the skin, an inflamed rash such as diaper rash; in the vagina, vaginitis, moniliasis, or yeast infection; and in or next to the nails, candidal onychomycosis or paronychia, respectively. It can also infect the esophagus (food pipe) and the digestive tract. In rare instances, when body resistance is low, *Candida albicans* enters the bloodstream and causes serious infection of the vital organs. Drug addicts, diabetics, and patients receiving chemotherapy are especially at risk. So are those whose natural defenses are weakened by certain drugs meant to suppress the immune system (such as are given to those who receive transplanted organs). Pregnant women are often susceptible to moniliasis, and babies passing through an infected birth canal may develop thrush.

Symptoms and treatment for the various forms of *Candida* infection follow:

- Vaginitis is characterized by a white or yellow discharge, with inflammation of the wall of the vagina and of the vulva (external genital area). A white, cheesy substance may cling to the wall of the vagina. Occasionally the infection will be passed to the woman's mate, causing irritation, redness, and soreness of the head of the penis and sometimes a slight discharge. Treatment is with an antifungal drug such as nystatin inserted deep in the vagina and if necessary applied to the entire region around the entrance to the vagina. Both sexual partners should use the medication when one has a recurring infection. Otherwise the disease may pass back and forth.
- Thrush appears as creamy white or bluish white patches on the tongue, which is also inflamed and sometimes beefy red, on the lining of the mouth, or in the throat. Treatment is with nystatin oral solution or drops five times a day until all patches have disappeared and then for a few days afterward.
- Diaper rash caused by *Candida* can be treated by keeping the baby dry with frequent diaper changes. In severe cases, rubber pants and disposable diapers should be avoided.
- Nail infections appear as red, painful swelling around the nail; later, pus develops (paronychia). After the area is treated with hot compresses and drainage, if necessary, and the nail cut back, an antifungal lotion is applied. The nail itself may be involved (appearing hard, yellow, and dull), making treatment more difficult and perhaps requiring long-term oral drugs.
- Systemic infection (when infection enters the bloodstream and affects the kidneys, heart, lung, eye, or other organs) can result in high fever, chills, anemia, and sometimes a rash or shock. Disease in the lungs can cause bloody sputum (mucus discharge); in the kidneys, blood in the urine; in the brain, seizures; in the heart, murmurs and valve damage; and in the eye, pain

and blurred vision. An antifungal medicine, is usually given intravenously (into the vein).

In all cases, the underlying condition that caused the outbreak of *Candida* needs to be removed, if possible. This may mean stopping the use of antibiotics or controlling diabetes. The same approach is used to prevent future infections.

See also Onychomycosis and Vaginitis.

Canker sores

Canker sores (technically known as aphthous ulcers) are inflamed tissue cavities or ulcers usually found in the mouth. They can be quite painful, often inhibiting eating ability. Even though up to one out of every four persons develops canker sores, they are not contagious.

Researchers differ about the cause of canker sores. One unconfirmed theory suggests that the sores are the result of an "autoimmune response," whereby the body develops antibodies to its own tissue. Other factors that have been said to trigger canker sores include fever, menstruation, fatigue, tension, or allergies. Some people get canker sores after eating certain foods. Poor dental hygiene, ill-fitting dentures, or injuries from stiff toothbrushes may also lead to the condition. All of the above may be contributing factors; however, the true cause of canker sores is unknown.

A canker sore begins as a small blister that occurs alone or in groups. It can be found almost anywhere in the mouth, such as inside the cheek and on the tongue, lips, or gums.

After the blister breaks, a small ulcer or cavity develops and enlarges until it becomes a bright red sore surrounding the whitish yellow cavity of the ulcer. This sore can last about 10 to 14 days before healing. Canker sores leave no scars. However, they often recur, sometimes every few weeks or months. They more frequently occur in women.

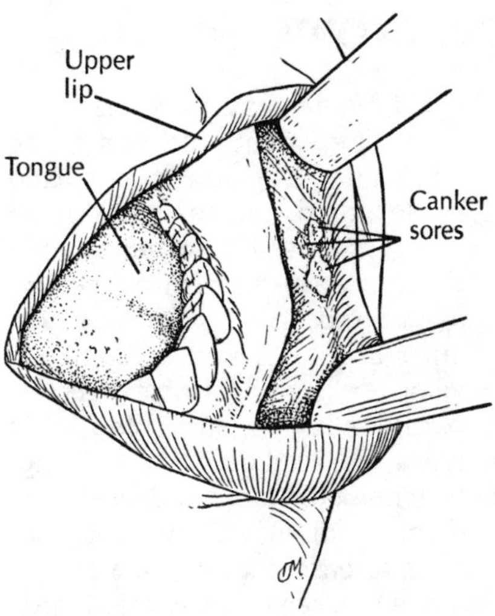

Canker sores are inflamed tissue cavities or ulcers usually found in the mouth, often inside the cheek.

Canker sores have no cure, but there are several treatments that may relieve pain. Some physicians prescribe the antibiotic tetracycline for canker sores. Treatment involves dissolving the capsule in an ounce of warm water and swishing the mixture in the mouth for five to ten minutes three or four times a day for five to seven days. Sometimes, therapy includes soaking a cotton wad in the solution and applying it directly to the sores.

There are also various over-the-counter preparations designed to reduce discomfort. However, they are of uncertain value, and you should always check with your doctor before using them.

People who have repeated attacks of canker sores should see a physician or dentist. Recurrence may be lessened by improving oral hygiene or by avoiding certain foods or other substances.

Carpal tunnel syndrome

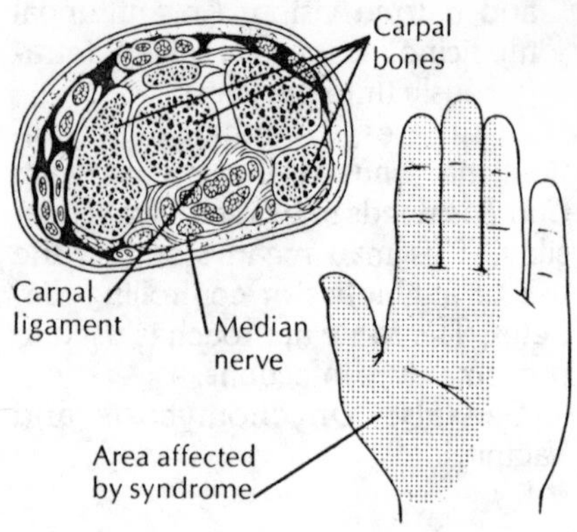

Carpal tunnel syndrome is weakness, pain, tingling, numbness or burning in the palm part of the thumb, and the index, third, and inner part of the ring fingers caused by entrapment of the median nerve within the carpal tunnel of the wrist. The carpal tunnel consists of the carpal bones of the wrist overlaid by the tough band of connective tissue called the carpal ligament.

Carpal tunnel syndrome is weakness, pain, tingling, numbness, or burning of the palm part of the thumb, and the index, third, and inner part of the ring fingers caused by an entrapment of the median nerve in the wrist. The condition most often affects women in their 30s, 40s, and 50s. It may develop or become worse because of work, such as scrubbing, that requires repeated grasping, twisting, or turning of the hand and wrist.

The condition, like any syndrome, is not a disease in itself but a collection of symptoms. The carpal tunnel consists of the bones of the wrist ("carpal" means "wrist") overlaid by a tough band of connective tissue known as the transverse carpal ligament. Inside the tunnel are the median nerve, its artery, and tendons that flex the fingers and thumb. Any swelling or thickening of tissue within the tunnel can cause the median (middle) nerve to be compressed between the tough band of carpal ligament and the tendons or other contents of the tunnel. The squeezed nerve, which controls the thumb, index finger, and third finger, cannot work as it should, and the symptoms of carpal tunnel syndrome result.

Pregnancy and other conditions that produce generalized swelling of body tissues may be a cause of carpal tunnel syndrome. So can localized swelling caused by a dislocation, sprain, or fracture of the wrist. Rheumatoid arthritis can cause inflammation of the sheaths (coverings) of the tendons causing compression. Other possible causes include inflamed wrist joint, benign (noncancerous) tumor, myxedema (tissue swelling caused by lack of thyroid hormone), tuberculosis, amyloidosis (a disease characterized by abnormal deposits in body organs of the protein amyloid), acromegaly (overgrowth of connective tissue), and diabetes mellitus. Aching pain may travel up the forearm and even into the shoulder joint, neck, and chest (this particular pain can usually be relieved by shaking the hand vigorously or dangling the arm loosely from its socket; occasionally such pains are caused by a compression of the median nerve in the forearm or upper arm). Other signs include an inability to make a fist, deteriorating nails, and dry and shiny skin over the involved surfaces. The pains may occur in both hands at the same time. They may be constant or may come and go and are increased by manual work or movement that flexes the wrist or palm. Weakness of the fingers occurs later than other symptoms and accompanies a wasting away of the muscle. Symptoms are usually worse at night and in the morning.

Diagnostic tests include tapping the wrist, which causes tingling in the area of pain if carpal tunnel syndrome is present, and forced flexion of the wrist, which may also reproduce the pain. X rays may be taken to reveal abnormalities of the wrist bones. Tests made to detect a delay in the conduction of nerve impulses are the most specific means of diagnosis.

Treatment is aimed first at relieving pressure on the median nerve. If soft tissue swelling is a cause, elevating the hand may eliminate the symptoms. It may help to keep the forearm in a splint at night, which holds the hand upward extending the wrist. If an inflammation (other than infection) inside the wrist is at fault, the carpal tunnel may be injected with cortisone. Other causes of the disease are treated appropriately.

The definitive treatment, to prevent permanent damage to nerves and muscles and to relieve symptoms, is surgery that releases the carpal tunnel ligament, relieving the pressure on the nerve. Muscle strength gradually returns following such surgery, but if the surgery has been delayed too long and muscles are severely deteriorated, full strength does not return. Symptoms usually disappear permanently shortly after the operation.

Cataract

A cataract is a clouding of the lens of the eye that results in obscured vision. Because people with cataracts see their environment as if they were looking through a waterfall, the condition is called cataract from the Greek word for waterfall.

Normally, the lens is clear. Its function is to direct light into the eye so that the eye can focus on objects at various distances more distinctly. However, if the lens becomes hazy, incoming light scatters and vision blurs.

The exact cause of cataracts is unknown. Aging may play a role in development of cataracts, but newborns whose mothers contracted German measles during pregnancy and some young people may also develop the condition.

Such conditions as diabetes (inability to use carbohydrates), glaucoma (increased pressure within the eyeball), or detachment of the retina (innermost layer of the eye) may lead to cataracts. In addition, injury to the lens, prolonged use of certain drugs, or high dosages of radiation (for example, prolonged exposure to X rays) may trigger the condition.

Although usually the condition is curable, in rare cases, cataracts can cause blindness. In addition, the shadowy lens prohibits a clear view of the interior of the eye. Because of this obstruction, a physician may not be able to detect other potentially serious eye disorders such as changes in the retina (innermost light-sensitive layer of the eyeball) or damage to the optic nerve (which transmits messages from the eye to the brain).

The main symptom of cataracts is painless blurring of vision, occurring most often in only one eye. During initial stages of development, cataracts can cause the person to experience glare in bright light since the clouded lens scatters rather than focuses incoming light. As the condition progresses, the lens becomes milky white, and vision worsens.

Successful treatment involves surgical removal of the affected lens followed by the wearing of special eyeglasses or contact lenses. With the aid of a microscope, a surgeon opens an area in the front of the eye and withdraws the lens. Local anesthetic eyedrops make the procedure relatively painless. After a few weeks of recuperation, an eye specialist prescribes special cataract eyeglasses or a contact lens to help correct the vision resulting from the removed lens. These aids are by no means perfect and require an adjustment period.

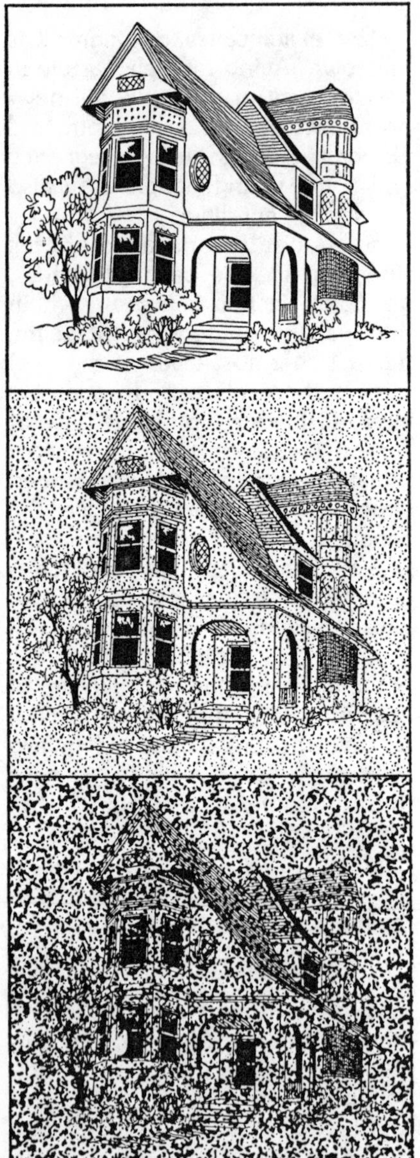

The main symptom of cataract is painless blurring of vision. Vision with early cataract may be close to normal (1). As cataract progresses, vision gradually blurs (2) and eventually may become extremely blurred (3).

More recently, many doctors recommend an intraocular lens (IOL) to be implanted in the eye after the cataract lens is removed. This lightweight plastic is relatively free from distortion and closer to normal vision than eyeglasses or contact lenses because it occupies the exact position of the natural lens. Nevertheless, not everyone can benefit from an intraocular lens. Doctors advise patients with glaucoma, detached retina, or eye disorders caused by diabetes to wear eyeglasses or contacts to restore vision.

Ninety-five percent of the surgery for cataracts is without complication. Restoration or substantial improvement of vision results after surgery in the majority of the cases. When vision remains unimproved, other disorders that were undetected because of the cataract may be causing the continued problem. Generally, however, cataracts can be successfully removed and the patient can resume a normal life.

Cautery

Cautery is the application of heat, electric current, or caustic chemicals to scar, burn, or cut the skin or tissues. The term has also been used to describe procedures using freezing techniques.

Cautery is an essential part of most major operations. As the surgeon's knife cuts through layers of skin and tissue, it opens a multitude of tiny blood vessels. These are immediately sealed by an assisting surgeon, using an electric instrument that burns just enough of the tissue to leave behind a tiny scar that prevents bleeding.

Cauterization may also be used to destroy unwanted tissue, as when polyps (noncancerous growths) in the colon are eliminated with an electric cauterizer. Cauterization may also be used in women to treat erosion (damaged tissue) of the cervix (the neck of the womb) to remove small polyps (growths) on it, or to prevent bleeding from small areas from which samples of tissue have been taken for laboratory analysis.

An example of chemical cauterization is the use of a silver nitrate stick inside the nose to stop a nosebleed. The caustic chemical causes the ends of the blood vessels to seal shut.

Cold cautery, or cryocautery, may be employed in cryosurgery (cold surgery) to treat Parkinson's disease, a disorder of the nervous system. Part of the thalamus, located in the brain, is destroyed by freezing it with an instrument containing super-cold liquid nitrogen. Today, however, this type of cautery is mostly done with electricity.

Celiac disease

Celiac disease, or celiac sprue, is a chronic disorder of the small intestine caused by sensitivity to gluten, a protein found in wheat and rye and to a lesser extent in oats and barley. The disorder causes poor absorption by the intestine of fat, protein, carbohydrates, iron, water, and vitamins A, D, E, and K. Removal of gluten from the diet normally brings improvement.

The basic cause is probably an inherited defect found mostly in people of northwestern European ancestry. For example, it affects one person in 300 in west Ireland, approximately one in 5,000 in the United States, and twice as many women as men. One theory about celiac disease has it that the body reacts to gluten and the related gliadin as if they were a virus or bacterium. When food containing gluten reaches the upper loop (jejunum) of the small intestine, antibodies in the intestinal wall are stimulated. In the process, for some unknown reason, the intestinal villi, which are hairlike projections through which food from the intestine is absorbed into the bloodstream, are destroyed. Destruction of the villi is almost total in the upper loop, less so in the rest of the small intestine. Poor absorption of food and water is the result. Another theory states that gluten/gliadin acts as a direct toxin or poison to the intestinal wall. One or both of these theories may be true.

Symptoms of celiac disease may begin in infancy when the child starts eating wheat cereal or other foods containing gluten. The child does not thrive, suffers painful bloating in the abdomen, and passes pale, foul-smelling, bulky stools. Failure to absorb enough iron produces anemia, a deficiency of oxygen-carrying red blood cells. Poor absorption of protein may cause edema (swelling of body tissues). There is little fat on the body. Growth may be stunted, signs of vitamin deficiency appear, and softening of bones may produce bone deformities and fractures. Sometimes the symptoms disappear in adolescence and reappear in adulthood.

Adults with celiac disease have many of the same symptoms, including bulky, foul-smelling stools, weight loss, vitamin deficiencies, swelling of body tissues, anemia, and bone pain. The disease may begin as late as age 60. It can also cause strange sensations in hands and feet, dry skin, eczema, acne, cessation of menstruation, mood changes, and irritability.

The most definite test for celiac disease is an examination under the microscope of a piece of tissue taken from the wall of the small intestine. (The sample is taken with the aid of a flexible tube with a cutting instrument at the tip that is inserted through the mouth into the intestine.) Several samples may be taken. The specimen from a celiac patient has almost no villi and appears as an alternating flat and bumpy surface with a disorganized network of blood vessels. Various blood tests, taken after the patient has eaten specific substances, reveal how well the intestine has absorbed these substances. In addition, blood tests may reveal low levels of protein, calcium, potassium, and sodium. Tests of stools reveal excess fat in the waste.

The primary treatment of celiac disease is to remove all gluten from the diet, which is easier said than done. Hot dogs, ice creams, commercial soups and sauces, candy bars, and all kinds of baked goods can be sources of gluten (even small amounts of gluten must be avoided). Many doctors refer the patient to a dietitian for detailed lists of foods to avoid and for advice in following a healthful diet, which should be high in calories and protein and low in fat. Vitamin and mineral supplements are given as needed. In stubborn cases, a cortisone drug may be given which will often result in improvement.

Recovery is most dramatic in children. For most patients, the outlook is good. In severe cases, complete return to normal bowel function and normal absorption may take months or may never occur. For that reason, and to rule out other diseases of deficiency or poor absorption, it is best to see a doctor as soon as symptoms appear. This is one ailment that is almost completely treatable.

Cerebral palsy

Cerebral palsy (CP) is a general term to describe various disorders of muscle control, caused by brain or nerve damage usually before or around the time of birth. The damage may result when brain tissue becomes starved for oxygen for whatever reason. It may result from separation and bleeding of the placenta (the organ that unites the unborn baby to the wall of the uterus and provides nourishment to the baby) in late pregnancy or from disorders caused by diabetes of the mother.

Symptoms of CP range from simple clumsiness or slight incoordination of muscles to multiple handicaps that prevent normal life and movement. Frequently, the brain damage that causes CP also causes mental retardation, epilepsy, hearing problems, visual defects, and learning and behavior disorders. However, some CP children are normal except for disordered muscle control.

There are four general types of cerebral palsy: spastic, athetoid or dyskinetic, ataxic, and mixed. Some 70 percent of people with CP are of the spastic type. They move stiffly and with great difficulty because their affected "spastic" muscles are constantly tense and tight. One arm and one leg may be affected, or both arms or both legs. Affected arms and legs appear thin and wasted, are weak, and are likely to twist and jerk. Walking on the toes, or with a "scissors" movement, is typical. When all four limbs are affected, the mouth, tongue, and palate may also be affected, interfering with speech, eating, and drinking and causing a constant drool.

Athetoid or dyskinetic CP accounts for about 20 percent of cases. Athetoid CP is characterized by continual slow, twisting movements of the fingers and hands during waking hours. Similar movements of the upper arm or legs and trunk may also occur. There may be sudden jerky movements as well. All of these symptoms are caused by damage to the basal ganglia, a mass of nerve-cell bodies at the base of the brain.

Ataxic CP results from damage to the cerebellum (lower brain) or nerves leading from it. Symptoms are weakness, lack of balance and coordination, tremor, difficulty with fine or quick movements, and a clumsy way of walking with feet wide apart.

Mixed CP occurs frequently. Often, spastic and athetoid types are combined. Ataxic and athetoid types are mixed less often.

In addition to the above disorders, about 25 percent of CP patients have convulsions — which usually can be controlled by anticonvulsant medicines.

Early diagnosis and treatment of cerebral palsy are vital if a child is to develop as fully as possible. Any baby who may have suffered brain damage around the time of birth should be watched carefully for signs of CP (such a baby may have been born nearly lifeless, or very small and premature, or undergone severe infection after birth). Possible signs of CP in a baby include twitching, convulsions, back-arching muscle spasms, partial paralysis of the face, and very late development of the ability to lift the head, sit, crawl, speak, stand, and walk. Although it is difficult to diagnose any particular form of CP in the first two years of life, parents should report any suspicion promptly to their doctor.

An important part of the doctor's investigation into possible CP is to discover if there is any other reason for the symptoms. Some of the same symptoms are caused by other conditions requiring surgery or other specific treatment. Still other conditions result from diseases, such as progressive cerebellar degenerative disease, which continue to worsen. (Although CP never disappears, at least it does not get worse.)

Treatment of a CP child requires many different elements. Ideally, it involves a physician working with a team of specialists in a special clinic, hospital, or other setting where their efforts can be coordinated. Someone with CP may need a series of medical diagnostic studies, psychological testing, speech therapy, physical therapy, special dental care, specially designed clothes, braces, corrective glasses, surgery, a hearing aid, special furniture, special schooling, and perhaps special institutional care. Occupational therapy can help the patient in self-care, including dressing, washing, and eating.

Because CP is a life-long condition, parents need to learn as much as possible about caring for a CP child. A good therapist will teach the parent how to continue the therapy at home. Every reasonable effort must be made to help the child become self-reliant. Parents can often get valuable advice and support from other CP parents and from professionals at the local chapter of the United Cerebral Palsy Association. Therapy for CP children and adults is provided at rehabilitation centers sponsored by the National Easter Seal Society for Crippled Children and Adults and by various other agencies.

Expectant mothers can guard against cerebral palsy in their unborn children by good prenatal care including an ample, well-balanced diet, rest, exercise, frequent check-ups, and avoidance of drugs and infections. During labor and birth, the doctor can keep track of the baby's heartbeat by use of a fetal monitor and if necessary operate quickly to save the baby from brain damage caused by oxygen starvation. Expectant mothers with difficult pregnancies should try to deliver their babies at a hospital with a newborn intensive care unit, directed by a certified M.D. specialist known as a neonatologist. Here, premature and ill babies can be watched closely and cared for by specially trained nurses and doctors using the latest methods.

Cerebrospinal fluid

Cerebrospinal fluid (CSF) is a clear, colorless fluid that surrounds the brain and spinal cord and cushions them against injury.

CSF is made up of water containing small amounts of minerals and organic substances (especially protein). It is continually being produced from blood in networks of capillaries (tiny blood vessels) known as choroid plexi, which are located in the ventricles (chambers) of the brain. About one pint is produced every 24 hours; approximately five ounces is circulating at any one time. From the two lateral (side) ventricles, the CSF flows into the third and fourth ventricles of the brain. It then passes into the space between the innermost and second layers of the tissue covering the brain, bathing the entire outer surface of the brain in fluid before passing downward around the spinal cord. Eventually the fluid returns upward, is absorbed into special tissue between the linings of the brain, and passes into the blood vessels.

Samples of cerebrospinal fluid, drawn from around the spinal cord by a needle inserted in the lower back region (lumbar puncture), can be valuable in diagnosing disorders of the brain and spinal cord. The samples may indicate a hemorrhage or blood clot in the brain, various types of meningitis (infection of the covering of the brain), a brain abscess, or a tumor of the brain or spinal cord.

Cesarean section

Cesarean section is the delivery of a baby by cutting through the abdomen and uterus and removing the baby through these incisions.

Two types of cesarean section are performed:

- In the classic cesarean, a verticle cut is made directly down the center of the uterus in its thick upper section. The incision on the skin of the abdomen is also made vertically and extends from the navel down to the pubic bone. This operation is generally used only if the baby is lying in an abnormal position or if the placenta (afterbirth) is located in an abnormally low position in the cavity of the uterus. With this type of cesarean, there is more bleeding than with the second method, it is more difficult to repair the incision, and the uterus is more likely to rupture during a future pregnancy. For these reasons, the classic cesarean is seldom used today unless there are specific reasons for its use.
- The lower segment cesarean is the more commonly performed operation. Here, the incision in the uterus is made in the lower, thinner section. This incision may be either a verticle cut or a curved, smile-shaped cut. For this operation, the incision on the skin may be either verticle down the middle or smile-shaped near the lower part of the abdomen.

About 10 to 20 percent of births in the United States are cesarean. They should be performed only by a skilled obstetrician, accompanied by an

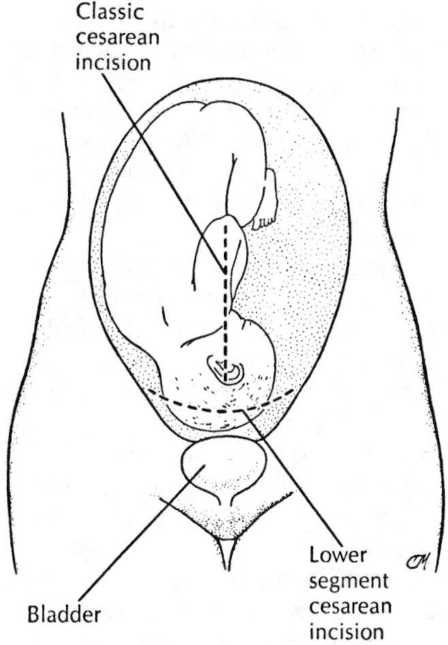

A cesarean section is the delivery of a baby by cutting through the abdomen and uterus and removing the baby through these incisions. The two types of cesareans are the classic and the lower segment; the incisions for each are shown here.

anesthesiologist to administer anesthesia to the mother and a pediatrician (specialist in care of children) to check the baby at birth. Cesarean section is performed when delivery of the baby is necessary and when a natural vaginal delivery would cause injury to either the mother or the baby. Antibiotics, better anesthesia, blood transfusions, and intravenous therapy have made cesareans much safer than in the past.

Some of the reasons for a cesarean section include:

- To save the baby's life when the umbilical cord (the unborn baby's supply line of oxygen and nutrients from the mother) is being pinched off during the birth process, or any other time the baby is not getting enough blood and oxygen to survive; this may be detected by abnormal heart rate patterns on the fetal monitor
- To prevent infection of the baby by dangerous bacteria in the surrounding (amniotic) fluid, or by a dangerous vaginal infection such as herpes
- To prevent injury to the baby during a breech birth, when the baby would emerge through the vagina buttocks or feet first rather than head first; many obstetricians believe that all breech births in first-time mothers and all premature breech births should be done by cesarean delivery
- To ease the birth or prevent injury when the baby is too large or the mother's pelvis too small for a vaginal delivery
- To deliver the baby if the mother fails to deliver after long labor
- To save the baby's life if problems with the placenta are cutting off blood supply to the baby
- To treat disease of the mother or baby that can be treated better if birth occurs rapidly
- To be safe if the mother has had a previous cesarean birth (the rule had been that any woman who has one cesarean must have cesarean sections on all following births; however, in recent years many vaginal deliveries have been performed successfully on women who had previous lower-segment cesarean sections).

Risks of a cesarean section include possible infection, bleeding, and dangerous blood clots that may get into the blood circulation. There is a small chance that the uterus will rupture during another pregnancy, before or during birth. The cesarean may be inconvenient for the mother, requiring her to stay in the hospital for five to seven days instead of going home with her baby in three days. She may not be able to see the baby for a number of hours after delivery if she has undergone general anesthesia. Breastfeeding may be difficult, if the mother is being given strong medications to relieve pain, which keeps her asleep for long periods of time. There is pain from the operation incision, and the mother's activity is restricted once she arrives home. It takes up to six weeks for complete healing of the incision. In addition, the extra expense for her and her baby is considerable. However, all of these costs are small if they save the baby from lifelong brain damage or save the life of infant or mother.

Chest pain

Chest pain is a major symptom in many disorders, including heart disease, indigestion, heartburn, and pleurisy.

In heart disease, chest pains may be the temporary discomfort of angina pectoris or the similar but more severe and long-lasting signs of a heart attack. In both cases the discomfort is felt as an aching or crushing sensation beneath the breastbone and may radiate into the left shoulder and arm. On some occasions it may also be felt in the back, throat, jaws, and teeth, or spread to the abdomen. In angina the discomfort typically is brought on by exertion and disappears in a few minutes with rest or with the taking of nitroglycerin. In a heart attack, the pain is usually much more intense and deep and is not relieved by nitroglycerin; in addition, the patient is restless, pale, and perspiring. When in doubt about a possible heart attack, call your doctor and go immediately to the hospital emergency room.

Often the symptoms of angina or even a heart attack, spreading to the abdomen, are mistaken for those of indigestion. Sometimes indigestion, ulcer pains, or a gallbladder attack will bring on angina, or be mistaken for a heart attack. Again, when in doubt about a heart attack, call your doctor and go to the emergency room.

Heartburn, felt as a burning pain beneath the breastbone, has nothing to do with the heart. It develops when some food from the stomach, mixed with digestive acids, backs up into the esophagus (the food tube from the mouth to the stomach). The acids burn the lining of the esophagus, producing pain. Heartburn may be treated by using antacids, by raising the head of the bed so that food is not as likely to back up when you are lying down, by avoiding foods like coffee and alcohol that stimulate acid production, or by taking drugs that help keep the esophagus outlet closed.

The chest pains of pleurisy, which may be sharp and stabbing or vaguely uncomfortable, may occur with every breath or only when the patient breathes deeply or coughs. The pains are caused by inflammation of the pleura, the membrane that surrounds the lungs and lines the chest cavity. The pains may appear only over the site of the infection or may radiate to the lower chest and abdomen.

Among other causes of chest pain are rib injuries, pneumonia, blood clot in the lung, inflammation of the tissue surrounding the heart, inflammation of the nerves supplying the chest wall, and tenderness of the chest muscle after injury or exertion.

It is important that you report to your doctor any prolonged or severe chest pain, since prompt evaluation and treatment may be lifesaving.

See also Angina pectoris, Heart attack, Heartburn, Indigestion, and Pleurisy.

Chicken pox

Chicken pox is an extremely contagious disease that is characterized by a blistery rash. It occurs most frequently in children between the ages of five and eight with less than 20 percent of the cases in the United States affecting people over 15 years old. Chicken pox is passed from one person to another so easily that almost everyone gets the disease at some time.

Chicken pox is caused by infection with the virus varicella zoster. The virus creates symptoms that can be mild or severe depending upon the infected person's age.

Anyone can contract chicken pox by touching either an infected person's blisters or anything that is contaminated by them. Chicken pox is also thought to be airborne since it may be caught from an infected person before the rash develops. Yet, some researchers contend that one or two spots from the disease may be present before the rash is recognized on the body. Another way to get chicken pox is by exposure to shingles, which is a nerve disorder caused by the same virus. The incubation period for chicken pox—the time between being exposed to the illness and actually showing symptoms—is 10 to 21 days. Chicken pox is contagious for about six to eight days after the rash appears.

The first symptom of chicken pox is usually a rash that can be very itchy. It begins as small, red spots on the trunk. Within hours, the spots become larger, fluid-filled blisters and begin spreading out from the trunk to the face, scalp, arms, and legs. Over the next few days, the blisters continue to fill with pus, burst, and then form a scab or crust. New spots appear periodically during a two- to six-day period. They may occasionally spread to the soles and palms. The rash may even affect the eyes, mouth, throat, vagina, and rectum.

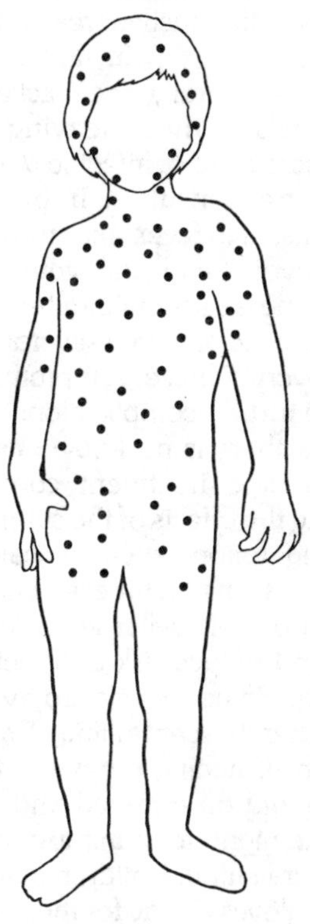

The first symptom of chicken pox is an itchy rash that begins as small red spots on the trunk. Within hours the spots begin spreading out from the trunk to the face, scalp, arms, and legs.

Another main symptom is a mild fever (101°F to 103°F) that rises and disappears as the rash comes and goes. Some children have a slight fever and feel sluggish a few days before the rash begins. However, this warning is more common in adults. Adults usually have higher fevers, a more severe rash, headaches and muscle aches, and they take longer to recuperate than children. Recovery from all symptoms takes ten days to two weeks.

Complications with chicken pox seldom develop in otherwise healthy people. The most common complication is infection of the blisters. The blister is scratched, and bacteria enter where the skin breaks. In some instances, the rash spreads to the eyes and causes pain and possible damage. Generally, the chicken pox rash heals without leaving scars unless scratched or infected. A doctor should be consulted if breathing problems, high fever, extreme drowsiness, severe headache, vomiting, or unsteadiness occur within the course of the disease or within several weeks of recovery. These symptoms may indicate further complications.

Since there is no known cure for chicken pox, treatment constitutes reducing the effects of the symptoms. Soothing lotion, such as calamine lotion, lessens itchiness. Baths in warm (not hot) water keep the skin clean and reduce risk of infection in the rash. Baths also destroy virus in water, thereby controlling spread of the rash. If itching is severe, fingernails should be trimmed and gloves worn at night to minimize unconscious scratching. Children may need to wear gloves all day for the duration of the rash.

Although it has not been proven that aspirin causes or promotes Reye's syndrome, a type of brain inflammation, it is recommended that aspirin not be given to a child with chicken pox. A doctor can suggest an aspirin substitute if needed.

Researchers are trying to develop a vaccine to prevent chicken pox, but there is nothing available as yet. Although almost everyone contracts the disease once, most people do not get it again. The same organism that causes chicken pox causes the body to manufacture antibodies to combat the virus. Antibodies prevent the disease from recurring. Nevertheless, the same virus may cause shingles later in life. Why shingles occurs in some people many years after they have had chicken pox is not understood.

See also Reye's syndrome and Shingles.

Choking

See Emergency first aid section at the end of this book.

Cholecystitis

Cholecystitis is an inflammation of the gallbladder. The gallbladder is a small pear-shaped organ that stores bile, produced by the liver, and releases it as needed to help digest food—particularly fats—in the small intestine. Cholecystitis may be either acute (sudden and severe) or chronic (less severe attacks that occur from time to time).

Acute cholecystitis in about 90 percent of cases is caused when the outlet of the gallbladder or the duct leading from it is plugged by a gallstone (a stone formed in the gallbladder from cholesterol, a fatty substance, and sometimes from calcium or bile pigments). Unless the stone becomes dislodged, inflammation and pressure build up behind it. In severe cases, the swollen gallbladder may not receive enough blood, resulting in partial tissue death and gangrene. The gangrene may perforate the gallbladder, causing bile to spill into the abdominal cavity. An abscess (collection of pus within a cavity) usually forms around the area of gangrene, and bacteria may infect the gallbladder fluid. Occasionally, the resulting leakage of infected bile produces a general infection (peritonitis) of the entire area around the abdominal organs. However, not all gallbladder attacks progress to this extreme; they may subside only to be repeated another time. Cholecystitis may also result from a blockage caused by enlarged blood veins in the common bile duct that the gallbladder shares with the liver. Rarely, infection may spread to the gallbladder from the nearby pancreas.

Acute cholecystitis often begins following a meal rich in fat (which requires more bile production), such as fried foods, chocolate, and cream. The individual may awaken in the middle of the night with indigestion, gas, and a sharp pain in the upper right quarter of the abdomen, which is often hard and tender to the touch. Pain may also appear in the middle of the abdomen and spread up to the tip of the right shoulder blade. The pain is steady and severe, gradually decreasing and finally disappearing in 12 to 18 hours unless there are complications. Vomiting is likely and provides some relief. There is little fever, unless the bile duct as well as the gallbladder is inflamed. If jaundice (yellowing of the skin, caused by bile pigment in the blood) is present, the symptoms are likely due to a gallstone blocking the common bile duct.

Radionuclide scanning confirms a diagnosis of cholecystitis (in this procedure, the patient takes in traces of radioactive material that travel to the affected area and radiate a picture onto the screen of a scanner). X rays and ultrasound, in which sound waves are bounced off internal structures to form an image of them, may also be used to locate gallstones.

Treatment of the acute attack consists of rest, intravenous feeding (from an IV bottle into the vein) but no food by mouth, painkilling drugs, and antibiotics if needed. Because attacks are likely to recur, however, the real solution is surgical removal of the gallbladder. This is done immediately if complications develop. Preferably, however, it is performed a few days after the attack has subsided. If the patient has another illness, that is best brought under control before the operation is performed.

Chronic cholecystitis is a continued inflammation of the gallbladder, with repeated attacks over time that are similar to but milder than those of acute cholecystitis. There are usually stones in the gallbladder; whether they develop before or after the emergence of the disease is unknown. The exact causes of chronic cholecystitis are not understood, although occasionally bacterial infection is the reason. Diet, heredity, and hormones appear to be involved, and the disease is more likely to affect women than men.

The pains of chronic cholecystitis commonly appear over the pit of the stomach and in the upper right quarter of the abdomen; they may be mild to unbearable. Pains usually come on suddenly and are normally steady, but may be separated by pain-free intervals of 15 minutes to an hour. The average attack lasts about an hour, although pains may disappear after 15 minutes or continue for several hours. Although the pains may appear together with nausea, gas, belching, and after eating fatty food, these indications may not be directly related to the disease.

Diagnosis of the disease is based on the symptoms and sometimes can be confirmed by X rays. The patient drinks a special chemical (designed to show on an X ray) that is absorbed by a normal gallbladder but not by an inflamed one. If the gallbladder does not show up in the X ray, the patient may have the disease. The doctor must make a careful investigation of other possible causes of the symptoms, including peptic ulcer (in the stomach or duodenum, the beginning of the small intestine), inflammation of the pancreas, and bowel disease.

The ideal way to treat chronic cholecystitis is to remove the gallbladder, together with any gallstones in the duct leading from the liver to the duodenum. If it is not clear that the symptoms are caused by gallbladder inflammation, or if the patient cannot withstand an operation, other methods are used. These include a low-fat diet (which lowers the need for bile) and weight reduction, plus antacids and other medications.

See also Gallstones.

Cholesterol

Cholesterol is a fatlike substance, found in all animal fats and oils. It is manufactured by the liver from saturated fats and is a basic ingredient in the formation of normal male and female hormones, Vitamin D, cell membranes, brain tissue, the sheaths that protect nerve fibers, blood, liver bile and other body substances. After the first six months of life, the liver can make all of the cholesterol the body needs—about 1,000 milligrams a day. However, the average American consumes about 600 milligrams a day of cholesterol from such sources as eggs and meat. Eating cholesterol–and also saturated fats, which are found in dairy products, animal fat, and oils such as coconut and palm — can raise the level of cholesterol in the blood. When the blood contains too much cholesterol, or when there is an inherited defect that interferes with the body's ability to use or process cholesterol and fats, the risk of heart attack and blood-vessel disease rises.

Hardening of the arteries (atherosclerosis), which causes most heart attacks, first begins with an injury to an artery wall. Normally a blood clot forms over the injury and heals it. But when there is too much cholesterol in the blood, cholesterol deposits itself in the wound and promotes the formation of a plaque. The plaque, made up of cholesterol, dead and dying cells, connective tissue, and a calcium cap, may grow to obstruct an artery. If the blockage is in one of the arteries nourishing heart muscle, it can cause a heart attack.

Normal levels of cholesterol in the blood are generally considered to be in the range of 100 to 250 or 280. However, many dietitians and doctors recommend keeping the cholesterol level below 200; a few researchers suggest that the healthiest range is 100 to 150, usually possible only on a vegetarian diet. Many studies have shown that heart attack risk rises almost in direct relation to the amount of cholesterol in the blood.

Not all people with high blood cholesterol levels, however, develop heart disease or hardening of the arteries. This seems to be due to the *kind* of cholesterol most of them have. They possess high levels of a fraction of cholesterol known as high-density lipoprotein (HDL), which transports excess cholesterol to the liver where it is eliminated. Some people have high HDL levels because of heredity. Exercise raises HDL levels, as does one or two drinks of alcohol a day. Cigarette smoking lowers HDL.

You can reduce the cholesterol in your diet by avoiding fatty meats, cutting back on eggs, and eating more fish and poultry, which contain less cholesterol and saturated fat than meats. Palm and coconut oils should be avoided because of their content of cholesterol-raising saturated fat.

Taking off excess weight, exercising regularly, and quitting smoking also help.

Chromosomes

Chromosomes are threadlike coils within the nucleus (core) of every living cell. There are 46 chromosomes in a human cell. Together, the chromosomes contain the "blueprint" or "genetic program" for the entire person. The set of instructions in each chromosome is written in a "genetic code." This is made up of chemical compounds arranged in a definite order on twisting ladder-like strands. Each strand contains thousands of genes, each of which is an instruction for a particular characteristic. Thus, there is a gene for blue eyes, another for black hair, another for blood type B. An error in a gene produces a genetic defect, such as an instruction for a cleft (hare) lip, or a genetic disease, such as juvenile diabetes (insulin-dependent), an inborn malfunction of the body's ability to convert sugar into energy.

In regular growth, when a cell divides into two new cells, each coiled chromosome separates into two identical chromosomes. The new cells thus have the same number of chromosomes and are exactly the same as the original cell.

In sexual reproduction the process is different. The 46 chromosomes form into 22 matching pairs—plus one pair of sex chromosomes that may or may not match (a male pair contains an X chromosome and a Y chromosome; a female pair contains two X chromosomes). Twenty-three chromosomes from the man's sperm cell join with 23 chromosomes from the woman's egg to form a new individual with 46 chromosomes. Since the fertilized egg is made up of individual chromosomes with genes from both parents, the resulting baby has a mixture of characteristics from both sides of the family.

See also DNA and Genes.

Circulatory system

See Blood, Blood vessels, and Heart.

Circumcision

Circumcision is the surgical removal of the foreskin, the retractable sleeve of skin covering the glans (the head of the penis). Among some religious groups, the operation is performed as a religious ritual on the eighth day following birth. In hospitals, it is usually done on the last day before a baby boy goes home. In any event, if it is to be done for nonmedical reasons it should be done in infancy and not later—when it is a more serious operation and might harm the child psychologically.

During the five-minute operation, which is done without anesthesia, the foreskin is carefully cut away. Dressing for the cut is petroleum jelly-soaked gauze applied to the incision. The incision heals rapidly, forming a dry scab that drops off after a few days. Although the incision should be kept as clean as possible, no other special care is necessary. Other than a few drops of blood that might be produced if the diaper rubs against the cut, there is no bleeding in a normal baby.

The decision for or against circumcision should be made by the parents before the baby's birth. There are two sides to the question. The operation became standard in American hospitals in recent decades as a cleanliness measure. In a young boy, the foreskin completely covers the head of the penis and cannot be pulled back very far. If the penis is not kept clean, urine and other substances can cause irritation of the glans and perhaps lead to infection between the foreskin and the glans. However, with normal care in cleanliness, this is not a problem. Even though the foreskin at first cannot be pulled back very far because of bands of tissue that bind it to the glans, it is necessary to wash only the part of the glans that can be uncovered comfortably at any one stage. Gradually the bands of tissue dissolve by later childhood when the foreskin can be pulled back completely.

It has been argued that circumcision prevents cancer of the penis and cancer of the cervix (neck of the uterus) in the sexual partner of the circumcised man and may help prevent venereal disease. However, there is no solid evidence to support these statements.

The strongest argument in favor of circumcision today, apart from religious circumcision, is to prevent a boy from feeling "different" from his father, brothers, friends, or schoolmates who are circumcised. In addition, it is a little more convenient to wash a circumcised penis.

Very seldom is there a medical reason to perform a circumcision. It should never be done in the first day of life, or if the baby is ill or premature. Furthermore, it should be delayed indefinitely if there is any abnormality of the glans or penis, so that the foreskin can be used later as graft tissue to repair the defect. It should not be done if the mother was taking during pregnancy or is taking while breast-feeding any medication that promotes bleeding, such as anticoagulants or aspirin, or if there is any family history of hemophilia or other bleeding disorders.

Risks of circumcision include local infection that may lead to significant hemorrhage and mutilation. Many medical authorities feel that there is no absolute medical reason for routine circumcision of the newborn. Adequate cleanliness and hygiene offer the same advantages of routine circumcision without the risks of the operation.

Parents, therefore, should consider all factors—cultural, religious, and physical—before making a decision about circumcision.

Cirrhosis

Cirrhosis is a disease in which the cells throughout the liver are progressively destroyed. They are replaced by nodules (swellings) containing normal new cells but also by much connective tissue that alters the structure of the organ. The flow of blood and lymph through the damaged liver is much less efficient, and eventually the liver fails.

Cirrhosis is the liver's attempt to rebuild itself and continue despite injury—from whatever cause. The injury may be a sudden and massive infection, as from hepatitis. It may occur in a less severe manner over months or years, as in chronic active hepatitis or in obstruction of the bile ducts within the liver. The latter process starts with inflammation, then scarring, then closure of the ducts. A similar condition is caused by obstruction of external bile ducts by a stone, scar, inborn defect, or tumor. The damage may be done over an even longer time, slowly and steadily, by alcohol abuse.

Alcoholism is by far the most common cause of cirrhosis. Once thought to be due to the poisonous effect of alcohol on the liver, its damage is now believed to result chiefly from malnutrition. Alcoholics get most of their calories from alcohol and so their diets are dangerously unbalanced. Lack of protein in the diet of an alcoholic, for example, casues scarring in a vital area of the liver. Other causes include:

- Some powerful medications—chemicals such as methotrexate, an anticancer drug; halothane, an anesthetic; and oxyphenisatin, a medicine used in enemas—may also cause liver damage
- Inborn errors in physical or chemical processes of the body
- Syphilis
- Passive liver congestion caused by a clot blocking the large (hepatic) vein carrying blood to the heart, or by an inefficient heart that cannot accept a normal flow of blood from the liver.

Frequently, cirrhosis is not suspected until it is well advanced, for it imitates many other diseases. Symptoms include a general weakness, a vague sick feeling, loss of appetite, loss of weight, and a loss of interest in sex. There may be a dull abdominal ache, nausea, constipation, or diarrhea. In a malnourished patient, the tongue may be inflamed. Many symptoms are the result of high blood pressure in the portal vein, which brings nutrient-bearing blood from the intestinal area to the liver where the blood is processed. In cirrhosis, the liver cannot handle a normal flow of blood, so the pressure in the portal vein rises. One result is that fluid from the blood is lost into the abdominal cavity. The fluid buildup may press against the diaphragm (the muscular wall separating the abdominal and chest cavities) and interfere with breathing. New blood vessels (collateral vessels) form to carry away the excess blood into the general circulation. There may be bleeding in the esophagus (food pipe) or stomach, when new collateral vessels burst under pressure. The patient may vomit blood. Serious, life-threatening hemorrhage may occur.

Other symptoms include an enlarged, firm liver and enlarged spleen; a mottled redness of the mound of the palm at the base of the thumb; "spider veins" on the skin of the upper body; loss of hair from chest and pubic area; diminishing testicles; and tingling sensations on the skin of the hands and feet.

Proof of cirrhosis of the liver is furnished by liver biopsy. A hollow needle is inserted through the skin and into the liver itself to obtain a tissue sample for analysis. Tissue from a diseased liver reveals destruction of cells and scarring. Other diagnostic procedures include radionuclide scanning (in this procedure, the patient takes in traces of radioactive material that travels to the liver and illuminates a picture of the organ onto the screen of the scanner). X-ray pictures are taken of the gallbladder and of bile ducts inside the liver and leading from it. Blood and urine tests reveal important clues, including bile pigments in the blood, low red blood cell count, vitamin and mineral deficiencies, and protein in the urine.

Treatment aims first to remove the cause of the original injury. Thus an alcoholic patient needs to stop drinking, is placed on a well-balanced moderate-to-high-protein diet, and is given larger than usual doses of multivitamins (supplemental vitamins include A, B complex, D, and K—which cannot be stored in the ill liver—and folic acid). If a stone is obstructing an external bile duct and thus causing liver damage, it can be removed. Fluids and salt are usually restricted, to prevent fluid buildup in the body.

Good care includes plenty of rest and frequent small meals rather than fewer large ones, to reduce the work load on the liver, and avoiding any infection that might cause new stress on the liver.

Many of the various causes of cirrhosis of the liver cannot be predicted and guarded against—but the major one can be. Drinking moderately or not at all is the best way the average person can reduce the risk of developing this serious disease.

See also Alcoholism.

Claustrophobia

Claustrophobia is an intense and unrealistic fear of being confined in an enclosed space, such as an elevator or small room.

The condition is a neurosis (nervous disorder) believed to be caused in the same way as other phobias (unreasonable fears). Although some scientists believe there may be chemical or physical causes of phobias that are yet to be discovered, this is not the prevailing view. Phobias, it is believed, are in each case substitute fears for an unconscious forbidden fear that the individual is afraid to face. The selection of the symbolic fear is by chance and may have happened because the person was exposed to the symbol—such as a small closed room — when the forbidden fear (such as hatred of a parent or a sex impulse) threatened the victim. By avoiding the symbol, the person avoids the pain of recognizing the true cause of the distress.

Commonly, the claustrophobic person becomes anxious even at the thought of being "trapped" in a small room or passageway. If the person unexpectedly has to face the phobia, as when caught in a stuck elevator, real panic may result.

Unlike some phobias such as a fear of mice, snakes, or spiders, which the average person seldom sees, claustrophobia can cripple one's vocational and social life. Enclosed spaces are part of the everyday environment, and so every effort needs to be made to overcome the phobia.

A therapist may be able to help the claustrophobic patient realize the source of the phobia and thereby try to reduce or eliminate it. If it still persists, the therapist may try to desensitize the patient to the phobia fear. Thus, the claustrophobic patient may be taught to enter small enclosed spaces to confront the fear time and again. The patient is taught relaxation techniques and may also use tranquilizers to quiet anxieties during the desensitization process.

Sometimes a phobia will disappear permanently without apparent reason. On the other hand, it may subside, disappear, and reappear time and again over the years. Although one or more extreme phobias may occur in the mental disease schizophrenia, a phobia is not in itself a sign of mental illness.

Self-understanding may be the best way to prevent phobias in oneself, if this can be achieved. The goal should be to face and acknowledge any hidden fears and channel them into constructive activity.

See also Agoraphobia and Phobia.

Cleft lip/cleft palate

Cleft lip and cleft palate, a defect in one of every 700 or 800 newborns, is characterized by a split running through all or part of the upper structure of the mouth. A cleft lip (or harelip) may be only a small notch near the center of the upper lip, or it may extend into the nostril. A cleft palate can be as minor as a split in the uvula, the little "finger" of tissue hanging down in the back of the throat. On the other hand, a cleft in the palate may divide the entire soft palate, the muscular tissue that roofs the rear of the mouth. In its most severe form, a cleft splits not only the soft palate but the entire hard palate (the bony roof of the mouth) and upper jaw, joining with a cleft lip. The cleft may even divide the palate into three parts, resulting in a split on either side of the nose, leaving a middle section of upper jaw and gum dangling.

Cleft lip happens in earliest pregnancy, soon after the fourth week when the baby's face starts to form. Bulges of tissue on either side of the face grow toward the midline to form the nostrils and lips. At about the seventh week they meet and join; if they do not, a cleft lip is the result.

A failure of development in the eighth week of pregnancy causes cleft palate. The palate is formed from two plates of tissue, which originally are on either side of the developing tongue. As the head and neck grow, the tongue moves downward and the tissue plates move into position and fuse into one—unless there is a mistake or weakness, which results in cleft palate.

The basic causes of cleft lip and cleft palate are not fully understood. There is obviously an inherited tendency toward the defects. More than one fourth of children with cleft lip also have a relative with a cleft. If parents without cleft defects have one child with a cleft, they have a 5 percent risk of having a second child with a cleft; if they have two children with clefts, there is a 12 percent risk of a cleft in future children. Perhaps some difference in the uterus, such as poor blood supply to the infant, combines with an inherited weakness to produce the error of development. Certain chemicals or medications,

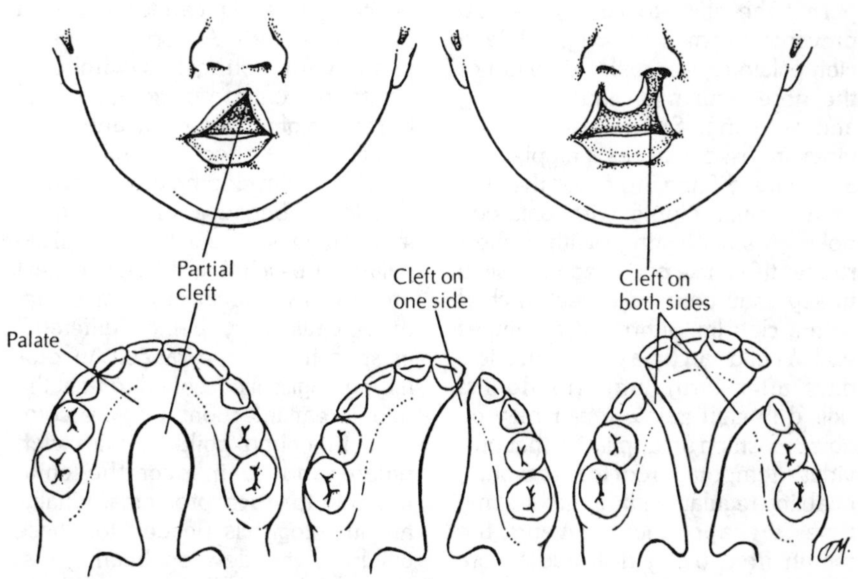

Cleft lip or cleft palate is a split running through all or part of the upper structure of the mouth. In its most severe form, the cleft may divide the palate into three parts, resulting in a split on either side of the nose and leaving a middle section of upper jaw and gum dangling, as shown on the right.

too many vitamins or not enough, and viruses have been suggested as possible causes of cleft defects.

Often cleft lip and cleft palate are associated with other birth defects. About one child in six who has a cleft lip, with or without cleft palate, has one or more other birth defects. A child who has only a cleft palate has up to a 50 percent chance of having another defect, such as joined fingers or toes, malformed ears, spina bifida, heart disease, or clubfoot.

Treatment of a patient with a cleft lip and/or a cleft palate requires the services of a specialized team. Such a group includes a pediatrician, orthodontist, speech therapist, plastic surgeon, psychologist, audiologist, and otolaryngologist. Treatment may take place at a specialized clinic or hospital center or may be coordinated by a pediatrician who brings in different experts as needed.

Before any treatment can begin, however, steps must be taken to permit the child to eat. A cleft lip prevents normal sucking, while a cleft palate causes milk to run out of the nose, and may cause choking and vomiting. Special feeding devices are used, such as a nipple with an enlarged flange to cover the cleft or a regular nipple with enlarged holes. A small syringe with a short rubber tube, like one used to baste a turkey, may be used to feed a child with a cleft lip, although sometimes such a child can breast-feed. In a few days after birth, an orthodontist skilled in cleft palate repair may be able to fashion an appliance that provides a temporary roof for the mouth, enabling regular feeding. At the same time, the appliance prevents the mouth from being distorted before the palate can be closed.

Surgery to correct a cleft lip is done in the first few days of life by some surgeons, because it will make the baby more acceptable to parents and make it easier to feed the baby by bottle. However, other surgeons delay the operation from two to eight months, so that surgery will not interfere with the growing bonds of affection between mother and baby (for one thing, the baby cannot breast-feed for six weeks after the operation) and to rule out other birth defects that might interfere with recovery.

Plastic surgery to correct cleft palate usually takes place in the second year of life. Some surgeons repair the soft palate first, when the child is between six and 18 months of age, and the hard palate much later—sometimes not until age five years. While early surgery helps the child's emotional and speech development, some surgeons wait because they are concerned that early surgery may cause distortion of growth in the middle third of the face. While waiting, the child wears an appliance that roofs over the mouth.

The problems created by cleft palate and cleft lip cannot be solved only by surgery. An orthodontist is needed for youngsters with cleft palate, not only to make appliances but to straighten teeth that are poorly positioned. A speech therapist aids the child in developing speech, which is altered because of missing or inadequate soft palate or artificial palate. A psychologist helps to treat emotional and social problems sometimes caused by being "different" in speech or appearance. An otolaryngologist is consulted to treat the middle ear infections that are common in young children with cleft palate and to inspect the child monthly for such problems. Finally, an audiologist is needed for those children who develop hearing loss because of middle ear infections. With proper care and encouragement and with modern plastic surgery, the average child with a cleft can make a good recovery.

Clubfoot

Clubfoot (*talipes*) is a common birth defect in which one and often both feet are fixed in an awkward, twisted position. The foot resists efforts to stretch or turn it back. In *talipes equinovarus,* the most frequent form, the foot points down and turns in while the front of the foot curls toward the heel. If not corrected, the condition worsens and interferes with walking. The person seems to walk on the ankle and the outside or inside edge of the foot.

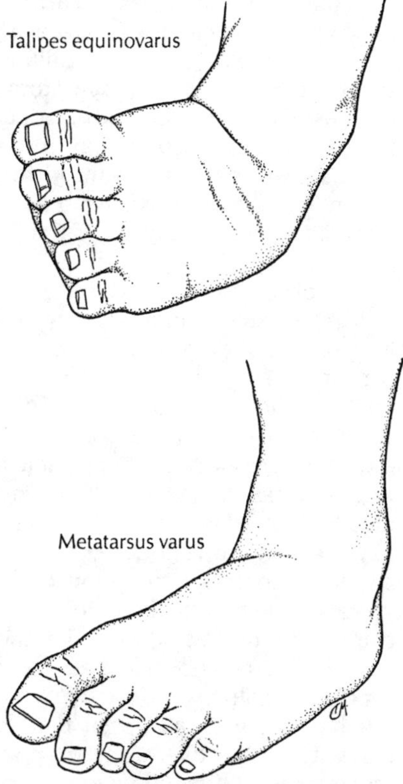

The most frequent form of clubfoot is *talipes equinovarus,* in which the foot points down and turns in with the front of the foot curling toward the heel. Related to clubfoot is *metatarsus varus,* in which the front of the foot turns inward. The condition is often called "pigeon toe."

The cause of clubfoot is unknown. However, it seems to involve heredity and something that happens in the womb to arrest development around the ninth week of pregnancy, when the baby's feet are being formed. Clubfoot may begin as a muscle abnormality. The Achilles (heel) tendon is shortened, the ankle and its muscles are deformed, and the heel bone is shortened and flattened to some extent.

Correction of clubfoot should begin as early as the first week of life, while the bones, muscles, ligaments, and tendons are soft and pliable. Usually the correction is done in separate stages, not all at once. In the talipes equinovarus form, the first stage is to uncurl the front of the foot away from the heel. The next is to turn the foot so that the sole faces outward. The third stage is to put the foot in a cast with the toes pointing up. This may require surgery to lengthen the Achilles tendon and to free the ankle joint.

Correction takes place in a series of small, painless, gradual adjustments. Typically, the therapist flexes and stretches the foot by hand and then fixes it in a cast in a partially corrected position. After a week or so the cast is removed, the foot is manipulated again, placed in a still better position, and a new cast applied. Sometimes, instead of making a new cast each time, wedges are placed inside the existing cast to adjust the foot. The entire casting process may take three months.

Once the correction is made, it must be followed up with exercises, devices which hold the feet in place at night while the baby is sleeping, and orthopedic shoes. A "night splint" often used consists of corrective shoes with soles joined by a flat metal bar that keeps the feet in exactly the right position.

Because clubfoot sometimes recurs, periodic checkups are necessary until the child becomes an adult. However, in most cases, the correction is completely successful and the individual can walk and run normally.

If early treatment has not succeeded, or if a child is not treated until age nine or ten, more extensive surgery is required. This is followed by several weeks with the foot in a cast. Usually this has satisfactory results. The foot is rather stiff, but this does not prevent the individual from engaging in the most active sports.

Somewhat separate from but related to true clubfoot is *metatarsus varus,* in which the front of the foot turns inward. Known as "apparent clubfoot," or "pigeon toe," this is a milder deformity that may not be diagnosed in the first several weeks. Unlike a true clubfoot, the apparent clubfoot can be moved easily into a correct position. Usually it can be corrected by manipulation, without the need for casts or surgery.

Colitis

Colitis is a general term meaning an inflammation of the colon (large intestine). It is usually a chronic (long-term) condition that is characterized by sudden attacks followed by periods of remission (relief). It should not be confused with irritable bowel syndrome (also called spastic or mucous colon), which is not an inflammation of the colon (although it can resemble colitis with symptoms such as diarrhea and abdominal pain) and which has been associated with emotional factors.

Frequently, the term colitis is used synonymously with an entity known as "inflammatory bowel disease." There are basically three diseases incorporated under this term: ulcerative colitis, granulomatous colitis (Crohn's disease), and ulcerative proctitis. Ulcerative colitis involves only the large intestine (except in rare instances). Granulomatous colitis may involve any portion of the food tract, including the mouth, and on occasion may not involve the colon. Ulcerative proctitis, the least serious, involves only the rectum, but can closely resemble ulcerative colitis in symptoms and appearance.

In some cases, the cause of colitis is unknown, although it can be a result of a bacterial infection or, in older people, lack of blood to the colon. It may begin slowly with abdominal discomfort, mild diarrhea or constipation, and a general feeling of being unwell. As the condition becomes more severe, symptoms such as abdominal pain or bleeding from the rectum may appear. If the disease appears suddenly, the patient may experience fever, bloody diarrhea, loss of appetite, and weight loss.

The diagnosis of colitis is based on a direct inspection of intestinal walls with the aid of a sigmoidoscope (or proctoscope), a lighted tube inserted into the colon through the anus, the opening to the outside of the body. A tissue sample of the intestinal wall may be taken to be examined for signs of infection. Other tests may be done to rule out other diseases or disorders of the colon.

Persons with a mild case of colitis can usually be treated at home and be permitted a normal diet. More seriously ill patients may be treated in the hospital with a special diet to allow the digestive tract to rest, replacement (often intravenously) of fluids and salts lost during episodes of diarrhea and/or bleeding, and medications, for example, antibiotics to treat an infection or cortisone (and other drugs) to treat inflammatory bowel disease. Those individuals with severe cases of colitis may require blood transfusions and perhaps even surgery to remove the inflamed portion of the colon.

See also Crohn's disease and Ulcerative colitis.

Color blindness

Color blindness is an inability to identify certain colors. By far the most common type is inherited red-green color blindness, which affects 8 percent of men and boys but only 0.5 percent of women and girls. Total color blindness, which is very rare, and pastel-shade blindness are believed to be inherited. Others, including blue-yellow blindness and red blindness, can be either inherited or acquired. Disease or injury of the retina, the light-sensitive tissue at the back of the eye, sometimes causes color blindness.

Color blindness results from a defect in the cone-shaped light-sensitive cells of the fovea, the tiny yellowish pit at the rear of the eye that is the eye's center for color and for close work. The cone cells — seven million of them — are much different from the 130 million rod-shaped cells in the rest of the retina, which register only in black and white. The cones are believed to contain bleachable pigments for red, green, and blue, colors which can combine to produce all of the colors of the spectrum. The pigments become more vivid or fade in response to colors that the eye sees. The changes of pigment produce tiny flashes of electricity that are carried by means of the optic nerve to the visual center of the brain. There, the electrical signals are combined into a full-color picture. In the color-blind person, for unknown reasons, the cones are effective in other ways but the process for one or more color pigments simply does not work right. No cure for the condition is known.

Why is red-green color blindness inherited by boys more often than by girls? The reason is that the defective gene for color blindness is carried in the pair of chromosomes which determines the sex of the child. In the female, who has two X sex chromosomes, the defective gene is almost always counteracted by a normal gene in the matching sex chromosome. In the male, with an X and Y sex chromosome, there is no matching normal gene in the paired chromosome to block the defect, and the boy is born color blind.

Red-green color blindness cannot be passed from an affected father to his sons. Nor will his daughters be color blind, unless the mother carries the same defective gene. However, all of the daughters are carriers of the defective gene, and the daughters' sons will have a 50 percent chance of inheriting it and being color blind.

Colostomy

Colostomy is the creation of an opening (stoma) in the wall of the abdomen to which an opening in the colon (ostomy) is attached. Thereafter, the contents of the colon are eliminated through the stoma instead of through the rectum and anus.

The operation may be permanent, as when some operations for cancer of the rectum eliminate the normal exit for the bowel, or it may be temporary, as in the surgical correction of Hirschsprung's disease. In this inherited disorder of newborns, the last portion of the bowel lacks specialized nerves and cannot move normally. The healthy portion of the bowel above this segment is connected to the stoma and drains into a special waist-band diaper for several months until the baby is strong enough for the second step of the surgery. This involves removal of the defective bowel portion and connection of the healthy portion to the anus, permitting normal bowel movements and elimination of the stoma.

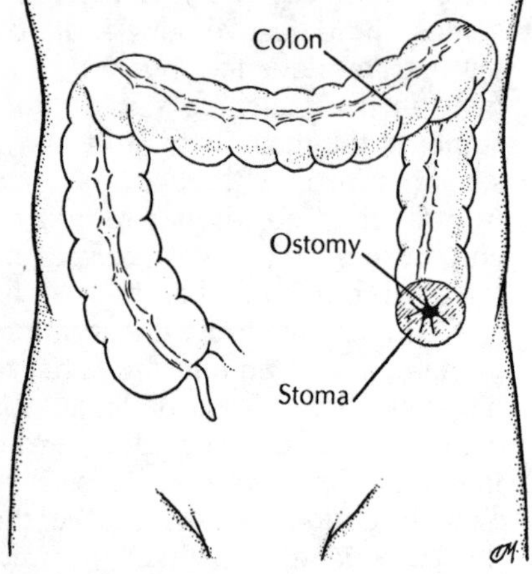

Colostomy is the creation of a stoma (opening) in the wall of the abdomen to which an opening in the colon (ostomy) is attached. The contents of the colon are then eliminated through the stoma rather than through the rectum and anus.

A permanent colostomy does not prevent a person from leading a normal life. After the stoma has healed, or even before, the patient is taught how to empty the colon once a day by using irrigations (enemas) and a special collecting device. By manipulating the diet it becomes possible to time a bowel movement occasionally. At first, patients wear a pouch over the stoma to collect any leakage from the colon. An adhesive is used to form a tight seal around the pouch's opening and the stoma, and a deodorant in the pouch controls odor. However, after a while many individuals with so-called "dry colostomies" need only wear a stoma cap or small gauze patch over the stoma to protect it and absorb mucus secretions. Physical activities can be resumed, with or without a pouch, including swimming, other sports, and sexual relations. The only exceptions are heavy lifting, which could cause a hernia through the weakened abdominal muscles, or any activity that could injure the stoma or abdomen, such as hard contact sports.

To avoid infection of the stoma or irritation of the skin around it, the patient needs to wash the surrounding skin area with mild soap and water each day, then rinse and dry it. Recently, special adhesive materials that protect and soothe the skin have become available. These are applied after cleaning the skin.

Support, encouragement, and practical advice from those who have undergone the operation are available through local chapters and the national headquarters of the United Ostomy Association.

See also Ileostomy.

Common cold

A simple, common cold is a collection of familiar symptoms signaling an infection of the upper respiratory tract, which includes the nose, throat, and sinuses.

Colds are self-limiting diseases, meaning that their symptoms last a certain length of time (or "run their course," as is often remarked) and then disappear without leaving lasting ill effects. A cold is a mild but commonplace disease, one contracted by adults about two to four times a year and by children six to eight times. Adults with children at home are more likely to catch colds than are those who do not live with children. Children are especially susceptible to colds because they have not yet developed immunity or resistance to the many viruses that can cause colds. Small children gradually build up immunity to viruses in their homes; then, when they go to school and have close contact with many other children, they have to combat new viruses. Similarly, adults who travel frequently or have a high number of close contacts outside their community are more likely than those leading more isolated lives to contract colds or encounter new cold viruses to which they are not immune.

A cold can be a minor irritation, but it can increase susceptibility for more serious conditions, especially in children, the very old, and the very weak. Pneumonia, an infection of the lungs, is probably the most serious. Ear infections, sinus infections, and bronchitis are other possible complications. Children sometimes develop croup, a few days after a cold, recognized by its harsh, barking cough that signals a swelling of the airways to the lungs.

At least five major categories of viruses cause colds. One of these groups, the rhinoviruses, includes a minimum of 100 viruses. A different combination of symptoms and possible complications can develop from each of these viruses. It is not known exactly how viruses spread, but it seems to be a combination of physical contact and the presence of both virus particles and moisture in the air. So a virus can spread from hand-to-hand contact, for example, or from the infected person's nasal passages and throat (by droplet), into the air or onto the skin of another person. Colds have an incubation period of 48 to 72 hours, meaning that it takes that long after the virus enters the body for early symptoms to appear.

Early symptoms of the common cold include stuffy or runny nose, sneezing, sore or scratchy throat, cough, and occasionally a mild fever. Usually, as the cold progresses, other symptoms may appear: burning or watery eyes, loss of taste or smell, pressure in the ears or sinuses, nasal voice, and tenderness surrounding the nose.

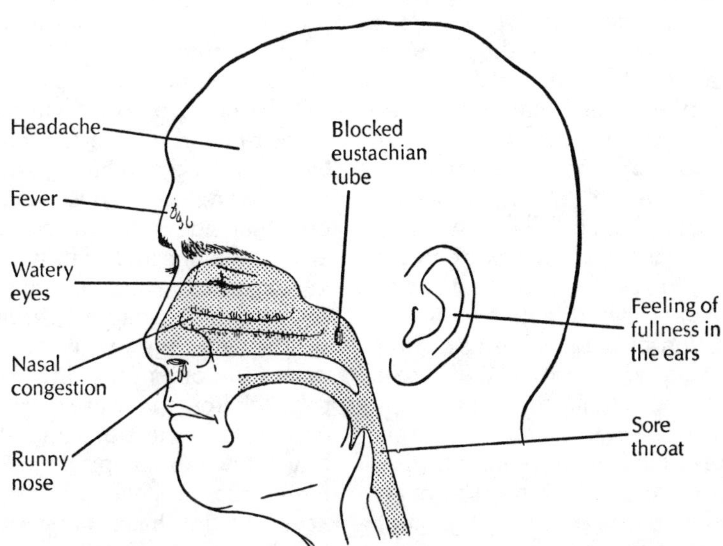

The symptoms of a common cold affect the upper respiratory tract, including the nose and throat.

Symptoms vary in type and severity among the various viruses, so a cold can begin with any symptom or combination of symptoms. Most colds last about a week, but about 25 percent of all colds last two weeks. Smokers and those with chronic respiratory diseases tend to display more severe symptoms, have longer-lasting colds, and develop complications more readily than do those who do not fall into these categories.

Since common colds are mild diseases, the physician, in diagnosing a cold, will actually be looking for symptoms indicating a complication more serious than the common cold. Material from the patient's throat or nasal passages may need to be tested for bacterial infections; a blood test may be recommended to check for mononucleosis, characterized by a long-lasting sore throat and swelling glands; or an X ray of the sinuses may be necessary if an infection of the sinuses (called sinusitis) is suspected.

Getting plenty of rest, drinking lots of fluids to prevent dehydration, and using a humidifier or vaporizer can help relieve the irritating symptoms of a cold. Nevertheless, the common cold cannot be cured, and no known treatment will actually hasten recovery. Many over-the-counter medicines and preparations are available that will at least ease the discomfort of a cold. However, it is best to take specific medicine only for the symptoms actually present and to carefully follow directions on the medication package. Overuse of an otherwise effective remedy can backfire and actually make the symptoms worse, and treating symptoms that are not there can complicate matters. For example, the overuse of an antihistamine or other drying agent for nasal congestion can make a cough more uncomfortable; or the use of a nasal decongestant for more than three days can cause more congestion because the blood vessels in the nose which have been constricted by the decongestant tend to relax in a rebound fashion after a few days' use of a decongestant, causing even more congestion. Anyone who is pregnant or has a chronic disease should check with a doctor before using cold preparations, even seemingly harmless over-the-counter drugs.

There is no known prevention for the common cold. Vitamin C has been said to help prevent colds, but many studies have shown that it has no measurable effect in this area. Avoiding exposure to viruses, when possible, may be the only means of avoiding the common cold.

See also Bronchitis, Croup, Infectious mononucleosis, Pneumonia, and Sinusitis.

Conception

Conception is the union of a sperm cell from the father with an egg from the mother to form a new life.

During the course of her life, the average woman produces about 350 to 400 eggs, or ova, one for each menstrual cycle. The two organs in which the eggs mature, known as ovaries, are located near the top and on either side of the uterus (womb), and are connected with it by ducts known as fallopian tubes. In the midpoint of the 28-day menstrual cycle of the average woman, an egg matures in one or the other ovary, is expelled from the ovary during a process called ovulation, and starts to travel down its fallopian tube toward the uterus, propelled by the waving action of tiny hairs, known as cilia, that line the tube. If the egg meets sperm cells en route, conception may occur.

Sperm cells—which look like tadpoles under a microscope—originate in the man's two testes, which are contained in a fleshy bag (the scrotum) that hangs beneath the penis. At the climax of sexual intercourse, an average of 300 million to 500 million sperm cells, floating in a teaspoonful of thick white fluid, spurt from the tip of the man's penis deep into the woman's vagina. Immediately the sperm start swimming forward, propelled by their long waving tails and aided by contractions of the muscles of the woman's vagina and uterus. The goal of the sperm is to swim through the cervix, into the uterus, and up one of the fallopian tubes to fertilize a new egg just released from the ovary that produced it. Even if all goes well, however, only one of the millions of sperm will succeed. Millions of sperm are killed by acid secretions of the vagina or cervix or are trapped by sticky mucus in the vagina (however, during the middle of the woman's menstrual cycle, when the egg is coming down a fallopian tube to be fertilized, the fluids are thinner, less acid, and less of a barrier; also there are alkaline chemicals in the fluid accompanying the sperm, which act to neutralize the woman's acids). Most of the remaining sperm fail to pass through the uterus and up one of the two fallopian tubes. During most of the woman's menstrual cycle, both tubes are empty and the sperm find nothing to fertilize. Only during a few days is an egg present in one of the tubes, and then it may be reached only by a few of the millions of sperm cells that began the journey. The sperm completely surround the egg, their thin long tails waving furiously in an attempt to force their pointed heads into the female cell. Finally one succeeds. The tail detaches, and the head moves toward the center of the egg. In seconds, a chemical change comes about in the egg that prevents the entry of any other sperm. Conception has occurred.

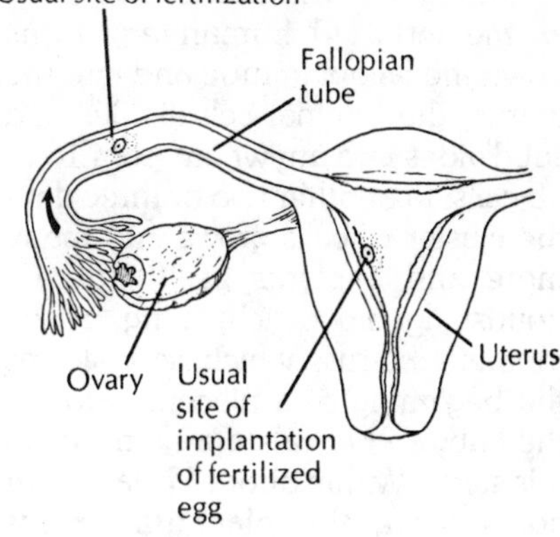

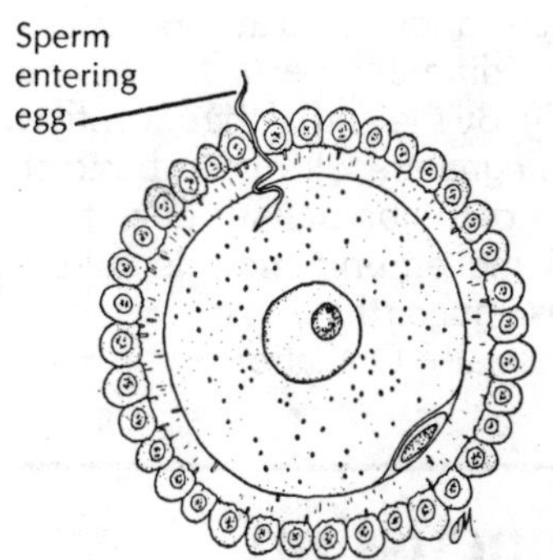

Conception is the union of a sperm cell from the father with an egg from the mother to form a new life. Once a month the woman's ovary releases an egg that travels through the nearby fallopian tube toward the uterus. If the egg meets sperm cells en route, conception may occur. Only one sperm can penetrate an egg.

Unlike all other cells in the body, the sperm and the egg each contain only 23 chromosomes (chromosomes are the chemical "blueprints" that together determine all of the inherited characteristics of the baby to come). All of the other cells contain twice that number, 46. But in the first 12 hours of conception, the 23 chromosomes from the mother and the 23 chromosomes from the father join to form a new nucleus of 46 chromosomes. This is the basic unit from which the new individual will come.

During the next four or five days, as the fertilized human egg drifts down the fallopian tube and into the uterus, the original cell divides and subdivides into anywhere from 16 to 48 cells. In another two or three days the cluster of cells grows into many more and implants itself into the nourishing blood-rich lining of the mother's uterus, which soon forms the beginning of a placenta around the baby-to-be, called an embryo at this stage. Within about 17 days after conception, the placenta begins blood circulation to the embryo, in which various cells are specializing to form different parts of the baby's body. By the end of the seventh week of pregnancy, all of the basic structures of the body have been formed, and the embryo now is called the fetus until birth.

See also Ovulation.

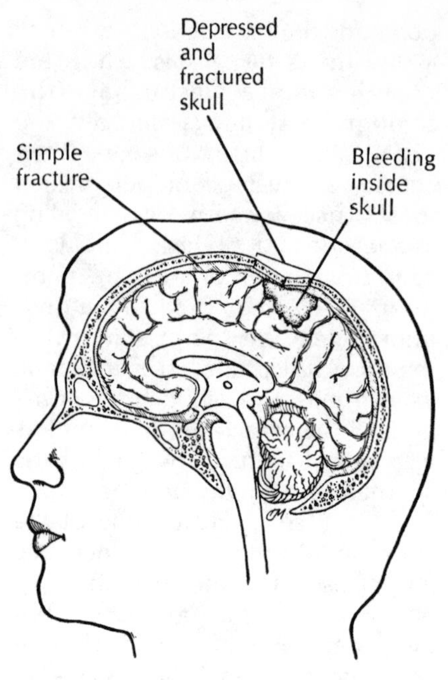

A depressed or fractured skull and bleeding between the covering of the brain and the skull should always be ruled out in an individual with a head injury. Neither of these conditions occurs in a simple concussion.

Concussion

Concussion is a mild injury to the brain, resulting in unconsciousness, caused by a violent jar or shock such as a blow to the head. The force of the shock causes the brain to strike against the inside of the skull and produce temporary brain swelling and malfunctioning. However, the shock is not enough to cause cerebral contusion (bruising of brain tissue) or hemorrhage or hematoma (bleeding between the covering of the brain and the skull, or inside the brain covering), which are much more serious disorders.

Unconsciousness is the chief symptom of concussion, often lasting only a few minutes or hours and never more than 24 hours (a longer period of unconsciousness or a deep coma indicates more serious brain damage). The patient may feel nauseous, irritable, "dragged out," dizzy, or suffer a severe headache, and these symptoms may continue for days or weeks after the accident and, on occasion, longer. Frequently, the individual cannot remember what happened just before the injury and later may not be able to recall anything in the first few hours or on the day following the concussion.

An accident serious enough to cause more than a concussion—that is, a cerebral contusion (bruising of brain tissue), laceration (cutting and tearing of nerve tissue, blood vessels, and brain covering), or edema (fluid buildup within or around the brain)—often shows symptoms other than those accompanying a simple concussion. Signs of serious damage to the brain—much worse than concussion—include partial paralysis of the body; arms and legs extended rigidly, with the jaws clenched; and unequal or pinpoint pupils of the eye.

A simple concussion usually requires no special care. The purpose of the doctor's examination is to determine if any more serious injury may have occurred. The patient is observed for level of consciousness, mental sharpness (if awake), and for proper nerve and muscle functions and reflexes. A head X ray may be taken to rule out a skull fracture (although most simple undepressed skull fractures are allowed to heal without treatment). If the patient acts strangely, out of character, or does not respond correctly to the tests, hospitalization and the services of a neurologist/neurosurgeon may be necessary.

Once a doctor has determined that a patient has had only a simple concussion, the patient may be allowed to return home without hospitalization. For the next 24 hours, the person is advised to relax and to take nothing stronger than an aspirin substitute (acetaminophen). It is best not to eat solid foods, following any vomiting (which is common after concussion). A parent, roommate, or spouse is usually asked to wake the patient every two hours during the night, and ask three questions: "What is your name? Where are you? What is my name?" If the patient cannot answer these questions, will not awaken, or has convulsions, he or she should be rushed to the hospital. In addition, certain other danger signals should send the patient back to the doctor and hospital immediately: a continuing or worsening headache, blurred vision, extreme or constant vomiting, unusual eye movements, twitching, a staggering way of walking, or any change of personality.

If none of these symptoms develop, the patient can resume normal activities after a day or so of rest.

Congenital hypothyroidism

Congenital hypothyroidism is a condition present at birth that leads to defective physical and mental development because of a deficiency of thyroid hormone. If untreated, a person born with congenital hypothyroidism grows to a maximum height of three or four feet, with a large flat broad head; short forehead; puffy wide-set eyes; broad, short, upturned nose; thick lips; large tongue protruding from a drooling mouth; narrow chest; potbelly; swayback; rough skin; dry hair; and severe mental retardation. In former times, these individuals were often found in the Alps and Pyrennes mountains and other inland areas where foods contain little iodine which is necessary for the body to produce thyroid hormone. The ocean is the basic source of iodine, so people living away from the ocean and its iodine-rich seafood are more likely to develop hypothyroidism.

Congenital hypothyroidism can result from a defect in development of a child before birth. The thyroid gland in the newborn child may be missing or underdeveloped, which may have been caused by a severe deficiency of iodine in the mother's diet during pregnancy. Rarely, congenital hypothyroidism is caused by an inherited absence of a body chemical needed to produce thyroid hormone. When hypothyroidism first occurs in children over age two, it is usually due to an inflammation of the thyroid gland resulting from an immune disorder. It can also be caused by disease of the pituitary gland or hypothalamus.

The symptoms of hypothyroidism need never develop in an infant.

Many states now require that the blood of every newborn be tested for thyroid hormone level, a test that can reveal hypothyroidism.

If a baby is not treated, the first symptoms of congenital hypothyroidism begin between age three and six months, or whenever the mother stops breast-feeding (breast milk contains tiny quantities of thyroid hormone). The baby is "too good," in the sense that he or she seldom cries (when the baby does cry, it is a strange hoarse cry), sleeps more than normal, is inactive, and thus is easy to care for. This behavior is a result of the baby's lack of thyroid hormone, which regulates the rate of body processes, and increasing mental retardation. The baby's movements are slow and awkward, and the child has feeding difficulties, is constipated, and develops jaundice (a yellowing of the skin produced by bile pigments in the blood—a result of poor liver function). The stomach protrudes, and a hernia may develop at the navel.

At this time the characteristic facial features of a child with hypothyroidism start to show: the thick tongue, which interferes with breathing; the wide-set eyes; turned-up nose; and also a dull expression indicating mental deficiency. The baby's heart beats slowly, resulting in poor circulation and cold skin. The hair is dry and dull. Teeth come in late and decay easily.

The child who develops hypothyroidism after age two is typically short and fat, with short legs and arms and a head that appears too large. Sexual development in an older child may be delayed.

Diagnosis of congenital hypothyroidism may include not only a blood test for thyroid hormone levels, but also administration of radioactive iodine, which normally would concentrate in the thyroid gland and reveal itself on the screen of a radiation scanner. Of course, if a child has no thyroid gland, that does not happen. X rays may also be used to detect delayed development of the skeleton, and an electrocardiogram may be ordered to reveal heartbeat patterns.

Treatment for congenital hypothyroidism is lifelong replacement of thyroid hormone with a synthetic substitute, ideally starting at birth. Those who receive the supplemental drug starting before the age of three months usually seem to grow and develop normally. Children born without a thyroid gland are even more at risk than those whose thyroid gland works poorly and if not treated by three months of age are retarded for life even though their growth is corrected.

Mothers-to-be can help prevent congenital hypothyroidism in their offspring by eating a well-balanced diet that includes iodine-rich foods like fish and by using iodized salt or an iodine supplement. At birth, the child's blood should be tested for thyroid hormone level.

See also Hypothyroidism.

Congestive heart failure

Congestive heart failure, often simply called "heart failure," is a condition in which the heart weakens and fails to keep the blood moving adequately. As a result, the supply of blood to the body's tissues decreases, lowering body efficiency and endurance. With poor circulation, the kidneys fail to remove enough water, salt and wastes from the blood. In addition, the kidneys, as a result of the decreased blood flow presented to them, also try to increase blood volume by retaining even more salt and water. As a result, blood volume increases, making more work for the already overworked heart, which may enlarge and beat faster in an attempt to satisfy the body's hunger for oxygen-rich blood. Veins distend with fluid and the balance of pressures between fluids inside and outside the veins shifts, which causes fluid that normally stays in the bloodstream to leak into surrounding tissue. This factor, reduction of forward blood flow, along with the backflow of blood and other factors are responsible for the accumulation of fluid in the lungs (called pulmonary edema) as well as for the swelling of the abdomen and legs often seen in patients with congestive heart failure.

The usual cause of congestive heart failure is a diseased heart that just cannot pump enough blood. The most common reason for that is severe coronary artery disease that decreases the flow of blood to the heart muscle. Coronary artery disease is largely responsible for a heart attack, which leaves non-working scar tissue that lowers the efficiency of the heart as a pump. However, other heart conditions can also cause congestive heart failure. Leaky or narrowed heart valves, due to a birth defect or rheumatic fever, can lead to heart failure. A large cardiac aneurysm, a bulge caused by the thinning of the wall of the lower left heart chamber (ventricle) that pumps blood out of the heart into the body, may weaken the heart's pumping ability.

Less frequently, the root of the problem is one of several different heart muscle diseases. Some are caused by poisons like alcohol (liquor), some by viruses, and others by the deposit in the heart tissue of iron or an abnormal body substance known as amyloid. Disturbances of the normal rhythm of the heart may also lead to failure.

Early signs of possible heart failure include unexplained rapid heartbeat, unusual fatigue during exertion, shortness of breath during stair climbing or other mild exercise, and inability to withstand cold. Attacks of shortness of breath and coughing when lying in bed that are relieved by sleeping with pillows under the back to tilt the chest are also early symptoms. Sometimes, a person is actually awakened by "air hunger" and must sit or stand to breathe more easily. These symptoms are caused by increased fluid pressure in the lung circulation. The relief obtained by assuming a more erect position is due to a shift of fluid (blood) volume to the lower half of the body, easing the burden of the heart. In advanced congestive heart failure, shortness of breath and, frequently, a severe cough with rusty or brownish-colored sputum (from blood) are common. There may also be swelling of the ankles and a feeling of fullness in the neck or abdomen.

Usually congestive heart failure can be diagnosed after a physical examination and on the basis of symptoms. However, a chest X ray is commonly taken to determine how much the heart has become enlarged by its overload and to see if fluid has accumulated within the lungs. In addition, an electrocardiogram (ECG), a tracing on a graph of the electric current produced by the contraction of the heart muscle, may reveal past heart attack damage and irregularities in the heart rhythm.

Treatment for congestive heart failure includes rest, oxygen, drugs (like digitalis) to strengthen the pumping ability of the heart, and medicine to prevent irregular heart rhythms. Diuretic drugs are given to help the kidneys remove more salt and water from the blood and thus decrease the amount of volume the heart must pump, and a low-salt diet is prescribed to prevent water buildup in the blood and tissues (salt tends to cause fluid to accumulate in the body). In more severe or chronic cases, a drug may be given to dilate or expand the blood vessels and thus make it easier for the heart to pump blood through them.

In some cases the original cause of the congestive heart failure can be corrected. Thus, bypass surgery may be performed on the coronary arteries to improve blood supply to the heart muscle. Surgery is also done to replace or correct a faulty heart valve, or to repair an aneurysm. Contributing factors to be controlled or eliminated may include high blood pressure, anemia, excess salt or alcohol intake, fever, overactive thyroid, and stress due to overexertion.

Congestive heart failure usually results from an already damaged heart; thus, the prevention of congestive heart failure rests on those good health habits that help prevent heart disease in general: a well-balanced diet with moderate or low intake of fats; weight control; plenty of exercise, rest, and sleep; avoidance of tobacco and excess alcohol; and periodic medical checkups to detect conditions such as high blood pressure that might eventually overload or injure the heart and thus lead to congestive heart failure. In people who already have congestive heart failure, control of the condition is much helped by eliminating salt and highly salted foods, avoiding overexertion, and adhering strictly to the prescribed program of medication.

See also Aneurysm, Bypass surgery, Heart attack, Heartbeat irregularities, Heart disease, Hypertension, and Rheumatic fever.

Conjunctivitis

Conjunctivitis, or pinkeye, is an inflammation of the conjunctiva. The conjunctiva is a delicate membrane that lines the inner surface of the eyelid and covers the exposed surface of the eye.

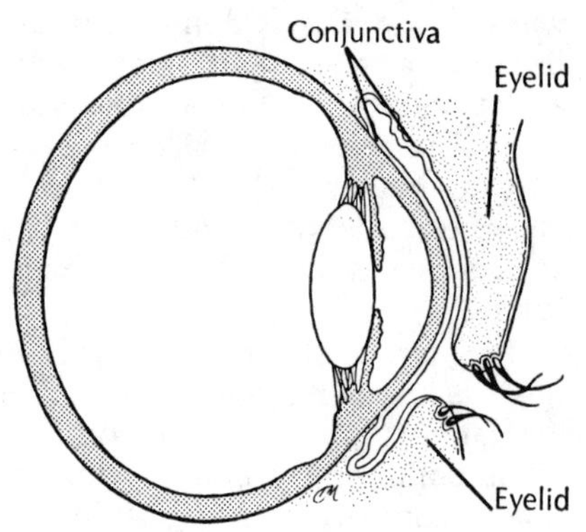

The conjunctiva is a delicate membrane lining the inner surface of the eyelid and covering the exposed surface of the eye.

Most cases of conjunctivitis result from disease-causing microorganisms such as bacteria, fungi, or viruses. Allergies, chemicals, dust, smoke, or foreign objects that irritate the conjunctiva may also lead to conjunctivitis. Swimming may also irritate the conjunctiva — either from chlorine in the pool or from contaminated water. Occasionally, a sexually transmitted disease can cause pinkeye if the eyes are rubbed after touching infected genital organs.

Children contract conjunctivitis most often. Measles, a viral disease, may be accompanied by the eye inflammation. In addition, those people, both children and adults, who have allergies, such as hay fever, or who work and live in areas where they are exposed to chemicals or other irritants are more susceptible to noninfectious conjunctivitis.

Conjunctivitis causes redness, a grating sensation, burning, itching, and perhaps light sensitivity. Sometimes, tearing or a discharge containing pus occurs. Symptoms can last a few days or up to two weeks.

Usually conjunctivitis produces no permanent damage. However, if left untreated, the infection can lead to more serious eye problems. Ulcers, or eroded areas, may form on the cornea (the transparent covering across the front of the eye). Should these ulcers persist, they can scar the eye and interfere with vision.

Treatment depends upon the cause and resulting symptoms of the conjunctivitis. If the inflammation is environmentally caused, simply removing the irritant may be sufficient to eliminate the condition. For more difficult cases, a physician may prescribe antibiotic, steroid, or combination eyedrops to be used several times a day as directed. Frequent use is necessary because drops tend to be washed away by the natural cleansing action of tears.

Sensitive eyes should be rested and shielded from bright lights. When the discharge glues the eyes closed, bathing them with warm water and wiping with a clean cloth will loosen eyelids.

A most important fact about conjunctivitis is that its infectious form is highly contagious. Individuals with infectious conjunctivitis should not share handkerchiefs, towels, or washcloths. If one eye becomes infected, you should not touch the clear eye after rubbing the infected eye to avoid infecting the second eye.

Constipation

Constipation is a condition in which the feces (stool) are hard and their elimination from the bowels is infrequent and difficult. This condition is often more uncomfortable than harmful, although occasionally a relatively sudden change in the bowel movements, involving prolonged constipation or extreme discomfort, can be a symptom of such serious illnesses as cancer, intestinal obstructions, disease or injury of the nervous system, and endocrine gland disorders.

It is important to remember, however, that it is not necessary to have a bowel movement every day. From three bowel movements per day to three per week is considered in the normal range.

Common causes of constipation are physical inactivity; lack of fiber or roughage in the diet; inadequate fluid intake; emotional stress, particularly depression; drug side effects; and the habit of postponing the bowel movement until some time after the urge has disappeared.

Conditions that often accompany constipation are difficulty and strain in producing a bowel movement, a full or bloated feeling, abdominal cramps, headache, gassiness, and hemorrhoids (swollen veins near the anus, the opening from the intestine to the outside of the body).

The treatment of constipation usually depends on its cause. In mild cases that are not related to other disorders, simple methods of recommended treatment include adding more fiber foods (such as bran, fruits, vegetables, and other forms of roughage) to the diet; drinking eight to ten glasses of water daily; increasing exercise; and developing good bathroom habits. This last recommendation may involve an attempt to have a bowel movement at the same time every day, usually 30 to 60 minutes after breakfast. Early morning is a good time because food that enters an empty stomach activates and increases normal intestine contractions; also, residue from the previous day's meals has moved by this time to the rectal area for elimination.

Laxatives and enemas are usually not recommended for treating simple constipation. Laxatives, in particular, should be used only when absolutely necessary because overuse can lead to irritation of the lining of the rectum, and, more importantly, dependence by the intestine to the point that it cannot function properly without laxatives. Frequent enemas can also lead to dependence.

Drinking plenty of water, getting adequate exercise, eating fibrous foods, and recognizing the urge for a bowel movement as soon as it is felt should be beneficial in promoting regular elimination and preventing constipation.

Contact dermatitis

Contact dermatitis is a type of allergy (an unusual reaction to or oversensitivity to an outside substance, called an allergen) in which the skin becomes inflamed in the area where it has come in contact with an irritant (called a contact allergen).

Contact dermatitis can be caused by soaps, detergents, shaving materials, shampoos, hair colorings or sprays, solvents in household cleaners, chemicals in foods and cosmetics, and certain plants such as poison ivy or poison oak. Photodermatitis (a skin inflammation caused by light) is a type of dermatitis that develops when certain ingested drugs, such as some antibiotics, sensitize the skin in a manner that causes a rash to develop on those skin surfaces exposed to the sun (this can also be seen in some unusual systemic disorders and in people with "true sun allergy").

The major symptoms of contact dermatitis are burning, swelling, severe itching, and stinging sensations on the area of the skin that has been exposed to the allergen. Blisters may form that ooze a clear fluid; a cloudy or yellow foul-smelling fluid indicates a bacterial infection.

Contact dermatitis is diagnosed by first identifying the allergen causing the trouble. In identifying this type of allergen, the process is somewhat simplified, because the location of the rash gives an important clue as to its identity. For instance, if the inflammation is on the scalp, the disorder may be assumed to be triggered by a shampoo, hair spray, or hair coloring. More specific identification of the allergen may be obtained from one of several tests available that pinpoint allergens in all types of allergies. These include scratch tests, in which a small amount of the suspected allergen is applied to a scratch on the skin; intracutaneous tests, in which a small amount of the allergen is injected in or under the skin; and the radioallergosorbent technique, a blood test in which specific antibodies produced by the body in response to the allergen are measured.

Once the allergen is identified, the best treatment for contact dermatitis is to avoid or remove the allergen from the patient's environment. Common sense precautions can be taken to remove the allergen from the patient's surroundings, such as switching brands of soaps or shampoos, wearing rubber gloves when using harsh detergents, and using unscented or hypoallergenic cosmetics. If the use of a drug cannot be discontinued despite a case of photodermatitis, sunscreens or adequate clothing to shield the skin from the sun's rays should be used when outdoors.

Steroid (cortisone) drugs, taken orally, help to relieve the itching of contact dermatitis; however, these are reserved for more serious cases. Topical (rubbed directly on the skin) steroids and antihistamines are more commonly used.

There is no actual preventive treatment for contact dermatitis, but those susceptible to one or more contact allergens can usually prevent outbreaks by using common sense and avoiding exposure to the allergen or allergens as much as possible.

See also Dermatitis.

Contraception

See Birth control.

Convulsions

See Emergency first aid section at the end of this book.

Corns

Corns are small, round mounds of firm, dead skin that form on or between the toes. Their hard, waxy core, which bores down into the skin and presses on the underlying tissue and nerves, can cause extreme pain. At times corns are associated with bursae (fluid-filled sacs), which can become irritated and result in bursitis.

Corns are caused by a great deal of pressure or friction on the toes (as are calluses, their basis), usually from ill-fitting shoes or high heels. Since the skin acts as the body's protector from the outside environment, corns form when the body attempts to protect the troubled area from more pressure by building up a mass of dead skin cells and secreting a hard substance called keratin. Sometimes people who have abnormal bone structures in their feet or some types of arthritis tend to develop corns. Generally, however, those who avoid high heels or tight-fitting shoes should be able to avoid corns. Usually regular in shape, corns can be

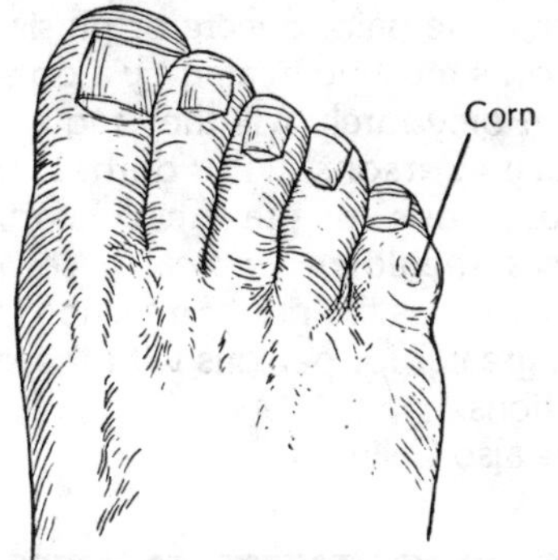

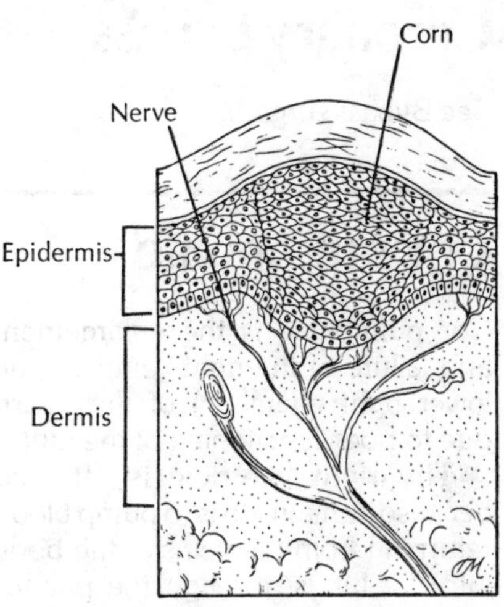

Corns are small mounds of dead skin that form on or between the toes. Their cores, formed in the epidermis layer of the skin, bore down on underlying tissue and nerves in the dermis layer, causing pain.

white, gray, or yellow, and usually form on the outside of the first or fifth toes, since that is where pressure most often occurs. Corns that form between the toes are called soft corns, since they are not as firm as other corns because of the moisture between the toes.

Corns are best treated by first eliminating the cause of the pressure. Over-the-counter preparations are available. These include padding to reduce the friction on the area, ointments, and medicated pads, which will soften and blister the skin layers, making them easier to remove and reducing the pain. Severe or persistent corns must be treated by a doctor, but only rarely will they require surgery. Persons with diabetes, atherosclerosis, or other circulatory diseases should *never* treat a corn themselves, as the risk of infection is much greater for persons with these conditions.

See also Calluses.

Coronary bypass

See Bypass surgery.

Cor pulmonale

Cor pulmonale is the enlargement and failure of the right ventricle (the lower right chamber) of the heart, due to poor functioning of the lungs.

The right ventricle is affected because its main job is to pump blood returning from the veins of the body into the lungs, through the pulmonary artery. When the lungs are not working properly — for example, when many of its capillaries (tiny blood vessels) have been destroyed or constricted by disease – not enough blood can get through the lungs. The blood backs up, its pressure rises, and it enlarges both the pulmonary artery and the now harder-working right ventricle. Blood pressure also rises in the veins leading to the heart.

In addition, because not enough blood is getting to the appropriate areas of the lungs and because of disease or destruction of the oxygenating units of the lungs called alveoli, the oxygen content of the blood decreases. This causes the bone marrow to produce more oxygen-carrying red blood cells, which in most circumstances would allow the blood to carry more oxygen. However, in this case it only makes matters worse, by thickening the blood which is then harder to pump. The result of the whole process is failure of the right ventricle to perform well.

In nearly six cases out of seven, the lung condition that has led to cor pulmonale is chronic obstructive pulmonary disease (COPD), which is a breakdown in breathing resulting from emphysema, chronic bronchitis, asthma, or a combination of these diseases. Some of the other causes are cystic fibrosis, recurrent blood clots in the blood vessels of the lung, loss of lung tissue because of surgery or injury, extreme obesity that prevents proper breathing, diseases of the nerves controlling the breathing muscles, or insufficient oxygen from living at high altitudes (chronic mountain sickness). Almost always the cause of cor pulmonale is a chronic, lifelong condition. One exception is acute (sudden and severe) cor pulmonale resulting from a massive blood clot in the lungs; the clot can sometimes be removed by surgery. Also more often an acute worsening cor pulmonale results from a severe infection of the breathing tract in someone with a chronic lung condition. Proper treatment usually can bring this under control.

Symptoms of right heart failure include increasing fatigue, drowsiness, fainting on exertion, ankle swelling, fullness in the neck and abdomen, enlarged neck veins, and an enlarged and tender liver. As in the more common left ventricle failure, the patient may wheeze; cough; find breathing difficult and painful (however, in pure right ventricle failure, there is no fluid in the lungs); and may at times be blue in the lips, nails, fingertips, and even the face from lack of oxygen.

X-ray or ultrasound pictures reveal the enlargement of the right ventricle and pulmonary artery. A markedly increased number of red blood cells that exceeds 50 percent of the blood volume is a telltale clue. Heartbeat patterns indicating right-ventricle failure can be seen on an electrocardiogram (ECG), which is a visual record of the electrical impulses of the heart.

Treatment for cor pulmonale is twofold to treat the heart failure and the lung condition at the same time. Heart failure therapy includes oxygen to make the patient more comfortable, to reduce the high blood pressure in the pulmonary artery, and to prevent a high red blood cell count. Salt and water restriction and diuretics (drugs that remove excess water from the blood) can reduce excess fluid in the tissues. Bed rest reduces the load on the heart.

In general, treatment of the underlying lung condition is much the same as it was (or should have been) before cor pulmonale occurred. The patient should not smoke. In most patients, smoking helped to cause the original condition, and smoking worsens the present condition. Once home from the hospital, the individual should regularly practice breathing exercises and may need oxygen and suction treatments to relieve symptoms. The patient should rest frequently, watch for signs of ankle swelling or other fluid buildup, avoid people with colds, and report early signs of infection for treatment.

You can help to prevent the lung condition leading to cor pulmonale by not smoking, by having periodic physical examinations including a test of lung function, and by seeking prompt medical treatment by a physician of any chronic cough or recurring respiratory (breathing) infection. It is especially important to observe these precautions if you come from a family that has an inherited tendency to certain chronic respiratory diseases such as emphysema and asthma.

See also Asthma, Bronchitis, Cystic fibrosis, and Emphysema.

Corticosteroids

Corticosteroids are hormones produced in the outer layer (cortex) of the adrenal glands, two small organs that lie atop the kidneys. (Hormones are chemical "messengers" manufactured by body cells and carried by fluids to another location, where they control a body process.) There are more than 30 corticosteroids. Together, they regulate processes throughout the body and are essential to life. They are divided into three groups: mineralocorticoids, glucocorticoids, and sex steroids.

Mineralocorticoids exert control on the distribution of body fluids and the sodium and potassium mineral salts dissolved within them. Without the mineralocorticoids, the tissues and blood become depleted of salt and water. The blood decreases in volume, causing a drop in blood pressure that can result in collapse of the blood circulation system (shock).

Glucocorticoids help regulate the body's use and reserves of sugars and proteins, among other complex metabolic processes. They assist various chemical processes throughout the body, and also participate in the inflammation response. (Cortisol, one of these hormones, is known for this effect. For example, as medication—called cortisone—it reduces the swollen joints of arthritis and can eliminate skin rashes.) Finally, these hormones also participate in the body's reaction to stress.

The sex steroids include androgens (such as testosterone, also produced in the male testes) and estrogens (also produced in the female ovaries). Men and women have both male and female hormones in their systems. However, the abundance of androgens in men produces beard growth, enlarged muscle development, and other male characteristics. In women, an abundance of estrogen produces feminine characteristics such as breast development.

Production of corticosteroids is under control of ACTH (adrenocorticotropic hormone), which is released by the pituitary gland located near the base of the brain. ACTH travels in the bloodstream to the adrenal cortex and stimulates the cortex to produce corticosteroids. The pituitary gland is regulated by the hypothalamus, a part of the brain.

See also ACTH, Adrenal glands, and Pituitary gland.

Cough

A cough is a normal reflex of the body to clear the airways. Coughing can result from inhaling dust, dirt, or irritating fumes; from breathing icy air; or from mistakenly drawing food into the airways. It can also be caused by mucus and other secretions from such respiratory disorders as the common cold, influenza, pneumonia, or tuberculosis. Persistent coughs (those that last more than two or three weeks) without other respiratory symptoms may, on occasion, suggest diseases of other organs, such as the heart. A cough may also be an early sign of congestive heart failure.

The type of cough—productive or nonproductive — partially determines how it should be treated. Productive coughs — those that produce fluid or mucus — are often caused by a lung infection When microorganisms attack the lungs, the lung tissue produces large amounts of secretions in defense. These accumulated secretions irritate the lungs, resulting in coughing that brings up fluid or mucus. A yellowish or reddish fluid in particular may indicate infection or other serious problems and requires a doctor's attention.

Nonproductive coughing does not bring up fluid. It occurs when secretions from nasal passages drip into the throat or when smoke, dust, pollen, or other irritants enter the respiratory system. Irritations such as foreign bodies or tumors may also cause a nonproductive cough, as can any inflammation of the airways and/or lung tissue, infectious or not. Another cause of nonproductive coughing is insufficient moisture in the air. The airways become dry and irritated, and coughing develops. This is particularly common in winter, when humidity is lowest. A humidifier or vaporizer that adds moisture to the air may provide more relief than any cough-suppressing drug.

Because coughing has the vital function of clearing the airways, it should never be totally suppressed. In fact, suppressing a cough in an individual with chronic lung disease may be dangerous. Furthermore, indiscriminate use of cough suppressants may mask important symptoms. However, controlling a cough that disrupts sleep or aggravates other conditions may sometimes be necessary. This may be accomplished by using a cough suppressant and/or an expectorant. A suppressant helps to inhibit the cough by depressing the cough center in the brain. An expectorant eases the discharge of mucus from the respiratory tract, thus perhaps shortening the course of the illness.

For other than the mildest cough with obvious causes and certainly for persistent coughs, a doctor should be consulted to determine the cause and to suggest appropriate treatment.

Coxsackie viruses

Coxsackie is the term for a group of viruses that cause a wide variety of usually brief illnesses particularly common to children. Together with two other groups of viruses that have been isolated from the gastrointestinal system, the echoviruses and the polioviruses, they are known as enteroviruses (entero means "intestine"). Coxsackie virus infections occur most often in summer and fall and can be spread by means of the mouth or infected human feces (solid waste). There are 24 group A coxsackie viruses and six group B coxsackie viruses. The following diseases are among those frequently caused by coxsackie viruses (some are also caused by other enteroviruses).

Herpangina. An epidemic disease in infants and young children, herpangina is marked by sudden high fever, headache, sore throat, vomiting, and grayish blisters or spots on the soft palate (rear roof of mouth), tonsils, or throat that become shallow ulcers and heal in three to six days.

Hand, foot, and mouth disease. Common in young children, this is similar to herpangina except that little blisters erupt over all of the mucous membrane in the mouth and also on the hands, feet, and sometimes in the diaper area.

Epidemic pleurodynia (Bornholm disease). Sudden, recurrent pains in the lower chest (or abdomen in 50 percent of the cases) signal the onset of this illness, often accompanied by fever, headache, nausea, abdominal tenderness, and sore throat. There may be muscle swelling of the involved area, which may be painful to the touch. Occasionally the disease spreads to cause pleuritis (inflammation of the membrane sac surrounding the lungs and lining of the chest cavity), pericarditis (inflammation of the sac around the heart), and, rarely, aseptic meningitis (see below).

Aseptic meningitis. This inflammation of the membrane covering the brain causes headache, pain and stiffness in the neck and back, fever, nausea, vomiting, drowsiness, a general sick feeling, and, rarely, muscle paralysis. Occasionally death results in newborns, but most patients recover in a week or so. Fatigue and irritability, however, may linger for months.

Paralytic disease. Various coxsackie, echo, and polio viruses produce a muscle weakness or paralysis that is similar to the paralysis of polio and is treated in the same manner. However, the paralysis is usually temporary.

Respiratory disease. Coxsackie and other enteroviruses appear to cause respiratory illnesses with head cold, fever, sore throat, and sometimes vomiting and diarrhea.

Rubella-like rash. A mild rash like that of rubella (German measles), but lasting longer, this usually occurs in epidemic form and only on the face, neck, and chest. Fever is common and meningitis can develop, but usually this is a mild disease.

Myocarditis and pericarditis. Heart failure in newborns may result from infection of the heart muscle by coxsackie or echoviruses transmitted to the baby before birth by the mother. Myocarditis (infection of the heart muscle) or pericarditis (infection of the sac around the heart) in older children and in adults may also be caused by a coxsackie virus, but patients usually make a complete recovery. (However, congestive heart failure can occur in the acute phase of these diseases.)

Although they produce a great deal of temporary discomfort, the coxsackie viruses generally do not cause lasting illness. In general the only treatment necessary is to make the patient as comfortable as possible, with plenty of liquids, bed rest, and lukewarm sponge baths and drugs such as acetaminophen to control fever until the illness has passed. Careful handwashing and proper disposal of human wastes can help prevent the spread of infection.

Crohn's disease

Crohn's disease (also known as regional enteritis or ileitis) is characterized by an inflammation of a section or sections of any part of the digestive tract – most often of the ileum (the last one third of the small intestine). The disease may first appear as patches of tiny ulcers in the innermost lining of the intestine, with swelling of nearby tissue. Eventually the inflammation extends through all layers of the intestine, which becomes thickened, hard, and brittle. Deepening ulcers, scarring, and swelling may obstruct the intestinal tract. Complications include abscesses (pus-filled cavities) and fistulas. Fistulas can be thought of as tunnels. They originate from inflamed bowel and commonly burrow out into and around the anorectal area where upon examination they are seen as openings in the skin. These openings are often infected and discharging pus. Fistulas can also occur from bowel to bowel, bowel to bladder and/or vagina, and bowel to abdominal wall.

Perforation of the intestine can also occur, leading to peritonitis (infection and/or inflammation of the lining of the abdominal cavity). This is marked by severe abdominal pain with a rigid abdomen and is most often an acute surgical emergency. On occasion, a small perforation will be unnoticed; the immune system will then "wall off" the area creating an abscess.

Malnutrition is also a very common complication of Crohn's disease, as areas of inflamed intestine cannot properly absorb nutrients. The incidence of cancer of the colon and rectum is also increased in patients with Crohn's disease.

The cause of Crohn's disease is unknown. However, research indicates that infection, immune disorders, or an inherited defect may play a part. There is some evidence of an increased incidence of Crohn's disease in Jews; blacks are least likely to develop the disease. The disease usually begins between age 15 and age 35, but can occur at any age.

Symptoms usually develop gradually, with spells of diarrhea (four to six stools a day, frequently bloody), low fever, weight loss, loss of appetite, general weakness, and steady or colicky pains in the abdomen, commonly on the right side. Milk, milk products, and coarse foods may make symptoms worse. The examining doctor, probing the abdomen and pelvis, may detect a tender mass of thickened or matted loops of intestine.

Occasionally an acute (sudden and severe) case resembles appendicitis, with sharp lower right abdomen pain, cramping, nausea, fever, and diarrhea. There may or may not be bloody stools. Also, an acute case can resemble infectious diarrhea.

The chronic form of the disease can occasionally be mistaken for other problems, such as irritable bowel syndrome. However, a barium X ray of the small intestine may reveal the characteristic pattern of narrowed bowel sharply differentiated from healthy bowel. X rays of the large intestine may show characteristic "skipped areas" or areas of disease interspersed with normal bowel. Fistulas are also commonly seen on X rays. The doctor may also inspect the inner lining of the large intestine visually, with a lighted tube (inserted through the anus) known as a sigmoidoscope (proctoscope), looking for patchy areas of inflammation and taking a sample of tissue (biopsy) from the lining for inspection under a microscope.

An acute case of bloody diarrhea occurring in young people may be caused by infection and be unrelated to true Crohn's disease. If so, complete recovery is possible, with no further attacks. Chronic Crohn's disease, however, is another matter. At present there is no cure for it. At times surgery is necessary to remove entirely a section of diseased bowel, drain an abscess, or eliminate a fistula. This relieves the condition for a time, but symptoms almost always recur and another operation may be necessary. Treatment of the disease is directed at making the patient as comfortable and functional as possible by reducing the symptoms. Disability may be mild or severe.

A diet rich in calories and vitamins with adequate protein is desirable, to compensate for the patient's poor absorption of food from the intestine. Individuals with severely inflamed or obstructed bowel may be placed temporarily on intravenous feeding or a special no-residue diet. Patients with anemia need supplements (such as iron, folic acid, or Vitamin B_{12}) and sometimes blood transfusions, and those with severe diarrhea or dehydration (loss of body fluids) may need intravenous fluids.

Cramps and diarrhea are frequently controlled by various medications that relax the bowel wall, while preparations such as psyllium may help to firm stools.

Antibiotics are used short-term to treat abscesses and infected fistulas. Sulfa/salicylate combination drugs may be used continually to curb inflammation and prevent acute episodes, particularly in disease involving the large intestine. In addition, a cortisone drug known as prednisone, taken by mouth, is a mainstay in treating flare-ups of symptoms.

Croup

Croup is a hoarse, barking cough that sometimes follows a cold or fever in very young children, most commonly those under the age of two years. A croup attack may occur only once for a short period and never reoccur, or it may linger or reappear when it seems to be gone.

Croup is caused by a viral infection of the larynx (voice box). The characteristic barking cough is produced when air forces its way through the child's swollen larynx. The air passageways in a child's throat are very narrow; therefore, when an infection causes swelling, there is little room for air to pass through, and breathing can be severely hampered. Also, the windpipe and the bronchi (the main breathing tubes that connect the windpipe and the lungs) may become blocked with mucus, further impairing breathing.

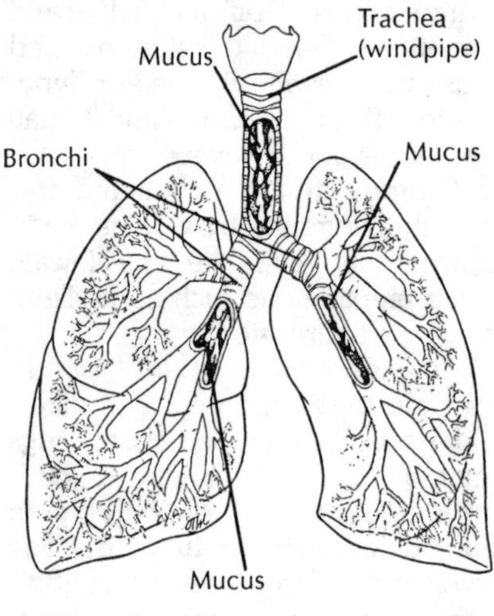

Croup can be complicated by mucus blocking the windpipe and the bronchi leading into lungs. This may lead to serious breathing problems and become a medical emergency.

The identifying symptoms of croup are a deep, barking cough and breathing difficulties, especially when breathing in. Sometimes a fever and hoarseness are also present. The child may gag while coughing, causing vomiting that usually relieves the cough. The coughing attack often occurs in the evening and usually lasts less than an hour.

Symptoms that indicate a worsening condition include blue skin and lips, drooling, and extreme exhaustion. When the croaking sound continues while the child is inhaling, a condition called stridor has developed. If any of these symptoms occur or if there are severe breathing difficulties, medical help should be obtained *immediately*.

Croup can be treated at home by first, and most importantly, calming the child. The barking cough, especially when accompanied by difficult breathing, can frighten anyone, especially a child, and this fear can only aggravate the symptoms. To calm the child, he or she can be asked to visualize what is happening in the throat; the child can picture the tubes to the lungs opening wide, allowing air to pass freely. Sometimes the child can be told to imagine a relaxing scene or to listen to a calming bedtime story. A relaxed child will respond much better to home remedies.

The goal is to relieve the cough by reducing the inflammation and swelling in the larynx. This can be accomplished by breathing in moist air from a humidifier or vaporizer, by leaning over a pan of hot water with a towel draped over the head, or by sitting in a steamy bathroom with a hot shower running. Moist air reduces the swelling and makes breathing easier. Of course, precautions should be taken to protect a young child from being scalded while taking part in these treatments, and the child should never be left alone.

Drinking extra fluids (not milk or orange juice) at room temperature is also recommended Cough medicine will not help, and may even harm, a child with croup, nor will putting a spoon or any other object into the mouth in an attempt to aid the breathing. In a severe case, drugs can be administered to control the inflammation in the throat; also, antibiotics can sometimes control the infections connected with croup.

It is not known why some children develop croup after a cold or fever and others do not; therefore, there is really no way to prevent croup.

Cushing's syndrome

Cushing's syndrome is a group of abnormalities resulting from an excess level of the hormones produced by the outer layer (cortex) of the adrenal glands, small glands that lie atop the kidneys. (Hormones are chemical "messengers" manufactured by body cells and carried by fluids to another location in the body, where they control a body process.) The hormones produced in excess are chiefly cortisol, which has many complex functions; other hormones that regulate the body's use of sugars and proteins; sex hormones; and a hormone that controls the distribution of fluids and salts in the body.

In most cases, Cushing's syndrome is caused by excess production of ACTH (adrenocorticotropic hormone), which is normally manufactured by the pituitary gland to stimulate the adrenal glands to produce hormones. This excess of ACTH can be caused by an ACTH-producing tumor (growth) in another organ, such as a cancer in the lung or pancreas; by overmedication with ACTH or cortisone drugs; by tiny nonmalignant ACTH-producing tumors on the pituitary gland; or by a nonmalignant (or occasionally malignant) cortisone-producing tumor on the adrenal gland. The effect of too much ACTH for whatever reason is an overgrowth of tissue in the adrenal cortex, resulting in overproduction of all its hormones. Since the hormones produced by the adrenal cortex regulate processes throughout the body and are essential to life, excess production causes widespread disorders.

Some of the most obvious signs of Cushing's syndrome are a "moon-shaped" face, caused by excess fluid in the tissues; a fat trunk but thin arms and legs; and fat pads over the shoulders and neck, producing a "buffalo hump." These abnormalities are all caused by excess deposits of fatty tissue in these locations. Purple stretch marks on the skin (usually of the abdomen); poor wound healing (caused by excess cortisone, which suppresses body defenses); easy bruising; hairiness, acne, and decreased or absent menstruation in women, because of increased male hormones; enlarged breasts in men, because of increased female hormones; muscle weakness; fractures in weakened bones; and emotional instability are also part of the syndrome. The development of diabetes and high blood pressure is also very common.

Diagnosis of Cushing's syndrome requires measurement of adrenal cortex hormones in the blood and urine. One clue is that in normal persons cortisol levels in the blood are high upon awakening but decrease during the day; in the Cushing's syndrome patient cortisol levels are high all the time. Various tests can determine whether the cause of the syndrome is a malfunction of the pituitary gland (in which case the disorder is known as Cushing's disease) or is a tumor on the adrenal gland or elsewhere. Tumors on the adrenal glands are located by X rays, ultrasound, and CAT scan (a technique using X rays of multiple and progressively deeper sections, yielding a more three-dimensional picture). CAT scans and other special X rays of the head can often locate tumors on the pituitary gland, which is located at the base of the brain.

Cushing's syndrome is treated by restoring a normal balance of hormones. This may involve surgery, X-ray treatments, or drugs. Tumors on the adrenal glands are removed by surgery. If there is a tumor on just one adrenal gland, the other gland usually shrinks and becomes hardly productive. Hormone supplements are usually given before surgery and must be taken for weeks or months after surgery until the second gland returns to normal function. In a rapidly worsening case of Cushing's syndrome, in which the adrenal cortex is greatly enlarged on both adrenal glands, one treatment is to remove both adrenal glands. This is usually a last resort. More commonly, however, other methods such as chemotherapy (drug treatments), X-ray treatments of the pituitary gland to weaken it and lower its output of adrenal-gland-stimulating ACTH, or removal of any adenomas (nonmalignant growths) on the pituitary gland may be tried first. If these measures fail, the adrenal glands are removed and the patient must take daily supplements of adrenal cortex hormones for the rest of his or her life.

If Cushing's syndrome is being caused by production of ACTH by a cancer in another part of the body, the cancer is located and removed, if possible. However, in most cases it is inoperable, in which case drugs to suppress production of the adrenal glands are given.

Cushing's syndrome is a very serious and possibly fatal disease unless it is detected and treated early. The outlook is best for those whose condition is caused by noncancerous growths and who receive early treatment.

Those who must take replacement hormones after treatment should carry a medical identification card and immediately tell their doctors about any infections, injuries, or stressful situations that might require an increase in hormone dosage. They should also report signs of underdosage, such as weakness, dizziness, or fatigue, and of overdosage, such as swollen tissues and rapid weight gain. Anyone whose adrenal glands have been removed must always take replacement hormones; stopping the use of these replacements for any length of time is fatal.

See also ACTH, Adrenal glands, Corticosteroids, and Pituitary gland.

Cyanosis

Cyanosis is a bluish coloration of the skin and mucous membranes. The abnormal coloration is easily seen in these areas, both because of their rich blood supply and their relative transparency. Usually it is a sign that the tissue is getting too little oxygen from the blood.

Blood rich in oxygen from the lungs is bright red. This is because of the red iron-containing pigment known as hemoglobin found in the erythrocytes, the disc-shaped red blood cells which carry oxygen. When blood passes through the blood vessels of the lungs, oxygen from the air in the lungs combines with the hemoglobin, which causes it and the blood to turn a very bright red. After the blood releases its oxygen to the cells of the body and picks up carbon dioxide and other waste products, the hemoglobin fades and the blood turns dark. However, if the lungs are not working well or for some other reason the red blood cells are not being oxygenated, the blood appears bluish, producing cyanosis.

Cyanosis is a sign of reduced air supply that can be due to such conditions as asthma, choking, pneumonia, and lung collapse. It can also be a sign of certain inborn heart defects, of severe heart failure, or of abnormally excessive production of red blood cells. It is seen most frequently in cold weather when lips, toes, and fingers turn blue from extreme cold, the result of sluggish surface circulation of the blood. This can be a normal phenomenon and does not indicate disease.

Cyst

A cyst is a sac or membrane containing a fluid or semisolid material. In normal anatomy, the term literally refers to a bladder, including the urinary bladder (which is why inflammation of that bladder is called cystitis) and the gallbladder (which is why the duct leading from the gallbladder is called the cystic duct and the gallbladder itself is called the cholecyst). However, most cysts are not normal. Cysts may form around a foreign body, such as a particle in the lung or the skin, or around a parasite. They may entrap an escaping body liquid, such as blood hemorrhaging into tissue or fluid leaking from a bursa (a sac containing lubricant for a joint). In the intestine, they may develop in a fold or pouch lining the intestinal tract. They may be enlargements of natural fluid-filled sacs such as a bursa. They may develop on the ovaries; ovarian cysts are abnormal, sometimes painful, but usually harmless and self-healing entities of the ovaries that usually occur in response to changes in a woman's menstrual cycle.

Perhaps the most common cysts are those of the skin and mucous membranes. A *sebaceous cyst* occurs when a sebaceous gland, the tiny oil gland at the base of each hair root, becomes plugged. Ordinarily this plugging just results in a blackhead, or a pus-filled pimple if the blackhead becomes infected. Occasionally, however, the pimple does not break and the swelling becomes entrapped beneath the skin. Sebum (oil from the sebaceous gland) continues to flow into the sac that forms in the cavity, and the cyst grows to the size of a marble or larger. Sebaceous cysts —which can occur on any part of the body where there is hair including the neck, scalp, and back—can easily be removed surgically if bothersome; however, if they become infected, they must be drained and removed. A type of tiny cyst known as *milium*, usually occurring on the scrotum, can simply be opened and drained. Larger cysts must be removed completely, or they will recur.

Mucous cysts which occur in the mouth, on the tongue, or on the lower lip are caused by plugged-up mucous glands and may grow to be the size of a pea or larger. They may be removed in the same manner as sebaceous cysts.

Traumatic epithelial cysts usually result from the trapping beneath the skin of a piece of skin, a blood clot, or foreign material because of some injury and may or may not need to be removed.

Cystic fibrosis

Cystic fibrosis is a serious hereditary disease characterized by abnormal secretions that affect many parts of the body, primarily the lungs, pancreas, and digestive tract.

When cystic fibrosis is present, the exocrine glands release abnormal mucus, sweat, or other secretions into the body. (The exocrine glands are those glands that secrete their solutions through various ducts and across membranes in order to transport vital chemicals throughout the body and to keep the membrane linings moist.) The most serious effects of cystic fibrosis occur when faulty mucous glands release an overly thickened, gummy mucus rather than the normal clear, free-flowing fluid. This thick mucus accumulates in the glands, causing swelling, forming cysts, and, more importantly, blocking various ducts throughout the body. This abnormal mucus secretion can affect many areas of the body. One of its most serious complications occurs when mucus in the lungs, which is normally present to sweep the lungs clean of bacteria and foreign particles, becomes thick and sticky, accumulating in the airways and creating a breeding ground for infection rather than preventing it. Consequent infections produce still more mucus, and the airways, already narrowed from the swelling, become even more clogged. Recurrent infections can lead to long-term breathing difficulties, and the condition becomes serious. Most patients die from respiratory failure caused by obstruction of the airways and by persistent infections.

Also affected by this disorder is the pancreas, the long, thin organ that secretes digestive juices through a series of ducts into the small intestine. These ducts can be blocked by the abnormally thickened secretions, preventing important digestive enzymes from being transported to the small intestine where they are needed to digest fats. Similarly, the reproductive system may show these effects of cystic fibrosis. Reproductive tract secretions are also thickened, so that mucus may block the pathway of the ovum (egg) and make it difficult for female patients to become pregnant. Likewise, about 98 percent of male patients are sterile because a duct through which the sperm normally travels is blocked by thickened mucus.

Heat exhaustion is another problem related to this disease, because of the large salt loss through excessive sweating.

Cystic fibrosis is caused when a gene (a unit in a cell that determines an inherited characteristic in the

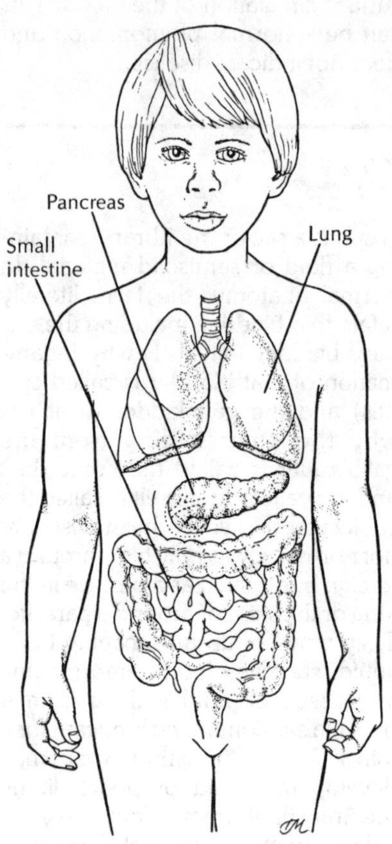

Cystic fibrosis is a disease characterized by abnormal secretions that affect many body parts, particularly the lungs, the pancreas, and the intestinal tract. In the lungs thick mucus hampers breathing and promotes infection. Thickened secretions can obstruct the ducts in the pancreas and block the passage of pancreatic digestive enzymes into the small intestine.

body) is defective and adversely affects the exocrine glands so that their secretions become abnormal. This defective gene is recessive, meaning that it must be inherited from both parents for the child to suffer from the disease. If the gene is received from only one parent, the child is a carrier but will not get the disease. About 5 percent of the white population in the United States are carriers, with much lower incidence in black and Oriental populations. Approximately one in every 400 marriages takes place between two carriers. A child of two carriers has a 25 percent chance of getting the disease, a 50 percent chance of being a carrier, and a 25 percent chance of being completely free of the defective gene.

The symptoms of cystic fibrosis may show up at birth or may not appear until adolescence. About 10 percent of babies are born with a plug in their intestinal tract which requires surgery, but this condition is not exclusive to cystic fibrosis.

Typically, children afflicted with the disease eat well but gain weight slowly and show signs of malnutrition because the fat in their foods is excreted from the body without being used; the pancreas has been prevented from releasing the enzymes necessary to digest fat, so digestive problems are common and stools are large and foul-smelling. In addition the patient usually has excessively salty sweat, a chronic cough accompanied by mucus discharge, rapid and difficult breathing, and fatigue and muscle cramps from salt loss. Sinusitis (inflammation of the air-filled cavities in the facial bones), nasal polyps (growths in the nose), and a barrel-shaped chest from overinflated lungs may also develop in some patients.

Many symptoms are indications of other, less serious, disorders, so unfortunately, cystic fibrosis cases often remain undiagnosed or undetected for some time while the disease progresses.

Diagnosis usually includes a physical exam, medical history, chest X ray, and sweat test to determine the patient's salt level. Most cystic fibrosis patients have excessively salty sweat, although salt level doesn't indicate the severity of the condition. Tests of the stool and digestive juices can show how well the pancreas is functioning.

Although cystic fibrosis cannot be cured, its symptoms can be relieved to some extent. Patients are advised to monitor their diet and health habits carefully: to reduce the fats in their diets; to eat very nutritious foods with high amounts of essential minerals and vitamins; to take salt tablets; to take pancreas enzyme tablets to aid digestion of fats; to take antibiotics, use aerosol mists, or receive vaccinations in order to fight specific respiratory diseases; to use mist tents; to exercise regularly; and to practice postural drainage (lowering the head below the chest) in order to help drain mucus from the clogged lungs.

There is no means of preventing cystic fibrosis today. Researchers continue to look for a reason why the defective gene causes mucus to become abnormal, as well as for a way to identify carriers of the gene. One new test may break some ground; it measures certain chemicals present in the amniotic fluid (the liquid that surrounds a fetus in the womb) so that an unborn baby with the gene can be identified. Meanwhile, scientific advances in this area have at least helped those afflicted to live more comfortably with the disease. Until the 1960s, few patients lived beyond the age of ten, but today those with cystic fibrosis can live to age 20 or 25 or beyond because of medical advances in managing the condition.

Cystitis

Cystitis is an inflammation of the urinary bladder; the term, however, is commonly used to mean bladder infection. Occurring in women much more often than in men, it is usually caused by bacteria that have invaded the urethra, the tube that transports urine from the bladder to the outside of the body, and entered the urinary bladder. Women are more susceptible than men because their urethras are so short (approximately one inch versus seven to eight inches in men), thus presenting less distance for the bacteria to travel. In addition, in women the external openings of the urethra, vagina (birth canal), and anus (intestine) are so close to each other that bacteria can easily migrate from one to another. Almost always the bacteria responsible are one of various types that normally live harmlessly in the human intestine, but which can contaminate or invade the area around the opening of the urethra and enter the bladder. Obstruction is also a common cause of urinary tract infection. When obstruction occurs, the bladder may not empty properly. The remaining urine in the bladder then creates a breeding ground for bacteria to multiply. Causes of obstruction can include tumors, stones, or an enlarged prostate gland (the male reproductive gland located at the base of the bladder surrounding the urethra).

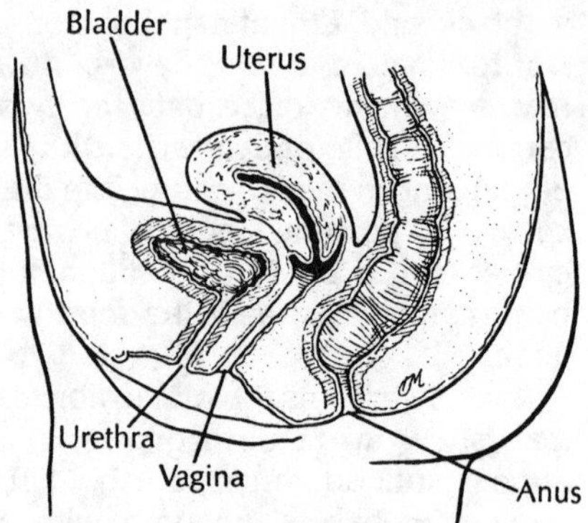

The female urethra is about one inch long, making it easier for infecting bacteria to invade the bladder.

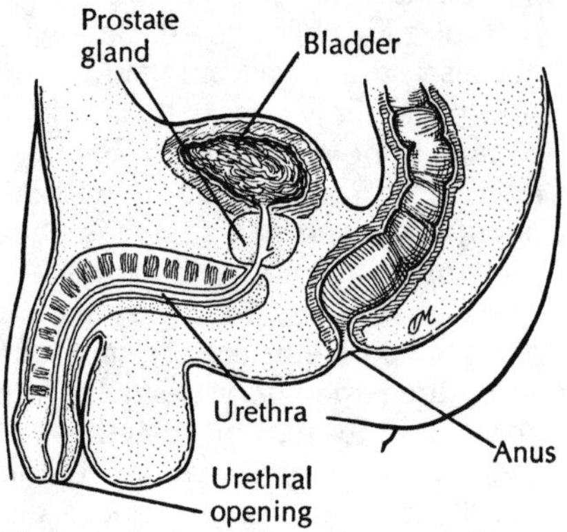

The male urethra is about seven or eight inches long, making a bacterial invasion of the bladder less likely than in a woman.

Besides blockage, the urethral lining may have a defect which allows bacteria to enter the tract. For example, frequent intercourse may traumatize the urethra, disrupting its lining and making it more susceptible to infection.

Cystitis in men is uncommon. When it does occur, the usual cause is an infection that has spread from an inflamed prostate gland or that has developed in the bladder because of an enlarged prostate. Bladder infections in men, unless from an obvious cause, usually require detailed evaluation such as a kidney X ray and possibly cystoscopy, an examination by means of a flexible lighted tube (called a cystoscope) inserted through the urethra.

Urethritis, an infection or inflammation of the urethra only, is common in both men and women and is usually acquired through sexual intercourse with an infected individual. Gonorrhea and nongonorrheal urethritis (in which the infectious agent, although acquired through intercourse, is different from that of gonorrhea) are the two most common examples of this. There are, of course, nonvenereal causes of urethritis also.

The symptoms of cystitis include a painful sensation or burning upon urination, a frequent and often urgent need to urinate (even awakening one at night), and occasional low back pain. These symptoms, along with bloody urine, are known as "hemmorhagic cystitis" and occur quite commonly in women. Although quite frightening, this is most often a minor, easily treatable condition. In men, however, bloody urine is not usually attributable to hemorrhagic cystitis and demands immediate investigation. With the exception of visibly bloody urine, all of the above symptoms can be present in urethritis which is also commonly accompanied by a discharge. High fever, chills, upper (usually one-sided) back pain with or without any of the above symptoms usually indicate a kidney infection (pyelonephritis) and demand the immediate attention of a doctor.

Along with the above symptoms and signs, the diagnosis of urinary infection rests on the urinalysis and culture. The presence of moderate to large amounts of white blood cells along with at least 100,000 colonies of any one bacterium in a culture, provides conclusive evidence of infection.

Not infrequently, it is difficult to determine which part of the urinary tract is infected, or if there is infection at all. In women, the opening of the urethra normally has some white blood cells and bacteria present. Therefore, in order to keep the urine specimen free from these contaminants, a midstream specimen is usually requested. The reason for this is that the first spurt of urine is thought to wash away the normal debris and the rest of the urine is now uncontaminated and provides a pure culture. For the vast majority of simple cystitis cases, this procedure is quite adequate; however, if a question exists as to the validity of the specimen or if for some reason the specimen must be absolutely free of contaminants, a catheter (thin, flexible tube) may be inserted into the bladder through the urethra. In women, this is an easy procedure and eliminates vaginal and/or anal (opening from the intestines) contaminants. If the catheterized specimen is free from pus and/or bacteria, the symptoms are of another condition—commonly vaginitis or urethritis. In a man, the procedure is somewhat more difficult and usually not necessary. If prostatitis is the suspected cause of the infection, the diagnosis is usually made by the physician inserting a gloved finger into the anus and directly feeling the gland. An infected prostate is usually quite tender and has a characteristic "boggy" feel. A specimen of prostatic fluid is usually obtained (by massaging the gland at the time of examination) through the urethra for culture.

Even with the above techniques, the differentiation between different sites of infection of the urinary tract is often not a simple matter and can have important implications as to treatment. The experience of the physician, the patient's history as to signs and symptoms such as discharge, recent intercourse, back pain, or fever, along with still more sophisticated diagnostic techniques all are important in making the correct diagnosis.

In difficult chronic cases of cystitis in both men and women, in which the cause of recurring infection may be an obstruction or drainage problem, contrast fluid may be placed into the bladder by means of a catheter and X-ray pictures taken of the bladder and of the urethra during urination. The X rays may detect narrowed portions of the urethra, stones, and incomplete emptying of the bladder (which promotes cystitis). The bladder might also be examined by means of a cystoscope — a flexible lighted tube inserted through the urethra. Most often these procedures are preceded by an intravenous pyelogram in which contrast material injected through a vein is eliminated by the kidneys, providing an X-ray picture of the kidneys, ureters (tubes from the kidneys to the bladder), and the bladder. From this anatomic abnormalities that increase susceptibility to urinary tract infection may be seen.

Treatment of first-time cystitis is by means of antibiotics by mouth for seven to ten days. Recently, large single doses of drugs have been found to work well in many cases. Recurrences may be treated in the same way if due to a different organism. If the same organism is causing the trouble, the condition may require larger doses of medication and/or treatment for up to four to six weeks. If the cystitis still persists, daily doses of medications may be necessary for up to six months. It is important that dosage instructions be followed exactly, because a person is vulnerable to a new infection or a reinfection of the same bacteria if the entire course of recommended drug therapy is not completed. Some individuals are prone to repeated episodes of cystitis or upper urinary tract infection. If an anatomic defect, such as a narrowed urethra, exists, dilatation (enlarging) may be needed. If stones are present, they may need to be removed surgically. If an infected prostate is the source of infection, antibiotics are usually tried first; surgery is a last resort. If no obvious reason for recurrent cystitis is found, the patient may be placed on low doses of antibiotics for long periods of time (this is called prophylactic—or preventive—therapy).

Women may be able to guard against recurrent cystitis by front-to-back wiping with toilet tissue and soap and water cleansing after each bowel movement. They should also try to urinate immediately after sexual intercourse to wash away infecting bacteria that might enter the urethra. Loose, absorbent underclothes allow evaporation and absorption of body fluids which help prevent infection. Both men and women should drink plenty of fluids and urinate frequently, completely emptying the bladder each time.

Cystocele

A cystocele is a protruding into the vagina of a portion of the urinary bladder. This is often a result of damage during childbirth of the wall of fibrous tissue that normally separates the vagina and the bladder. This may happen during the birth of a baby of any size. However, women who have never delivered a baby may also develop a cystocele. A cystocele may not appear until menopause, when the damaged or weak area weakens further, permitting the rear and base of the bladder to protrude into the vagina. At the same time, or separately, there may also be a bulging into the vagina of a portion of the rectum (final part of large bowel) or small intestine or urethra (the tube through which urine leaves the body). There may also be a prolapse of the uterus (in which the uterus drops through the vagina and in very severe cases protrudes from the vagina opening).

The bladder's protrusion into the vagina creates a pool of stale urine in the bladder which cannot be easily emptied and which becomes a breeding ground for bacteria. Cystitis (inflammation/infection of the bladder) with its symptoms of painful and difficult urination often results. A woman with cystocele may feel a fullness in the vagina and may find it difficult to empty her bladder completely (she may be able to do this by urinating a second time). However, many women with cystocele have no symptoms at all. Diagnosis is made by examining the inside of the vagina where a bulge can be seen in front of the cervix (the neck of the womb that protrudes into the vagina). Also, if a catheter inserted into the bladder after urination can draw out more than two ounces of left-over urine, a cystocele is definitely suspected. A special X ray in which dye is inserted into the bladder will reveal the bulged-out section of bladder.

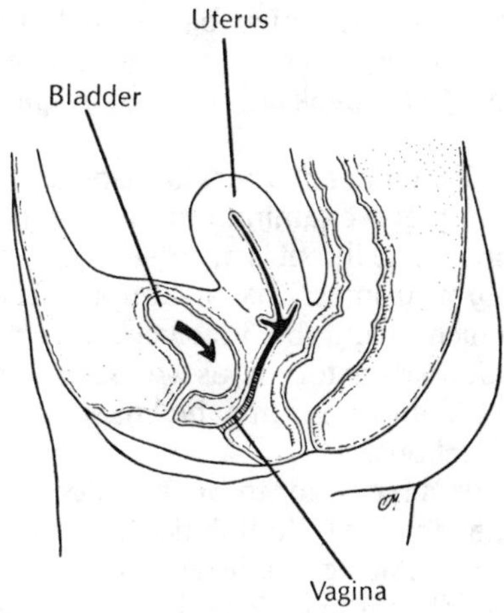

A cystocele is a protrusion of the urinary bladder into the vagina.

The preferred treatment for cystocele is surgery to repair the damaged wall and put the protruding section of bladder back in its original place. A pessary (a device inserted into the vagina to support the vagina and reduce the cystocele) may be used in women who refuse or cannot withstand surgery. A cystocele does not always require treatment. However, if frequent bouts of cystitis occur, some form of treatment will be necessary.

See also Cystitis, Prolapse, and Rectocele.

D

D and C

See Dilatation and curettage.

Deafness

Deafness is a term to describe complete or partial loss of the ability to hear. There are four main types of deafness.

Conductive deafness. This type of deafness is caused by a defect in the external or middle ear, which prevents normal transmission of sound. It may be present at birth as the result of an inherited defect, an accident in development, or an infection of the baby in the womb. It may be produced by an injury that perforates the eardrum or that breaks up the linkage of the three tiny bones – hammer, anvil, stirrup—that normally transmit sound from the eardrum through the middle ear to the inner ear. Inflammation of the middle ear, a condition known as otitis media, is another important cause of conductive deafness. Infection from an upper respiratory (breathing) tract ailment such as strep throat or flu can produce a buildup of pus in the middle ear so great that it ruptures the eardrum. Also, a plugged-up eustachian tube (the tube leading from the back of the throat to the ear) may trap fluid in the middle ear, creating temporary deafness. Conductive deafness in the middle and later years is most often caused by otosclerosis. In this inherited condition, new spongy bone grows over the stirrup bone, preventing it from vibrating when sound travels to it through the hammer and anvil bones.

Sensorineural deafness. Known, less accurately, as nerve deafness, this type of hearing loss occurs because of damage to the bony structures of the inner ear, to the auditory nerve carrying sound messages to the brain, or to the hearing center in the brain itself in the temporal lobe. It may be due to a head injury during birth, the effects of a woman's rubella infection on her unborn baby, a skull fracture affecting the inner ear or the auditory nerve, fever, bacterial or viral infections such as mumps or meningitis, tertiary (final stage) syphilis, Meniere's disease, cancers, multiple sclerosis, a hemorrhage or blood clot occurring in the inner ear, drug side effects, normal aging, prolonged or repeated exposure to intense noise, or edema (fluid buildup) caused by a thyroid deficiency. Most sensorineural deafness is not nerve deafness, the popular term for it. It is usually sensory deafness, caused by defects not in nerves but in the structure of the inner ear, especially in the fluid-filled cochlea and its organ of Corti which contains sensory cells that code sound waves into electrical impulses to be transmitted to the brain.

Mixed deafness. This is a combination of conductive and sensorineural deafness and is common.

Functional deafness. This form of deafness is that which occurs without any organic defect of the hearing system or of the brain.

People with pure conductive deafness simply need louder volume to hear all sounds. Those with defects in the inner ear can hear low sounds more easily than high sounds, and some sounds may be distorted. When there is damage to the temporal lobe, the hearing center in the brain, the person may be able to hear sounds, but has trouble recognizing them and understanding words (this problem can also occur with the other types of deafness).

Testing for hearing loss is important for all ages, but especially for infants. Many times, partial deafness in a baby is not discovered until the child fails to learn to talk — a direct result of the hearing loss. Babies who have been born prematurely or ill, or whose mothers had certain viral infections such as rubella during pregnancy, are in special need of testing. Although at present inborn hearing defects usually cannot be corrected, deaf children can be helped to deal with their handicap. Starting very early, they may be fitted with hearing aids, may be instructed in lipreading or sign language, and are taught to speak although they cannot hear.

When hearing loss is suspected, a complete examination of the ear, nose, and throat is necessary to identify any infections or abnormalities which might be involved. Infected adenoids or tonsils, as well as sinus or nasal infections may be linked to ear infections.

It is far easier to prevent deafness than to cure it. Antibiotics have made it possible to eradicate most of the middle ear infections that have been the major source of conductive hearing loss in children. Sometimes the middle ear problems are eliminated by treating allergies that cause the eustachian tubes to close up, or by removing infected adenoids. Nerve deafness caused by continued exposure to intense industrial noise, gun shots, rock music, or aircraft engines may be avoided by wearing ear plugs or other ear protectors. Some lost hearing may return after several months of relief from intense sound. Drugs that can cause hearing loss, including some antibiotics and certain diuretics (drugs that remove water from the blood), need to be used with care by medical personnel, and signs of hearing loss noted.

Surgery to correct conductive hearing loss includes middle ear operations to replace the stirrup bone or all three tiny bones with tissue or synthetic material, to repair a punctured eardrum, and to clean out a chronic middle ear infection.

A hearing aid can help to restore hearing loss in many people. It should only be purchased, however, after thorough testing of the hearing by a specialist in audiometry, who can advise on the need for a hearing aid and on the type to buy. Classes in lipreading and listening can also be helpful.

See also Ear infection.

Defibrillation

Defibrillation is a technique to correct the fibrillation of the heart, a disorder marked by very rapid disorganized twitching or trembling of the heart muscle in place of the normal beat. Fibrillation produces a condition called cardiac arrest, in which no heartbeat, pulse, or blood pressure can be detected. Death or permanent brain damage follows within a few minutes unless this condition is corrected, or unless first aid measures maintain blood circulation and breathing until help can arrive.

The most common cause of fibrillation of the heart is heart attack. When this happens, certain parts of the heart will start contracting independently of the normal heartbeat. Other causes of fibrillation are severe electric shock and prolonged exposure to extreme cold.

Correction is by means of an electric defibrillator. A pair of metal paddles is placed on the patient's chest and a single jolt of direct-current electricity from the defibrillator is directed into the heart to shock it back into its regular rhythm. The shock stops the independent action of individual muscle fibers and allows the natural pacemaker of the heart to take over again. Once the heartbeat is restored, other measures are taken. A drug such as lidocaine is injected to prevent further fibrillation. An intravenous tube is inserted to drip sodium bicarbonate (to neutralize acids in the blood) and defibrillating medication into a vein. A breathing tube is passed down into the lungs, attached to a mechanical pump that forces air in and out of lungs. Then the patient is taken to a hospital cardiac intensive care unit, where electric instruments constantly keep track of the patient's condition and sound an alarm if danger threatens. An electric defibrillator is close at hand if needed in an emergency.

Electric defibrillation is also used to restart a heart which has been stopped for purposes of heart surgery.

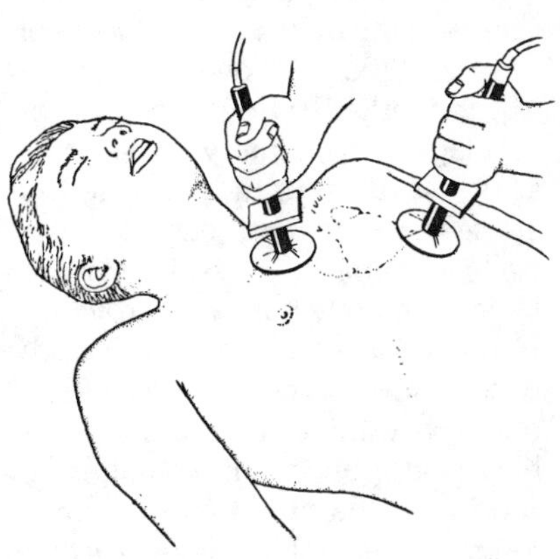

To correct fibrillation—the disorganized twitching or trembling of the heart muscle in place of its normal beat—a pair of metal paddles is placed on the chest, and a single jolt of electricity from the defibrillator is directed into the heart to shock it back into its normal rhythm.

Degenerative diseases

Degenerative diseases are conditions in which certain body tissue deteriorates, that is, changes to a less effective form. The change may be chemical or structural, or it may result from the deposit of an abnormal substance in body tissues. These changes may severely affect the normal functions of that tissue.

Certain degenerative diseases result from inherited deficiencies or defects. Others are produced by infection, disorders of the body's immune system, poisonous chemicals, or repeated injury. Many are associated with advancing age, with normal "wear and tear." Most can be helped by treatment but cannot be cured or reversed.

Among the most important degenerative diseases are the following:

- Osteoarthritis (degenerative joint disease), the most common form of arthritis especially over the age of 40, is marked by deterioration of cartilage in the joints, with resulting stiffness and joint pain. Many causes have been suggested, especially continued stresses over the years, but none has been proven.
- Multiple sclerosis, a progressive destruction of myelin, the fat-like outer covering of certain nerve fibers in the brain and spinal cord, produces many different symptoms of central nervous system disorder. The disease mainly strikes those in their 20s and 30s, continues over many years, and may be fatal. Its cause is unknown, but an immune system disorder is suspected, as are an inherited factor and an unknown virus.
- Atherosclerosis, or "hardening of the arteries," produces fatty, fibrous, calcium-topped patches on the walls of blood vessels—especially those feeding the brain and heart. Sometimes the patches—or plaques, as they are known—completely obstruct a blood vessel, and the tissue formerly nourished by the vessel dies for lack of oxygen. In the brain, the result is a stroke; in the heart, a heart attack. The dead brain cells and dead heart muscle are replaced by scar tissue—another degenerative change.
- Emphysema is a degenerative disease of the lungs. It is marked by destruction of the walls of many of the tiny air sacs (alveoli) in the lungs, and a ballooning out of the air spaces remaining, making the lungs less effective and breathing difficult. Recurrent inflammation of alveolar walls irritated by cigarette smoke, sometimes combined with an inherited enzyme deficiency, is the principal cause of emphysema. Emphysema is chronic and the leading cause of death from respiratory (breathing) disease in the United States.

See also Arthritis, Atherosclerosis, Emphysema, and Multiple sclerosis.

Dehydration

Dehydration is a condition in which the body or certain body tissues suffer from lack of water.

Tissue dehydration may occur in dry climates and during the winter heating season: extremely dry air causes the rapid evaporation of water from the skin and from the mucous linings of the respiratory (breathing) system. The results are discomfort and sometimes cracking of the skin, unless it is protected by natural lubrication or lotions, and increased susceptibility of the respiratory system to infections.

Dehydration of the entire body can be life-threatening. Illnesses that produce diarrhea and vomiting are common causes of dehydration, since both of these conditions expel excessive body fluids. Cholera, which results in extreme diarrhea and vomiting, can kill through dehydration. Other causes of dehydration include diabetes; kidney disease; excess diuretics (drugs which remove excess water from the blood); liver disease resulting in an accumulation of fluid in the abdominal cavity; inflammation of the abdominal cavity, resulting in fluid accumulation; and burns. Tissue beneath a burn swells with body fluid. If the burn covers much of the body, the buildup of fluid in burn tissue draws considerable water from the blood. This can decrease its volume so much that circulation to the outer parts of the body collapses. This is shock.

Symptoms of dehydration in addition to thirst include sudden weight loss; rough, dry skin; dry mucous membranes; rapid heartbeat and low blood pressure; lack of energy; and weakness. In an extreme case the patient is in shock, with pale skin; bluish lips and fingertips; rapid and shallow breathing; and a weak, rapid, irregular pulse. Blood tests reveal a thickening of the blood because of decreased water content.

Treatment of mild to moderate dehydration is to have the patient drink more water with some salt added. However, if the individual suffers from vomiting or diarrhea or is unconscious, it may be necessary for medical personnel to administer saline solution (salt water) intravenously (through the vein). The intravenous method is always used in severe cases of dehydration. The goal is to replace totally the lost fluid within 48 to 72 hours, together with the valuable mineral salts that have also been lost.

Delirium

Delirium is a confused mental state marked by disorganized or incoherent speech and hallucinations (imagined perceptions believed to be real). Often the person is unaware of time or place; is fearful, excited, and restless; and suffers from delusions. The heartbeat is rapid, the pupils of the eyes are dilated (enlarged), and sweating is common.

The condition can occur because of fever, disease, injury, poisons in the system, or mental disease. It may result from the sudden withdrawal of alcohol or another drug upon which the individual has become dependent; from liver, kidney, or heart failure; or from deficiencies in certain B vitamins or thyroid hormone. It can also be caused by pressure on brain tissue or a bruising or bleeding of brain tissue.

Delirium often develops rapidly and fluctuates in severity. The patient usually cannot remember what has happened during the delirious period and does not recall past events well. Depending on its cause, delirium may last from hours to weeks. Partial or complete recovery depends on the nature, severity, and treatability of the underlying cause.

Treating the underlying disease or condition is the first step in treating delirium. In the meantime, the patient should be cared for patiently and sympathetically in a quiet, relaxed, simple environment. Every effort should be made to keep the patient in touch with reality.

Deoxyribonucleic acid

See DNA.

Depression

Depression is a psychological condition characterized by prolonged sadness, combined with other negative mood symptoms, such as loss of interest in others, in work, and in recreation; indecisiveness and inability to concentrate; anxiety; apathy; loneliness; lowered self-esteem; and self-blame.

Deep sadness or depression is a normal reaction of an emotionally healthy person to discouraging life events such as loss, separation, death of a family member, and disappointment. It is probably a protective reaction, enabling you to withdraw from everyday concerns long enough to sort out your feelings and prepare yourself for a new approach to life.

Temporary depression can also occur because of normal chemical changes in the body. Two examples are premenstrual depression and postpartum (after childbirth) depression, both thought to be linked to female hormone activity. In addition, certain drugs, including oral contraceptives, reserpine (used to lower high blood pressure), alcohol, and some sedatives, may cause a side effect of depression in some people. Certain infections including influenza, viral hepatitis, infectious mononucleosis, and tuberculosis can depress one's mood, as can a deficiency of Vitamin B_{12}, an over- or underproduction of hormones by the outer layer of the adrenal gland, or various diseases of the nervous system.

Normal depression, which is a reaction to a specific disappointment or loss, is temporary. It can be helped by the support of family and friends or simply by the passage of time and by steps the person takes to change his or her life situation. Medication is not usually necessary, nor is any other treatment. However, a visit to a physician can provide valuable assurance that the depression is not abnormal.

Severe depression is another matter. Unlike normal depression, which is sometimes called *reactive* depression because it is a reaction to a specific circumstance, this disorder does not have an obvious cause. Also, the reaction is out of proportion to the seeming cause, and it may continue for weeks or months.

The causes of severe depression are unclear. Loss of a parent at an early age or growing up in a cold, critical, unstable, or unfriendly family setting may make it hard for a person to deal with life's losses and disappointments. A certain type of deepest depression, melancholia, may be caused by a chemical deficiency and is sometimes treated with the medication lithium carbonate. Finally, a small percentage of severe depression is linked to mental disease.

The symptoms of severe depression include crying spells, slow speech, agitation, hopelessness, helplessness, withdrawal from usual activities, recurring thoughts of death and suicide, and irritability. (Some of these symptoms also occur in moderate depression, to a lesser degree.) Early awakening, insomnia, fatigue, loss of appetite, weight loss or gain, loss of sexual desire, and imagined pains are also common. Depressed patients with certain mental diseases may hear voices accusing them of unpardonable sins, see visions of coffins or dead relatives, believe that others are watching or persecuting them, and suffer delusions that they are terribly worthless, sinful, or incurably ill.

Diagnosis of severe depression can be complicated. Some depression is "masked." The person is "smiling on the outside, crying on the inside" and may not even realize his or her depressed mental condition. Instead, the depression is expressed in physical symptoms, such as headaches or backaches that have no physical cause. In addition, the person may seem to have lost all emotion, including the ability to take pleasure in anything.

The examining physician needs to rule out any possible physical causes of the depression, such as that induced by disease, deficiencies, or medication. Drug abuse and alcoholism may be involved—but perhaps as results rather than causes of the depression. Schizophrenia and other mental disorders must be considered.

Sometimes periods of deep depression alternate with periods of elation, high hopes, grandiose ideas, and overactivity. This is known as a manic-depressive condition. When in the manic state, the person is overwhelmingly confident and inexhaustible, racing from thought to thought. Eventually, however, the mood changes to blackest despair.

Treatment for depression does not usually require hospitalization. Exceptions are those cases in which the patient is suicidal, in a stupor, agitated and out of touch with reality, or physically deteriorated as a result of the depression. Hospital treatment for the first three types of cases may involve treatment with drugs known as antidepressants or may include four to eight treatments of electroconvulsive therapy (ECT). In ECT, the patient is put to sleep with a general anesthetic and electric current is passed through the brain. This results in a seizure like that of epilepsy. After a brief period of drowsiness, the patient is often alert and in a clearer state of mind than before the treatment.

Most severe depression, however, can be handled out of the doctor's office with drugs, psychotherapy (counseling by a psychiatrist or psychologist, or preferably a combination of the two), with office visits once or twice a week at the beginning of treatment and fewer later if improvement occurs. It is extremely important to find professionals who are not only knowledgeable, but also reassuring and encouraging, as well as trusted by the patient. Elaborate psychotherapy over a long period of time is often not called for unless there is a serious personality disorder. If the depresssion is a secondary result of a serious physical illness, individual reassurance and support groups may provide the best help.

Lithium carbonate is used to treat manic-depressive illness both in its extreme form and its more moderate form, known as cyclothymia. In the latter type, the person alternates between brief periods (usually days) of gloom and elation.

Suicide is a major risk in depression and should especially be guarded against when the person seems to be recovering from the depression but is still feeling "low," when anniversaries of landmarks in the person's life occur, and in the days preceding menstruation.

Depression is the most common form of emotional disorder. It should not be disregarded and often can be reduced or eliminated with proper support and treatment.

See also Electroconvulsive therapy.

Dermatitis

Dermatitis is an inflammation of the skin. There are many different kinds of dermatitis, and a great variety of causes. Some of the more common varieties include the following.

Contact dermatitis. This is a skin inflammation caused by a substance that has touched the skin. This may be a harsh chemical or a detergent or soap that directly irritates. On the other hand, the substance may produce an allergic reaction that can appear five or six days after the contact or, less commonly, after years of repeated use. Common causes of allergic contact dermatitis are poison ivy, chemicals in shoes and clothing, metal watchbands and rings, antibiotic salves, and cosmetics. There are also cases in which a substance, such as a shaving lotion or cosmetic, produces a "photoallergic" reaction when the skin under the substance is exposed to sunlight.

Eczema. This inflammation of the skin is marked by blisters (when severe), redness, fluid in the tissue, oozing, scales, crusts or scabs, burning or itching, and sometimes dryness. There are several different forms of eczema. One of the more common types is atopic dermatitis. This is a continuing, itching skin inflammation whose victims often have a family history of allergic diseases such as asthma or hay fever. Typically, it begins in infancy, subsides by age three, and may reappear by age ten or 12. Foods such as wheat, milk, eggs, and substances such as pollen or fur often bring on symptoms and, if so, must be avoided.

Seborrheic dermatitis. This is a scaling and inflammation of the scalp and sometimes the face or other parts of the body. This is the cause of dandruff in adults and cradle cap in infants.

Nummular dermatitis. Coin-shaped patches of blisters that later ooze liquid and crust over mark this condition, which usually is accompanied by dry skin and itching. Most often it appears on the legs and sometimes the buttocks and trunks of middle-aged people.

Localized neurodermatitis. This condition is characterized by thick, sharp-bordered scaly breaks in the skin, with little blisters. This is a temporary condition caused by habitual scratching of an insect bite or other irritation of the skin and is corrected by covering the area and stopping the scratching. In the case of an itch in the area around the openings of the vagina and colon, however, warts, pinworms, hemorrhoids, infections, or certain diseases may be the cause.

Chronic dermatitis. This often occurs on the hands or feet, and may simply be the result of continued irritation, especially by contact dermatitis. It is marked by thickened skin, inflammation, and scaling. Sometimes it is caused by excessive hand washing and by soaps or detergents accumulating under rings. Fungus infections of the feet occasionally spread to the hands, producing inflammation.

Exfoliative dermatitis. This condition produces a shedding of skin all over the body, together with hair loss. The entire skin surface is red, scaly, and thickened. The cause is unknown in most cases, but it sometimes occurs following a lesser dermatitis or as a side effect of a drug. Hospitalization is frequently necessary because the condition can threaten life. A first step is to consult a doctor about stopping or changing all medications.

Stasis dermatitis. This stubborn skin inflammation of the lower legs is usually the result of poor blood supply to the area. There is redness, mild scaling, and a brown discoloration of the skin. If the condition is neglected, the skin swells and may become infected or affected by ulcers (eroded skin sores).

Because there is such a bewildering variety of skin diseases and because some can be dangerous if neglected, it is important to seek medical care for any dermatitis. In general, this care usually begins with very simple measures. Dry skins need lubricating agents, while moist or oily skins require powders or other drying substances. Inflamed skin is treated with soothing creams; cool, wet dressings; or baths.

Hardened dried skin may be peeled off with strong substances. If possible, the cause of the dermatitis is sought out with the patient's help and eliminated. Cortisone creams are often used to make the patient more comfortable by reducing inflammation, although continuous use is not usually recommended. Antibiotics are employed promptly to eliminate any infections that arise, before they can spread to other parts of the body. Patients need to resist the constant temptation to scratch itchy areas or remove scabs, because that can simply prolong and even worsen the trouble. In addition, while cleanliness is desirable, some patients need to be told to reduce hand washing and the number of baths they take, because they are washing away natural oils designed to protect the skin. Along the same lines, patients should not use more medication than the doctor recommends, or leave it on longer than directed. Overmedication of skin diseases is worse than undermedication.

See also Contact dermatitis.

DES

DES (diethylstilbestrol) is an artificial (man-made) estrogen (female sex hormone) used to treat a variety of disorders.

The drug was popularly prescribed to prevent miscarriage from the early 1940s until it was found to be ineffective and was banned for this use by the Food and Drug Administration in 1971. It is now linked to an increased incidence of adenocarcinoma—a rare cancer of the glandular cells of the reproductive organs—in daughters of the several million women who took DES to prevent miscarriage and other pregnancy complications. Recently, testicular cancer in male offspring was also associated with maternal DES use.

Although experience has shown that the chance of developing a malignancy is small, children exposed to DES before birth run a higher than average risk for benign (noncancerous or precancerous) growths and for structural changes involving the reproductive organs (vagina, cervix, and uterus in women; penis, testicles, and urinary tract in men) as well as for infertility problems. These abnormalities usually appear after puberty, generally in the late teens to early 30s, years after the exposure.

Because of these potential problems, DES should not be taken by a woman who is pregnant or suspects that she is pregnant. DES may be used safely in nonpregnant women to treat a variety of disorders including certain vaginal conditions and estrogen deficiency that may occur at menopause or after the surgical removal of the ovaries. DES may also be used as a post-coital contraceptive (the so-called "morning-after pill"). Since DES is a hormone that may produce a variety of effects on the body, its use must always be supervised by a physician.

Recently, DES has been shown to be effective in some patients in reducing the growth of advanced prostate cancer in men and certain forms of breast cancer in both sexes.

Although the incidence of serious

complications is small, physicians strongly advise that individuals who were exposed to DES because it was taken by their mother should be routinely examined to detect any developing abnormalities.

Detached retina

A detached retina is a condition in which the retina separates from its attachment to underlying tissues in the eye. Normally, the retina – the delicate, light-sensitive lining of the inner eyeball—is firmly attached to an underlying structure called the choroid. If fluid collects between the retina and the choroid, the retina may partially or totally detach. Fluid from the vitreous cavity – the fluid-filled space within the eye—may penetrate beneath the retina because of a small hole in the retina. Fluid leaking out of certain blood vessels in the eye may also penetrate beneath the retina to cause detachment.

Cataract surgery, severe myopia (nearsightedness), and injury can cause retinal detachment. Although injury can be the primary cause of this condition, it is more likely to accelerate a detachment that has already begun. Conditions that increase susceptibility to retinal detachment are inflammation or tumors of the eye, high blood pressure, and vitreous hemorrhaging.

Symptoms of detachment—at the onset – include seeing floating dark spots or flashes or streaks of light, or experiencing a blurring of vision. As the condition progresses, a curtain or veil seems to fall over part or all of the field of vision.

The detached retina can be treated by using a laser to fuse the retina to the choroid. It can also be treated through the use of diathermy (repair using heat), cryotherapy (repair using extreme cold), or microsurgery (surgery using a microscope). Left untreated, the detachment will enlarge and can, in extreme cases, lead to the loss of sight.

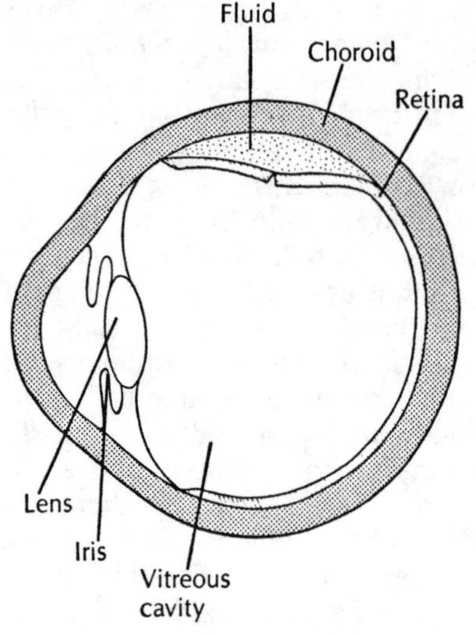

A detached retina is a condition in which the retina separates from its attachment to underlying tissues in the eye. Normally, the retina—the light-sensitive lining of the inner eyeball—is firmly attached to an underlying structure called the choroid. If fluid collects between the retina and the choroid, the retina may partially or totally detach. Fluid from the vitreous cavity may penetrate beneath the retina because of a small hole in the retina. Fluid leaking out of certain blood vessels in the eye may also penetrate beneath the retina to cause detachment.

Diabetes mellitus

Diabetes mellitus, often called sugar diabetes, is a condition in which the body is unable to process properly carbohydrates (sugars and starches), which are the body's major source of energy.

Normally, digestion causes these carbohydrates to release a form of sugar called glucose into the blood.

As the blood glucose level rises, the pancreas gland located in the upper abdomen is stimulated to secrete the hormone insulin. Insulin acts to reduce the sugar content in the blood by transporting glucose from the blood to body cells where it is used for fuel or to the liver where it is stored until needed for fuel.

When the pancreas produces insufficient insulin or the body cannot use the insulin it manufactures, diabetes results. Sugar concentrations accumulate in the blood as glucose circulates throughout the body without being absorbed. Eventually, the kidney filters sugar from the blood, and urine (the fluid mixture of water and waste products) carries the excess blood sugar from the body.

There are two major forms of diabetes. Type I, or insulin-dependent, diabetes results from a defect of unknown origin in the islets of Langerhans, the part of the pancreas that produces insulin. This form of diabetes can develop in very young children.

With Type II, or insulin-independent, diabetes the pancreas functions adequately, but the body is unable to use insulin efficiently. Sometimes, a shortage of insulin-receptor cells (sites throughout the body where interaction of sugar and insulin occurs) allows the insulin to float in the bloodstream without working properly. Obesity often contributes to the problem as excess fat cells displace insulin-receptor cells.

Since Type II appears most often in adults over the age of 40, this form may evolve from a gradual slowing of insulin production within the pan-

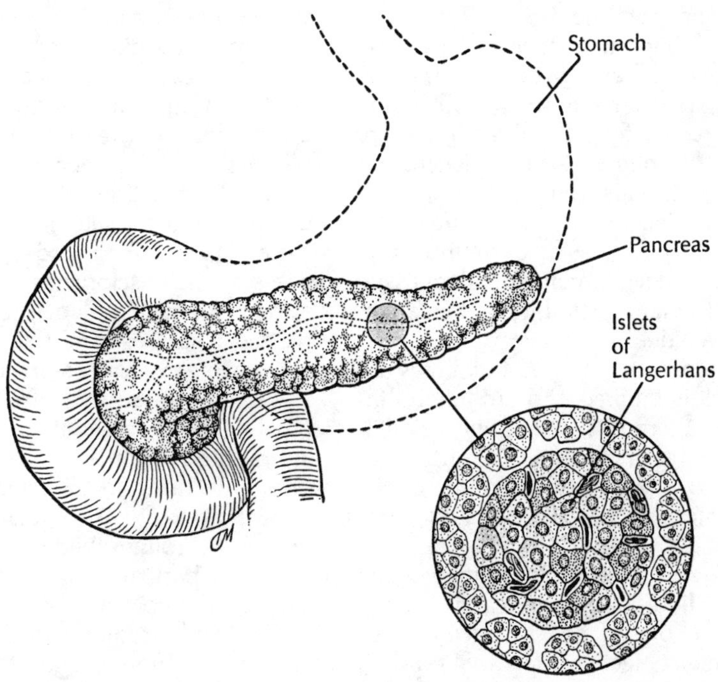

The islets of Langerhans in the pancreas secretes insulin, the hormone that helps the body cells absorb sugar for fuel. One type of diabetes may result from a defect in the islets of Langerhans, causing decreased production of insulin.

creas. In addition, other disorders of the endocrine system (glands that secrete hormones into the bloodstream) may cause hormonal imbalances that disturb insulin-sugar regulation.

Research shows that people who have Type II diabetes in their families have a greater tendency to acquire the condition. Women are more likely to be affected, but chances of developing Type II for all adults doubles with every decade past 40 years.

In some women, pregnancy triggers diabetes. The disease usually subsides after childbirth. However, women who show signs of diabetes during pregnancy and deliver babies weighing over ten pounds have a greater risk of diabetes later in life.

Even though patients with diabetes can usually control the condition, untreated diabetes can lead to serious complications. Extremely high blood sugar levels place great strain on other organs. Diabetes may trigger atherosclerosis, hardening and narrowing of arteries that carry blood throughout the body. Insufficient blood supply contributes to heart attack; stroke; kidney disease; eye disorders, such as retinopathy; impotence; gangrene, death of tissue due to inadequate blood circulation; or even death.

Symptoms of Type I diabetes are excessive thirst and urination, fatigue, altered vision, fainting, irritability, and slow-healing cuts and bruises. Weight loss may occur despite constant hunger and voracious eating.

The same symptoms may signal Type II diabetes, or no symptoms may show at all. Physicians frequently detect this form when they perform routine examinations or tests for other problems.

Should no symptoms be obvious, doctors can diagnose diabetes by analyzing blood and urine samples for elevated sugar concentrations. They may also test blood for extra insulin and urine for excess ketones. Ketones are the end products of breaking down fat for energy. Since people with diabetes do not use sugar normally, their bodies burn fat for fuel and eliminate the ketone end products in the urine.

Both forms of diabetes mellitus require a treatment plan that maintains normal steady blood glucose levels. Once blood sugar levels are under control with insulin injections, diet, or medication, a person with diabetes can usually lead a normal life.

Type I, or insulin-dependent, diabetes requires injections of insulin to regulate blood sugar levels evenly all day. If blood glucose concentrations rise, the body may signal an imbalance by displaying symptoms of weakness, fatigue, and thirst. These symptoms mean that increased insulin is needed. However, if blood sugar levels become too low, an insulin reaction sets in, causing dizziness, hunger, fatigue, headache, sweating, trembling, and—in severe cases — unconsciousness. A quick remedy for this problem is to eat simple sugar, such as candy.

Ideally, a doctor can prevent these fluctuations of sugar levels by coordinating the type and timing of insulin injections with meal content and energy output. A special diet is important to balance daily insulin injections. Young children with diabetes, in particular, need sufficient calories to grow and develop normally. Insulin requirements for persons with Type I diabetes differ widely among individuals. Some patients may maintain balanced blood sugar levels with one insulin injection taken before breakfast. Other patients may require several insulin injections per day. Furthermore, insulin requirements may change as the patient grows older, undergoes surgery, becomes pregnant, or develops another unrelated illness.

Most people with Type II, or insulin-independent, diabetes can regulate their condition by proper diet. Sometimes, oral antidiabetic drugs, which work by stimulating the pancreas to produce more insulin, may be prescribed. However, there is some evidence that these drugs may be no more effective in controlling diabetes than diet alone. In addition, some investigators feel that these drugs may increase the incidence of death caused by cardiovascular diseases; however, this has not been fully proved.

A controlled diet is critical for diabetes control. Overweight individuals need to lose weight. Thereafter, emphasis is on eating balanced meals that will sustain recommended weight. Fats need to be limited to reduce chances of atherosclerosis, and the diet should be low in simple sugars. The diet should include plenty of fibrous roughage, such as is contained in fruits, vegetables, and whole grains; fiber in the diet has been shown to reduce or slow sugar absorption in the digestive tract. Your doctor can provide a medically approved diet plan with food exchanges that allow flexibility with regular family meals and dietary needs.

With either type of diabetes, follow-up is important to plan diet, determine changes in insulin dosage, and retest blood and urine for blood sugar levels. Careful control of blood sugar levels can enable a person with diabetes to lead a normal life.

See also Ketosis and Retinopathy.

Dialysis

Dialysis is the removal of wastes and other undesirable substances from the blood by means of a membrane that is selective in what it allows to cross. In the healthy body, this task is performed by the kidneys. In a patient suffering from temporary or permanent kidney failure, however, this can be done with an artificial kidney machine and is known as hemodialysis. Two plastic tubes, one connected to an artery and one to a vein, are implanted in the patient's arm or leg. During dialysis, which can take three to five hours per treatment, blood from the artery tube enters the machine and comes into contact with a thin, (commonly cellophane) membrane. Wastes from the blood pass through the membrane into circulating fluid on the other side. The blood cells themselves, along with other protein elements, are not allowed across the membrane. The cleaned blood is then piped back into the patient through the vein tube.

Another method is called peritoneal dialysis. Here, the individual's own peritoneum (lining of the abdominal cavity) is used as the membrane. A sterile plastic catheter (tube) is passed into the abdominal cavity and a solution of glucose (a sugar) and mineral salts is periodically injected into and withdrawn from the cavity. The fluid comes into contact with delicate blood vessels in the peritoneum. Because of the difference in concentration of certain elements in the blood and the fluid, fluids and wastes from the blood are caused (by complex biologic principles) to pass through the peritoneal membrane wall into the dialysis liquid, which is withdrawn and replaced by a new liquid. The passage of material from one side of a membrane (the blood side) to the other (dialysis fluid side) is based on the same principles of the above mentioned hemodialysis.

A new method called continuous ambulatory peritoneal dialysis has greatly lowered the cost of dialysis and made it more convenient. It can be done at home by the patient without the complex equipment and the skilled supervision that has made machine dialysis so expensive. A tube is surgically implanted in the patient, just below the navel. About every four to five hours and just before bedtime, the patient empties a bag of fresh dialysis fluid into the abdominal cavity through the tube and drains out the old fluid. This insures that fluid remains in the cavity, soaking up waste from the blood, while the patient sleeps or goes about usual daily activities. The procedure takes about 30 minutes each time but enables the patient to be independent and mobile.

See also Kidney failure.

Diaphragmatic hernia

Diaphragmatic hernia (also called hiatus hernia) occurs when a portion of the stomach protrudes above the diaphragm, the muscular wall separating the chest and abdominal cavities, into the chest. Normally, the esophagus (the passageway from the throat to the stomach) passes through a tight muscular collar that prevents the stomach from squeezing up into the chest cavity. However, if the collar is too large or relaxes, a *sliding hiatus hernia* may occur. When sliding hiatal hernia exists, pressure in the abdominal cavity, perhaps caused by obesity, pregnancy, tight clothing, bending or other position changes, coughing, or straining causes the top part of the stomach to slide (herniate) through the opening. Along with the stomach, a pouch of the peritoneum (lining of the abdomen) also protrudes through the opening. This condition is very common, especially in women and older people, and seldom causes trouble or needs correction.

However, there is a second, relatively uncommon, dangerous type of diaphragmatic hernia known as a rolling or paraesophageal hernia. In this type, the junction of the esophagus and stomach retains its normal position (unlike a sliding hernia) while a portion of stomach along with part of its peritoneum rolls up (through the opening in the diaphragm) alongside the junction. The danger here is that the herniated section may become trapped in the chest with its blood supply choked off, thereby causing death of stomach tissue. Bleeding is also a common complication. Although dangerous, this condition causes no symptoms (such as heartburn) and is usually found by accident on X rays taken for other purposes. The only symptom, if occurring at all, is usually a sense of fullness in the chest after eating. Because of the potential complications of the paraesophageal hernia, many authorities recommend surgery, even in the absence of symptoms. This is exactly opposite to the recommended treatment for the sliding hernia where surgery is reserved for only the most severe cases.

Surgery for the paraesophageal hernia involves entering the abdomen and pushing the herniated portion of stomach back into its proper position while removing the hernial

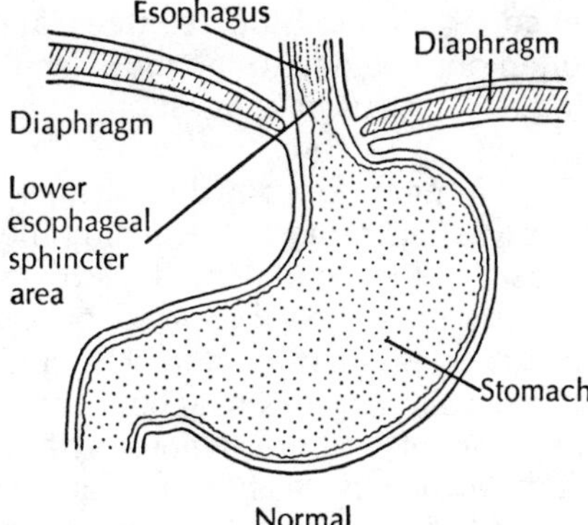

Normal

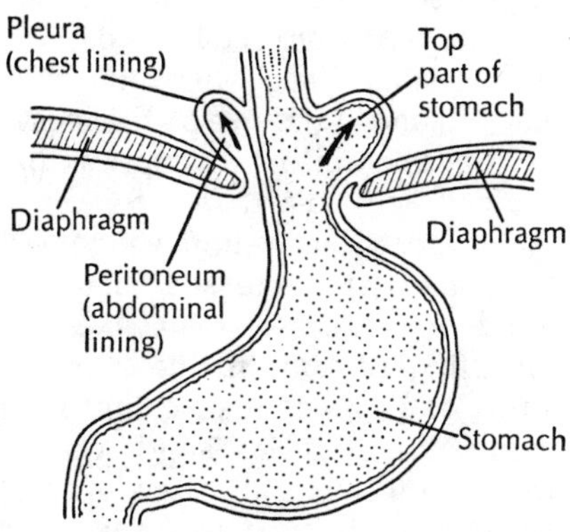

Sliding hernia
(entire gastroesophageal junction
moves upward)

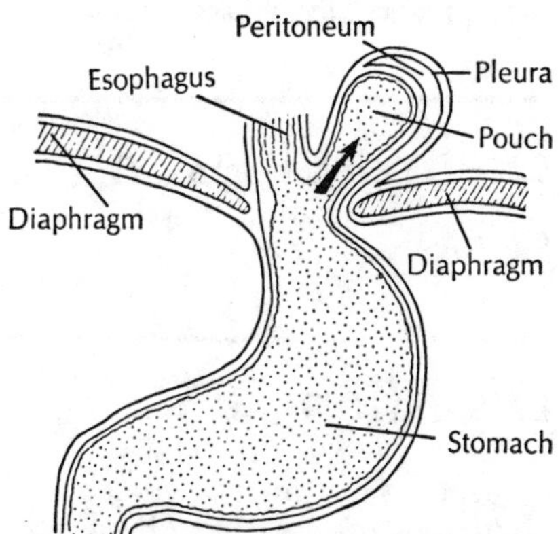

Paraesophagel (rolling) hernia (gastro-esophageal junction is in normal location)

A diaphragmatic hernia occurs when a portion of the stomach protrudes above the diaphragm, the muscular wall separating the chest from the abdomen. The two primary types are a sliding hernia and a paraesophageal hernia shown here.

sac of peritoneum around it. After this, the muscular collar of the diaphragm is tightened by stitches. Surgical treatment of the sliding type is much more varied, but in general is aimed at restoring functional ability of the lower esophageal sphincter (the muscular valve that keeps stomach contents from regurgitating upward).

Until recently it was believed that a sliding hernia in and of itself caused the stomach to regurgitate food containing harsh stomach acid into the esophagus, producing the symptom of heartburn. Heartburn is a burning sensation perceived in the chest, usually in the area underneath the breastbone. It can occur at any time, particularly after eating and is usually made worse by reclining or belching, or by increased pressure in the abdomen. It is now believed that the presence of diaphragmatic hernia alone does not cause heartburn. Heartburn and regurgitation result from a loss of functional ability of the valve (the sphincter) at the bottom of the esophagus.

See also Heartburn.

Diarrhea

Diarrhea is abnormally frequent and excessively liquid bowel movements. This is often the body's defensive attempt to rid itself of irritating or toxic substances. It is a symptom that accompanies many disorders, both mild and serious.

There are two basic types of diarrhea: acute (or short-term) diarrhea, the more common form, which comes on quickly and usually lasts no more than two or three days, although it can last as long as two weeks; and chronic (or long-term) diarrhea, which may also appear suddenly but lingers for many weeks or months with symptoms either constantly present or appearing and disappearing.

Both acute and, particularly, chronic diarrhea can become a serious problem because of the excessive loss of body fluids and salt (called dehydration) as well as loss of nutrients. It may also be a symptom of a disorder such as inflammatory bowel disease (Crohn's disease, ulcerative colitis).

The reasons for the consistency of the stool in diarrhea are complex. In an infection, the intestine may pour out massive quantities of fluids and salts in response to a bacterial toxin (poison) or other irritant. In inflammatory bowel disease, protein, blood, and mucus are lost through the inflamed lining of the colon, taking large quantities of water along. Other disorders speed up the normal movement of the colon, thereby not allowing time for absorption of fluids. Yet another type of diarrhea is caused by poor absorption of a type of sugar (called lactose), which draws fluid out of the colon. Finally, many diarrhea conditions are combinations of these biologic mechanisms.

Other causes of diarrhea include changes in the diet, drugs taken for other disorders (particularly antibiotics which upset the bacteria balance of the intestine), stress and food allergies.

The symptoms often experienced with diarrhea are the characteristic loose and frequent bowel movements as well as nausea, cramps or pain in the abdomen, gassiness, fatigue, and fever.

Diagnosis of the cause of this problem will require a report to the doctor concerning the patient's normal diet, emotional state, and recent changes in the daily habits. In addition, a sample of the bowel movement may be examined for color, consistency, odor, chemical content, and presence of blood. Stool cultures are often done to determine the offending microorganism if infection is suspected.

Treatment for diarrhea usually involves removing or correcting the cause of the condition. If diarrhea lasts for more than three days or is a recurring problem, a doctor should be consulted, as this may be a warning sign of a more serious illness. Antidiarrhea medications can be prescribed for particularly bothersome or persistent diarrhea, but these are to be used only with caution, particularly in some infections where they may prolong the course of the illness.

The discomfort of occasional bouts of acute diarrhea, however, is usually treated with simple remedies: adequate rest; increased intake of liquids to replace lost fluids; a diet consisting of light meals, perhaps soups or broth at first, eaten more frequently; and, as solid food is added to the diet, the avoidance of irritating foods such as bran, fruits and vegetables, fried foods, coffee, and alcoholic beverages.

See also Crohn's disease, Dehydration, and Ulcerative colitis.

Diethylstilbestrol

See DES.

Digestion

Digestion is the process whereby the body converts food into basic substances that can either be absorbed in the bloodstream as nutrients or passed out of the body as waste. This breakdown and assimilation occurs within the digestive tract, a convoluted tube over 30 feet long lined by a mucous membrane that aids in absorbing nutrients. The tract includes several hollow organs — mouth, esophagus, stomach, small intestine, and large intestine (colon) — each of which has a specific function in digestion. Muscles of these organs move the food through the system while mucus lubricates the tract and prevents irritation. Solid organs—the liver, gallbladder, and pancreas—also are critical in digestion.

Food first enters the digestive tract through the mouth. In the mouth, the jaw and teeth chew the food into smaller pieces that are mixed with saliva, a secretion of the salivary glands in the mouth. Saliva moistens food for easier swallowing and contains an enzyme (a special protein) that begins breakdown of starches.

From the mouth, food passes down the throat and into the esophagus, (a muscular tube) through which it is conducted to the stomach. The stomach is a large pouch or sac in the abdominal cavity where food is combined with acid and digestive juices secreted by gastric glands within the stomach. The food becomes semifluid so that it can pass into the small intestine.

In the first ten inches (duodenum) of the small intestine, food is broken down further with additional digestive juices from the liver and pancreas. This process further separates nutrients and allows for their absorption into the bloodstream, which takes place in the remainder of the small intestine.

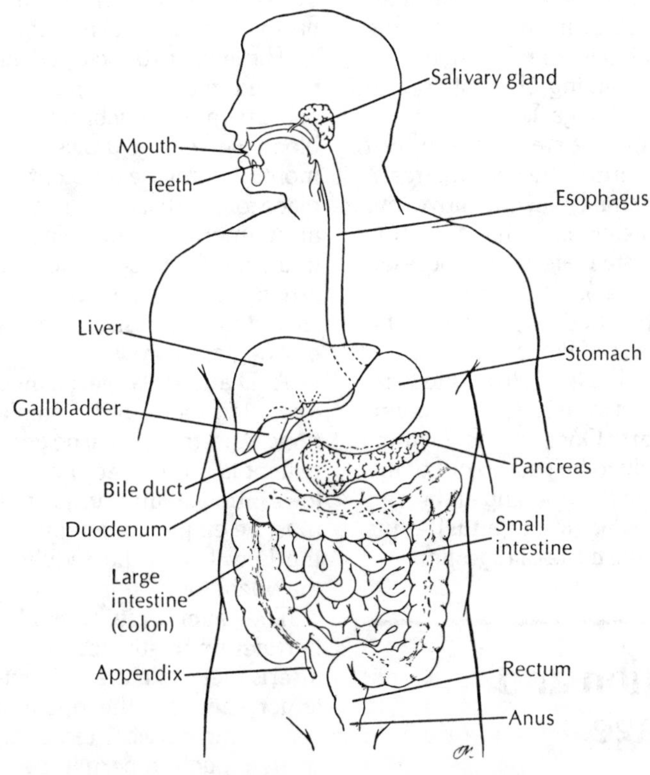

The digestive system includes the mouth, esophagus, stomach, small intestine, large intestine, liver, gallbladder, and pancreas, each of which plays a specific role in digestion.

Aiding digestion is the liver, an accessory organ of digestion. The liver produces bile that is necessary for absorption of fat in the small intestine. The liver also functions to purify and remove some wastes from the blood, as well as to produce and store glucose and to process many drugs.

The gallbladder on the underside of the liver is another organ that provides an indirect digestive function. The gallbladder stores the bile manufactured by the liver. As bile is needed, the gallbladder contracts and releases the fluid into the small intestine.

Other digestive juices required by the small intestine to digest and absorb food, particularly fats and starches, come from the pancreas, an organ located just under the stomach. The pancreas also secretes insulin and other hormones into the blood. Insulin is the hormone responsible for aiding absorption and use of glucose (sugar).

Whatever substances are not assimilated into the bloodstream through the small intestine move into the large intestine. Within the large intestine, waste material is processed into stool (feces). At this point, too, water is absorbed to preserve the body's balance of fluids.

The left colon then stores the fecal matter until its transfer to the rectum, its lower part. Once in the rectum, waste is ready to be passed out of the body through the opening at the end of the digestive tract (anus), thus completing the cycle of digestion.

Dilatation and curettage

Dilatation and curettage, also called a D and C, is the surgical scraping of the lining of the uterus after the cervix (neck of the uterus) has been dilated (expanded). This minor procedure is often done to diagnose disease of the uterus (such as cancer) or to correct extreme or prolonged bleeding. It is also used to perform an abortion and may be employed after a miscarriage (an involuntary expulsion of an unborn baby—before it is able to live on its own — from the uterus) to remove any remains of tissue, thus lowering the risk of hemorrhage and infection. Dilatation alone may be performed to enlarge the passageway out of the uterus. This might be done in the case of a severely narrowed cervix to eliminate painful menstruation caused by restricted flow of menstrual fluid. For treatment of this problem, multiple dilatations may be necessary since the cervix will often again become narrow after several months.

The lining to be scraped, known as the endometrium, consists of a mucous membrane richly supplied with blood vessels. It grows anew each month to provide a potential nesting place for a fertilized egg and forms an attachment to the placenta that nourishes the baby-to-be. If no fertilization occurs, the endometrium is shed during menstruation and a new one begins to grow.

A D and C is performed in an operating room under sterile conditions. Anesthesia may be general (the patient is put to sleep) or local. The lower bowel and urinary bladder must be empty; an enema (to empty the bowel) may be required before the operation.

The patient rests on her back with her feet up in stirrups. The surgeon inserts metal dilators of progressively larger sizes into the opening of the cervix, the cervical canal, until it is open enough to permit the insertion of the surgical instruments. An alternate method of cervical dilatation employs a small tube of dried seaweed that is left in the cervical canal for eight to 24 hours. As the seaweed absorbs moisture from the cervical canal, it expands and enlarges the canal.

A curette, a scraping instrument designed for this purpose, is used to remove endometrial tissue. Special forceps may also be used to remove tissue.

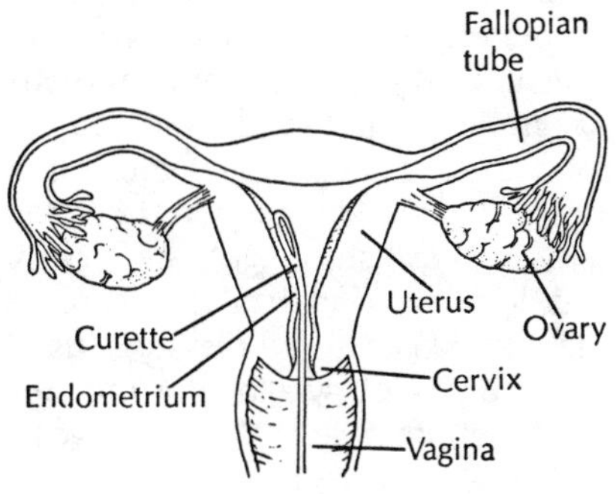

Dilatation and curettage (D and C) is the surgical scraping of the lining (endometrium) of the uterus after the cervix has been dilated (enlarged). The procedure is done with a curette, a special scraping instrument.

The principal risks of a D and C are hemorrhage, infection, and perforation (puncture) of the uterus. The latter is more possible during pregnancy because the uterus is especially soft and thin at that time.

When the operation is finished, an absorbent pad is placed over the entrance to the vagina. Following the operation, the pad is checked every 15 minutes for two hours, and excessive bleeding reported to the physician.

Mild painkillers should be enough to control discomfort from the operation. If there is pain in the abdomen that cannot be relieved in this way, or that is continuous or sharp, it should be reported immediately. Some difficulty in urinating may be expected immediately after the procedure.

In most cases, the patient stays in bed for one to two hours following surgery but then may resume normal activities. Most women return home several hours after the operation or the next day. Many daily activities can be resumed immediately, and in a week all normal physical activities may be resumed. Sexual intercourse should not be attempted, however, until after the next visit to the doctor, when the doctor can determine if and when sexual relations can be resumed.

Diphtheria

Diphtheria is a sudden, severe, and highly contagious disease that primarily affects the tonsils, upper airways, and larynx (voice box) and is marked by formation of a membrane on the infected tissue. Complications can include inflammation of the heart (myocarditis), sometimes resulting in heart failure, and temporary neuritis (nerve inflammation). Diphtheria-type bacteria also infect skin wounds, but cannot invade intact skin.

Diphtheria is caused by a bacterium known as *Corynebacterium diphtheriae,* which is transmitted through the air or otherwise on droplets of moisture from the throats and noses of infected persons. It is most common during the colder months when schools are in session and people are in closer contact. Frequently, the bacteria are transmitted by carriers — people who have no symptoms and do not even know they harbor the disease. The incubation period (the time between exposure to the infection and appearance of the first symptom) is only one to seven days. Diphtheria bacteria destroy the outer layer of the mucous membrane of the throat or larynx;

the slush of dead cells, bacteria, and white blood cells remaining coagulates to form the membrane that is the chief sign of the disease.

Symptoms include a mild sore throat, hoarseness, a rasping cough, pain on swallowing, and a mild fever. Children may be nauseous, vomit, and have chills and headache as well as fever and other symptoms. The membrane that forms is typically tough, adheres tightly, and causes bleeding if removed. It appears in patches and can vary from yellowish to grayish green or dirty gray (the most common color). Some people have little or no characteristic membrane. If the membrane extends from the throat to the trachea (windpipe), larynx, or bronchi (air tubes in the lungs), it can become detached and obstruct the passage partially or completely, choking off the air supply. Signs of this life-threatening emergency are rapid breathing, shrill breathing sounds, and blue lips and fingertips. A narrowed air passage is also caused by edema (swelling of fluid-filled tissue) in the lining of the larynx and throat.

Treatment is with diphtheria antitoxin (a solution of refined and concentrated protective antibodies taken from the blood of horses that have been immunized against the poisons created by the diphtheria bacteria). This should be done at once, after a skin test to determine that the patient is not allergic to horse serum (blood fluid). (A patient who is found to be allergic is desensitized with great caution by a series of diluted doses of antitoxin.) After the antitoxin is given, antibiotics such as penicillin or erythromycin are given for at least a week to eliminate the diphtheria organisms. The patient remains isolated (no visitors) until two cultures (24 hours apart) of the nose, throat, or other involved area indicate that the infection is gone.

Because of the possible severe or even fatal complications of diphtheria, patients with symptoms need to be placed in a hospital intensive care unit for complete rest and careful attention. There must be constant observation for signs of airway obstruction, along with access to facilities for performing an immediate tracheostomy (creation of a hole in the neck to breathe through), to pass an air tube down into the lungs and to supply oxygen as needed. Frequent checking of the heart and nervous system is needed to identify complications. In severe cases, these can include heart irregularities, cardiac arrest (heart stoppage), and early and late nervous system disorders such as swallowing difficulty caused by paralysis of swallowing muscles due to inflammation of their nerves.

Those who have been close contacts of the patient and who have not been immunized should receive throat cultures and be immunized with vaccine. These people should be watched carefully for the development of symptoms and be given antitoxin should symptoms occur. Another approach is to give antitoxin immediately (after allergy is excluded). In people who have been immunized, a booster of vaccine will be sufficient. All contacts of patients with diphtheria should have cultures done of their nose, throat, and/or open wounds. Carriers of diphtheria should be given seven to ten days of an appropriate antibiotic (usually erythromycin) and recultured. If the organism is still present, another course of drug therapy is given. If this fails, tonsillectomy may be needed.

Fortunately, widespread immunization has made diphtheria a rare disease. To maintain this status, children should be immunized in a series of shots beginning in infancy.

See also Immunizations.

Diverticulitis

Diverticulitis is the inflammation and/or infection of little sacs or pouches (diverticula) that have ballooned out through the walls of the colon (large intestine). The pouches form when the inner lining of the colon is forced under pressure through weaker spots in the colon's muscular layer. The existence of the pouches (as a condition, not a disease) is referred to as diverticulosis.

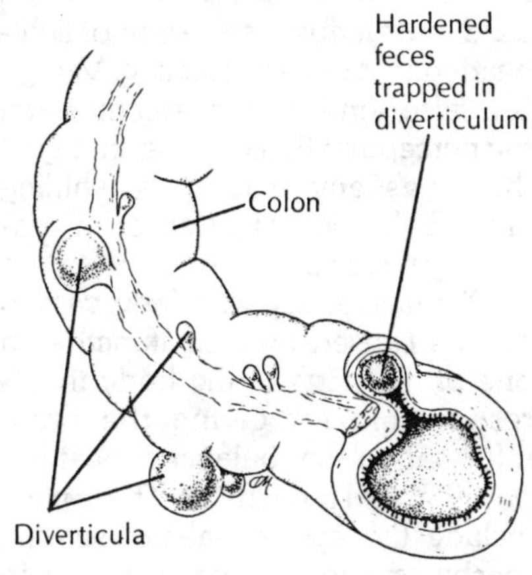

Diverticulitis is the inflammation of the small pouches (diverticula) that have ballooned out from the colon wall due to the condition called diverticulosis. The inflammation often develops when a mass of hardened waste material (feces) becomes trapped in a diverticulum, reducing the blood supply to the pouch wall and making it more susceptible to infection from bacteria in the colon.

Diverticulosis may be present in about one third of the people over 60 in the United States, and both its incidence and the frequency of complications increase with age. One theory as to the cause of diverticulosis is that abnormal movement of the colon (possibly because of too little bulk in the diet) produces intense pressure that forces intestinal lining through the weak spots in the muscular layer. Most people with simple diverticulosis have no symptoms. Occasionally, however, a pouch next to a blood vessel may ulcerate, causing it to bleed. If the vessel is an artery, severe bleeding can result, seen as bleeding from the anus (the exit of the colon). Shock and possible death may result if the condition is not treated.

It has been estimated that about one fifth to one fourth of the people with diverticulosis may develop the symptoms of diverticulitis. Diverticulitis develops when a mass of hardened waste matter (called a fecalith) forms in a pouch and reduces the blood supply to the thin walls of the pouch (by means of pressure against the wall), making them more liable to infection by the bacteria of the colon. The inflammation that follows can lead to perforation, abscess (an enclosed sac of pus around the perforation), or infection of the lining of the abdominal cavity (peritonitis). Not infrequently, the inflamed section of bowel attaches to the urinary bladder or vagina, burrowing out from the colon to create a fistula (channel) that leaks infection into the other organ. Repeated inflammation can cause thickening of the wall of the colon, narrowing the colon and causing partial or sometimes total obstruction.

Symptoms include intermittent cramping pains and tenderness, usually in the lower left abdomen but sometimes in other areas of the lower abdomen in which case the pains may resemble those of appendicitis. Pain that worsens during urination may indicate that the inflamed colon is attached to the bladder. Stool (feces) and/or air in the urine may indicate a colon-to-bladder fistula. Constipation or constipation alternating with diarrhea is common. Fever is usually present with acute attacks.

The diagnosis of diverticulitis usually is made if there is a history of pain in the left lower quadrant (quarter) of the abdomen accompanied by fever and a change in bowel habits. A physical examination may reveal a mass in the left lower quadrant along with extreme tenderness. After the acute episode has subsided, the examining doctor may insert a proctoscope (a lighted tube) through the anus and up the colon to see if there is any evidence of cancer that might be causing the symptoms. A barium (X-ray contrast fluid) enema and X ray is usually done to further rule out cancer of the colon and to locate diverticula, obstructions, and fistulas.

Treatment of severe diverticulitis begins with bed rest in a hospital and intravenous (in the vein) feeding with nothing by mouth (to give the intestine a rest). Antibiotics are given if there is fever or other evidence of an infection. If peritonitis (inflammation and/or infection of the lining of the abdominal cavity) develops, it may be necessary to operate. The inflamed section of the colon may simply be cut out and the remaining sections joined, or, more often, a temporary colostomy (in which the colon empties through an opening in the abdominal wall to the outside) may be necessary. Later, after all inflammation and infection has subsided, this is reconnected to the remaining colon or rectum.

A diet with plenty of bulk appears to be a way to avoid diverticulosis, the pouching that precedes diverticulitis. Those people who have developed diverticulosis should eat a relatively high-fiber diet. Supplements, such as psyllium, which increase bulk, may be recommended to move the stool through the colon at a normal rate.

See also Colostomy.

Dizziness and vertigo

Dizziness and vertigo are sensations of disorientation and distorted perception. Occasional episodes are not serious, but recurrent dizziness or vertigo can be symptoms of a variety of disorders, particularly those involving the eye, ear, or nervous system.

Dizziness and vertigo are sometimes confused with one another. Dizziness is an uncomfortable, distorted, or unsteady sense of the environment; the word *dizziness* is often used to describe a sensation of lightheadedness or a faint feeling. Vertigo is a false sense of movement, often the perception that one is spinning or that one's environment is whirling around. Vertigo is often accompanied by nausea.

Dizziness and, particularly, vertigo can be caused by a malfunction in one of the parts of the body that is responsible for giving the brain information on balanced posture, position, and movement. These parts include the eye, a balance-sensing mechanism in the ear, and certain areas of the brain. Thus, balance can be disturbed by any injury, impairment, or disorder involving the eyes, ears, and certain areas of the brain, as well as the nerves leading to these areas. A wide variety of problems such as injury to the head, ear infections, and migraine headaches can display dizziness or vertigo as their symptoms. Also, occasional mild upsets to the body can cause dizziness (but usually not vertigo), including such harmless factors as being overheated, overtired, tense, or nervous, as well as standing up too quickly after lying or sitting for some time.

Dizziness is characterized by feelings of unsteadiness, swaying, lightheadedness, weakness, faintness, and, at times, nausea and vomiting. Vertigo is marked by feelings of spinning and may be associated with unsteady walking; a tendency to veer to one side while walking and, in severe attacks, falling down; paleness; sweating; and continuous rapid eye movement.

Simple cases of dizziness can be easily avoided. Getting up slowly after lying or sitting, leaving overheated rooms to get some fresh air, eating a balanced diet, and getting adequate rest should all help to prevent common episodes of dizziness. Recurrent dizziness, however, should be investigated.

True vertigo, on the other hand, may be a sign of physical disease that can range from an inflammation of the balance mechanism in the ear (labyrinthitis) to a brain disorder. Frequently, however, no cause will be found, and the vertigo is treated symptomatically with drugs. In all cases, any episode of true vertigo should be reported to a physician.

DNA

DNA (deoxyribonucleic acid) is the basic building block of chromosomes, the microscopic bodies in cells that hold the genetic information that determines the characteristics of the cells. Each human cell has 46 chromosomes, which together contain the hereditary "blueprint" for the entire person and instructions for operating that particular cell. The blueprint or instructions in each chromosome comprise the "genetic code." The code is contained in DNA, an amazingly long, thin, spiraled, ladderlike structure made up of six compounds. Two of the compounds are a sugar and a phosphate, which form the sides of the ladder. Each rung is made up of a pair of two of the other compounds. The composition of these rungs and the order in which they follow each other determine the genetic makeup of the chromosome.

Each strip of DNA containing the instructions for a particular characteristic, such as blood type A, blond hair, or brown eyes, is known as a gene and may be made up of hundreds or thousands of rungs on the DNA ladder. The DNA within each chromosome may contain thousands of genes, each of them a portion of a ladder containing tens of millions of rungs.

When the cell, in the process of growth, divides itself, the DNA ladder splits apart down the middle; each side of the ladder then forms a duplicate of itself on the other side to create a complete new ladder.

In a somewhat similar fashion, sections of the DNA ladder split apart to direct body functions, such as the creation of a chemical the body needs to repair a cell. In this case the half-ladder combines with each of its complementary chemicals, except for one substitute, to create a new strand known as ribonucleic acid, or RNA. RNA is much like DNA except that it is only one side of a ladder. The RNA strip made from DNA is known as "messenger" RNA because it carries a code of instructions, travels to another part of the cell and acts as a template (like a mold or pattern) to form the chemical substance the body needs.

See also Chromosomes and Genes.

Down's syndrome

Down's syndrome is a congenital (present at birth) disorder characterized by moderate to severe mental retardation and a variety of physical abnormalities.

Down's syndrome is caused by an error in the fertilized egg before it divides. Normally, each cell in the human body has 46 chromosomes—the genetic "blueprints" that determine the characteristics of the person and that carry instructions for performing all body processes. The cells in someone with Down's syndrome, however, have an extra chromosome, for a total of 47. This difference, in ways yet unknown, causes all of the unusual characteristics of Down's syndrome. In 95 percent of cases, the condition is called trisomy 21 (because the extra chromosome is attached to the 21st pair of chromosomes), and the mistake is one that apparently could happen to anyone. In 5 percent of cases, the syndrome is called a translocation, and the defect apparently is inherited.

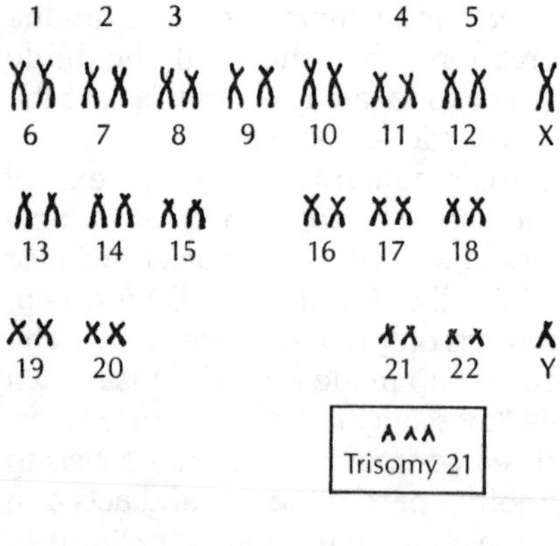

Normal chromosomal makeup of the human cell is 23 pairs (22 pairs plus a pair of the sex chromosomes—X or Y) as shown is this diagram. In a person with Down's syndrome, however, there is an extra number 21 chromosome (trisomy 21, as shown in the box) resulting in a total of 47 chromosomes. This extra chromosome is responsible for the collection of symptoms known as Down's syndrome.

Down's syndrome (also called mongolism) is marked by somewhat slanted eyes in small sockets; a small, short head, flattened in back and front; a nose flattened at the bridge; a thick tongue; short hands, feet, neck, trunk, arms, and legs; a single rather than a double crease across the top of the palm; flabby arms and legs, with poor muscle tone; a wide gap between the first and second toes; retarded physical and mental development, with an average IQ of about 50 but ranging up to 80; and various deficiencies throughout the body. A child with Down's syndrome also usually has a poorly functioning thyroid gland (which regulates metabolism, the rate at which the body uses energy) and pituitary gland (which regulates other glands including those responsible for growth, maturation, and reproduction). About one third are born with heart defects, and both the skin and mucous membranes are especially susceptible to infection.

Despite these handicaps, children with Down's syndrome are known for their sweet and lovable dispositions. Slower to walk, talk, and learn, Down's syndrome children can benefit from attending special nursery schools and play groups for retarded boys and girls. Most can attend public school in classes for the mentally trainable mentally handicapped; some can handle the work in classes for the educable mentally handicapped and eventually can perform at about the third-grade level. When they become adults, they will not be able to live independently but may be able to hold a simple, routine job, perhaps in a sheltered workshop.

Prospective parents can reduce their chances of having a Down's syndrome child by starting their families early. A 20-year-old mother has only one chance in 2,000 of producing a child with Down's syndrome, while at age 35 the chance is one in 300, at age 40 is one in 100, and at age 45 is one in 40 live births. The age of the father also has some bearing on the risk, but not as much as the mother's age. Diagnosis of Down's syndrome can be made between the twelfth and thirteenth week of pregnancy, by testing samples of amniotic fluid that surrounds the unborn baby and contains cells shed by the baby.

Drowning

See Emergency first aid section at the end of this book.

Dysmenorrhea

Dysmenorrhea is the term for painful menstruation. It occurs most commonly in teenagers and in women who have never been pregnant.

There are two types of dysmenorrhea. Primary dysmenorrhea is a recurring condition usually beginning shortly after the onset of menstruation in a young girl. Secondary dysmenorrhea develops later in life after a woman has been menstruating for some time.

The cause of primary dysmenorrhea is thought to be the release of prostaglandins (substances which stimulate uterine contractions) from the lining of the uterus shortly before a menstrual period begins. The resulting contractions will constrict blood vessels in the uterus, causing pain in the same way that a decrease in blood supply to the heart results in chest pain. The reason for this excessive production of prostaglandins is not known. Secondary dysmenorrhea is usually secondary to—that is, a result of—other reproductive problems, such as fibroid tumors, a narrow cervix, or endometriosis (the displacement of tissue from the lining of the uterus to the outside of the uterus).

The major symptoms of both types of dysmenorrhea are cramps or pain in the lower abdomen, possibly extending around to the back. Nausea, vomiting, diarrhea, headache, fatigue, and nervousness are mainly associated with primary dysmenorrhea. These symptoms usually appear at the beginning of or slightly before the menstrual period, and may last several hours or several days.

Diagnosis will include a complete physical exam as well as medical and menstrual histories. If the symptoms are present from the onset of menstruation at puberty, primary dysmenorrhea is usually the diagnosis. If symptoms have appeared suddenly in a woman who has menstruated for some years, secondary dysmenorrhea can be assumed and further diagnostic evaluation of the reproductive organs may be necessary to determine the disorder that is causing the dysmenorrhea. Ultrasound examinations, in which sound waves bounce off internal structures forming a visual image of them, or X rays may help in determining the underlying disorder.

Dysmenorrhea is not a serious condition, but it can be annoying, uncomfortable, and even incapacitating. Since secondary dysmenorrhea usually indicates that another affliction is present, treatment should always be sought for this condition.

Recently, primary dysmenorrhea has been treated successfully with nonsteroidal anti-inflammatory drugs (including ibuprofen, naproxen sodium, meclofenamate sodium, diflunisal, and mefenamic acid) which, when taken just before a period is to begin, act to suppress the release of prostaglandins and thereby reduce the contractions that are causing pain.

Secondary dysmenorrhea is treated by correcting the problem that is causing it; for instance, endometriosis can be treated with hormone therapy or surgery, thus relieving the source of the dysmenorrhea.

Home remedies often help to ease menstrual pain and relieve pressure. These include a hot water bottle or heating pad placed on the abdomen; hot baths; and lying on the back with the knees bent. Also, interestingly, childbirth may relieve dysmenorrhea problems, possibly because of the enlargement of the cervix (mouth of the uterus) or destruction of some nerve fibers in the uterus.

See also Premenstrual tension and Prostaglandins.

Dyspareunia

Dyspareunia is difficulty or pain for a woman during sexual intercourse. This may be caused by a resistant hymen (the membrane that partially or completely covers the opening to the vagina); or inflammation or injury of the vagina, urethra (the urinary tube), vulva (the lips and other structures around the opening to the vagina), or the anus (the opening of the large intestine). It can be the result of scar tissue forming around an episiotomy (a surgical cut to enlarge the opening of the vagina before childbirth) or surgery to repair the vagina. Other organic causes include tight muscles in the area around the vagina, an "hourglass" contraction of the vagina, a divided vagina, inflammation of the cervix (the neck of the uterus), prolapsed (fallen) uterus, infected fallopian tubes (which lead from the ovaries to the uterus), and endometriosis (in which bits of tissue from the lining of the uterus grow outside the uterus on various organs in the pelvic cavity, including the ovaries and fallopian tubes).

Inadequate lubrication of the vagina is a common cause of dyspareunia, as is an unconscious tightening of the vaginal muscles—perhaps the result of fear, unreadiness, or unwillingness to perform the sex act, or other psychological reasons. Improperly fitted or improperly lubricated birth control devices (condoms or diaphragms) and an allergy to contraceptive spermicides are other causes.

Treatment for dyspareunia is correction of any underlying disease, injury, or structural defect if such a problem exists. For some couples, psychological or psychiatric counseling is helpful in removing psychological barriers to sexual intercourse that may result in dyspareunia.

Water-soluble lubricating jelly (*not* petroleum jelly), obtainable in any drugstore, provides a good vaginal lubricant. Estrogen creams can be used along with water-soluble jelly to restore lubrication to a dry vagina after menopause. Soothing anesthetic creams and temporary avoidance of intercourse can relieve the soreness of dyspareunia.

Dyspepsia

See Indigestion.

Dyspnea

Dyspnea is a sensation of "air hunger." It is usually accompanied by difficult, labored breathing and discomfort. Dyspnea is a symptom that occurs in many different diseases. It may be caused by lack of oxygen being delivered to the tissues, as in severe anemia; by failure of the heart to keep up with the needs of the body, as in heart failure; as well as by extreme exercise.

Dyspnea may be the result of obstruction of the airways, such as the narrowing of air passages that occurs in asthma, or by restricted capacity of the lungs, as in chest deformities. Emphysema (in which many of the lung's small air sacs have been weakened or destroyed) is also commonly associated with dyspnea. It can also occur because of fluid in the lungs, as in pneumonia or congestive heart failure. Here, the access of oxygen into the air exchange units of the lungs (known as alveoli) is blocked by the fluid, thereby preventing oxygenation of the blood.

A nighttime form of dyspnea is called paroxysmal nocturnal dyspnea, in which the patient awakens gasping for breath and can only breathe by sitting up or standing. Usually this is caused by congestive heart failure.

Another type of dyspnea is psychogenic (originating in the mind) or hysterical hyperventilation (excessive breathing), caused by anxiety. This excessive breathing leads to exhaling too much carbon dioxide, which makes the blood too alkaline. This produces light-headedness, numbness and tingling of the hands and toes, and sometimes fainting. (Breathing into a paper bag restores the carbon dioxide balance.) This condition is harmless.

Signs of dyspnea include noisy breathing; an anxious, distressed expression; dilated nostrils; gasping; protruding abdomen; expanded chest; and blue lips and fingertips.

Treatment involves treating the condition causing the dyspnea, including the anxiety responsible for psychogenic hyperventilation.

See also Anemia, Asthma, Congestive heart failure, Emphysema, and Pneumonia.

E

Ear infections

The ear, which is responsible for both hearing and the body's sense of balance, can become infected in any one of its three parts—the inner ear, middle ear, or outer ear. However, most commonly, ear infections settle in the middle ear. The medical term for middle ear infections is otitis media.

Ear infections are much more likely to affect children than adults; those most susceptible range from ages six months to six years. Children who contract ear infections in their first year are more likely to have chronic (long-term) ear infections later in life, and by the age of eight, almost every child has had at least one ear infection.

Inner ear infections are rare, but they may result from middle ear infections and can lead to permanent ear damage. The inner ear has two parts: the labyrinth, the semicircular canals that act as the organs of balance; and the cochlea, which converts sound into nerve impulses and transports them to the brain.

Outer ear infections are basically skin infections, are seldom serious, and can be treated by cleaning, sometimes, with antibiotic or steroid ointments or drops. The outer ear includes the pinna (the visible ear), and the outer ear canal.

Middle ear infections usually clear

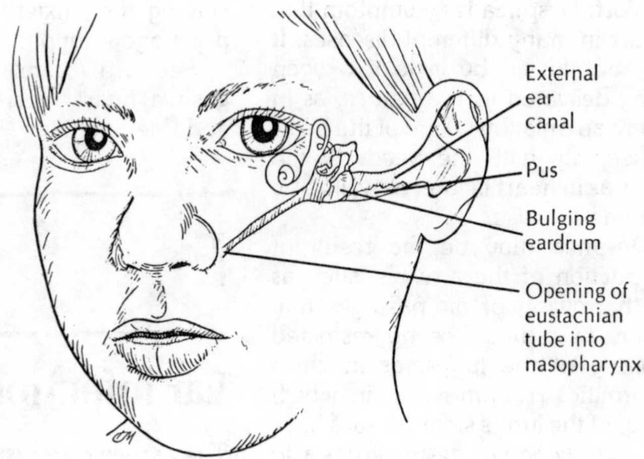

A middle ear infection may cause the eardrum to bulge out and even rupture. In the event of a rupture, pus may leak into the outer ear canal. A middle ear infection may follow a nose or throat infection that migrates to the middle ear through the eustachian tube.

up quickly, but the more serious or persistent infections can lead to a variety of serious complications: temporary or permanent hearing loss, infection of the semicircular canals in the inner ear, facial paralysis, brain abscess, meningitis (infection of the covering of the brain), and infection of the mastoid bone, located behind the pinna. The middle ear includes the eardrum and the three tiny bones — the hammer, anvil, and stirrup — that vibrate and convey sound into the inner ear.

Middle ear infections develop when viruses or bacteria in the nose or throat travel to the ear through the eustachian tube, which connects the middle ear to the nose and throat. The middle ear also can become infected when infection spreads from a severe outer ear infection or injury.

Middle ear infections can be recognized by severe throbbing pain in the ear; fevers up to 104° or 105° F (101° or 102° F in adults); hearing loss; and possibly dizziness, nausea, vomiting, or sore throat. Eardrums may bulge out or may even burst, oozing blood and pus into the outer ear and relieving the pain. Symptoms may worsen over hours or days. A child too young to talk may seem ill or feverish or may pull on an ear, indicating an infection.

Ear infections are diagnosed by an inspection of the eardrum. If it is red and swollen or bulging out, middle ear infection can usually be confirmed.

Middle ear infections are usually quickly eliminated when they are treated with an antibiotic, often a form of penicillin, as well as with, at times, decongestants. If a virus infection is present, however, antibiotics are not used, since viruses do not respond to antibiotics. If the eardrum is bulging out and the pain is severe, the doctor may make a small cut in the eardrum (called a myringotomy) to relieve the pressure. If the eardrum bursts, the outer ear must be kept clean to prevent infection from spreading.

Improved antibiotics have lessened the need for surgery, but the infected tissue, in rare cases, may need to be surgically removed. However, it should again be emphasized that this is seldom necessary because of modern, improved antibiotics.

Ear, nose, and throat

The ear, nose, and throat are interconnected, and for this reason they are often grouped together in the field of medicine. Because they are joined, infection in one structure may spread into one of the others.

Ear. The ear is the organ of hearing consisting of three parts: the external ear, middle ear, and inner ear. The pinna, or external ear, traps sound waves and directs them into the ear canal through the eardrum into the middle ear.

In the middle ear, sound waves vibrate through three tiny bones called the hammer, anvil, and stirrup. Vibrations continue into the inner ear, where the cochlea transforms the sound waves into nerve impulses. These impulses then travel to the brain through the auditory nerve.

A eustachian tube in the middle ear connects the ear with the nasopharynx, the upper part of the throat opening into the nose. This tube allows air pressure in the middle ear to equalize with pressure outside the body, thus helping to prevent a ruptured eardrum. However, the eustachian tube also provides a passageway for infecting microorganisms to enter the middle ear from the nose or throat.

Besides functioning as the organ of hearing, the ear also provides signals to the brain about the position of the body. Semicircular canals (or labyrinth) within the inner ear serve as the organ of balance by detecting motion of the head and feeding this information to the brain.

Nose. The nose is a specialized structure with two nostrils, or external openings. The nose serves dual functions as organ for the sense of smell and as an entry to the respiratory system.

When the nose works as the organ of smelling, nerve receptor cells within the nose detect odor and transmit signals to the brain through the olfactory nerve. The sense of smell also enhances the sense of taste. The ability to smell is more refined than the ability to taste; therefore, when a cold blocks nasal pas-

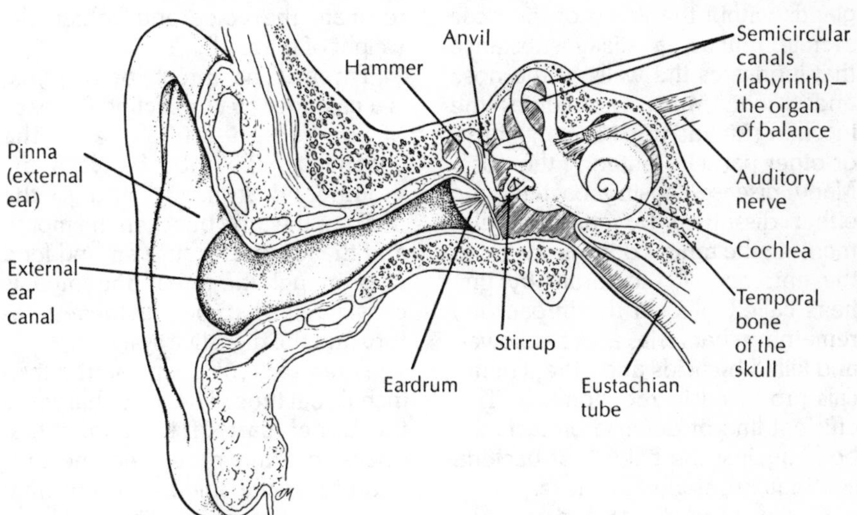

The ear is a complex structure that is responsible for the sense of hearing and for the body's sense of balance.

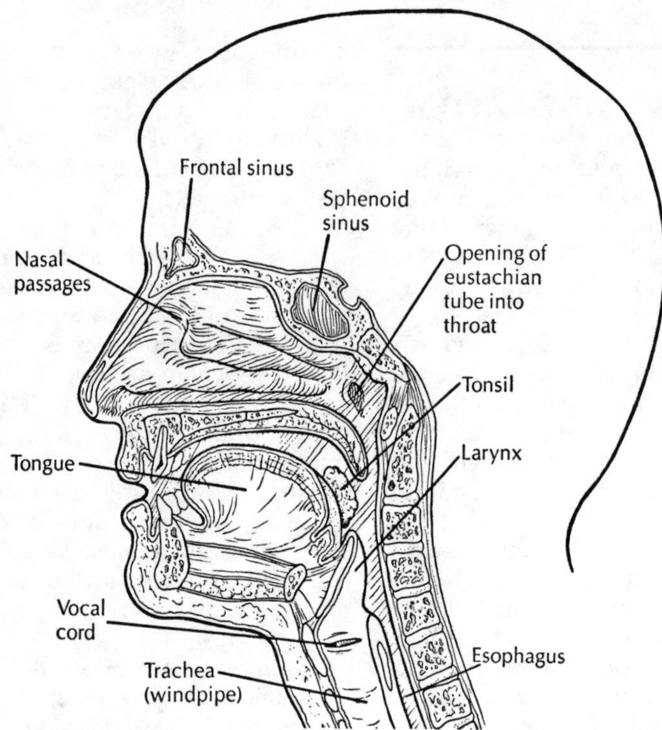

The ear, nose and throat are interconnecting structures.

sages, food may seem bland and tasteless.

As an organ of breathing, the nose moisturizes incoming air and filters out any foreign materials. Small glands within the lining of the nose secrete mucus, a sticky substance that lubricates the walls of the nose and throat. Mucus humidifies the incoming air and traps bacteria, dust, or other particles entering the nose. Many disease-causing bacteria are either dissolved by chemical elements in the mucus or transported to the entrance of the throat by tiny hairs called cilia. In the throat, any remaining bacteria are swallowed and killed by acids and other chemicals produced in the stomach. This efficient line of defense protects the body against the billions of bacteria continually entering the nose.

Connected to the nose are sinuses. Sinuses are cavities lined with mucous-secreting glands and filled with air located in certain facial bones. There are four groups of sinuses—frontal, sphenoid, ethmoid, and maxillary. Their purposes are to resonate the voice and lighten the weight of the skull.

Throat. The throat, or pharynx, is a passageway connecting the back of the mouth and nose to the esophagus, the tube between the mouth and stomach, and to the trachea, the tube between the mouth and the lungs. Because air and food pass through the throat, the throat is considered a part of both the respiratory and the digestive systems.

Three sections comprise the five-inch throat tube. The nasopharynx is the upper part of the throat that opens into the nose, and the oropharynx is the middle portion that opens into the mouth. The lower section of the throat, or laryngopharynx, connects the other sections with the larynx, or voice box.

Within the throat are two small tissue masses called tonsils. Tonsils help fight disease by destroying bacteria that enter the throat. This can be a formidable task, since disease can easily spread from the nose and ears to the throat.

Echoviruses

See Coxsackie viruses.

ECT

See Electroconvulsive therapy.

Ectopic pregnancy

Ectopic pregnancy is a pregnancy in which the fertilized egg develops outside the uterus. Usually it occurs in either of the two fallopian tubes which each extend some four-and-a-half inches from the ovaries (egg-producing organs) to the uterus and through which the egg travels from the ovary to the uterus. In that case it is also known as a *tubal pregnancy.* However, on rare occasions the pregnancy starts to develop in the ovary, on the cervix (neck) of the uterus, or attached to the outside of a nearby organ in the abdominal cavity. (The ovary is not directly connected to the fallopian tube. There is a slight gap between them, which sometimes permits an egg to escape into the abdominal cavity.)

The usual cause of an ectopic (out of place) pregnancy is an obstruction or narrowing of the fallopian tube that prevents the egg from passing

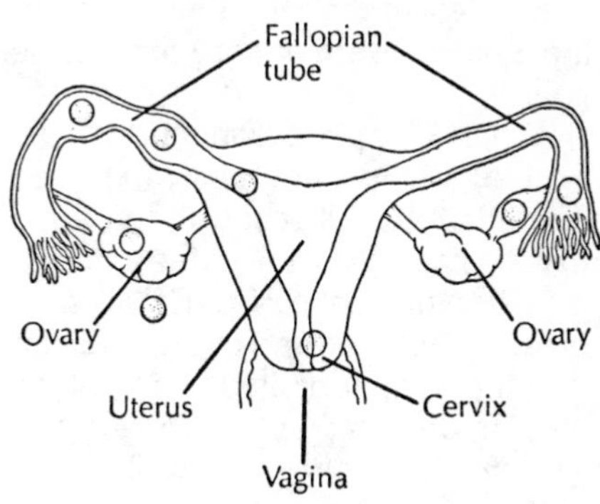

An ectopic pregnancy is one in which the fertilized egg develops outside the uterus, most often in the fallopian tubes, but also in the ovary, on the cervix, or attached to another organ in the abdominal cavity.

downward through the tube to the uterus. The obstruction or narrowing is usually the result of inflammation or scarring from an infection, such as gonorrhea, but it may also develop after abdominal surgery or because of a growth such as a pelvic tumor. Tubal infections caused by numerous other bacteria can occur after miscarriage or childbirth or during the use of an IUD (intrauterine device). If these infections are severe, blockage of the tube may result.

An ectopic pregnancy may be fatal unless it is promptly treated. The danger is that it will not be detected until it has ruptured (broken) the tube enclosing it, causing massive bleeding. Pregnancies located in other areas such as the ovary and cervix can invade large nearby blood vessels and cause massive bleeding.

Symptoms of ectopic pregnancy usually begin from two to four weeks after a woman misses her menstrual period. She may be bothered by sharp, continuous pains on one side of her pelvis (lower abdomen) and by slight bleeding from her vagina. The examining doctor may discover a tender swelling on one side of the pelvis. Movement of the uterus (during a pelvic examination) may cause pain.

When ectopic pregnancy is suspected, the patient is hospitalized immediately. Ultrasound pictures may reveal the outline of the expanding mass. In most cases, there is slow bleeding from the end of the fallopian tube into the abdominal cavity, which may be detected by inserting a hollow needle through the wall of the vagina beneath the cervix and drawing off blood. With rapid bleeding, which usually does not occur until after the sixth week of the pregnancy, the patient may suffer from sudden sharp pains in the lower abdomen, from backache, low blood pressure, fainting, and even shock (collapse of circulation to the outer parts of the body). The diagnosis is confirmed by inserting a laparoscope (a lighted tube) through a small cut into the abdominal cavity to detect the ectopic pregnancy visually.

Treatment for ectopic pregnancy is surgical removal of the pregnancy. When the pregnancy is in a fallopian tube, the entire tube and sometimes the ovary must be removed. However, it is sometimes possible to remove the pregnancy and reconstruct the tube.

A woman who has had one ectopic pregnancy has a 15 percent chance of having a second one. This does not mean that she should not try to become pregnant again—but that when she does try, she should be especially watchful for symptoms of ectopic pregnancy, and she should see her physician immediately so that the location of this pregnancy may be determined.

Eczema

See Dermatitis.

Edema

Edema is the accumulation of excessive amounts of fluid within the body's tissues. It is a symptom, rather than a cause, of many other conditions that can be minor or serious.

The fluid that accumulates comes from the blood. Normally, there is a constant exchange of body fluid between the blood vessels and other body tissues. The blood removes any extra fluids and carries them to the kidneys where they are excreted. Edema occurs when that exchange does not function properly, either allowing too much liquid to leave the blood vessels or too little fluid to enter the blood vessels from body tissues. A change in pressure within the blood vessels because of heart disease, high blood pressure, blocked or damaged vessels, or kidney problems may trigger an imbalance in fluid exchange.

Mild edema is common before menstruation and during pregnancy when the blood volume increases. Excess weight, tight clothing, and hot weather may also lead to edema. Edema occurring under these circumstances is normal and should not be a cause for alarm.

Edema can be confined to a small area of the body or become generalized. Some forms are more noticeable than others, depending upon their cause and location. For example, the swelling that appears around a splinter in the skin is edema. However, generalized edema results in widespread body swelling and puffiness, usually first noticed in the fingers and feet. The most serious forms of edema occur within the internal organs of the body. Heart disease, for example, may result in internal edema of the heart and lungs, causing swelling that puts tremendous strain on these organs, even to the point of becoming dangerous.

Simple or temporary edema may be relieved by decreasing salt intake, since the sodium in salt causes the body to retain fluid. More severe or internal edema may be treated with a diuretic, a drug that stimulates the kidneys to produce more urine and thus rid the body of excess fluid. Edema that is symptomatic of an underlying disorder will often disappear with management of the condition.

Controlling weight gain, eating a balanced diet low in salt, and wearing loose clothing may prevent milder forms of edema. Any prolonged edema not attributable to causes such as hot weather or menstruation needs investigation by a physician to determine the cause.

See also Electrolyte balance.

Electroconvulsive therapy

Electroconvulsive therapy (ECT) is a treatment procedure in which an electric current is passed through the brain to create a convulsion of the central nervous system. Based on the belief that electric shock breaks down disturbed mental patterns, ECT is used chiefly in severe depression and manic-depressive illness (alternating periods of depression and elation). Occasionally, it is employed to arouse a schizophrenic patient from catatonia (an unresponsive state).

Prior to treatment, the patient is examined, given appropriate laboratory tests, and may undergo an electroencephalogram (brain wave test) to detect any brain injury that might be related to the condition. Such an injury would rule out the use of ECT. Usually ECT is given early in the morning, because the patient must not have had anything to eat or drink for eight hours before treatment. The patient is put to sleep briefly by an anesthetic given intravenously (into a vein). Electrodes are placed on one or both sides of the head and electric current administered. The seizure that results lasts from five to 20 seconds. Recovery is rapid; after half an hour or an hour of drowsiness the patient is usually alert and willing to talk. Some temporary memory loss is common, and headaches sometimes occur. However, the use of general anesthesia has prevented spinal injuries and the anxiety that used to precede shock treatments. It is said that serious complications of ECT arise in less than 1/10 of 1 percent of all cases.

A usual course of ECT treatments is two or three times a week for three to four weeks. A faster method, in which the patient's heart rate is monitored with an electrocardiograph, employs repeated surges of electric current in one to three sessions.

See also Depression and Schizophrenia.

Electrolyte balance

Electrolyte is a term that refers to a substance that can conduct an electrical current when dissolved in a solution. In medical terms, electrolyte balance refers to the concentrations of separate electrolyte substances in the blood. The common electrolytes in the human blood are sodium, chloride, potassium, calcium, bicarbonate, phosphate, and magnesium.

The levels and balance of electrolytes in the body are intimately related to the levels and balance of fluid or water in the body. If fluids are lost from the body (for example, in severe vomiting or diarrhea), electrolytes contained in the fluids are also lost. On the other hand, electrolytes and fluids can accumulate in the body, as in the case of kidney failure when the kidneys shut down and fluid and its electrolytes build up in the blood and body tissues. In either of these cases, the electrochemical environment in the body that ensures proper cell function is upset. An excess of fluid in the body (so much that it spills into the tissues causing swelling) is called edema; an abnormally low fluid level is called dehydration.

See also Dehydration and Edema.

Embolism

An embolism occurs when some part of the circulatory system is either partially or completely blocked by some obstructing mass that has traveled through the system. The occurrence of an obstruction is called an *embolism* while the mass causing the embolism is called an *embolus.*

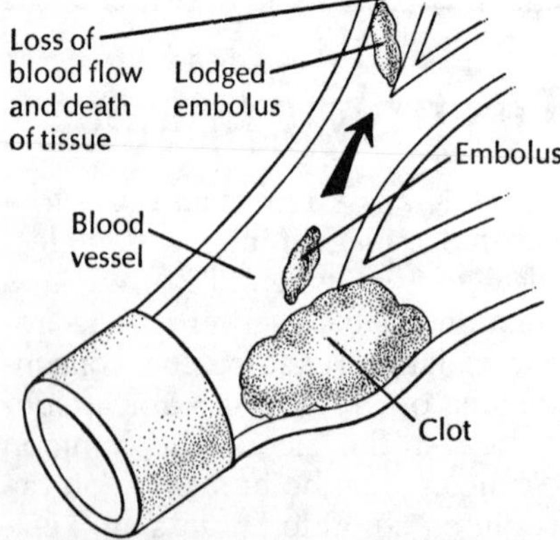

An embolus is a piece of a clot that has broken off and traveled through the circulatory system. The embolus will usually lodge downstream causing loss of blood flow and death of tissue in the area nourished by that vessel.

Emboli (the plural of embolus) are classified in three major groups:

- Solid emboli, which are made up of a variety of substances, such as clumps of tissue, tumor cells, or pieces of blood clots
- Liquid emboli, which are made up of globules of fat or amniotic fluid (fluid in which the fetus is bathed during pregnancy)
- Gaseous emboli, which are made up of the different constituents of air.

Emboli are further categorized according to the location of the blockage:

- Arterial emboli, which originate either from the heart or the artery itself, travel downstream, and prevent the flow of fresh blood to whatever area or organ is being supplied
- Paradoxical emboli, which originate in the venous system and pass over into the arterial system (this usually occurs because of defects in the walls separating the chambers of the heart)
- Pulmonary emboli, which block vessels in the lungs
- Coronary artery emboli, which block coronary arteries of the heart
- Cerebral emboli, which usually originate in the heart or the carotid arteries in the neck leading to the brain (these are a major cause of stroke).

Emboli have a variety of causes, depending on the specific type. The most common cause is the breaking away of a blood clot from within the heart or blood vessels. Arterial emboli commonly originate in the heart itself, because of plaques or accumulations on the heart's valves, from blood clots on the walls of the heart, or within an aneurysm. An arterial embolus can also originate from a plaque or clot within the artery itself. Fat emboli can develop from injury to the bones (particularly the long bones of the leg) or from damage to cells in fat tissue. Air emboli can develop (rarely) if a very large amount of air is admitted during an intravenous (into the vein) infusion or as a complication of surgery, especially in operations on the neck or the chest. In these cases, air enters vessels that are open because of the surgery. However, the oxygen in air is not the only gas involved in gaseous emboli. When divers ascend from high pressure levels in the water to normal pressure levels too quickly or when aviators (in planes without cabin pressurization) climb from normal pressure levels to low pressure levels, there is always the possibility of nitrogen bubbles arising in the bloodstream because of too rapid decompression. If any of these gaseous emboli find their way into the central nervous system, the result can be catastrophic.

An arterial embolism deprives the affected area of its blood supply, which can cause damage or death of the area. An embolism in a brain artery may produce the symptoms of a stroke. In an embolism in the leg, the area beyond the blockage – if totally or nearly totally deprived of blood–becomes white and painful. If the obstruction is not relieved, death of tissue will ensue.

Emboli resulting from blood clots are often treated with a variety of anticoagulants (agents that inhibit normal clotting mechanisms in the blood). Common anticoagulants such as heparin and warfarin do not actually dissolve clots, but instead prevent additional clots from forming and embolizing. There are newer drugs that do dissolve clots, but their use is restricted to special situations. If an embolism is in an available location, such as in an artery in a limb, and tissue is threatened, surgery to remove the clot is the preferred method of treatment to save the limb. In cases of massive embolism to the lung (usually from deep veins in the legs) where life is threatened, surgery can also be attempted. In addition, if an individual has clots in the deep venous system of the lower half of the body and for some reason (for example, a recent hemorrhage in the brain or other vital organ) anticoagulants cannot be prescribed, blocking devices such as clips can be placed on or in the main vein (inferior vena cava) receiving blood from the lower body to prevent emboli from reaching the lungs.

See also Pulmonary embolism and Stroke.

Emphysema

Emphysema is a chronic, progressive lung disease. Emphysema develops when the small air passages leading to the air sacs (alveoli) in the lungs become distended and the walls dividing the sacs themselves are injured or destroyed. This leads to the creation of lung tissue that is essentially nonfunctioning. Emphysema is commonly associated with chronic bronchitis, which is a condition in which the airways become inflamed, causing specialized cells within them to secrete a great deal of mucus. The inflammation and swelling, along with mucus plugging, result in a great deal of obstruction to air flow and cause air to become trapped.

As the disease progresses, many complex changes take place, ultimately leading to a diminished amount of oxygen in the blood frequently associated with an increased amount of carbon dioxide. Also, as the lung tissue deteriorates and loses its elasticity, changes also occur in the blood vessels carrying deoxygenated blood to the lungs for a fresh supply of oxygen. The net effect of all of this

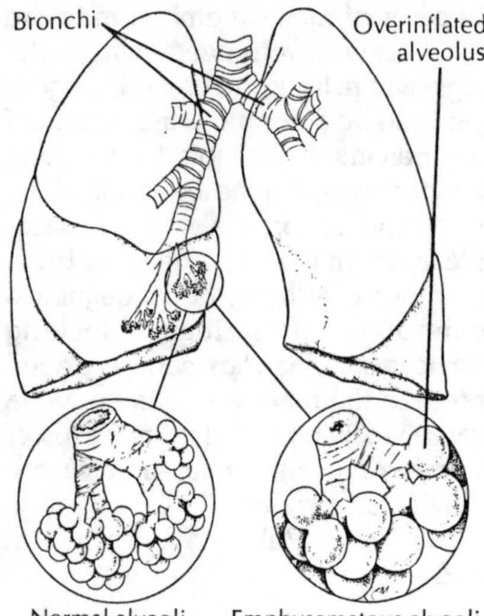

Emphysema is a chronic disease in which the tiny air sacs (alveoli) of the lungs become overinflated with trapped air.

is that the right side of the heart, which is responsible for collecting deoxygenated blood from the veins of the body and pumping it through the lungs, must now work much harder. As the process continues, the right heart muscle is weakened by this extra work and becomes less able to pump blood into the lungs. The blood "backs up" causing increased back pressure in the veins. This, in turn, causes the exodus of fluid into the tissues, and the result is severe swelling of the feet, ankles, and legs. If this right-sided heart failure (also known as cor pulmonale) is very severe, distention of the abdomen with fluid will also occur.

External factors that irritate the lungs, such as tobacco smoke and air pollutants, are commonly linked to emphysema, but no one single cause has been determined. Emphysema does not stem from viruses or bacteria, as do some respiratory diseases. However, it is often aggravated by a case of bronchitis (an inflammation of the bronchial passages) or any lung infection.

In a minority of cases, emphysema may result from a genetic deficiency or an inherited lack of a blood protein that may lead to loss of elasticity in the lung's air sacs.

Those afflicted with emphysema are usually white males over the age of 50, although females are becoming equally susceptible because of increased smoking among women during recent years.

Emphysema is characterized by one major symptom: shortness of breath. Patients may also have a persistent, racking cough, which either brings up mucus or is overly dry. Patients experience difficulty in breathing, often taking twice as many breaths as others to get enough oxygen. It has been found that advanced emphysema sufferers exert tremendous amounts of energy just to breathe. They also tire quite easily and require more calories to maintain their weight than does a normal individual. Many patients may develop an enlarged, rounded "barrel" chest from over inflated lungs and overdeveloped chest muscles used in breathing. Lips, ear lobes, skin, and fingernails may become tinged blue from lack of oxygen in the blood.

Emphysema is usually diagnosed by several procedures, since no one single test exists to pinpoint the condition. Doctors may administer breathing tests to measure the amount of air being inhaled and exhaled, but this will not reveal the disease in its early stages. A blood test may be given to determine the patient's red blood cell count; when emphysema exists with diminished oxygenation of the blood, the body will produce more red blood cells in order to carry more oxygen throughout the system, so an emphysema patient's red blood cell count may be high because of this compensation. A chest X ray may be taken to search for specific changes in the lungs that may point to advanced stages of the disease, but a chest X ray will not actually diagnose early emphysema. Emphysema is thus diagnosed by a collection of findings.

There is no known cure for emphysema, nor is it reversible. However, the progress of the disease can be checked by removing irritants, particularly cigarette smoke. Patients are encouraged to drink large amounts of fluids to help thin out the mucus that is blocking the airways. Adequate rest, a balanced diet, and moderate regular exercise are recommended. Vaporizers, humidifiers, and air conditioners help to moisturize and filter the air. Patients can learn to use their chest and abdominal muscles (with the help of a therapist) in such a way as to breathe more efficiently.

Several drugs may aid the emphysema patient. They act to loosen mucus secretions or to relax and expand the air passages. Antibiotics are sometimes prescribed if infection exists. In advanced cases, oxygen may need to be administered continuously. However, an emphysema patient must be particularly careful to use only the amount of oxygen prescribed. Too much oxygen can suppress the drive to breathe in some patients, thereby causing respiratory failure and possibly death. In addition, sedatives and sleeping medications should be avoided by patients with severe emphysema as these can also lead to a dangerous slowing of breathing.

Emphysema is a very serious condition. However, with the help of modern treatments, breathing aids, and medications, patients can lead a reasonably comfortable life. It is, however, necessary for these individuals to stop smoking and avoid air pollutants as much as possible.

See also Bronchitis and Cor pulmonale.

Encephalitis

Encephalitis is an inflammation of the brain. The term is usually used to describe an infectious process caused by bacteria, parasites, vaccines, and, most often, viruses. Noninfectious agents such as poisons (lead), metabolic abnormalities due to liver or kidney failure, and tumors can cause "encephalitis-like" conditions.

Viruses may cause encephalitis either as a primary disease or as a secondary complication of an infection. Some of these viruses are mosquito-borne and afflict humans only in warm weather when mosquitoes are in season. Many cases of encephalitis occur as complications of viral infections, such as measles, mumps, chicken pox, rubella (German measles), and other infections. These cases usually develop five to ten days after the onset of the original illness but can develop up to six weeks afterward.

Encephalitis may be associated with meningitis (infection of the layers of tissue that cover the brain and spinal cord) with evidence of brain disturbances such as alterations in mental state, personality changes, seizures, and paralysis. Edema (fluid buildup) in the brain is present and there may be petechial hemorrhages (small red bleeding spots) scattered throughout parts of the brain and spinal cord. As with meningitis, fever, headache, vomiting, a general feeling of illness, and a stiff neck may be the first symptoms to appear.

Prompt diagnosis and supportive treatment are essential in any case of encephalitis, or suspected encephalitis. Even patients who have been seriously or critically ill with encephalitis often recover. One problem of diagnosis is differentiating encephalitis from bacterial menin-

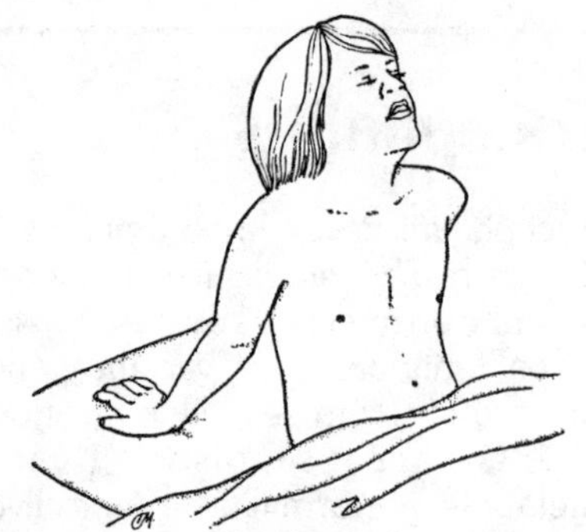
Encephalitis is characterized by fever, a severe headache, and sometimes a stiff neck.

gitis and other similar ailments. Even with ideal circumstances for diagnosis, the encephalitis virus is commonly not identified in many cases. Viruses can sometimes be isolated directly from cerebrospinal fluid or from the tissues. Since many forms of encephalitis, such as the mosquito-borne forms, have important public health implications, blood is often drawn whenever encephalitis is suspected and sent to local departments of health who can supply more precise diagnoses.

Early recognition and treatment of a form of encephalitis called herpes simplex encephalitis with a medication that inhibits the reproduction of viruses reduces the chances of death and neurologic impairment significantly. However, the drug should be given before coma and/or paralysis set in for maximal effectiveness. There is no other known antiviral agent that is effective in cases of encephalitis. Supportive therapy involves bed rest and maintaining fluid balance to avoid dehydration (loss of body fluids).

See also Meningitis.

Endocarditis

Endocarditis is the term used to describe an inflammation of the endocardial layer of the heart. The heart is made up of three cellular layers; the endocardium (innermost layer), myocardium (middle, muscular layer), and epicardium (the outermost layer). The endocardium lines all of the chambers and valves of the heart, and its cells are continuous with those of blood vessels leaving the heart.

Endocarditis is divided into two forms, infectious and noninfectious. Infectious endocarditis usually occurs in people with congential (inborn) or acquired defects in the walls and/or valves of the heart. An example of the former would be a hole in the wall between the different chambers of the heart. Examples of an acquired defect are heart valves damaged by rheumatic fever and damage that may result from the use of non-sterile needles by drug addicts who inject intravenously. For complex reasons, these anatomic or structural abnormalities are more susceptible to infection. Bacteria probably circulate through the bloodstream of all people at some time or another. However, certain procedures such as dental work (fillings, extractions, cleaning, gum surgery) lead to significant bacteremia (the presence of large amounts of bacteria traveling through the bloodstream). The bacteria somehow rest on these abnormal areas in the heart and cause inflammation and/or infection that serves as a foundation for the collection of platelets, strands of clotting material (fibrin), and other debris of the circulatory system. The clump of material that forms is referred to as a "vegetation."

Abnormal heart valves or walls can be infected with microorganisms from any site in the body that contains a high amount of bacteria. People with abnormal heart valves, prosthetic (artificial) valves, and other structural abnormalities must be given antibiotics before and after any procedure (dental work, surgery of the urogenital or large intestinal tract, opening of an abscess) likely to disperse bacteria. Fungi and yeast *(candida)* can also cause endocarditis but usually in people with other serious diseases and depressed immune function. The antibiotics serve either to prevent or at least lessen the number of microorganisms passing through the bloodstream, thereby lessening (significantly) the chance of developing endocarditis.

Infectious endocarditis is a serious systemic disease with a wide spectrum of symptoms and signs. Patients may complain of fevers, weakness, and weight loss. Anemia (deficiency in red blood cells) may also be present. Pieces of the vegetations may break off and embolize to (travel to and lodge in) other areas of the body, for example, the brain causing a stroke, or to the kidneys causing microscopic blood in the urine, among other problems. If the infection of a valve is particularly intense or if a prosthetic valve is involved, the valve may actually have to be surgically replaced.

The diagnosis of infectious endocarditis is made by the history and physical examination along with appropriate laboratory data. Blood cultures (taking of blood and placing it into special materials designed to support bacterial or fungal growth) are the mainstay of diagnosis. Once the infectious agent is isolated, appropriate antibiotics can be administered. Antibiotic administration is by the intravenous route (at least at first) and usually for long periods up to six to eight weeks.

Prevention of infectious endocarditis involves having knowledge of abnormalities in one's heart and taking the proper antibiotics prior to and after dental and many surgical procedures.

Noninfectious endocarditis can be associated with many different diseases. Endocardial inflammation with consequent changes causing some loss of function of the heart is one form. Another is the formation of valvular vegetations that are sterile, but nonetheless can embolize and cause serious damage. Treatment of these conditions depends on the underlying disease process.

Endocrine system

The endocrine system is a set of glands that release hormones into the bloodstream. Hormones are chemical messengers that direct cell activity in various parts of the body. They also coordinate operations among the different cell groups.

Endocrine glands are so named because they secrete hormones internally (endo) into the bloodstream. No ducts transport the chemicals. In contrast, exocrine glands send secretions outward (exo) through tubes or ducts (for example, sweat glands produce fluid that flows to the skin's surface through tubes or ducts).

Several glands with different functions comprise the endocrine system. However, all endocrine glands come under the control of the pituitary, or master, gland. The pituitary gland lies at the base of the brain. Its job is to receive messages about the need for a particular hormone and secrete either the hormone or substances that cause the manufacture and release of a hormone in response. For instance, if there is a need for more thyroid hormone, the pituitary is stimulated to secrete thyroid-stimulating hormone that causes the thyroid gland to increase production. By triggering responses throughout the endocrine system, the pituitary gland controls many body functions, including growth, response to stress, and energy regulation.

The gland directly responsible for body energy regulation is the thyroid gland. The thyroid is located in front of the throat above the top of the breastbone. It consists of two main sections or lobes on either side of the trachea (windpipe) that are connected by a narrow band of tissue called the "isthmus."

Behind the thyroid glands are the parathyroid glands. Parathyroid glands control calcium levels in the blood by secreting parathyroid hormone.

The other glands in the endocrine system are located within the abdominal cavity. Specialized cells in the pancreas, produce two hormones needed to maintain stable blood sugar levels in the body. Insulin helps body cells utilize glucose for energy, thereby regulating the amount of sugar in the bloodstream. To balance this action, the hormone glucagon stimulates the liver to release its stored sugar into the blood, thus raising the blood sugar level.

The pancreas also functions in digestion of foods. Other cells in the pancreas produce special chemicals called enzymes that are secreted directly into the small intestine through ducts. These enzymes help break down food (particularly fats and starches) in the small intestine.

This varied activity of the organ means that the pancreas functions as both an exocrine and endocrine organ.

Other glands critical to normal body functions such as fluid balance, reaction to stress, and reproduction are the adrenal glands. Each of the two adrenal glands lies above a kidney. The adrenal glands have two distinct parts: the cortex (outer layer) that secretes steroid hormones and

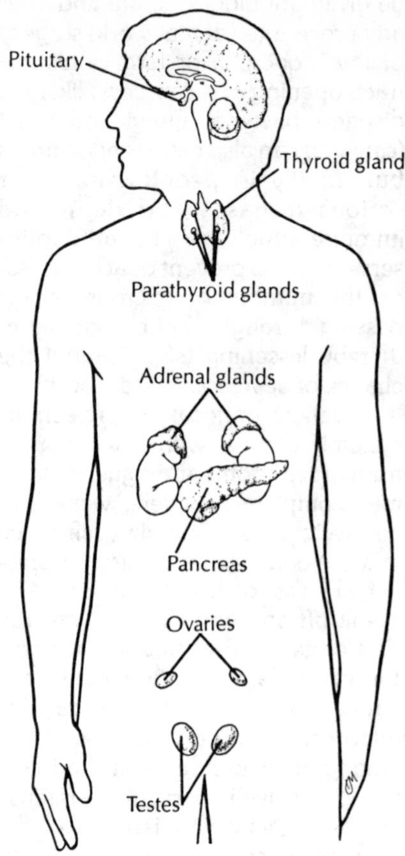

The endocrine system is composed of glands that release vital hormones into the blood.

the medulla that secretes adrenaline and noradrenaline. Adrenaline and noradrenaline are responsible for the changes in heart rate, blood pressure, and level of usable glucose (sugar) that are necessary to cope with stress. In addition, adrenal glands in both men and women produce small amounts of the sex hormone known as androgens (male) and estrogens (female).

The primary responsibility for hormone production for the reproductive system is with the testes (male sex glands) and ovaries (female sex glands). Testes are two oval-shaped organs in the scrotum, the external pouch of skin behind and under the penis. They produce sperm and male sex hormones that provide male sex characteristics of penis development, body hair growth, voice changes, and increased muscle mass. Two ovaries in the female pelvis secrete the hormones estrogen and progesterone which govern the development of secondary female characteristics including ovulation (monthly release of egg from ovary), breast development, and body hair growth.

The endocrine system has a large influence on the way we feel and act. In turn, our energy and other needs in any given situation set the activity of the endocrine system. This feedback relationship is crucial in maintaining our general well-being.

See also Adrenal glands, Diabetes mellitus, Pituitary gland, and Reproduction.

Endometriosis

Endometriosis is a condition in which tissue from the lining of the uterus detaches itself and grows elsewhere in the abdominal cavity outside the uterus. It occurs only in women during the childbearing years, especially in women between the ages of 30 and 40.

Endometriosis develops when the tissue that normally lines the uterus (called endometrial tissue or the endometrium) displaces itself and grows on the outside of the uterus, on the ovaries, the intestine, or anywhere else in the abdomen. The endometrium normally thickens and swells during each menstrual cycle in preparation for possible pregnancy, then breaks down and flows out of the body during menstruation if no pregnancy occurs. When endometriosis develops, the displaced endometrial tisssue continues to swell and bleed each month, but it has nowhere to flow. The body responds to the presence of this accumulated blood by building scar tissue around it that builds up month after month, finally leading to the formation of blood-filled pockets or cysts (often called "chocolate cysts") on the affected organs.

The exact cause of endometriosis is not known, but several conditions are thought to lead to its development: menstrual blood may flow backwards through the fallopian tubes and into the abdominal cavity, but the reason for this is not known; the cervix or vagina may be blocked

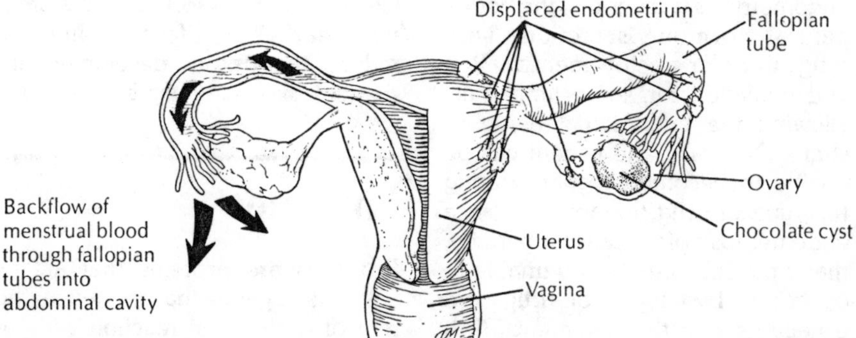

Endometriosis is a condition in which tissue from the lining of the uterus detaches itself and grows elsewhere in the abdominal cavity, such as on the ovaries, the fallopian tubes, the outside of the uterus, or anywhere in the abdominal cavity. Sometimes endometriosis patches form blood-filled sacs called "chocolate cysts."

so that the menstrual blood cannot flow out normally; or surgery or another condition may lead to the displacement of some tissue from the uterus.

The symptoms of endometriosis are pain during, immediately before, or immediately after the menstrual period; pain during intercourse; discomfort in the lower urinary tract or intestine; irregular or excessively heavy menstrual flow; bleeding from the rectum; blood in the urine; and infertility. These symptoms may vary from person to person. Some women may experience all of these symptoms, while others may experience only one or two.

Endometriosis is diagnosed with a complete medical and menstrual history. Two pelvic examinations may be performed, one during menstruation and one between periods, to determine the changes in the reproductive area during the cycle. The doctor may also perform a laparoscopy, in which a small, lighted tube is inserted into the lower abdomen through a tiny incision; any displaced tissues can usually be seen through the tube.

Treatment of this disorder involves halting the condition, reducing the pain, and restoring normal menstruation and fertility. The best way to halt endometriosis is to modify the body's natural hormone secretions with drugs in order to stop menstruation and ovulation for some time, thus allowing the endometrial tissue to shrink. Naturally, the patient will be unable to become pregnant during this type of drug therapy, but since endometriosis often causes infertility, many patients are already unable to conceive. Two types of drugs are usually used in this treatment. Birth control pills as well as several other medications that modify female hormone secretions are sometimes prescribed in high enough doses to stop menstruation and ovulation. However, an excessive dosage often brings with it undesirable side effects such as nausea, fluid retention, and the possibility of blood clotting.

A new synthetic hormone called danazol creates a condition similar to menopause, causing menstruation and ovulation to stop and the endometrial tissue to shrink almost immediately, but without some of the side effects associated with hormonal drugs. However, danazol can be expensive and in some cases is not effective.

If drug therapy is unsuccessful, surgery may be necessary, involving either the removal of scar tissue and endometrial tissue or, in advanced cases, the removal of the uterus and ovaries (called a hysterectomy), rendering the patient permanently sterile.

There are no specific measures that will prevent the development of endometriosis, but pregnancy and breast-feeding often have a beneficial effect on this condition because, in interrupting the menstrual cycle, they prevent the buildup of tissue. Childbirth enlarges the cervix, which may be beneficial in the prevention of endometriosis. The disease is seen more often in women who have postponed childbearing until their late 20s or 30s, so becoming pregnant earlier in life may help to reduce the risk of developing endometriosis in later years.

Enzymes

Enzymes are proteins that act as catalysts (agents that influence the rate of a chemical reaction without being themselves affected) for chemical reactions that occur in the body. The number of enzymes and their specific functions in the body are numerous. Enzymes work by speeding up the rate of a chemical reaction without being used up in the reaction.

Enzymes are produced within cells and act either within the cell or outside the cell in other parts of the body. Enzymes are absolutely essential for the proper functioning and development of the body. A deficiency, failure to perform, or overactivity of an enzyme can lead to many disorders, some of which are potentially serious.

The names of enzymes usually end in *-ase.* Their names also indicate the substance with which they react. For example, the enzyme lactase catalyzes the breakdown of lactose, a sugar present in milk, and thus aids in the digestion of milk.

Epilepsy

Epilepsy is a disorder characterized by sudden surges of disorganized electrical impulses in the brain, which lead to seizures.

There are several categories of seizures; they can be so mild as to go almost unnoticed or so severe that, if untreated, they can cause serious harm.

Epilepsy is usually divided into two categories: idiopathic (cause unknown) and acquired (cause—such as brain tumor or old injury—able to be determined). Up until the age of 35, idiopathic epilepsy is a very common cause of seizures. After age 35, however, a thorough diagnostic workup to exclude a cause is needed. Acquired epilepsy can be due to a multitude of causes, such as cerebral palsy, brain tumor, infection of the central nervous system, and malformations of blood vessels.

Idiopathic epilepsy, although by definition of unknown cause, has several consistent attributes. It occurs with highest frequency between the ages of two and five years and again at puberty and tends to run in families.

The symptoms of epilepsy vary according to the type of seizure experienced. A seizure is a term used to describe an attack of epilepsy. Not all seizures are convulsions. A convulsion involves the nerves that control movement and is characterized by jerking, spastic muscle movements. It is also marked by alterations in sensation and consciousness; in fact, loss of consciousness is common.

Seizures are classified according to the symptoms experienced. In the past, classifications were *grand mal* (big sickness), *petit mal* (little sickness), psychomotor, and focal. Current classifications separate seizures into partial or generalized types, depending on the extent of the brain's involvement.

The four current classifications and their symptoms:

- Simple partial seizures, confined to small areas of the brain, are experienced by feeling a tingling sensation in the arm, finger, or foot; perceiving a bad odor; seeing flashing lights; or speaking unintelligibly. The patient remains conscious.
- Complex partial seizures include episodes of "automatic behavior," in which the patient remains conscious but sits motionless or moves or behaves in a strange, repetitive, or somehow inappropriate way.
- Generalized convulsive seizures have a number of symptoms: the patient may cry out, stiffen and fall to the ground unconscious, lose urinary and bowel control, and have muscle spasms or thrashing movements that cause the limbs to jerk. Spasm of the jaw muscles can cause tongue biting. After the convulsion the patient falls into a deep

sleep, and will awaken dazed, often with a headache and no recollection of the seizure. Several warning signals (called the aura) may precede this type of seizure, among them headache, sleepiness, yawning, or tingling in the arms or legs.

- Generalized nonconvulsive or absence seizures, usually experienced by children, are characterized by periods of staring into space, rhythmic blinking, and what appears to be daydreaming. The patient remains conscious but is totally unaware of the seizure. This type of seizure may be mistaken for a short attention span or a learning disability in school.

Epilepsy is diagnosed by observing the symptoms and by using an electroencephalograph (EEG), which measures the electrical activity of the brain and gives a visual record of brain impulses. In this way, abnormal electrical discharges can be detected if they are present in the brain. However, an abnormal EEG in the absence of symptoms is by no means proof of epilepsy, nor does a normal EEG rule it out.

Non-medical treatment of an epileptic seizure should be limited to preventing injury and keeping the patient comfortable by loosening clothing or placing a pillow under the head. The patient should not be left face downward or in any position in which vomit can be swallowed or inhaled. *Never* should an attempt be made to pry open the mouth or insert any object into the mouth of a convulsing individual.

Anticonvulsant drugs are used to control epilepsy, and the majority of epileptics nowadays are well controlled. Patients who tend to have seizures following emotional or physical stress may also benefit from tranquilizers.

Epilepsy cannot be cured, but it can usually be controlled with a program of anticonvulsant drug therapy. After two to five years of drug control of idiopathic epilepsy, the dosage is sometimes decreased and, occasionally, when enough time has elapsed during which no seizures have occurred, medication can be discontinued.

Epilepsy cannot actually be prevented, but once the seizures are controlled by medication, epileptics can lead normal lives—hold jobs, raise families, drive cars, and so on—in the same way that victims of high blood pressure or diabetes can learn to live with their disabilities.

Episiotomy

An episiotomy is a surgical incision into the tissues surrounding the opening of the vagina during childbirth in order to make the delivery easier and to avoid extensive tearing of the tissues. The advantage of the procedure is that it substitutes a controlled surgical incision for excessive stretching and tearing of all the tissues. The incision itself is easier to repair later than a tear or break in the tissues would be.

Episiotomy is often performed for women who are having their first baby. With subsequent pregnancies, episiotomy may not be necessary, since the tissues surrounding the vagina have often been stretched sufficiently by the first delivery to allow an easy second delivery.

The most common type of episiotomy is a midline incision made with surgical scissors from the midpoint of the vaginal opening directly downward toward the rectum. This type of incision carries one important risk: during the birth it might extend into the anal sphincter (the ring of muscle surrounding the opening

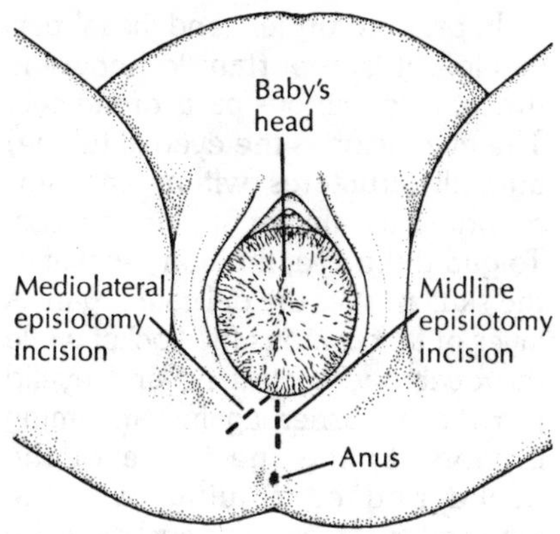

An episiotomy is done to make childbirth easier and to avoid tearing of tissues. The most common type of episiotomy is a midline incision from the midpoint of the vaginal opening directly downward toward the anus. Some doctors, however, prefer an incision at an angle, called mediolateral episiotomy.

from the intestine) or the rectum itself; however, it can be repaired easily and will eventually heal itself. To avoid the risks of entering the rectum, some physicians prefer the mediolateral episiotomy in which the incision is made at an angle, thus avoiding the rectum and anal sphincter.

Extrasystole

An extrasystole is a contraction (beat) of the heart caused by a stimulus or impulse somewhere in the heart other than in the sinoatrial node, the natural pacemaker of the heart. In some ways, the condition is like a "stray" signal or "static" in an electrical circuit.

While the immediate cause of an extrasystole is a "stray" signal telling the heart muscle to contract, the real causes lie elsewhere. For example, strenuous activity, especially if there are existing heart problems, can trigger extrasystoles, which, in turn, may trigger an episode of heart arrhythmia (abnormal rhythm and rate of the heart beat) that leads to more serious complications. Coffee, nicotine, and certain drugs, as well as anxiety and sudden shocks or frights, are thought to play a role in extrasystoles. It is important to note, however, that extrasystoles also occur in normal hearts and, in these cases, are quite harmless and do not necessarily indicate underlying heart disease.

The symptoms of extrasystoles are familiar to anyone who has ever been startled and found that his or her heart "skipped a beat." The extrasystole sometimes presents itself as an extra beat and sometimes as two extra beats. On other occasions, there will be a beat followed by a long silence, then a couple of quick beats. Some people experience a feeling of giddiness, shortness of breath, and weakness, with momentary feelings of blacking out. These symptoms, if prolonged and particularly if associated with a loss of consciousness, usually indicate that a sustained arrhythmia (alteration of the normal rhythmic contraction of the heart) is occurring, which should be reported to a doctor.

While physicians have for years debated the importance of extrasystoles, recent thought on the subject has led to a reassessment of the seriousness of the phenomenon. Many sudden deaths may be attributed to severe cardiac arrhythmia that was itself triggered by ventricular extrasystoles in patients with severe underlying heart disease.

One method of documenting the occurrence and nature of extrasystoles is continuous ambulatory electrocardiographic monitoring. The patient in whom arrhythmias are suspected is hooked up to a monitor the size of a portable cassette tape recorder which he or she carries for a certain period of time. A diary is furnished so that the patient can record his or her activity and symptoms. The patient is usually told to perform the normal routine activities during the test. After a specified time period, usually 24 hours, the monitor is taken off and the tape translated into a continuous electrocardiographic record. This record allows a definite diagnosis to be made as to the presence and type of arrhythmia. Treatment can then be prescribed on the basis of concrete evidence.

See also Heartbeat irregularities.

Eye

The eye is the organ of sight. This complex structure works by capturing light and transforming it into impulses that the brain can interpret as images. These visual images give individuals information about their environment.

In order to understand visual perception, it is important to know the functions of various parts of the eye. The eye includes the eyeball (globe) and all structures within and surrounding its almost spherical mass. To guard the eye, the bony socket of the skull nestles the delicate organ. A layer of fat cushions the socket while the eyebrow, eyelashes, and eyelid provide a barrier against incoming irritants. Lining the inside of the eyelid and continuing over the exposed surface of the eyeball is the conjunctiva, a thin protective membrane. Tears (watery secretions) released from the lacrimal (tear) glands moisten the conjunctiva and keep the eyeball clean.

Light first enters the eye through the three outer layers of the eyeball. The cornea is a transparent covering over the area that admits the light. The sclera is the white of the eye

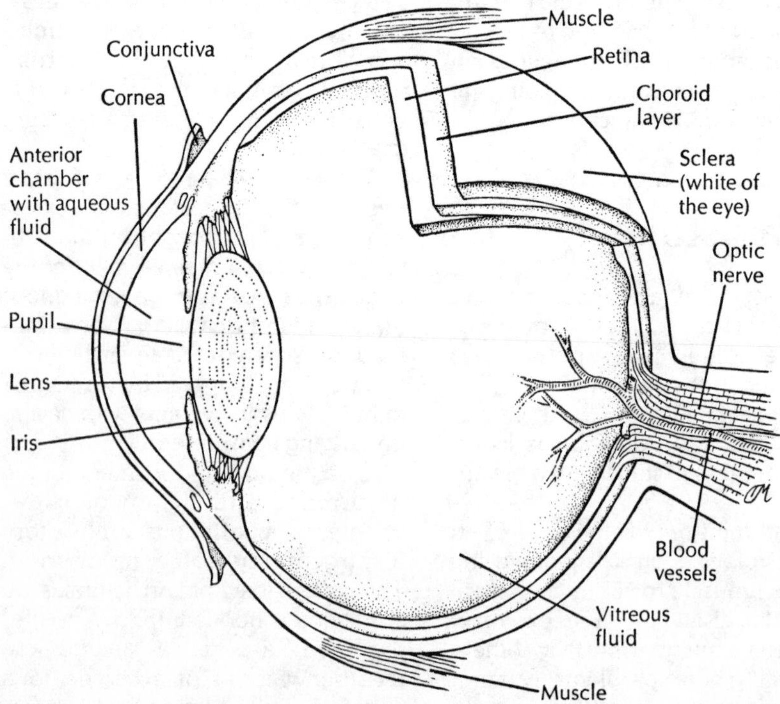

The eye is the organ of sight.

(actually the tough, outer covering of the globe), and the choroid membrane contains blood vessels to nourish the eye.

Light enters the eye first through the cornea. Behind the cornea is a pigmented (colored) structure called the iris. The iris surrounds an opening known as the pupil. The iris changes the size of the pupil depending on the amount of light present in the environment. If the surroundings are relatively dark, the pupil is enlarged to admit more light; if the environment is bright, the pupil is made smaller. Behind the iris is the lens, a transparent body held in place by elastic muscular-type tissue. The shape of the lens is changed to accommodate the light and to focus on objects at varying distances.

Between the cornea and the lens is a space, the anterior chamber, filled with a substance called aqueous humor (fluid). Aqueous fluid contains nutrients that nourish the cornea and the lens. The fluid also allows light rays to pass through the area easily.

Another chamber of the eyeball behind the lens holds vitreous humor. This clear jelly is surrounded by the retina, the innermost layer of the eyeball. In the retina are the sensitive nerve endings that convert light focused from the lens into electrical impulses. These impulses are then transmitted to the brain by the optic nerve, which extends from the rear of the eyeball to the brain.

F

Fainting

Fainting is a temporary loss of consciousness and is often the result when the body attempts to supply extra needed blood to the brain. Fainting can be a symptom of a relatively mild condition (such as hunger) or a serious disorder (such as arrhythmia — or heartbeat irregularity).

When the brain experiences a temporary reduction of its blood supply, the body reacts defensively by, in effect, causing itself to fall down, thus bringing the head to the same level as the heart thereby minimizing the effect of gravity that favors pooling of blood in the lower extremities. The net effect of this is an increase in the amount of blood coming back to the heart which allows the heart to pump blood to the brain more easily.

Fainting can be caused by an interference with any one of several internal mechanisms that protect and maintain the brain's blood supply by working against gravity and its tendency to allow blood to pool in the lower parts of the body. An example of one of these mechanisms is the "muscle pump." The muscles of the legs, when in motion, act to squeeze the veins in the legs thereby actually forcing the column of blood up toward the heart. If a person stands motionless for a long period of time without using these muscles, pooling of blood in the legs takes place, reducing the amount available to the brain. This reduction frequently causes fainting or loss of consciousness. In addition, the ability of the heart to increase its rate and force of contraction when under stress is another built-in protective mechanism.

These protective functions are impaired by a variety of causes, among them certain conditions such as an overheated or crowded environment; emotional stress; hunger; extreme fatigue; various drugs, particularly some high blood pressure medications; as well as certain diseases, including anemia, hypoglycemia (low blood sugar), heart disease, and blood loss.

The symptoms that usually precede actual fainting are lightheadedness; confusion; spots before the eyes; white or grayish coloring of the face; cold, moist, or clammy skin; and, at times, nausea and vomiting.

Fainting is treated by taking several simple steps to make the person more comfortable. The patient should be lying down, preferably with the feet higher than the head (to help blood return), the clothing loosened, and plenty of fresh air to breathe. Recovery should occur within a few seconds of fainting, but a sense of disorientation may linger for several minutes. Spirits of ammonia and smelling salts are not usually recommended for fainting, as they may be ineffective or may cause vomiting.

Recurrent fainting should be reported to a doctor, as more testing may be needed to diagnose another disorder that is causing the fainting.

Fainting can be prevented by lying down, preferably with legs up, or hanging the head down between the knees and breathing deeply as soon as any of the warning symptoms are noticed. These precautions help to lower the brain to the level of the heart, thus increasing the blood supply to the brain.

Fatigue

Fatigue may be physical or mental exhaustion, an overwhelming feeling of weariness, or a lack of energy and enthusiasm for even pleasant activities. It is a symptom of a vast number of diseases and disorders.

Fatigue should not be confused with weakness, which is an actual, physical loss of strength.

Fatigue and tiring rapidly with minimal activity are often the first or one of the early signs of an approaching illness. It is a warning signal of a variety of diseases and disorders: the common cold, influenza, hepatitis, infectious mononucleosis, and other infectious diseases; heart disease; lung disorders such as emphysema; some gland diseases; anemia and nutritional deficiencies; and some diseases of the nervous system. Overwork, either physical or mental, may also cause fatigue, as can psychological disorders or emotional stress.

The symptoms of fatigue can include nervousness, anxiety, depression, irritability, headache, diminished sexual function, and difficulty in concentrating. When fatigue is due to psychological problems, sleep disorders are common associated symptoms, including insomnia, as well as frequent nighttime and early morning waking.

Fatigue is best treated by treating the physical disorder or psychological problem that is causing it. Some types of fatigue, particularly that due to physical overexertion, can probably be prevented by getting adequate exercise and rest, as well as eating well-balanced meals and finding ways to cope with stress and overwork.

Fertilization

See Conception.

Fever

Fever is an abnormally high body temperature, a common symptom accompanying a number of infections and disorders.

A fever is present when the body temperature rises above the normal range of 98.6° F to 99.6° F; that is, if the body temperature is more than 101.5° F when measured with a rectal thermometer, 100.5° F when measured with an oral thermometer, or 99.5° F when measured under the arm, it is considered abnormal.

Fever is a symptom of illness and often appears to be an undesirable condition, but in fact fever acts as a defense mechanism for the body when it is being attacked by a bacterium or virus. Fever occurs when a regulatory center in the brain, whose job it is to maintain a constant body temperature regardless of the surrounding environment, responds to an illness or infection such as the common cold or influenza and sets the body temperature higher as a means of killing the invading microorganisms. It is thought that the microorganisms cannot survive these higher temperatures.

Infections are the most common cause of fever. But a fever can also be a symptom of heart attack, some forms of cancer, and disorders in the portion of the brain that regulates temperature such as stroke, brain tumor, or brain injury.

The early signs of fever include chills or hot flashes, flushed skin, increased pulse and breathing rates, headache, and aching muscles or joints. A slight fever may show none of these symptoms, a high fever may result in delirium or convulsions, and a prolonged fever may cause weakness and dehydration (excess loss of body fluids).

Treatment of fever depends on its severity, duration, and cause. Immediate emergency medical treatment should be sought if fever is more than 105° F (although fever is usually higher in very young children) or if convulsions have occurred. A doctor should be consulted if a fever is high (103° F to 104° F, lasting for 12 to 24 hours); if a moderate fever (101° F to 102° F) lasts for several days; if the body temperature fluctuates widely; or if the fever disappears, then returns several days later, usually signaling a new or additional infection.

The goal of treating a fever is actually to diagnose and treat its cause. Merely lowering a mild fever may do more harm than good, as it reduces the protection that the fever may be providing in fighting off the infection; it may also mask a fever when its cause is unknown or disturb the natural course that would have been taken by the underlying illness, thus hindering diagnosis. Therefore, treating a fever should never be confused with treating its cause.

However, at times fever does need to be lowered to keep the patient comfortable and to prevent weakness and dehydration that can result from prolonged fever. Increasing fluid intake and taking aspirin or an aspirin substitute such as acetaminophen will lower a fever; tepid, not cold, baths and comfortable but not overly warm clothing and blankets will help to lower the fever but also keep the patient from feeling chilled.

It should be noted that any drug treatment for fever, especially for children, should be undertaken only after consulting with a doctor. For instance, although it has not been proven that aspirin causes or promotes a disorder called Reye's syndrome, it is recommended that aspirin not be given to children with chicken pox or influenza.

See also Reye's syndrome.

Fever blisters

Fever blisters, also called cold sores, are fluid-filled blisters that appear on the border of the lips and on or around the nose. They are the result of a very contagious virus that has affected most of the population at one time or another.

The virus that causes fever blisters is a type of herpes simplex virus, and it enters the body most often in the mouth or nose areas where skin is easier to penetrate.

At first, characteristic blisters may or may not result. Antibodies (protective substances) in the body defend against the invading virus. When inactive, the virus withdraws to a nearby nerve, where it remains until stress to the body or a diminished capacity to fight off infection triggers a recurrence. When the virus reactivates, it overruns the body's protective system and progresses back along the nerve to the general area of original infection.

Factors that seem to favor the appearance of blisters include fever, colds, menstruation, skin injury from dental work, excessive sun and wind exposure, and emotional stress. Cold sores can return every few weeks for several weeks or not at all.

Initially, the virus may present no symptons, so some people are unaware of infection. For others, the infection begins with numbness and tenderness in the affected area. Then small fluid-filled blisters appear. These blisters break, encrust, and heal within one to two weeks without leaving a scar.

Occasionally, excessive pain or swollen lymph glands develop. These symptoms may indicate a secondary bacterial infection that needs a doctor's attention.

Other complications can be more serious. *Herpes simplex keratitis* is a painful viral infection of the cornea (transparent covering) of the eye that can result in blindness if not treated. When inflamed eyes accompany fever blisters, a physician should be consulted immediately. In addition, steroid (cortisone) medication or cream should not be used near eyes during a herpes attack without consulting a doctor, since these preparations can encourage spread of the virus to the eye.

Other serious complications can occur in infants and extremely ill patients who contract herpes virus if the infection travels to the lungs, brain, or other internal organs.

Treatment involves relieving symptoms since there is no known cure for fever blisters. Some over-the-counter remedies may relieve pain and help dry blisters. Topical corticosteroid creams, however, should not be applied unless prescribed by a physician; the possibility of spreading infection may increase if the corticosteroid depresses the immune response.

Healing time can be shortened by certain newer prescription drugs, if they are used early in the development of the disease.

Fibrillation

See Defibrillation.

Fibrocystic disease of the breast

Fibrocystic disease is a condition in which benign (noncancerous) lumps form in the breast, either temporarily or for the duration of the childbearing years.

This condition is not dangerous in itself, but it has been found that women with certain forms of fibrocystic disease are two to four times more likely to develop breast cancer than other women. To complicate matters, the constant presence of these benign lumps makes it difficult to detect any new, possibly more dangerous, growths.

The exact cause of fibrocystic disease is not known. However, the tendency to develop it may be inherited. Also, it is seen more often in women who have never breast-fed a child, but the reason for this is not known.

The most noticeable symptoms of this disorder, obviously, are the lumps, which may take the form of either solid masses or fluid-filled sacs called cysts. Large cystic lumps near the surface may be moved about freely, unlike cancerous lumps that are usually firmly attached to surrounding tissue. Changes in the body's hormone secretions during the menstrual period tend to increase slightly the size of the lumps and cause additional pain, but the cysts reduce in size following the period. Other symptoms may include a slight discharge from the nipple as well as persistently heavy and tender breasts, not only before and during menstruation, as is commonly seen in healthy breasts, but all the time.

Diagnosis will include a physical exam and, possibly, one of two additional procedures: mamography (breast X ray) or diaphanography, an examination of the breast tissue by shining a light through the translucent tissue. Either of these procedures will determine whether the lumps are fluid-filled cysts or solid masses. If they are found to be solid, a biopsy (the removal of a small piece of tissue for analysis) may need to be performed in order to detect the possibility of cancerous cells.

Fibrocystic disease often requires no treatment. In some cases lumps may disappear in a few months. However, cysts which are unusually large or particularly bothersome may be drained of their fluid by the insertion of a hollow needle in a procedure called aspiration. If there are many small lumps or continuous development of new ones, other forms of treatment may be necessary to prevent the formation of cysts. Birth control pills may be prescribed, as they act to equalize the amount of hormones present in the body during the monthly cycle; however, birth control pills have also been found to cause cysts in some women. Large doses of Vitamin E have also been effective in treating this disorder.

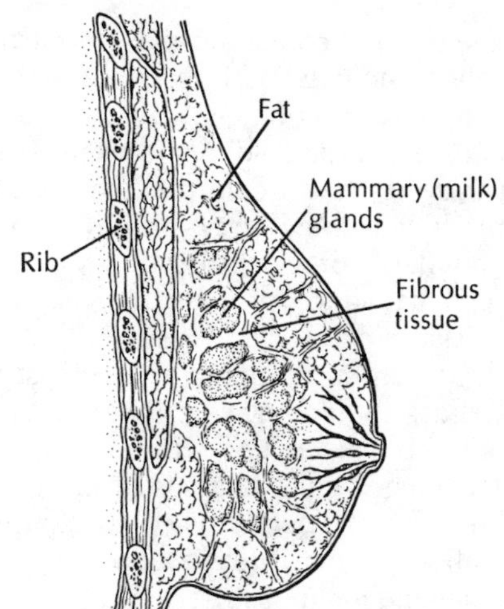

There is some fibrous tissue in the normal breast to support the milk glands.

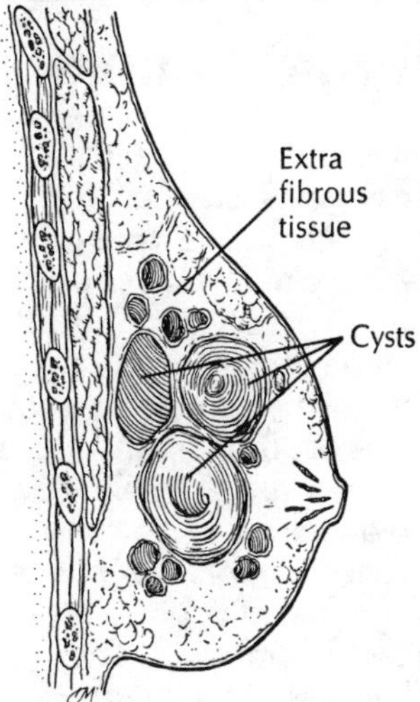

In the fibrocystic breast, there is extra fibrous tissue and solid or fluid-filled lumps (cysts).

Relieving or preventing fibrocystic disease may be promoted by discontinuing or drastically limiting the intake of nicotine and a chemical called methylxanthine, found most commonly in coffee, tea, cola, chocolate, and some cold medications. It is thought that both nicotine and methylxanthine may promote the growth of fibrocystic tissue.

Because of the greater risk of breast cancer with certain forms of this disorder, women with fibrocystic disease should have a physical exam at least twice a year, report any new growths or enlargements of existing lumps, and perform a self-examination of their breasts each month following the menstrual period.

See also Cancer and Mastitis.

Fibroid tumors

Fibroid tumors are solid, noncancerous growths composed of smooth muscle fibers and connective tissue that appear in and on the uterus. They are thought to be the most common abdominal tumor, found in about 25 percent of all women over the age of 30 and more often in black women. Cancer rarely develops in fibroid tumors.

These tumors vary in size and shape, usually grow slowly, and cause few problems. They may grow in the walls of the uterus or out from the uterus; only rarely, they may appear on the cervix; and occasionally they fill the entire uterus, push through the cervix, and appear in the vagina.

Sometimes fibroid tumors do cause complications. If they become very large, they may press on surrounding organs (for instance, on the intestine or bladder, which may result in constipation or frequent urination). If they extend into the uterus, heavy and prolonged menstrual periods may result. If pregnancy occurs, the tumors tend to enlarge and may cause complications as the unborn baby grows.

The cause of fibroid tumors is not known, but their growth seems to be related to estrogen, a female hormone, since these tumors rarely appear before puberty and tend to recede by the menopause years. They most commonly appear in the middle to late reproductive years, when the body's estrogen level is at its peak.

Fibroid tumors may occur along with other disorders, such as endometriosis (the displacement of tissue from the lining of the uterus to outside the uterus) or pelvic inflammatory disease (an infection of the fallopian tubes).

The symptoms of fibroid tumors are dysmenorrhea (pain during menstruation); a gushing or flooding of menstrual flow; occasionally, abdominal pain (although pain is not usually a symptom unless a complication develops, such as a twisting of the tumor, cutting off its blood supply and causing severe pain); and, if the tumor is advanced, a noticeably enlarged abdomen. Sometimes these tumors display no symptoms and are simply discovered during a routine physical exam.

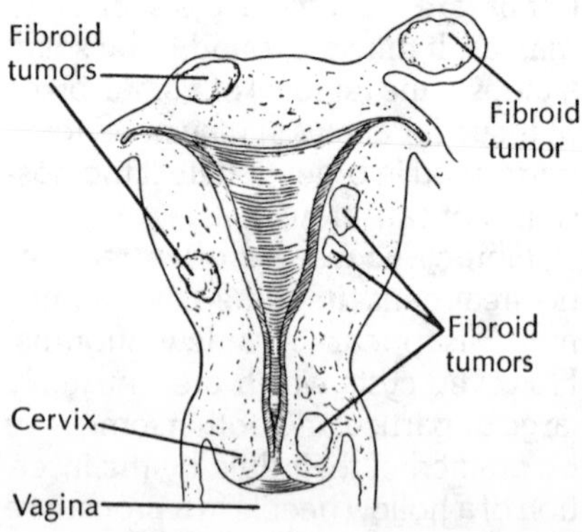

Fibroid tumors are solid, noncancerous growths that can grow within the walls of the uterus or may grow out from the uterine wall on a stalk.

Diagnosis begins with a physical examination and may include curettage (scraping the uterus walls) or endometrial biopsy (removal of some tissue from the lining of the uterus) to test for cancer. X rays as well as ultrasound (a technique that uses sound waves to outline internal structures) may also be used to view the location and nature of the tumor.

Fibroid tumors may require no treatment at all, other then regular checkups with the doctor. Those that are causing complications may require one of two types of surgery: the removal of the tumor (called a myomectomy), recommended for women in their early reproductive years whose symptoms are somewhat mild and who desire a future pregnancy; or the removal of the uterus (called a hysterectomy), usually recommended for older women or for those who do not want to become pregnant, as this operation makes pregnancy impossible.

See also Dysmenorrhea, Endometriosis, and Pelvic inflammatory disease.

Fistula

A fistula is any abnormal, tube-like passage or channel within a body tissue or tissues, usually between two internal organs, or leading from an internal organ to the body's surface. A fistula is sometimes created by surgery for diagnostic or therapeutic purposes. Others occur as the result of injury or congenital (present at birth) defects.

A fistula may develop at virtually any body site. One very common type of fistula is the anal fistula that usually develops as the result of a break, or fissure, in the wall of the anal canal or the rectum (leading from the intestine to the outside of the body) or because of an abscess (an enclosed cavity of pus) in the area. Another common type of fistula is the vaginal fistula, which may follow a difficult labor and childbirth. This fistula is between the bladder and the vagina, causing urine to leak into the vagina. In another type of vaginal fistula, between the vagina and rectum, feces escape through the wall of the rectum into the vagina. Another fistula, the intestinal type, extends from the bladder to the intestine and allows urine to leak from the bladder into the intestines. Fistulas at other sites in the body can be caused by tuberculosis actinomycosis (a type of fungal infection), diverticulitis, or another disease.

Each type of fistula can produce its own peculiar set of symptoms, depending on its location, its size, and its depth. Typical symptoms are pain in the affected region and an abnormal discharge through the skin–particularly if the fistula affects the anus or vagina–which can be seen on examination of these areas. Often the fistula itself is a site of frequent infection and discomfort. The anal fistula usually has recurrent abscesses and constant watery discharge.

In almost all cases, surgery is recommended as the only effective treatment. Vaginal fistulas are frequently corrected following childbirth, and the surgery is nearly always successful. In the case of anal fistulas, surgery is recommended unless severe diarrhea, active ulcerative coilitis, or enterocolitis is present, in which case the healing of the surgical wound would present many problems and complications. Usually these infections are treated before surgery is scheduled.

Avoiding injury to body tissues is probably the only specific preventive measure against the occurrence of fistula. Prompt diagnosis and treatment will lessen the possibility of secondary infections and abscesses.

Fluoride

Fluoride is a compound of fluorine, a chemical element. Fluorine is found in soil and is necessary to plant life and to the formation of teeth and bones in animals, including humans.

In the human body, traces of fluoride are found in the bones, the teeth, the thyroid gland, and the skin. However, it has been found that larger amounts of fluoride than are naturally present in the teeth will help prevent and/or reduce tooth decay.

The best source of fluoride for prevention of tooth decay is fluoridated drinking water. Water with a fluoride content of one part per million is considered safe and effective, especially if given to children while their teeth are developing. The maximum benefit is obtained when the child drinks fluoridated water daily from birth until the permanent teeth are complete (between the ages of ten and 13). However, if fluoride intake is excessive before the permanent teeth erupt while the tooth enamel is forming, the enamel may become stained and mottled. If the teeth have erupted, this staining and mottling cannot occur.

There has been some controversy over the fluoridation of drinking water. Most health scientists today believe that a fluoride level of about one part per million does not damage either teeth or other body tissues. Some dentists report that fluoridation prevents dental diseases other than cavities, such as periodontal diseases (diseases of the gum and bone supporting the teeth) and abnormal positioning of the teeth. Many physicians and researchers also find that fluorides may play a significant role in the treatment and prevention of osteoporosis, an abnormal thinness and brittleness of the bones, common in women after menopause and in both men and women over the age of 65. One recent study of over 1000 persons age 45 and older shows that osteoporosis is less frequent in those who have lived most of their lives in areas where the drinking water has a high fluoride content. There was also significantly less arteriosclerosis (hardening of the arteries often because of calcium deposits) in these persons, suggesting that fluorides help keep calcium deposited in the hard tissues of the body and not in the soft tissues. It would seem, therefore, that fluorides play an important role in preventing osteoporosis and arteriosclerosis, two of the main diseases of aging.

Opponents of fluoridation point to the long-range and unknown effects of adding fluoride to the water supply and to infringements on freedom of choice in imposing this "compulsory medication" on scores of children and adults. Supporters counter these charges by pointing out that fluorides are not medications but preventives, used in the same way that chlorine is used to kill bacteria in water supplies. Fluorides, they also assert, are normally found in teeth and bones as well as in water, and other methods of consuming fluorides are more costly and less effective in the long run than obtaining them from one's water supply.

See also Tooth decay.

Fontanelles

Fontanelles are the gaps between the bony plates of an infant's skull. The largest and most noticeable of these gaps is the "soft spot" on top of the head and toward the front, which lies between four bone plates. There is also a groove that runs like a center part toward the back of the head, where a much smaller soft spot is located. The fontanelles serve two purposes. During birth, they permit the head to adapt without injury to being squeezed as it passes through the birth canal. After birth, they permit the brain to grow. During the first two or three years of a child's life, the skull plates grow toward each other until they meet, covering the soft spots. However, the plates do not fully knit together until shortly before adolescence, when the brain stops growing.

The baby's soft spot is supported by tough membrane and does not have to be treated more delicately than any other part of the head. It is normal for it to be slightly depressed, to tense up when the baby cries, and to pulsate in rhythm with the heartbeat. (Contrary to what many believe, the pulsation is not that of an artery directly beneath the soft spot. Instead, it is caused by changes in the pressure of cerebrospinal fluid, which surrounds and protects the brain and spinal cord.)

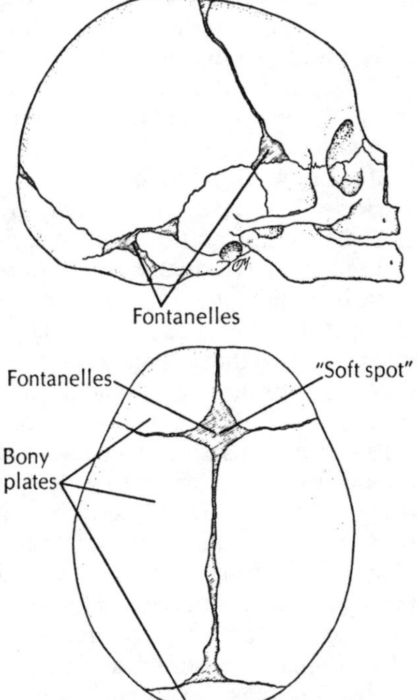

Fontanelles are the gaps between the bony plates of an infant's skull. Fontanelles permit the head to adapt without injury to being squeezed during birth, and after birth they allow room for the brain to grow. Eventually, the bones meet and knit together.

Food allergy

A food allergy is an allergic reaction to a specific food and most often occurs in children. (An allergy is an unusual reaction or oversensitivity to an outside substance, called an allergen.)

A food allergy needs to be distinguished from a food intolerance. A food intolerance exists when contaminants such as bacteria or chemicals are present in the food, or when the body lacks the certain natural chemicals called enzymes needed to digest the food. A food allergy exists when the body's immune system actually manufactures antibodies as a reaction to the food. This food then becomes an example of an ingestant allergen (an allergy-causing substance that is swallowed or eaten). Any food can become an allergen, but the foods most commonly found to cause allergic reactions are milk, eggs, shellfish and other fish, peanuts, chocolate, strawberries, and citrus fruits.

The symptoms of a food allergy most commonly occur in the digestive tract: cramps, nausea, vomiting, and diarrhea. Other signs may also be present: hives, rash, headache, nasal congestion, or even anaphylactic shock (a very serious reaction that can be fatal, characterized by breathing problems, hives, collapse of blood vessels, and sometimes vomiting, diarrhea, and cramps).

Food allergy is diagnosed by having the patient maintain a detailed record of all foods eaten as well as of the times when symptoms appear. Elimination trials may also help diagnose the allergen; the patient eliminates one food at a time from the diet to see if the symptoms disappear. In addition, several tests are used to detect all types of allergens: scratch tests, in which a small amount of the suspected allergen is applied to a scratch on the skin; intracutaneous tests, in which a small amount of the allergen is injected in or under the skin; and the radioallergosorbent technique, in which specific antibodies in the blood are measured.

There is no way to treat or prevent a food allergy other than to avoid eating the food. Fortunately, children usually outgrow these allergies.

See also Allergy and Anaphylactic shock.

Fracture

A fracture is a break in a bone or a cartilage, and it can be one of several different types.

The most common fractures are the closed fracture, the comminuted fracture, the complicated fracture, the composite fracture, the greenstick fracture, the impacted fracture, and the open fracture.

- Closed fracture–one in which the skin is not broken
- Comminuted fracture–one in which the bone is broken into several pieces
- Complicated fracture–one in which significant injury has been done to internal organs, blood vessels, or nerves
- Composite fracture–one in which there are multiple breaks in the bone
- Greenstick fracture–one in which only one side of the bone is broken and the bone is not severed
- Impacted fracture – one in which the ends or fragments of bone are jammed together
- Open fracture–one in which the broken end(s) of the bone pierces the skin.

Most often, fractures are caused by direct violence, such as a blow from a heavy object. They can, however, be the result of an indirect cause. A fall on a hand, for example, may result in a fractured collarbone. There are also pathological fractures, in which disease softens the bone and leads to a break.

Among the symptoms of a fracture are pain, swelling, loss of strength, abnormal movement, and a grating sound caused when the broken pieces of bone rub together. Shock (collapse of the circulatory system) may also occur with a severe fracture if large amounts of blood are lost.

Bone fractures are treated by closed (nonsurgical) or open (surgical) reduction. Reduction is a procedure in which the broken bone is manipulated, for example, by pulling or bending, so that the ends will be in the best position for healing. The pieces of bone are often held together by pins, metal plates, and rods, some of which are left in the body and others of which are removed after healing has taken place. Most fractures are treated through closed reduction. However, open reduction may be required when damage to bones, joints, ligaments, tendons, or other internal parts is severe or extensive.

Fractures are common among children and older people. Children have relatively soft, elastic bones. For this reason, their breaks may be

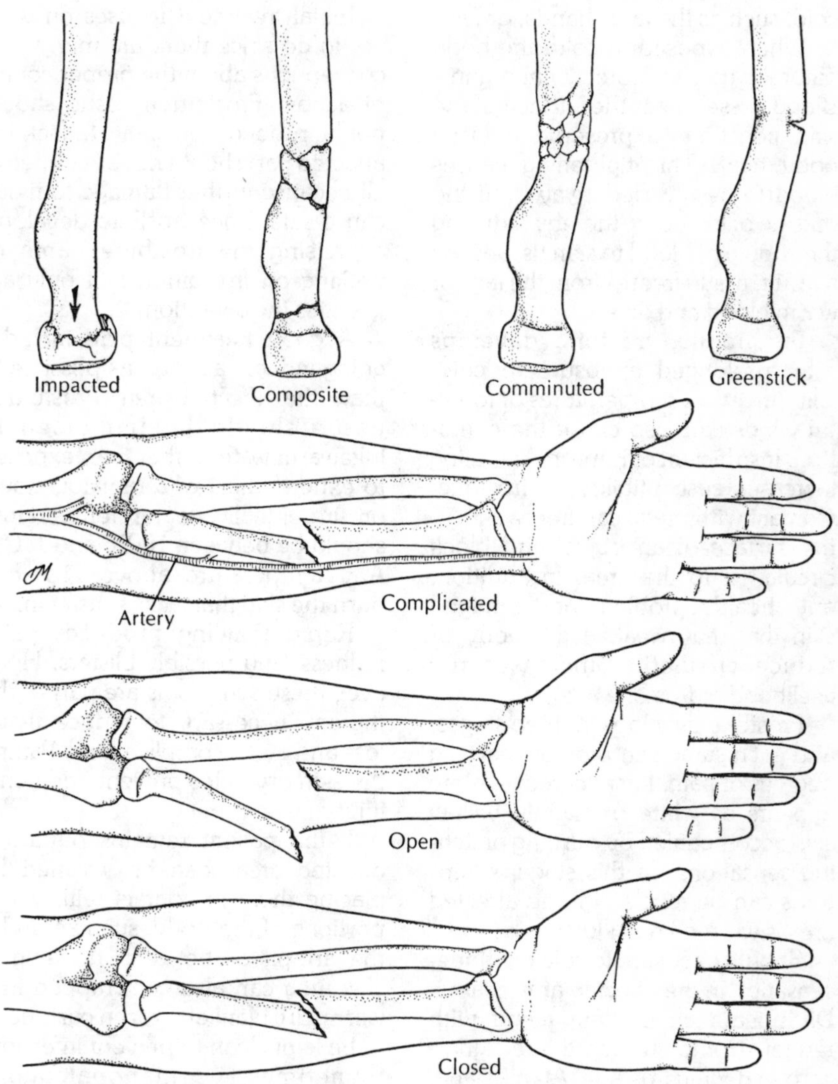

A fracture is a break in a bone and can be one of several types as shown here.

incomplete, that is, they may be on only one side of the bone. Older people have brittle bones that tend to break easily. Hip fractures are particularly common among the elderly. Among the more serious consequences of fractures are the possibility of infection and the possible damage done to the nerves, blood vessels, and internal organs near the fracture.

Frostbite

Frostbite is damage to skin tissue resulting from exposure to low environmental temperatures. The condition can affect any part of the body, but more often those areas involved have the poorest blood circulation and greatest exposure to cold, such as the face, hands, or feet.

When exposed to cold, the body naturally tries to protect vital organs. Blood vessels near the surface of the skin constrict to preserve internal body heat. This tightening causes blood to be diverted away from the outside of the body, thereby reducing the supply of blood to skin tissues. As a result, tissue freezes from the lack of warm blood and dies.

Frequently, frostbite develops after prolonged exposure to cold. Extremely low temperatures or forceful winds can also cause the condition. Insufficient or improper clothing increases susceptibility to frostbite. Contact with metal can freeze skin to the surface of an object and block circulation to the area. In addition, any health problem or damaged skin that may weaken the body or reduce circulation increases the likelihood of frostbite.

Frostbite develops in three stages, and each stage can produce varying degrees of pain. First degree frostbite appears as white or slightly yellow skin accompanied by burning or itching sensations. In this stage, symptoms can be reversed if the affected area is warmed quickly.

Should exposure to cold continue, sensation in the affected area ceases. Disappearance of pain along with reddened and swollen tissue signals second degree frostbite. At this stage, warming the area may produce blisters and skin peeling. Blisters may persist for weeks, and tenderness may linger for months.

Skin with third degree frostbite becomes waxy and hard. By this stage, skin tissue dies and the affected portions may show edema (collection of fluid in tissues). Severe frostbite can damage muscles, tendons, and nerves. Blood clots may form in small blood vessels and inhibit circulation. In turn, blockage causes death of tissue (gangrene).

Initial treatment focuses on what *not* to do since there are many misconceptions about the proper course of action. Frostbitten tissue should not be rubbed with snow. In fact, the affected part should not be rubbed at all because further damage to tissue can result. Once frostbite develops, exercising the frostbitten area or walking on frostbitten feet only aggravates the condition.

A good treatment plan includes going indoors as soon as possible to thaw the affected area. Frostbitten tissue should be immersed in lukewarm water rather than exposed to extreme heat of a radiator, stove, or fire. Ideally, water temperature should be between 100°F and 110°F. Any temperature above 110° can burn the skin that lacks sensation.

Rapid thawing produces pain, redness, and possibly blisters. However, these symptoms are part of the therapy necessary to reduce tissue loss and avoid complications. Patting the skin dry helps prevent additional injury.

If the patient remains outdoors, affected areas can be warmed by placing them in contact with warm portions of the body, such as under the armpit or between the thighs. The area can also be wrapped in a warm, dry blanket. Frozen parts need to be kept clean to prevent infection. Sometimes, warm nonalcoholic drinks aid circulation. Nevertheless, affected people should not smoke because smoking constricts blood vessels.

Once frozen tissue rewarms, the patient should elevate the extremity to promote increased blood circulation and maintain the skin at room temperature. Most cases of frostbite require a doctor's consultation. The physician may prescribe medication to prevent infection or formation of clots in blood vessels.

The best prevention of frostbite is

to wear adequate clothing to protect the skin. Feet, hands, and parts of the face need covering since these areas are likely to have the poorest blood circulation and are the most exposed. When weather is unusually cold or windy, remaining indoors or keeping outside trips short to limit exposure is recommended.

See also Gangrene.

G

Gallstones

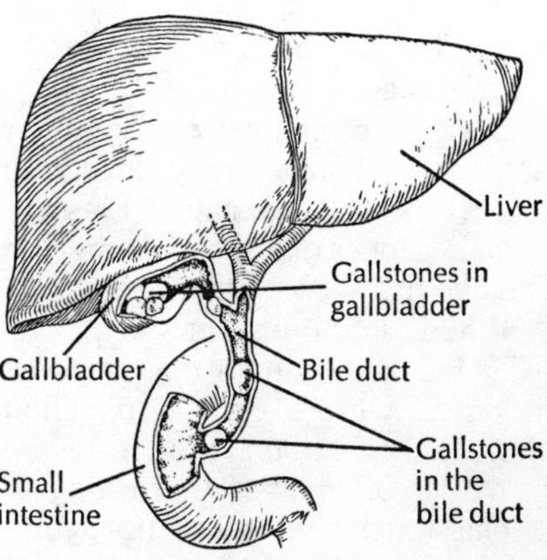

Gallstones can form in the gallbladder or bile duct and cause inflammation of the gallbladder or even liver damage if they block the flow of bile from the gallbladder to the small intestine.

Gallstones are hardened masses that consist mainly of cholesterol, a substance regularly found in animal fats, blood, bile (fluid produced in the liver and stored in the gallbladder that is required for fat absorption in the small intestine), the liver, and other tissues. The stones form in the gallbladder or in the bile duct leading from the gallbladder into the small intestine, where food is digested and nutrients absorbed into the blood.

When bile contains excessive amounts of cholesterol in comparison to other ingredients, the unnecessary cholesterol separates from the solution and forms stone-like masses. Unfortunately, these stones cannot be prevented by controlling cholesterol intake in the diet. Cholesterol from food passes into the blood, and there is no relationship between cholesterol levels in the blood and cholesterol levels in the bile.

In addition to concentrated bile and bile salts, several other factors contribute to the formation of gallstones. Eating too much fat, infection, liver disease, and forms of anemia can lead to gallstones.

Pregnancy, obesity, or diabetes can also increase the risk of gallstones. Overweight people who frequently lose and gain large amounts of weight seem more susceptible to gallstones, as do women who have had two or more children. Although reasons are unclear, twice as many women as men over age 40 develop gallstones.

By themselves, gallstones often produce no signs of disease. About half the people with gallstones have no symptoms. Symptoms that do appear are usually chronic (long-term) in nature, causing discomfort and pain in the upper abdomen, indigestion, nausea, and intolerance of fatty foods. Sometimes stones pass through the bile duct into the intestines to be excreted naturally.

However, symptoms can occur if the stones lodge in the bile duct. In an acute gallbladder attack, a sharp pain often on the right side of the upper abdomen may travel to the back and under the right shoulder blade. Frequently, the pain develops suddenly after a meal and leads to fever, chills, vomiting, and possibly jaundice (yellowing of the skin and whites of the eyes caused by excess bile pigment). These symptoms occur after a stone that was previously free-floating in the gallbladder becomes trapped in the bile duct.

Serious complications of liver damage or jaundice may develop if stones block the flow of bile. Pressure from the stones may also inflame and damage nearby organs.

When gallstones remain in the gallbladder, the organ may become inflamed with a condition called cholecystitis, which causes severe pain 30 to 60 minutes after eating.

Gallstones that show no symptoms may be detected by an X ray of the gallbladder called a cholecystogram. A cholecystogram is taken after the patient swallows a tablet containing dye which outlines the gallbladder and any stones that may be present. Some physicians use ultrasound rather than X ray; ultrasound is a procedure in which sound waves bounce off internal body organs and construct a visual image.

For acute attacks of gallstones with severe and prolonged symptoms, doctors recommend a cholecystectomy (surgical removal of the gallbladder). This treatment is one of the most common forms of abdominal surgery. Many doctors even suggest removing a gallbladder containing stones that is not causing symptoms to avoid future complications.

As an alternative to surgery, some researchers are investigating a drug to dissolve cholesterol gallstones. There is also some experimentation being conducted to see if gallstones can be dissolved with localized forms of high-intensity radiation.

See also Bile and Cholecystitis.

Gamma globulin

Gamma globulin is a protein containing antibodies in the blood. Gamma globulin is developed by the body in response to invasion by harmful agents, such as bacteria, viruses and toxins. Its purpose is to react chemically with the invading agent and destroy it, thus providing immunity. Almost all antibodies produced in the body's defense system are gamma globulin molecules.

Gamma globulin preparations are derived from the blood of another person or animal and contain preformed antibodies made by that person or animal. The preparations are widely used for the prevention, modification, and treatment of many kinds of infectious diseases. This type of gamma globulin is usually injected and contains almost all the known antibodies circulating in the blood. It can provide a passive (borrowed) immunity lasting up to about six weeks.

In cases of hepatitis, for example, gamma globulin injections are especially useful, since human blood gamma globulins do not transmit hepatitis. Not only is gamma globulin given to the hepatitis patient, but to all household members and other persons who have been in direct contact with a case or cases of infectious hepatitis. Persons with a high risk of exposure to hepatitis, such as hospital staff members and persons traveling in areas where hepatitis is prevalent, should receive a dose of gamma globulin every four to five months to maintain the preventive effects.

Measles can be prevented in many cases by the administration of gamma globulin injections within five days of exposure. The injections are especially important for children under three years, for pregnant women, for tuberculosis patients, or for those with impaired immune mechanisms. Often even if measles is not prevented, a less serious case will result; however, gamma globulin is of no use once the symptoms appear.

Similarly, chicken pox can be prevented or its seriousness modified if gamma globulin is given within five days of exposure.

Gamma globulin can also be used as a diagnostic tool: one important symptom of multiple sclerosis, for example, is that the proportion of gamma globulin in the patient's cerebrospinal fluid is altered in about 60 percent of the cases, especially those that are long-lasting. This is an especially important finding, since this is the only definitive known lab test for multiple sclerosis.

Gangrene

Gangrene is a term that refers to the death of body tissue, often in a considerable mass. It is usually associated with the loss of blood, and hence nutrient supply, and followed by bacterial infection and decomposition of the tissue. Although it usually affects the extremities of the body, gangrene can sometimes affect the internal organs—in which case it may be followed or attended by pain and general collapse.

There are three major types of gangrene: moist, dry, and gas gangrene. Moist and dry gangrene both result from the loss of blood circulation. Dry gangrene usually refers to tissue death that occurs without bacterial decomposition, so that the tissues become dry and shriveled. In moist gangrene, on the other hand, the tissue death is accompanied by decomposition resulting from bacterial action. The third type, gas gangrene, occurs in wounds infected by anaerobic (able to live without air) bacteria, which break down tissues by producing gas and toxins. Each of the types has its own specific causes and symptoms.

Moist gangrene is usually caused by a sudden stoppage of blood to a certain body site, usually resulting from burning by heat or by acid; from severe freezing; from a physical accident that destroys the tissues; from a tourniquet that has remained on too long; or from a clot or other blockage. At first, tissues affected by moist gangrene are the color of a severe bruise and are swollen and often blistered. The gangrenous infection is likely to spread rapidly as toxins are formed in the affected tissues and absorbed.

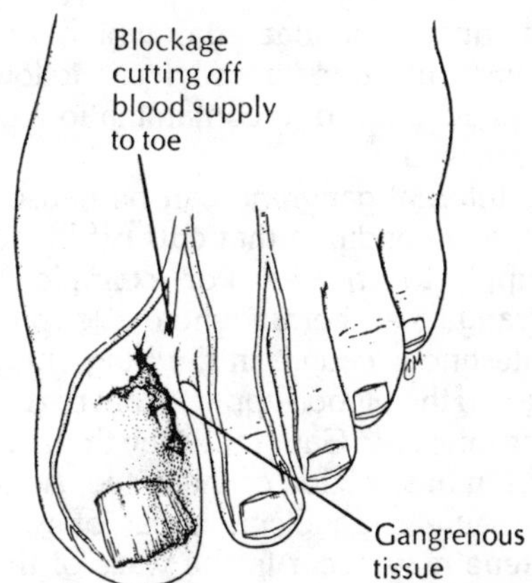

Gangrene is the death of body tissue usually caused by lack of blood circulation to an area. It often affects the extremities, such as a toe, and is characterized by breakdown and decomposition of tissue.

Dry gangrene, on the other hand, usually occurs gradually and results from a slow, gradual reduction of blood flow in the arteries. As mentioned earlier, there is no bacterial decomposition; the tissues simply become dry and shriveled. This type of gangrene occurs only in the extremities. It may occur as a secondary effect of arteriosclerosis in the elderly, of advanced stages of diabetes, or of Buerger's disease (an inflammatory condition that affects the blood vessels of the limbs, primarily the legs, leading to an inadequate blood flow to the affected part and eventually to gangrene).

Gas gangrene is often caused by dirty wounds that become infected by anaerobic bacteria, which are commonly found in soil. It can follow rapidly after dirt contamination of deep wounds.

Internal gangrene can be caused by any condition that cuts off blood supply to an area. For example, a strangulated hernia where a loop of intestine is caught in the bulge may cut off the blood supply to that part of the intestine. Gangrene may then occur in that section of the tissue. Also, in acute appendicitis, areas of gangrene may occur in the walls of the appendix with rupture of the appendix through the gangrenous area. In severe cholecystitis, inflammation of the gallbladder usually associated with gallstones, gangrene can develop in areas where the stones compress the mucous membrane cutting off the blood supply.

In all these instances, the gangrene is secondary to—a result of—another primary infection.

Moist gangrene is characterized by a purplish-red, bruised color, by swelling and, often, by blisters. Dry gangrene is marked by gradual shrinking of the tissues, which first grow cold and lack a pulse, then turn brown, then black. Usually there is a sharp "line of demarcation" where the gangrene stops due to the fact that the tissue above and below this line is continuing to receive plenty of blood. This type of gangrene is sometimes called *mummification* of tissue because of the dry, shriveled, dark appearance.

The symptoms of gas gangrene are swelling; paleness of skin; and a thin, not foul, discharge—the gas and foul smell come later in the progression of this form of the disorder. It is an acute, painful condition in which the muscles and tissues under the skin literally become filled with gas and a thin, bloody discharge.

Treatment of moist and dry gangrene usually involves simple drainage and cleaning out of the area, along with medication such as penicillin and other antibiotics. Gas gangrene is also treated with cleaning of the wound and either penicillin or tetracycline antibiotics. The effectiveness of antibiotic therapy seems to depend on the time elapsed between injury and/or infection and the point where the treatment begins.

In the case of gangrene such as the form caused by deterioration in the blood supply of the elderly or gangrene associated with appendicitis, hernia, diabetes, or Buerger's disease, the treatment begins with the diagnosis and treatment of the underlying condition.

Preventing gangrene in an open wound begins with cleanliness. All dirt and particles from an open wound should be removed as soon as possible, and alcohol, hydrogen peroxide, or tincture of iodine should be applied. If a tourniquet must be used in cases of excessive bleeding, it should be loosened for about one minute in every ten-minute interval in order to keep fresh blood circulating in the tissues. Burned skin requires careful, antiseptic handling in order not to become gangrenous. Frostbite also is dangerous because the freezing impairs circulation, and skin is tender and easily broken. Frostbitten skin must be handled with great care to avoid gangrenous infections.

See also Frostbite.

Gastric bypass

See Bypass surgery.

Gastroenteritis

Gastroenteritis is an inflammation of the lining of the stomach and the intestine.

Gastroenteritis can be caused by bacteria or viruses; by allergic reactions to certain foods or to certain drinks; by infectious diseases, such as typhoid fever or influenza; by food poisoning; by overconsumption of alcohol; or by certain drugs.

Symptoms include headache, nausea, vomiting, diarrhea, and gas pains in the stomach and the intestine. Often, the individual will feel that gas is "caught" in certain portions of the intestine. On occasions, the intestines will seem to cramp, producing severe pain.

The first task in treating gastroenteritis is to identify the cause or causes of the inflammation. Blood tests and cultures for viruses or bacteria may be done. If the problem is caused by an allergic reaction, the source of the reaction may be identified by allergy tests. Antibiotics can be administered for bacterial infections. A variety of medicines (many nonprescription) can ease the effects of stomach cramps and gas pains. Diarrhea may necessitate replacement of lost water. If the patient is a victim of heart disease, lost fluid (and resulting imbalances in the electrolyte and fluid balance) may cause irregular heartbeat.

Maintaining a clean kitchen, eating in restaurants where the kitchens are kept clean, washing fresh foods thoroughly, and cooking foods carefully are all safeguards against bacterial and viral infections. Identification of allergy-causing foods and moderation in alcohol consumption also help prevent gastroenteritis if these are the causes of the problem.

Genes

A gene is the basic unit of hereditary characteristics in the cell. A gene is a component of DNA which, in turn, is a component of chromosomes. Chromosomes are threadlike coils within every living cell that contain the "blueprint" or "genetic code" for the cell. This code is contained in strands of DNA, which is the basic building block of chromosomes and which is composed of genes. Each gene is an instruction for a particular characteristic. (It has been estimated that each cell contains about five feet of coiled DNA strands and each strand carries about 100,000 genes.)

It is the genes, then, as part of the structure of the DNA, that determine both what a cell is and how it works. It is as if a computer program not only told the computer what to do but helped to form the machine itself.

Consequently, cells that are coded to develop into tissue for the human liver, for example, do so because that is what their genetic coding tells them to do. Cells that give rise to bone tissue do so because that is what their genes tell them to do. The same goes for blue eyes, long fingers, brown hair, and all the other characteristics that an individual human body exhibits.

Each cell in the human body contains 46 chromosomes, made up of genes. The only exception to this rule are the sex cells—the ovum and sperm—each of which contain only 23 chromosomes. When these sex cells unite, as in the fertilization of the ovum by a sperm, the result is the full complement of chromosomes with genes that are donated by both parents. Since each parent donates only 23 chromosomes (half of the genetic coding that makes each parent a unique individual), the resulting offspring is a blending of a portion of each parent's genetic material.

The traits that genes give rise to are called *dominant* or *recessive*. A recessive gene usually carries a trait that does not appear because it is overridden by a dominant gene. Eye color provides an example. Usually, when one parent has brown eyes and the other parent has blue eyes, the offspring will have brown eyes. This means that for this particular union of genetic material, brown eyes are a dominant genetic characteristic, while blue eyes are recessive. Of course, it does not always work this way, and sometimes a child will have green or hazel eyes from a union of brown-eyed and blue-eyed parents. Furthermore, the brown-eyed child may have inherited the recessive blue-eyed trait. If, in the future, the brown-eyed person's recessive blue-eyed trait combines with another recessive blue-eyed trait in creating a new individual, the two recessive traits may override the brown-eyed trait, and the new individual will be blue-eyed.

Genes sometimes mutate. This means that for some reason (a malformed gene, the effects of toxic substances or disease, radiation, or even —as some have speculated—a chance collision between a gene and a cosmic particle), the offspring will exhibit physical or mental characteristics that are not evident in either parent. The same is true in the case of recessive genes: sometimes, a gene that is normally recessive will show up in offspring when least expected. It can be as simple a phenomenon as, for example, a deformed ear that is shared by a grandparent but by no other member of the family.

The discovery of the structure of the DNA molecule has opened a new era in biological research, the most recent branch of which is called genetic engineering. In this field, through complex procedures and high technology, researchers hope to be able to eliminate diseases such as cancer by altering the genetic coding of the human body and its immune system.

See also Chromosomes and DNA.

Genital warts

Genital warts (condylomata acuminata) are small growths caused by a virus that appear on the external genital organs and are considered to be a sexually transmitted disease. (A sexually transmitted disease, also known as a venereal disease, is a highly contagious illness spread primarily through direct sexual contact.)

If left untreated, genital warts can grow quite large, causing discomfort during sexual intercourse, urination, and bowel movements. They tend to be seen more frequently in uncircumcised men than in those who have been circumcised. Pregnancy may make them grow faster, but they usually shrink after the baby is born. However, they may become so large that they block the birth canal, making a cesarean delivery necessary. The wart virus can also be transmitted from a mother to her child during birth, but there is no evidence that it causes any serious complications in infants, as do some other sexually transmitted diseases.

Genital warts are caused by direct sexual contact with an infected person. About 60 percent of all those exposed to them will develop the disease. However, the warts will not appear until six weeks to eight months after the initial exposure.

The only symptom of genital warts are the warts themselves, appearing most frequently on the penis, vagina, anus (opening from the rectum to the outside), and, less commonly, in the mouth or on the cervix (neck of the uterus). They are soft, moist, and pink, appearing alone or in clusters; cluster formations tend to resemble cauliflower in their uneven, puffy appearance. They are seldom painful, but they can be irritated by sexual intercourse.

Genital warts can usually be diagnosed by a simple physical examination because their appearance is so distinct. If there is any doubt, a sample of tissue from the wart can be tested to rule out other disorders such as cancerous growths or the swelling that often accompanies syphilis, another sexually transmitted disease.

Genital warts are treated with a drug called podophyllin, applied directly to the warts, then washed off several hours later. More than one application may be necessary. Podophyllin is toxic in large quantities, however, so very large or troublesome warts are often removed by cryotherapy (a process in which liquid nitrogen freezes the growths off) or by heat treatments which dry out and destroy the warts.

A person who has developed genital warts or any other sexually transmitted disease should abstain from sexual activity until all tests have indicated that the disease is no longer present. A case of genital warts, as well as all sexually transmitted diseases, requires that every sexual partner of the infected person also be examined and treated, if necessary.

Genital warts can be prevented, obviously, by avoiding sexual contact with someone who has the disease. However, since this cannot always be possible, it should be remembered that the chances of contracting these diseases increase with the number of different sexual partners a person has; therefore, limiting the number of partners may decrease the chances of developing this disease.

Gilles de la Tourette's syndrome

Gilles de la Tourette's syndrome is a childhood disorder marked by intense tics (twitchy, repetitive movements of certain muscles) which may be either single or multiple. It begins, generally in boys, around the age of seven or eight years. At first the tics are simple: facial twisting, blinking, grimacing, shoulder shrugging or twitching. Later the tics progress to vocal tics accompanied by psychological involvement.

The causes of Gilles de la Tourette's syndrome are unknown. It is still disputed whether the disorder is of physical or of psychological origin.

The symptoms of Gilles de la Tourette's syndrome are at first limited to the muscles in the face, head, neck, and shoulders. At first, and often as the first symptom, there are incomprehensible gasping or breathing noises from the larynx (voice box) as if the patient were barking, wheezing, or gasping for air. As the tics spread to the shoulders and arms, there are shoulder shrugs and twitches, and twistings of the neck and arm.

Next, vocal tics, such as grunting, sniffling, snuffing, shouting, and "barking" sounds, begin to develop. As the vocal symptoms worsen, the patient begins to exclaim in a loud voice words or phrases with obscene meanings or common "swear words." Echolalia (repetition by the patient of all that is said to him or her, almost automatically) is often seen. The patient will seem to "fixate" on a word or phrase and repeat it over and over with increasing speed. Often, too, the individual will spasmodically and automatically repeat or mimic the actions of those around him or her.

The symptoms of Gilles de la Tourette's syndrome tend to come and go, especially as the patient approaches puberty and adulthood. Tics that are very violent during waking hours often stop during sleep. Some tics are intensified by emotional upheavals. Unlike most movement disorders, Tourette tics are often suppressed in school or social settings and expressed more often when the patient is alone or with family members. In some cases, the tics are capable of being suppressed by voluntary control. The excessive swearing, however, unlike many of the other Tourette symptoms, only appears in the presence of others. Some patients attempt to cover it up by coughing, thus developing another tic. Often symptoms decrease in adult life and disappear, but return during a period of stress. Mental activity remains normal.

Diagnosing Tourette's syndrome is often difficult, since the early stages often resemble common childhood tics seen in many young school-age children. Also, early and middle-stage symptoms are difficult to distinguish from certain brain conditions, which can produce similar symptoms. However, Gilles de la Tourette's syndrome can often be diagnosed with some assurance as the course of the illness unfolds.

Tourette's syndrome can be treated with medications starting with small doses and increasing the dosage until the tics are controlled. Often a combination of drugs is used, depending on the individual case. Group psychotherapy can be helpful in some cases, although it seems to be of limited use in most. In extreme cases, leukotomy, or surgical interruption of nerve fibers of the frontal lobe of the brain, is considered.

At present there are no known preventive measures for Tourette's syndrome.

Glaucoma

Glaucoma is an eye disorder that results from increased pressure within the eyeball. The pressure builds up because fluids within the eyeball are unable to circulate and drain normally.

Although glaucoma is understood to be a problem with the eye's fluid-regulating mechanism, its precise cause is unknown. In the healthy eye, aqueous fluid in the anterior chamber of the eyeball remains under gentle pressure. When the delicate fluid balance changes, internal pressure rises in the eye. This buildup produces damage to the sensitive structures and nerve endings within the eye.

Depending upon the type of defect in the fluid-regulating system, one of two primary forms of glaucoma results. *Chronic,* or *open angle,* glaucoma develops when pressure elevates gradually and normal fluid drainage slows but is not obstructed. *Acute,* or *closed angle,* glaucoma occurs when pressure mounts suddenly and forces the iris (colored portion of the eye) into an angle joining the cornea (transparent covering across the front of the eyeball that helps focus light), thereby blocking fluid drainage from the anterior chamber of the eye.

Both forms of glaucoma are more common in adults over 40 years of age. Statistics show that people with glaucoma in their families have greater risk of acquiring the condition, but inheritance has not been proven. Some evidence suggests that glaucoma may be linked to long-term use of certain drugs, especially steroids that can alter body fluid levels. Glaucoma can also follow other eye disorders such as infections, injuries, or cataracts.

Chronic glaucoma begins with no noticeable symptoms. Vision deterioration is so gradual and painless that this form of glaucoma has been termed the "sneak thief of sight." Sometimes, peripheral, or side, vision loss slowly progresses as central vision remains normal. As the disorder advances, other symptoms that may be intermittent or constant include foggy or blurred vision; difficulty in adjusting to brightness and darkness; and slight pain in or around the eye, usually on one side. The one symptom indicative of chronic glaucoma is the perception of a faint white circle or halo surrounding a light. This halo is most visible in the dark while looking at a distant light.

Acute glaucoma brings sudden and severe symptoms of extreme eye pain and abrupt vision blurring. Frequently, the pain can be so intense that it causes nausea and vomiting.

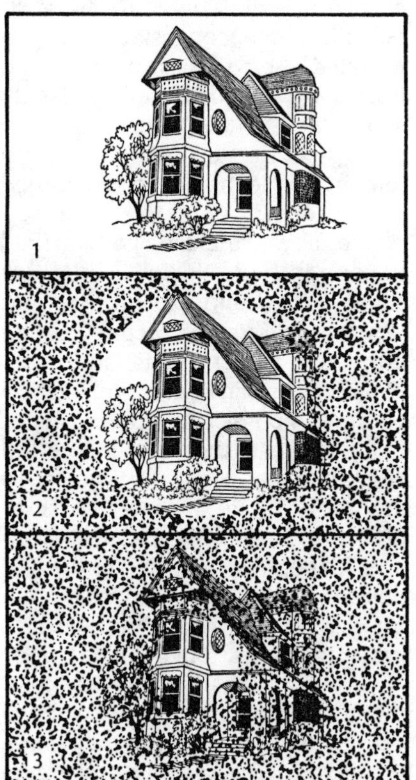

Untreated glaucoma can cause progressive loss of vision. View 1 is what is seen if glaucoma is properly treated and there is no vision loss. View 2 shows some loss of side vision that occurs with untreated glaucoma. View 3 shows serious loss of side vision with advanced untreated glaucoma.

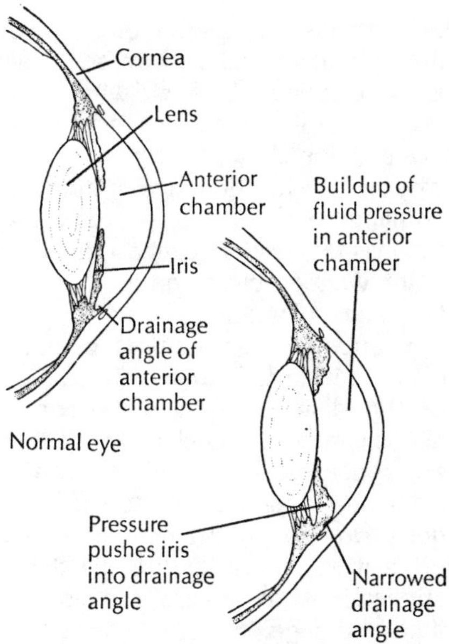

In acute glaucoma, normal drainage may be obstructed by a sudden elevation of fluid pressure which pushes the iris into the angle of the eye where the iris joins the cornea.

Fortunately, acute glaucoma is rare, but when it does occur, medical attention is needed immediately to prevent permanent blindness. Usually, however, the symptoms are so severe that medical help is promptly sought.

If left untreated, glaucoma can lead to partial or complete vision loss. However, if diagnosed early, treatment can usually halt the problem. Because chronic glaucoma gives no warning signs, it is particularly important that persons over the age of 40 be tested for glaucoma every two or three years. In addition, physicians recommend that people with family history of the disease be screened every year and possibly before the age of 40.

Glaucoma testing is a simple procedure. First, eyedrops anesthetize the eyeball. Then, the doctor places a pressure gauge on the front surface of the eye to measure the amount of pressure within. In addition, the doctor inspects the interior of the eye through a special instrument that allows a view of the angle where the iris and cornea meet. This part of the examination shows whether there is blockage in the drainage system or damage to the optic nerve. Side vision is also tested by measuring the point where objects enter the patient's field of vision.

Glaucoma treatment is usually effective if started early in the course of the disease. Acute glaucoma needs surgery to quickly restore the eye's draining system. Chronic glaucoma responds well to medications. Oral drugs work by decreasing production of eye fluid, while daily applications of eyedrops promote fluid drainage. Some medications constrict pupils of the eye, which can be misconstrued as a symptom of drug overdose. Consequently, many glaucoma patients carry an identification card with their medical history in case of emergency.

There is a new type of eyedrop called beta blocker which reduces production of eye fluid without altering the size of the pupil. However, beta blockers can affect heart rate and narrow breathing passages, making these drugs unsuitable for patients with heart or lung disease.

Although chronic glaucoma responds to medication, some patients (less than 5 percent) require surgery to open new pathways for fluid drainage. Laser therapy is the most current surgical technique under investigation. Here, the laser, or intense light beam, generates enough heat to alter tissues and cells in order to stimulate better fluid drainage.

The best way to prevent serious complications of glaucoma is periodic screening for early diagnosis. If glaucoma is diagnosed, attention to prescribed treatment procedures is required.

Glomerulonephritis

Glomerulonephritis is an inflammation of the capillaries (tiny blood vessels) in the filtering units of the kidneys, called glomeruli, where wastes are drawn from the blood to form urine. The disease can be caused by an infection in the kidneys, but most often it is due to an allergic or immune response to infections in other parts of the body, particularly streptococcal infections such as strep throat, or to drugs or poisons in the bloodstream. The immune response occurs as an inflammation of the capillaries in the glomeruli. The capillaries become congested and surrounded by blood cells and pus. Fluid builds up in surrounding tissue, sometimes causing the kidney to enlarge. Protein, which should remain in the blood, is discharged into the urine by the diseased glomeruli, and there is a general fluid buildup in body tissues. These two signs—fluid buildup (edema) and albumin (a form of protein) in the urine—are the two chief indicators of the disease first described in 1827 by English physician Richard Bright. (The disease used to be called Bright's disease, but doctors today are more likely to refer to it as glomerulonephritis from "glomeruli"; "nephro," referring to the kidney; and "itis," meaning inflammation.) If the disease continues to progress, the tiny arteries in the kidney become thickened and scarred so that some can no longer carry blood. The parts of the kidney they serve shrink and change. The eventual result of this process over many years may be total kidney failure. However, the great majority of patients with acute glomerulonephritis recover within one to two years. Only 5 to 20 percent develop chronic cases.

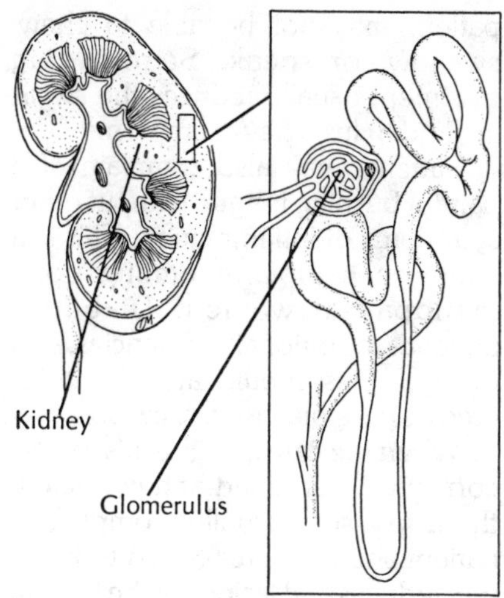

Glomerulonephritis is an inflammation of the tiny blood vessels of the glomeruli, the kidney's filtering units that draw wastes from the blood to form urine.

Although many different kinds of infections can lead to glomerulonephritis, including pneumonia, bacterial infection of the heart, secondary syphilis, malaria, hepatitis, and measles, by far the most common cause is streptococcal infection of the throat, tonsils, or skin.

Symptoms of glomerulonephritis begin one to six weeks after an initial infection such as strep throat. The patient has headaches, a mild fever, a puffy face, pain in the area between the ribs and the hip, and decreased urine output. The urine may be bloody or coffee-colored. Shortness of breath may occur, together with increased heartbeat and a rise in blood pressure. A urine test for protein and red blood cells confirms the diagnosis. In extreme cases, the bloated condition of the body from accumulated fluids can cause the symptoms of heart failure, including rapid heartbeat, heart enlargement, and congestion of the lungs.

Treatment consists of bed rest until one to two weeks after tests of blood, blood pressure, and of the urine reveal that the kidney is back to normal. Sodium (salt) and protein may be restricted or even forbidden for a time. Fluids are restricted until the output of urine returns to normal. Heart failure is treated with restriction of salt and water and use of oxygen and the drug digitalis. Any infection is treated promptly with antibiotics.

If the disease is still present after one to two years, it may be considered chronic. Typically, the damage to the kidney continues to progress, but so slowly that the patient is without symptoms except for evidence in the urine including protein and red and white blood cells. A normal life may be possible for 20 or 30 years until the kidney can no longer function. At that time, replacement with a kidney transplant or periodic cleansing of the blood with a dialysis machine is necessary for life.

Guarding against infection, injury, and fatigue can help prevent flare-ups of the disease. Intake of protein may have to be limited, depending upon how the kidney is working. Plenty of fluids and normal activity are desirable, but strenuous exercise should be avoided, to prevent fatigue.

Glossitis

Glossitis is an acute or chronic inflammation of the tongue. It may exist either as a primary disease or as a symptom of another disease or disorder.

The causes of glossitis can be either *local* or *systemic*. Local causes include immediate irritants such as jagged or broken teeth; badly-fitting dentures; poor oral habits; biting of the tongue (such as during convulsions); irritants such as alcohol, tobacco, hot or spicy foods; or even mouthwashes, toothpastes, or breath fresheners. Local infections, burns, and injuries may also produce glossitis symptoms. Systemic causes may include certain vitamin deficiencies (especially Vitamin B deficiencies, such as in pellagra), anemia, generalized skin diseases such as erythema (redness of the skin because of capillary congestion), and syphilis.

Glossitis symptoms vary widely, ranging from simple redness of the tip and edges of the tongue (if the cause is pellagra, anemia, or irritation from smoking or a tooth with a rough surface) to painful ulcers and whitish patches. In the later stages of pellagra, the entire tongue may be fiery red, swollen, and ulcerated. In iron deficiency and pernicious anemia, the tongue is pale and smooth. Painful ulcers on the tongue may indicate herpes lesions, tuberculosis, a streptococcal infection, or other diseases. White patches suggest candidiasis (a type of yeast infection), syphilis, or simple mouth breathing (which dries out the mucous membrane of the tongue). Very smooth and painless areas may be what is called geographic tongue, or "benign" glossitis. Hairy tongue usually has no symptoms and often follows antibiotic therapy, a high fever, excessive use of certain mouthwashes, or a simple reduction in saliva secretion. Tiny brown growths on the tongue usually come from tobacco stains or from certain bacteria; the treatment is to stop smoking or otherwise correct the underlying cause and also to "brush" the tongue with a toothbrush.

Severe acute glossitis, which can result from local infection, burns, and injury, can cause tenderness and pain sufficient to make the tongue protrude from the mouth into the back of the throat—creating the danger of airway obstruction and even suffocation. In severe cases, the patient may not be able to chew, swallow, or speak. Steroid drug treatment usually reduces the swelling and helps relieve symptoms.

Patients may also complain of a painful burning tongue without other symptoms of inflammation. This is a common complaint among postmenopausal women. Diabetes, anemias, nutritional deficiencies, and malignancies should all be considered as possible primary causes.

When the cause of glossitis can be correctly determined and corrected, the response is usually prompt. The patient should be reassured to know that redness and lesions of the tongue are usually harmless and respond well to treatment. Such complaints as ulcers and "hairy tongue," however, often recur periodically; ulcers that do not respond to treatment after a week or so should be biopsied (have a sample of tissue taken to be examined under a microscope).

In treating glossitis, specific causes, such as jagged teeth or ill-fitting dentures, should be corrected. Irritants, including hot or spicy foods, tobacco, alcohol, mouthwashes, and toothpastes should be avoided once they are identified as the source of the trouble. A bland or liquid diet, preferably cool or cold, will often have a soothing effect. Good oral hygiene is indicated in all cases.

Symptomatic relief for large lesions include rinsing the mouth with a medicated mouthwash before meals. Topical anesthetics, such as lidocaine and benzocaine, applied to the lesions, can give relief. Patients with complaints of painful burning should be tested for Vitamin B_{12} deficiency and to rule out more serious ailments, such as diabetes and anemias.

Prevention of glossitis involves avoiding all irritants to the tongue and mouth as well as correcting nutritional and vitamin deficiencies and treating all primary infections that produce glossitis as a secondary symptom.

Goiter

Goiter is an enlargement of the thyroid gland, characterized by a swelling at the front of the neck. It may be caused by a lack of dietary iodine which is necessary for the production of thyroid hormone. In this case, the thyroid gland enlarges in an attempt to produce more hormone. When this happens, the cells in the gland enlarge, but do not increase in number. If iodine deficiency is minor, the condition is usually confined to young women. Men and school-age children are affected if the iodine deficiency is severe.

Goiter was at one time common in areas where there is a lack of iodine in the soil and water. Since the ocean is the basic source of iodine, inland areas were the most deficient (in the United States, the Great Lakes region was such an area; in Europe mountainous inland regions in the Alps often had inhabitants with iodine deficiency). In recent times, however, iodized table salt has solved this problem.

Some forms of goiter are associated with an overactive thyroid gland, that is, the diseased thyroid produces more hormone than the body needs. In this case, the symptoms accompanying the swelling in the neck include nervousness, weight loss, bulging eyes, rapid heartbeat, and occasionally high blood pressure. Sometimes a person with goiter shows signs of an underactive thyroid, such as sluggishness, weight gain, dry skin and hair, and fatigue. Often, however, the only symptom of goiter is the swelling in the neck.

The chief objective of goiter

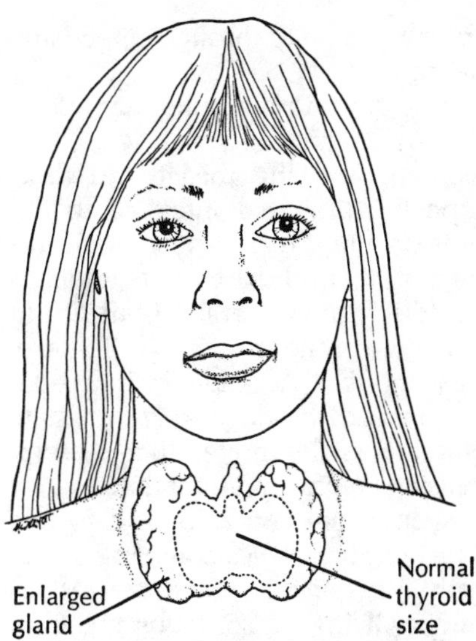

Goiter is a swelling in the neck caused by an enlarged thyroid, whose cells have enlarged to produce more thyroid hormone.

treatment is reduction of the swelling. The first step is usually to suppress the thyroid gland's overfunctioning. If the goiter is caused by simple iodine deficiency, small doses of iodine can be given. Sometimes, administering synthetic thyroid hormone, in an attempt to halt the gland's increased efforts to produce the natural hormone, will reduce the enlargement. If treatment is started early enough, surgery to remove enlarged portions of the gland can be avoided. On the other hand, while surgery is not usually advised, it is sometimes necessary in cases in which the size of the goiter interferes with normal breathing by pressing on the windpipe.

See also Hyperthyroidism and Hypothyroidism.

Gonorrhea

Gonorrhea is the most frequently reported sexually transmitted disease, also known as venereal disease. It is a highly contagious infection spread primarily through direct sexual contact.

Gonorrhea predominantly affects the penis in men, the vagina in women, and the throat and anus (opening from the intestine to the outside) in both sexes. Left untreated, it can lead to a generalized blood infection, sterility (inability to conceive children), arthritis, and heart trouble. Additionally, in men it can spread throughout the prostate gland and the male duct system, causing painful inflammation.

Gonorrhea can also lead to eye infections if the eyes come in contact with the genital secretions—for instance, if the person rubs the eyes after handling the genital organs. Moreover, it can infect the eyes of a newborn during birth and cause blindness as the baby moves through the birth canal; most states, however, require that a few drops of silver nitrate or penicillin be placed in the eyes of all newborns to prevent this possibility.

Gonorrhea is caused by a bacterial infection and is spread by direct sexual contact with an infected person.

In females, this disease may exist entirely without symptoms, but in many cases it is marked by a discharge from the vagina and urethra; frequent, painful urination; cloudy urine; vomiting; and diarrhea. Gonorrhea often leads to pelvic inflammatory disease (PID), which, in turn, often causes sterility. (PID results when an infection in the lower reproductive or urinary tract moves to the fallopian tubes, forming scar tissue and blocking the tubes, thereby preventing conception. Its symptoms are lower abdominal pain, fever, chills, and vaginal discharge.)

The symptoms of gonorrhea in men are a yellowish discharge from the penis within two to ten days of exposure to the disease, accompanied by painful and burning urination.

Gonorrhea of the anus is marked by an often bloody or mucus-filled discharge from the anus and pain during bowel movements. Gonorrhea of the throat may have no noticeable symptoms or may reveal itself only by a scratchy, sore throat.

Diagnosis is accomplished by taking a "smear" (sample) of the dis-

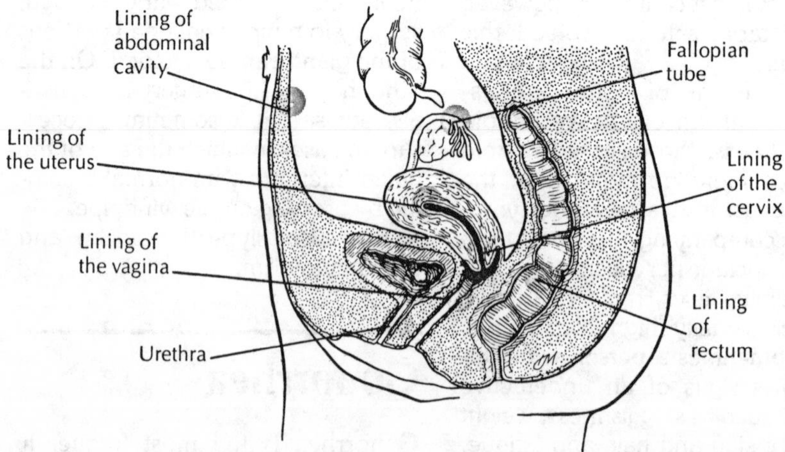

In females, an untreated gonorrhea infection may spread to various sites in the pelvic area as shown causing pelvic inflammatory disease and perhaps sterility.

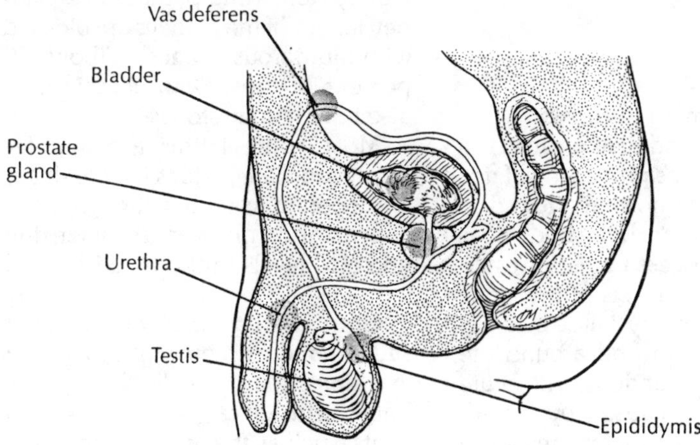

In males untreated gonorrhea may involve the prostate gland, the male duct system (including the epididymis, which connects the testis to the vas deferens, and the vas deferens, which conducts the sperm cells to the urethra), the bladder, and the urethra.

charge, examining it under a microscope to identify the gonorrhea bacterium, and confirming the diagnosis with a culture of the smear in which the sample is placed in a special substance that encourages the growth of bacteria.

Gonorrhea is usually treated with penicillin, either injected or taken orally. A synthetic antibiotic is prescribed for those who are allergic to penicillin or who have contracted a penicillin-resistant strain of gonorrhea.

While under treatment, the patient should abstain from sexual activity until further tests have confirmed that gonorrhea is no longer present. This is usually done one week after treatment begins and sometimes again two weeks later. If signs of the disease are still present, drug therapy can be reinstated with the same antibiotic at higher dosages or perhaps with a different antibiotic.

Another sexually transmitted disease called nongonococcal urethritis (NGU) sometimes occurs simultaneously with gonorrhea, but NGU is not affected by penicillin. So if symptoms persist after treatment for gonorrhea, it may be that the gonorrhea is cleared up but NGU also is present and should be treated with another antibiotic, often tetracycline.

Treatment of gonorrhea, as well as of all forms of sexually transmitted disease, requires that every sexual partner of the infected person also be examined and treated if necessary. In addition, men being treated for gonorrhea should avoid alcoholic beverages, as it has been recently shown that drinking may increase the chance of developing an inflammation of the urethra.

Gonorrhea can be prevented, obviously, by avoiding sexual contact with someone who has the disease. However, since this is not always possible, it should be remembered that the chances of contracting the disease increase with the number of different sexual partners a person has, so limiting the number of partners may be beneficial in preventing gonorrhea as well as other sexually transmitted diseases.

See also Nongonococcal urethritis and Pelvic inflammatory disease.

Gout

Gout is a form of recurrent acute arthritis whose underlying cause is a defect in the body's processing of uric acid, a chemical normally found in the blood and urine. If the body does not properly process uric acid resulting in high blood levels of uric acid, the uric acid may crystallize and become deposited in and around the joints and their tendons. An acute attack of gout is caused by the affected joint's inflammatory response to the deposits of crystals.

The high levels of uric acid can also lead to deposits in areas of the body other than the joints, most notably the skin and the kidneys. Uric acid deposits in the skin take the form of white lumps under the skin, most often appearing in the rims of the outer ear, the hands, the feet, and the elbows. Uric acid deposits in the kidneys may lead to the formation of kidney stones and perhaps even kidney failure (if the kidneys are blocked with numerous stones). About 20 percent of those with chronic gout also have kidney stones.

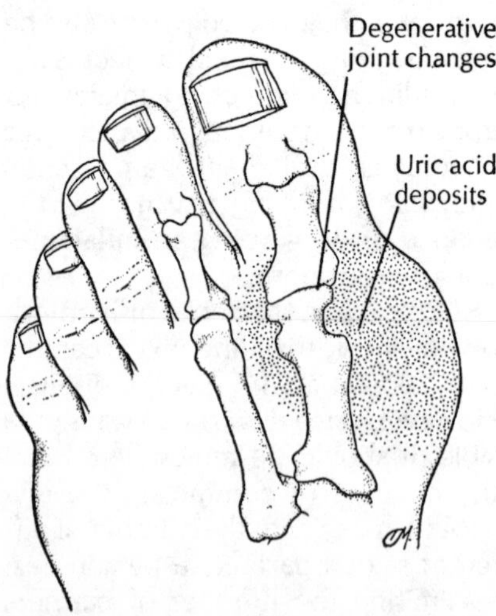

Gout is an extremely painful condition caused by an excess of uric acid in the blood that leads to deposits of uric acid crystals in the joints. The big toe joint is commonly affected, and changes within the joint can occur if the condition is not treated.

Most gout victims are middle-aged men. Rarely does the condition affect young women, although it can appear after menopause when the uric acid levels in the blood tend to increase.

Gout usually first appears as a sudden and extremely painful attack in a single joint, usually the big toe. Later attacks can involve several joints, such as the ankle, knee, wrist, and elbow. The pain commonly begins at night during sleep and may occur without warning or may be preceded by excessive alcohol consumption or unusual exercise earlier in the day. The pain grows in intensity and is often described as throbbing or crushing. Inflammation follows with swelling, warmth, redness, and tenderness over the affected joint. Sometimes the pain is so severe that the individual cannot tolerate the weight of a sheet over the joint. Other symptoms that may accompany the joint pain and swelling include fever, rapid heartbeat, chills, and an overall feeling of being unwell.

The first attacks usually last only a few days, but if the disorder goes untreated, later attacks may last for weeks. Symptoms eventually disappear, and joint function returns to normal between attacks. As the disease progresses, the periods of remission become shorter and shorter as more and more attacks occur each year.

The treatment of gout is twofold: (1) to relieve the symptoms of an acute attack and (2) to prevent attacks from occurring. The drug colchicine has traditionally been used to relieve a gout attack, but now—although colchicine is still used—nonsteroidal anti-inflammatory drugs are more often prescribed to relieve the inflammation and pain. These drugs are quite effective, but do have side effects so they should be used under close medical supervision.

Once the acute attack is under control, prevention of future attacks is the main goal. This can be done with the drug allopurinol, which interferes with the formation of excess uric acid and thus prevents the deposits of uric acid crystals in the body. Allopurinol usually has to be taken for long periods of time to maintain normal blood levels of uric acid. There are also other drugs, called uricosurics, that speed up the excretion of uric acid by the kidneys. These drugs, however, cannot be used if there is known kidney damage.

H

Hay fever

Hay fever is a type of allergy (an unusual reaction or oversensitivity to an outside substance, called an allergen) in which the membranes of the nose react to an inhaled substance. For this reason, this substance is called an inhalant allergen.

Hay fever may be caused by a variety of environmental substances, but acute (short-lived), seasonal attacks are usually allergic reactions to pollen (the allergen). Most often, spring attacks are reactions to tree pollen; summer attacks are reactions to grass pollen; and autumn attacks are reactions to weed pollen. Chronic (year-round) hay fever may be an allergic reaction to a number of other substances, including pet dander (scales of dry skin on pets), certain fibers, feathers, dust, and molds.

The symptoms of hay fever are usually the same, regardless of the allergen causing the irritation. Common symptoms include itching of the nose and roof of the mouth; a thin, watery discharge constantly draining from the nose; itchy, watery eyes; sneezing; headache; irritability; a feeling of exhaustion; insomnia; loss of appetite; and, in advanced cases, coughing and wheezing.

Hay fever, as well as other allergies, is diagnosed by identifying the allergen. This is done by taking a medical history and reviewing the patient's environment, daily habits, and recent changes in lifestyle. Skin tests and blood tests may also be taken. These include scratch tests, in which a small amount of the suspected allergen is applied to a scratch on the skin; intracutaneous tests, in which a small amount of the allergen is injected in or under the skin; and the radioallergosorbent technique, in which specific antibodies (developed in response to suspected allergens) in the blood are measured.

A severe case of hay fever may be best treated by a change in environment; that is, removing or reducing the allergen causing the trouble. Those reacting to weed pollen may need to move to a more urban, less pollinated location; those allergic to household dusts may have to dust and wet mop more frequently; those reacting to pets or fibers in carpeting, stuffed furniture, or draperies may need to remove these allergens from the household. In addition, many hay fever sufferers would benefit from the installation of an air conditioner, which should help keep pollen and dust levels in the home to a minimum.

Several medications are available for the hay fever sufferer: oral antihistamines, which fight the histamine that is released by the body as a reaction to the forming antibodies; corticosteroids, which reduce swelling; eyedrops, which relieve itching and redness; and desensitization shots, which cause the body to develop its own immunity to the allergen.

There is no actual method of preventing hay fever, but precautionary measures such as those discussed above may help at least to relieve some of its discomfort.

See also Allergy.

Headaches

A headache is a symptom, not a disease. A headache is rarely the symptom of a serious illness, but severe or frequent headaches can be exhausting and can affect daily life.

There are three basic types of headaches. Vascular (pertaining to blood vessels) headaches occur when blood vessels in the head enlarge and press on nerves causing pain. The most common vascular headache is the migraine. Another common type of headache is the muscle contraction headache that results when the muscles of the face, neck, and/or scalp contract and tighten. A tension headache is an example of a muscle contraction headache. The third common kind of headache is the traction or inflammatory headache. These headaches are caused by pressure within the head, ranging from a minor condition like sinusitis to a more serious problem such as a brain tumor.

A more detailed description of each type of headache follows.

Migraine headache. A migraine, or vascular headache, occurs when the blood vessels in the head enlarge and press on the nerves, causing pain. However, one theory about migraine headaches says that they result when the blood vessels first overreact to outside stimuli by constricting and thus blocking blood flow to parts of the brain; this may cause the visual impairment and numbness that often accompany a migraine. The blood vessels then become full of blood and press on surrounding nerves, causing pain.

Women are more prone to migraines than are men, and a certain personality type—compulsive, perfectionist, excessively neat, and very success-oriented—seems to be more susceptible to this kind of headache.

A number of physical and emotional factors may contribute to migraine headaches. Migraines may be triggered by a sharp reduction in caffeine intake or by allergies to certain foods or food additives (among them chocolate, fatty foods, alcohol, citrus fruits, monosodium glutamate, and nitrates). Emotional stress can also cause migraine headaches, as can drinking, smoking, or an interruption in routine eating and sleeping habits (all of which may be responsi-

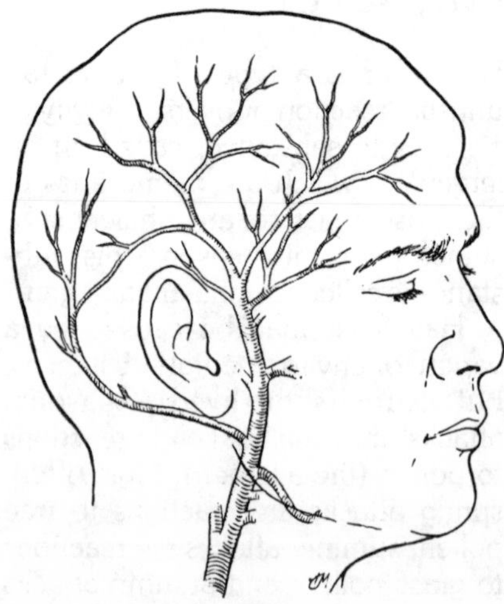

These blood vessels are the ones that are usually involved in a vascular-migraine headache.

ble for "week-end" headaches suffered by some patients). Cyclical, seasonal, or emotional factors, such as menstruation, for instance, may be associated with migraine. A tendency toward having this type of headache may also be inherited.

The predominant symptom of a migraine headache is a sharp, pulsating, incapacitating pain on one or both sides of the head. Pale, sweaty skin; nausea; and sensitivity to light may accompany this pain.

Warning sensations (called an aura) may indicate an approaching migraine headache. Before the pain appears, some individuals may see flashing lights or "shooting stars," hear noises or smell fragrances, or feel a tingling sensation in the limbs.

Cluster headaches, a form of migraine most commonly experienced by men, occur in groups or clusters of up to six a day, lasting for weeks or months. Their symptoms are intense pain on one side of the head, teary eyes, and runny nose. Drinking and smoking may aggravate these headaches.

Vascular headaches are diagnosed by a careful review of the circumstances surrounding the headaches as well as by a physical exam to rule out any other disorder that may be causing them. Elimination tests may be done to identify the exact cause of migraines suffered by people who seem to react to certain foods or changes in eating and sleeping habits. In an elimination test, all the substances that are suspected to be causing the trouble are eliminated, then reintroduced one at a time, to determine the one causing the headaches.

Treatment of a migraine already in progress usually consists of a drug therapy program chosen from a variety of painkillers, sedatives, and special drugs to combat migraine. For the occasional migraine sufferer, tranquilizers and sedatives may relieve some of the discomfort experienced during an attack.

Prevention of migraines is possible with several types of medication. The most commonly prescribed is ergotamine, which constricts the blood vessels and thus prevents the swelling that causes pressure on the surrounding nerves. This drug is usually taken to stop an approaching migraine, so it has no effect on the "aura" symptoms some patients experience. Also, antidepressant drugs, taken in small doses, may prevent migraines in a patient who experiences them regularly.

A more recent development in migraine treatment is the use of the drug propranolol, a beta blocking drug. This drug works in the body to block what are called the beta effects, one of which causes blood vessels to enlarge. Because propranolol blocks the enlargement of blood vessels, it has been used to prevent, but not treat acute attacks of, migraine headaches.

Muscle contraction headache. Muscle contraction headaches occur when muscles of the face, neck, or scalp contract and have spasms.

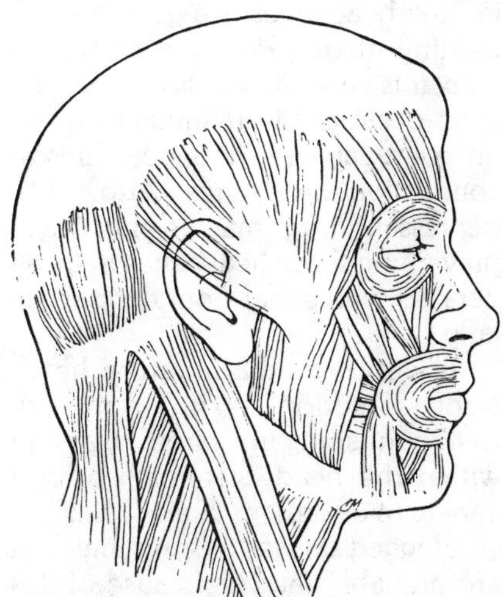

A muscular contraction headache usually involves these muscles.

These headaches usually occur following a specific event that has caused the muscles to tense. The tension is then translated into physical discomfort in the form of a clenched jaw, aching neck, and squeezed muscles in the face and head.

Muscle contraction headaches can also be brought about by abnormalities in the eyes, neck, teeth, or jaws, or by poor posture—especially by holding the head at an awkward angle while reading, driving, or watching TV, for example.

The major symptom of these headaches is a tight, squeezing pain in the forehead, jaws, or around the back of the head or neck. This constant, dull pain usually occurs on both sides of the head.

Diagnosis involves a review of the events that have led up to the headache as well as a physical examination to rule out any other disorder that may be causing it. A psychological examination may also be conducted to detect any emotional problems that may be contributing to the headaches.

Eliminating the tension or correcting the physical problem that is causing the headaches is a good start in treating them. Painkillers, muscle relaxants, and tranquilizers may be used occasionally (although not on an everyday basis) to treat muscle contraction headaches. Also, antidepressant drugs may be effective in preventing these headaches in those persons who suffer from them regularly.

Traction or inflammatory headache. Traction or inflammatory headaches occur when pressure within the head, stemming from a variety of disorders, causes pain.

Clogged sinuses or sinus infection are probably the chief cause of this type of headache. Sinuses are the cavities lined with mucous membrane within the facial bones. When mucus, which normally flows freely through the sinuses and drains out the nose, cannot properly drain, it collects in the sinuses and causes excess pressure on the surrounding tissues, leading to headache.

Other causes of traction or inflammatory headaches include aneurysm (a bulge in a blood vessel) or a brain tumor, both of which press directly on the brain; high blood pressure, which causes blood to rush through the vessels with too great a force, resulting in pressure in the head; infections, which inflame sensitive tissue; or fever, which may enlarge the blood vessels and cause excess pressure.

The symptoms of inflammatory headaches are a dull, aching pain, often occurring early in the day, accompanied by a feeling of pressure in the head. The pain is heightened by sneezing, coughing, bending over, or doing anything that increases the amount of blood in the head.

This type of headache is diagnosed by determining first whether sinus problems are causing it; if not, the doctor may order X rays; a CAT (computerized axial tomography) scan, which shows a cross-sectional picture of the brain; or an EEG (electroencephalogram), which records electrical activity in the brain. These tests can detect the presence of a tumor, aneurysm, or abnormality in the brain.

Inflammatory headaches are treated according to their cause. Those triggered by a sinus infection can usually be treated with painkillers or with antihistamines and decongestants, which dry out and help the sinuses to drain. Headaches resulting from more serious disorders such as brain tumor, brain abnormality, or aneurysm, will almost certainly require surgery.

Prevention of these headaches is

possible if the cause is as simple as a sinus infection. Of course, the correction of a more serious disorder that has caused the pain should also prevent future problems with traction or inflammatory headaches.

Heart

The heart is a hollow, muscular organ that is the basis of the circulatory system that maintains blood circulation throughout the body. The organ lies behind the sternum, or breastbone, between the lungs; and its size in most adults approximates that of a clenched fist. A normal heart can beat from 60 to 90 times per minute. A heartbeat is the rhythmic contraction of heart muscle pumping blood.

Blood passes through four chambers in the heart separated by valves. Valves control movement of blood among these compartments. First, blood flows from the veins into the right atrium or upper right chamber. The fluid continues down to the right lower compartment, or right ventricle. From this chamber, the blood is pumped into the lungs to exchange carbon dioxide (waste product from cells) for oxygen (element necessary for cell life). This rejuvenated blood then returns to the heart into the upper left chamber, or left atrium, which pumps the blood down into the lower left chamber, or left ventricle. From here, the left ventricle forces blood away from the heart through the aorta (main artery or passageway that extends through the chest and abdomen) to arteries that carry the blood to all the tissues of the body.

Heart attack

A heart attack (or myocardial infarction) occurs when an area of the heart muscle is damaged or dies because a coronary artery has been blocked and the oxygen-rich blood supply to that area of the heart has been drastically reduced. The damaged muscle tissue of the heart is replaced with scar tissue, which

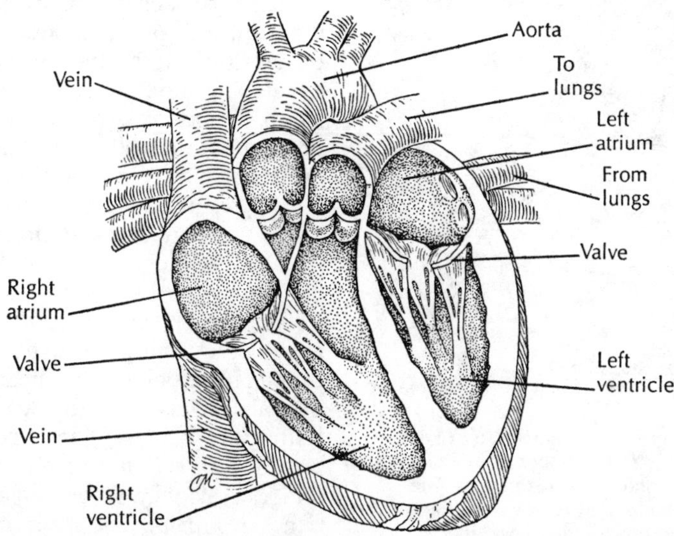

The heart is a hollow, muscular organ that is divided into four chambers. Valves between the chambers control the movement of blood between the chambers. The heart acts as a pump to maintain the circulation of blood.

affects the heart's future performance.

Although the chances of surviving a heart attack are now better than ever and complete recovery is common, heart attack or another form of circulatory disease is still the number one cause of death in the United States. Heart attacks that do not result in death often lead to serious complications: shock; cardiac arrhythmia, marked by an irregular heartbeat; or congestive heart failure, in which the heart cannot pump enough blood to meet the body's needs and fluid accumulates in the lower parts of the body.

Heart attack is caused by the total blockage of a coronary artery by a blood clot (thrombus) or by atherosclerosis, a disease in which the artery linings become gradually clogged and, finally, completely blocked by various fatty deposits, thus shutting off blood flow to the heart. Other healthy arteries that are not clogged may be much narrower and therefore unable to deliver the extra oxygenated blood needed by the heart during emotional stress or physical exertion. So damage to the heart results.

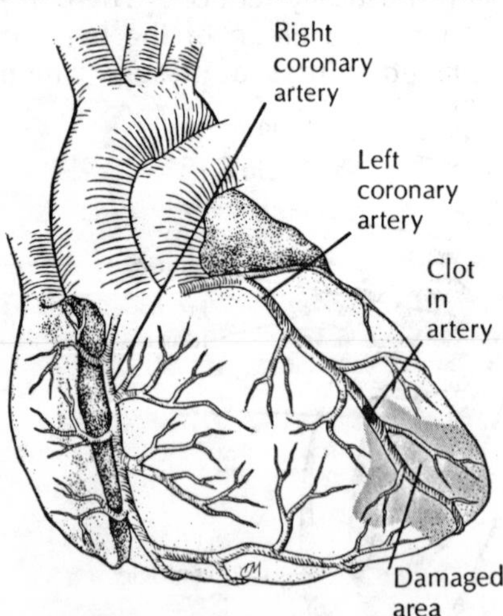

A heart attack occurs when an area of the heart is damaged or dies because of a reduction in the blood supply to that area. The reduced blood supply results when the coronary artery supplying the area is blocked by a blood clot or advanced atherosclerosis.

A number of physical and environmental factors, other than a thrombus or atherosclerosis, can increase the chances of heart attack: hypertension (high blood pressure) increases the resistance in the blood vessels, making the heart pump harder to push blood through; excessive cholesterol in the blood increases the likelihood of developing atherosclerosis; and birth control pills, especially those taken by women over the age of 35 or by smokers, have been linked to the increased incidence of heart attack.

Smoking, stress, improper diet, and lack of exercise have also been associated with the increased risk of heart attack. Smoking acts to constrict the arteries and reduce the blood flow to the heart muscle; stress puts an extra demand on the heart's need for blood; a diet high in saturated fats (fats that are usually solid at room temperature, including those animal fats found in butter and meats) has been found to increase the serum cholesterol level in the blood and thus the chances of developing atherosclerosis; and the lack of moderate, regular exercise prevents the development of collateral circulation. Collateral circulation is the system of smaller blood vessels that bypass a blocked artery and increase the blood supply to the area that the blocked artery serves.

The major symptom of a heart attack is a crushing pain in the middle of the chest, behind the breastbone; the pain can also extend down one or both arms. Fatigue, heavy perspiration, dizziness, difficulty in breathing, and, occasionally, fever, may accompany this pain. The pain may be somewhat similar to that experienced from angina pectoris (chest pain), but the pain of a heart attack is more intense, will not be relieved by nitroglycerin, and will not go away within a few minutes, as angina pain will. Also, a heart attack may take place during sleep, which is rare for angina pain.

Heart attacks range from very mild, signaled only by a slight discomfort, faintness, and nausea, to very serious, which can be accompanied by cardiac arrest (when the heartbeat completely stops) or ventricular fibrillation (when the normal, steady heartbeat is reduced to a useless quivering that prevents blood from being pumped to the body).

Heart attack is diagnosed by the electrocardiograph (ECG), which measures the electrical impulses produced by the heart; a diseased heart will show a record of disturbed patterns because the impulses must travel around the damaged area. A test for an increased white blood cell count may also be done, as the body's immune system will increase its number of white blood cells in order to carry away dead tissue in the damaged heart. Other blood tests may be taken to measure certain proteins in the blood that signal damaged heart muscle, although these tests may not show results until 24 to 72 hours after the attack.

The best and only treatment for heart attack is to rush to a hospital for emergency medical treatment as soon as an attack is suspected. More deaths could be prevented if heart attack victims did not delay going to a hospital. Studies have shown that, on the average, heart attack victims wait three hours before seeing a doctor.

In almost every case, hospitalization will be necessary following a heart attack. Treatment in the hospital will probably include care in the cardiac care unit (CCU), with limited physical activity at first and a gradual return to normal activities. In some cases, surgery to bypass the major obstructions in the arteries may be necessary.

A variety of medications are used to treat heart attack patients: anticoagulants, which thin the blood and prevent clots; digitalis, which establishes a steady heartbeat; antiarrhythmics, which inhibit irregularities in the heartbeat; diuretics, which reduce strain on the heart by removing excess water from the blood; antianginals, which diminish chest pain; sedatives, which relax the body; and beta blockers, which ease the strain on the heart by decreasing its work. Beta blocker drugs have been found to be especially effective in preventing additional heart attacks in those who have survived the first heart attack. (Nevertheless, beta blockers should be used only with great caution by asthma sufferers, as these drugs can cause spasms in the air passages and subsequent breathing difficulties.)

Lifestyle changes will also help heart attack victims. Patients will be expected to stop smoking, perhaps lose weight, and partake in regular, moderate exercise.

Prevention of heart attack begins with sensible health and dietary habits. Those who do not smoke, do not overeat or overindulge in saturated fats, and do not take birth control pills, but do exercise regularly and eliminate as much stress as possible from their lives are much less likely to become heart attack victims. Those who have already suffered one or more heart attacks can possibly prevent further attacks by changes in their living habits along these lines.

In the event of an attack, obtaining immediate medical attention can prevent death. A person with a suspected heart attack should not hesitate in going to the nearest hospital.

See also Angina pectoris, Beta-adrenergic blockers, Bypass surgery, and Heart attack in the Emergency first aid section at the end of this book.

Heartbeat irregularities (arrhythmia)

Heartbeat irregularities (called arrhythmia) are defined as any deviation from the normal, steady beating of the heart, which is responsible for regular circulation of the blood throughout the body.

Minor irregularities in the heartbeat are common, but more serious arrhythmias can lead to fainting, angina (chest pain), or heart attack. The most devastating heartbeat irregularity is called ventricular fibrillation. This occurs when the normally steady pumping of the heart is reduced to a useless quivering, preventing the heart from pumping sufficient blood throughout the body. Ventricular fibrillation often occurs after a heart attack or some other serious injury, such as a severe electric shock, and it must receive immediate emergency medical attention or it can be fatal.

Arrhythmias are usually caused by damage to the heart muscle or to a small mass of specialized heart tissue called the sinus node. The sinus node, the natural pacemaker of the heart, is responsible for establishing and maintaining a healthy, steady heartbeat.

Heartbeat irregularities can also be caused by improper use of drugs (drugs prescribed for arrhythmia can actually cause it if dosage is too high); excessive smoking (the nicotine in cigarettes slows the heartbeat); or consumption of large quantities of caffeine (the high amounts found in coffee, tea, chocolate, cola, and some cold medicines may overstimulate the heart).

Heartbeat irregularities may also develop as a result of congenital damage (present at birth) to the heart; a poorly functioning left ventricle (the lower chamber of the heart that pumps blood into the arteries); high blood pressure; or a previous heart attack in which the resulting scar tissue interferes with the nerve impulses governing the heartbeat.

Some heartbeat irregularities have no noticeable symptoms. Others will be signaled by light-headedness, fainting, a pounding heart, dizziness, and chest pain.

Arrhythmias are diagnosed primarily with the electrocardiograph (ECG), which records the electrical impulses made by the heart's beating. A normal heart will produce a record of regular peaks and valleys; an arrhythmic heart will show an uneven pattern. Another method of diagnosing heartbeat irregularities is the injection of radioactive isotopes or X-ray contrast dyes into the bloodstream; in this way, the regular or irregular movement of blood through the heart can be traced.

Occasionally, an arrhythmia is so mild that no particular treatment is required. But most irregularities are treated with medication, defibrillators, or pacemakers. All of these methods act to steady the irregularities and maintain a healthy, steady heartbeat.

Medications commonly used include digitalis, which slows the heartbeat; beta blockers, which correct extra beats originating in the lower chambers of the heart; and various antiarrhythmics, which act on specific problems of the heartbeat.

A defibrillator is a device applied to the chest which electrically jolts the quivering heart that is suffering from ventricular fibrillation back into a normal pattern of beating.

For those whose arrhythmia is caused by a faulty sinus node, an artificial pacemaker may be implanted in the heart. A pacemaker is a tiny electrical device powered by a small generator which, when implanted in the chest, acts to steady an abnormal heartbeat. Once inserted under the skin and threaded through a vein into the heart, it takes over the job of regulating the heartbeat by sending out electrical impulses similar to those emitted by the heart. Some pacemakers only go into action when the heart fails to beat after a specified time period; others completely take over the heart's job and are set to beat at a constant rate, usually about 72 times per minute.

Lifestyle changes will probably be recommended to patients suffering from heartbeat irregularities; they may need to quit smoking, lose weight, exercise more regularly, and reduce their caffeine intake. These precautions may also be taken in an effort to prevent arrhythmias.

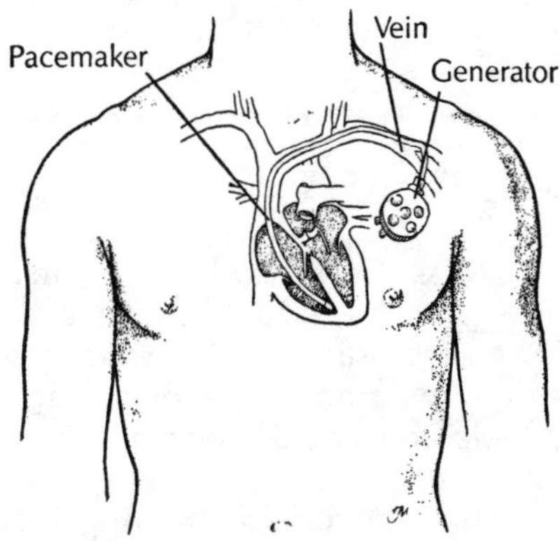

A mechanical pacemaker, a tiny electrical device powered by a small generator, can be used to correct heartbeat irregularities in those persons whose natural pacemaker is defective. The pacemaker is inserted into the chest and threaded through a vein until it rests within the heart. The generator is then sewn under the skin.

See also Defibrillation and Extrasystole.

Heartburn

Heartburn is an uncomfortable, burning pain felt behind the lower part of the breastbone, sometimes extending up into the upper chest or lower neck. Despite its name, it is not caused by pain in the heart or by a heart attack. In fact, heartburn is often triggered by simple digestive upsets, although an occasional severe case may be a symptom of a more serious disorder such as peptic ulcer.

Heartburn occurs when the acid digestive juices and partially digested food from the stomach back up into the lower esophagus (the passageway between the mouth and stomach) and irritate its tissues.

Heartburn most often develops ten minutes to one hour after eating. It may be caused by overeating; smoking; lying down or bending over after eating, which allows the backup of stomach acids and food into the esophagus; alcoholic drinks; coffee; spicy or highly seasoned foods; acidic fruits or fruit juices; and aspirin. Heartburn is a common problem during pregnancy because the growing baby presses on the stomach and esophagus, encouraging digestive juices to move up toward the throat; these cases of heartburn usually disappear after childbirth.

The major symptom of heartburn is the characteristic burning sensation behind the breastbone and up toward the throat; it may be accompanied by gassiness, belching, and an uncomfortable, tight feeling in the chest.

Heartburn can usually be relieved by merely standing or sitting upright or by drinking milk or something soothing to the stomach. Nonprescription antacids may also be helpful in more severe cases (but not in the presence of kidney disease, because one of the ingredients in antacids may interfere with kidney function). Any persistent, uncontrollable, or severe heartburn should be reported to a doctor, as it may be a sign of a more severe condition such as peptic ulcer.

Heartburn can often be prevented by avoiding spicy, acidic, or other troublesome foods as well as coffee or alcoholic beverages if they seem to trigger it. Eating smaller meals more frequently and refraining from smoking at mealtimes are also beneficial in avoiding heartburn. Sleeping with the back and head propped up on pillows may prevent stomach contents from flowing into the esophagus.

Heart failure

See Congestive heart failure.

Heart murmurs

Heart murmurs are extra whishing sounds—over and above the regular "lub-dub" sound of the heartbeat—made as blood flows through heart chambers and valves. They can be heard in many healthy people, especially children, teenagers, and pregnant women, and in these cases are considered innocent or functional because they are a normal sound caused by the blood rushing through the heart.

On the other hand, heart murmurs can be a symptom that first alerts a doctor to the possibility of a heart condition or disease. These abnormal murmurs come from vibrations or turbulence in the bloodstream. They are called organic or structural heart murmurs and can be caused by blood being forced through narrowed or obstructed heart valves, a defect in the heart walls, or valves that do not close completely and allow blood to seep back into the upper or lower heart chambers.

Heart murmurs can be congenital (existing at birth but not hereditary) or acquired because of rheumatic fever, atherosclerosis, syphilis, or other ailments. They can only be detected by physical examination. A doctor listening to the heart, either directly or through a stethoscope, can usually distinguish any extra sound and identify whether or not it signifies a serious problem by its quality, intensity, location, and timing.

A person with a functional or innocent heart murmur can live a completely normal life. If the heart murmur is organic or structural, the doctor will order tests (chest X ray, electrocardiogram, ultrasound, cardiac catheterization, echocardiogram, or fluoroscopy) to evaluate the extent of the condition and prescribe appropriate treatment.

Heat rash

Heat rash, or prickly heat, is a mild skin condition that produces an itchy, burning sensation. It is found most often in infants and overweight people who have overlapping folds of fat.

When skin surfaces press together, sweat ducts that carry secretions from the sweat glands to the skin's surface become temporarily blocked. Normally, these sweat glands work along with blood vessels to regulate the body's heat. If the blood temperature rises, the brain triggers a reflex in the sweat glands to encourage secretion of sweat. Sweating reduces body temperature by releasing sweat to the surface of the skin where it evaporates and cools the skin. If sweat cannot reach the skin's surface, it may break through its duct wall and remain trapped in an inner layer of the skin where it can cause inflammation and a rash.

Heat rash can result any time the body needs to perspire. Most often, hot weather or exertion triggers the reaction. However, tight clothing or overdressing may compound the problem.

Heat rash in infants may be caused by immature sweat glands that cannot transport large amounts of perspiration to the surface of the skin. The sweat stays in the skin, thereby producing the same irritation.

Usually heat rash, or miliaria as it is known medically, appears on moist parts of the body where skin surfaces can touch, such as on the neck, under arms, or between legs. Infants can show the rash under a tight-fitting diaper. The rash looks like tiny, pinhead-sized red pimples, and it can cause itching and a prickling or burning sensation.

Heat rash is sometimes confused with a condition called chafing because the symptoms are similar. However, chafing is caused by friction between the two surfaces rubbing together and not by obstructed sweat ducts.

Under extreme conditions, the warm, moist areas where heat rash develops can become breeding grounds for microorganisms that cause secondary infection.

Treatment and prevention of heat rash involve reducing or eliminating the stimulus for sweating. The affected person needs to stay in a cool environment and refrain from exertion. Cool showers followed by thorough drying can also help, as can

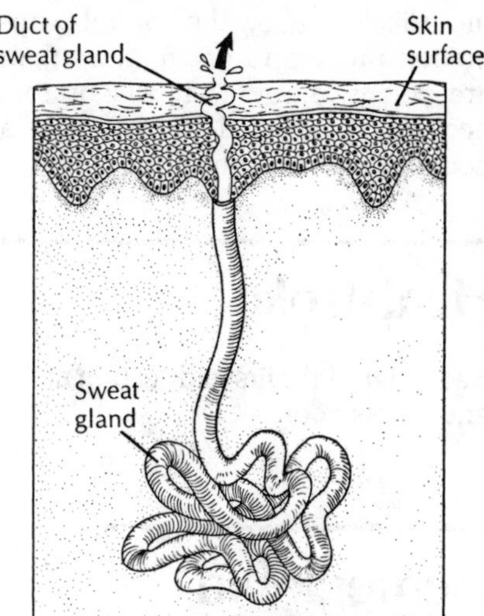

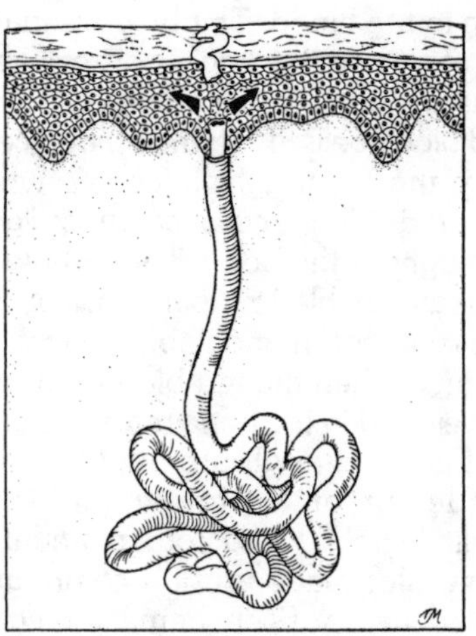

A sweat gland normally releases sweat through its duct onto the skin's surface. When perspiration cannot reach the skin's surface, perhaps because of folds of fat or tight clothing, heat rash results. When this happens, the sweat may break through the wall of its duct and become trapped in an internal layer of skin, causing inflammation and rash.

wearing light, loose-fitting clothes. Once sweating stops, the rash may disappear in a few hours.

Babies who suffer from heat rash can be bathed in plain water and dried thoroughly. Cloth diapers are more likely to allow the natural evaporation process to occur more than are paper diapers. If discomfort becomes prolonged or extreme, a doctor should be consulted.

Heatstroke

See Emergency first aid section at the end of this book.

Hemoglobin

Hemoglobin is the pigment (colored agent) in the blood that carries oxygen in the blood. The blood is made up of plasma (the liquid portion), various elements, white blood cells, and red blood cells. The white blood cells help the body fight infection, while the red blood cells carry oxygen throughout the body. The red blood cells are enabled to do this task by the presence of hemoglobin, which is formed when the red blood cells are developed in the bone marrow.

Each hemoglobin molecule is made up of a protein molecule (called *globin*) and four pigmented molecules made up of a compound called *heme.* Each heme molecule has one atom of iron; there are four heme molecules in a single molecule of hemoglobin, hence a single molecule of hemoglobin has four atoms of iron. This structure makes it possible for one hemoglobin molecule to join with four oxygen molecules to form a substance called *oxyhemoglobin.* This reaction is also reversible, thus enabling hemoglobin to pick up oxygen while the blood is in the lungs and deposit oxygen in the cells after the heart has pumped oxygenated blood into the circulatory system.

The blood of males usually has more hemoglobin per unit volume than that of females (14 to 16 grams per 100 milliliters of blood for men, but only 12 to 14 grams per 100 milliliters of blood for women). If the blood contains less than 12 grams of hemoglobin per 100 milliliters, it is considered below normal and the person with such blood is diagnosed as being anemic.

Hemoglobin disorders occur when there is a change in its chemical structure, thus reducing its oxygen-carrying or oxygen-releasing capabilities. One condition, called Bart's disease, for example, occurs when the internal composition of hemoglobin has a high attraction for oxygen, so that the hemoglobin can pick up and carry oxygen, but cannot readily give it up and release it to the body cells. Cancer of the bone marrow can also cause changes in hemoglobin, either in its composition or in its production. Because the pigmented portion of hemoglobin is made up of iron, a lack of iron in the diet also affects hemoglobin functions.

In addition to hemoglobin deficiencies, there are also conditions in which there is too much hemoglobin in the blood. For example, while an anemic person has less than 12 grams of hemoglobin per 100 milliliters of blood, a person suffering from polycythemia often has counts of more than 17.5 grams of hemoglobin per 100 milliliters of blood. It should be noted that the anemic person may or may not have a shortage of red blood cells, and (although the name implies differently) a person suffering from polycythemia does not necessarily have too many red blood cells. The problem is in the amount of hemoglobin the red blood cells carry, not in the number of red cells.

See also Anemia and Polycythemia.

Hemophilia

Hemophilia is a hereditary bleeding disorder in which the blood's clotting process does not function properly. Blood normally contains several factors that enable clotting to occur. These are designated coagulation factors I through XIII. In the most common form of hemophilia, classical hemophilia or hemophilia A, factor VIII is deficient. In this case, factors I through VII function adequately, but the clotting process is interrupted by a lack of sufficient amounts of factor VIII. Hemophilia B is the other form of the common hemophilias, although it occurs significantly less often than hemophilia A. Hemophilia B is caused by a deficiency of factor IX. Hemophilia B is also known as Christmas disease.

Hemophilia is inherited as a sex-linked recessive trait. This means that the condition appears almost exclusively in males, but the trait is carried only by females. In other words, a woman can carry the disease and pass it on to her sons without being affected herself. This is because the defective gene appears in one of the chromosomes that determine sex—the X chromosome, which is the female sex chromosome. Males carry the sex chromosomes X and Y and females carry two X chromosomes. Thus a male who inherits a defective X chromosome does not have a normal X chromosome to counteract the defect. A female, however, may have a defective X chromosome but her other normal X chromosome means that she will not develop the disease but that she can pass her defective X chromosome on to her sons who will have the disease. If she passes the defective chromosome to her daughters, they, too, will be carriers but not have the disease. Similarly, a male hemophiliac will pass his defective X chromosome to his daughters who will be carriers. However, he passes on only his normal Y chromosome to his sons who therefore cannot develop the disease. A woman can be a hemophiliac only if her mother is a carrier and her father is a hemophiliac; in this case she inherits two defective X chromosomes.

Although affected males are born with the disease, the onset of symptoms is variable. Milder cases may not be readily apparent. Usually the symptoms of hemophilia begin during early childhood. When a cut in the skin occurs or an injury is suffered, the bleeding may be substantial and prolonged. In severe cases, spontaneous internal bleeding may occur without any obvious cause. Blood in the urine may result from internal bleeding. Pain is also a symptom when the bleeding occurs internally, between muscles and into joints. The course of the disease may result in irreversible damage to the joints, which, in turn, results in greater pain and in limitations in movement.

If a child has any of these symptoms, or if there is known hemophilia in the family history, a physician should be consulted. The physician will order laboratory tests to diagnose the disease. The most common test for hemophilia is called partial thromboplastin time (PTT), a one-stage clotting time test. Additional laboratory tests may be ordered in certain cases. In addition, today genetic testing can detect if a woman is a carrier of hemophilia with increasing accuracy. Treatment of hemophilia has undergone dramatic changes over the past several years. The treatment has become more scientific and effective. Plasma, the fluid portion of blood, contains more of factor VIII and IX than whole blood. For patients with hemophilia A, the plasma of an individual donor can be quickly frozen by a special process, slowly thawed, and separated into portions rich in factor VIII. This product is called cryoprecipitate. It can be prepared later for intravenous (into the vein) administration. However, cryoprecipitate has the disadvantage of requiring hospital availability for storage and preparation. Also, since cryoprecipitate is prepared from the plasma of a single donor, the amount of factor VIII is variable.

Treatment of hemophilia A has been further advanced by a process of rapid freezing and dehydration (removal of water) of plasma, called lyophilization. Freeze-dried concentrates are prepared and packaged, yet can be readily dissolved by a single mixing procedure. (This process is similar in concept to the convenience of freeze-dried coffee.) This concentrate is particularly efficient for home use in comparison with cryoprecipitate. The concentrate quickly stops the bleeding. Nevertheless, infection may result from the donors. The recipient of concentrate is placed at increased risk for infection compared to the recipient of cryoprecipitate. Whereas the latter is prepared from a single donor, the concentrate is prepared from thousands of donors. Hepatitis, a serious infection of the liver, is an example of disease that may be transmitted from a donor. Very recently, a new condition, acquired immune deficiency syndrome (AIDS), which is thought to be carried in the blood, has developed in several hemophiliacs treated with concentrate. This syndrome increases susceptibility to serious infection. Scientists are continuing to investigate the risks and benefits of concentrate compared to cryoprecipitate for hemophilia A.

Treatment of hemophilia B involves the use of fresh or stored plasma. Concentrate is also available for hemophilia B and is known as prothrombin complex concentrate.

Hemorrhage

Hemorrhage is the technical term for bleeding, often referring to substantial blood loss or uncontrollable bleeding, either externally or internally. The effects of and damage from hemorrhage depend on the part of the body that is bleeding and the total amount of blood that is lost. Hemorrhage can be a symptom of a number of serious, sometimes fatal, disorders.

Hemorrhage occurs when blood vessels are torn or broken. In normal situations, blood clots within seconds or minutes, stopping the blood flow. However, when serious injuries or other disorders are involved, the body's normal blood-clotting function may be inadequate or malfunctioning; if blood loss is not quickly stopped, death may result.

When the blood-clotting mechanism is temporarily inadequate (usually caused by serious injury), external hemorrhage results; when the blood-clotting mechanism has been disrupted as a result of some disorder (including hemophilia, peptic ulcer, cancer, or diseases involving the stomach, kidney, or urinary tract), internal hemorrhage may result.

Severe external hemorrhage displays the following symptoms: rapid pulse; dizziness or faintness; collapse; shock; a drop in blood pressure and a rise in pulse rate; and pale, cold, clammy, or sweaty skin.

Internal hemorrhage may also show symptoms, even if the bleeding is slight. Black, tarry stools may signal bleeding in the intestinal tract from a peptic ulcer or cancer of the colon; blood in the vomitus indicates bleeding in the stomach; and blood in the urine means bleeding is occurring in the kidneys or urinary tract.

Blood in the stool, urine, or vomitus should always be reported to a doctor at once, as should external bleeding that occurs frequently or that cannot be stopped within minutes or hours, depending on the severity of the wound.

Treatment for internal hemorrhage involves correcting the cause of the bleeding, possibly with surgery. External hemorrhage is treated by applying pressure to the wound with a sterile bandage (or, in an emergency, just pressing it with the fingers) until the bleeding stops. If bleeding cannot be stopped, the patient will almost certainly be hospitalized, where lost blood can be replaced with blood transfusions or damaged blood vessels can be surgically tied off and sealed.

See also Bleeding in the Emergency first aid section at the end of this book.

Hemorrhoids

Hemorrhoids, often called piles, are enlarged veins inside or just outside the anal canal, which is the opening at the end of the large intestine. As veins swell, they cause severe inflammation and discomfort.

In most cases, hemorrhoids are the result of individual toilet habits whereby some people postpone normal bowel functioning. Habitual postponement of bowel movements can lead to loss of rectal function and undesirable straining during elimination. Straining irritates veins and slows the flow of blood, thereby contributing to swollen or inflamed veins. Postponing bowel movements may also cause stools retained in the bowels to lose moisture. When feces become dry and hard, the added strain of constipation encourages hemorrhoids.

Diet plays a major role in the development of hemorrhoids. A diet containing a high proportion of refined foods, such as white flour and sugar, rather than foods with natural roughage increases the likelihood of constipation and, therefore, the likelihood of hemorrhoids.

Another source of hemorrhoid irritation comes from pressure on the veins from diseases of the liver or heart or from a tumor. Pregnancy also contributes to the development of hemorrhoids because the enlarged uterus increases pressure on the veins. Moreover, prolonged pressure from pushing during labor and delivery can inflame the area. Although women appear to develop hemorrhoids during pregnancy, recent research suggests that they probably had the condition prior to pregnancy.

Hemorrhoids seem to be more prevalent in some families. However, this tendency has been attributed more to similar dietary and personal habits than to any inherited physical characteristics.

Hemorrhoids may take years to develop and almost always result in irritating symptoms. The first signs of hemorrhoids include itching and some discomfort during and after bowel movements. Continued straining during elimination will eventually produce slight swelling of the lining of the anal canal. This swelling may not be noticed until hard stools scrape the anal lining and cause slight bleeding—an early clue that a hemorrhoid may have developed.

With prolonged straining, a portion of the anal canal may jut out of the anus during a bowel movement. At this stage, the elastic connective tissue is still strong enough to pull the hemorrhoid back into the anal canal unassisted, so the individual may not notice the growing problem. However, with persistent pressure, the protruding tissue may remain outside the anus after a bowel movement and need to be manually returned to the anal canal. Once outside the anal canal, the hemorrhoid creates a dull aching sensation.

A more involved problem develops when the hemorrhoid is difficult or impossible to return, and permanent swelling at the anal opening interferes with elimination. Then the patient may postpone bowel movements in an effort to avoid pain. Instead of helping, this intensifies the problem, because it leads to constipation that aggravates the hemorrhoid.

To diagnose a hemorrhoid, a physician inspects the anal canal, often with special instruments. An anoscope (short, lighted tube) inserted into the anus can reveal the condition of the rectal lining. A sigmoidoscope, which is a longer instrument, shows a view of the inner area of the colon.

Painful hemorrhoids can be treated at home by applying cold water compresses directly to the anal area for five to ten minutes until pain is relieved. Some people reduce pain by taking hot baths. Over-the-counter preparations cannot cure hemorrhoids, but they can relieve itching and swelling. Should symptoms worsen after application of any remedy, its use should be suspended and a doctor consulted. Chemicals in these preparations may produce an allergic reaction. Nonirritating laxatives may also be occasionally useful in softening stools.

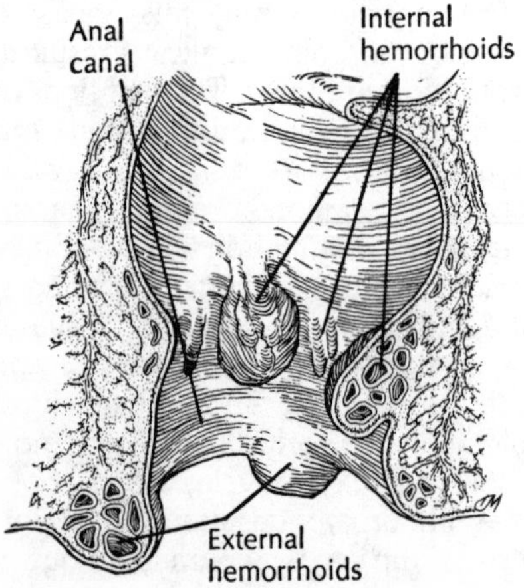

Hemorrhoids are enlarged veins inside (internal) or protruding from (external) the anal canal. These swollen veins cause itching and pain which may be accompanied by bleeding.

In the early stages of hemorrhoid development, adjustment of personal habits may prevent progression of the condition. A bowel movement should never be delayed, once the urge is felt. During bowel movements, straining should be avoided. A diet including plenty of roughage—natural grains, fresh fruits, and vegetables—softens stools and helps prevent constipation.

For severe cases of hemorrhoids, a doctor may recommend a surgical procedure called hemorrhoidectomy to remove dilated portions of the affected veins and tie off the remaining parts of the vein. A newer procedure called cryosurgery removes the hemorrhoid, but with less pain and fewer postoperative complications. With this technique, the hemorrhoid is frozen with an extremely cold probe. As the frozen tissue dies, the hemorrhoid falls off within several days. Physicians perform cryosurgery in their offices within a few minutes. The only postoperative symptom is a slight watery discharge for a few days.

Another technique used to eliminate internal hemorrhoids is rubber band ligation. Here, the doctor ties off the hemorrhoid's blood supply with a special instrument. This procedure causes the hemorrhoid to die and drop off within three to nine days. The physician performs the procedure in the office, but there is one drawback. Only one hemorrhoid can be treated per visit. Once the hemorrhoid dies, brief spotting of blood and minor itching may occur.

Hepatitis

Hepatitis is a viral infection of the liver that is characterized by jaundice, a yellowing of the skin and whites of the eyes. The disease is caused by several viruses, but the most common virus strains of hepatitis are hepatitis A, or infectious hepatitis, and hepatitis B, or serum hepatitis.

Both strains enter the body as minute organisms and attack cells in the liver. Hepatitis A passes through the digestive tract and is transmitted from person to person by contaminated food or water or through the stools of an infected person. This form may occur as epidemics in places where sanitation is poor and sewage contaminated. Incubation, the time between exposure to the disease and the appearance of symptoms, is between 14 to 40 days. Sometimes, hepatitis A is so mild that symptoms never appear, but the infected person can still transmit the disease as a carrier of infection.

With hepatitis B, the virus enters the bloodstream, either from transfusion of contaminated blood or from contaminated needles, especially among drug users. Hepatitis B begins more gradually than does hepatitis A, so the disease may be present 40 to 180 days before the onset of symptoms. In addition, the virus can live in almost all body fluids, including saliva, semen, urine, and tears. This allows hepatitis B to be transmitted by sexual contact or by more casual contact such as sharing toothbrushes or razors.

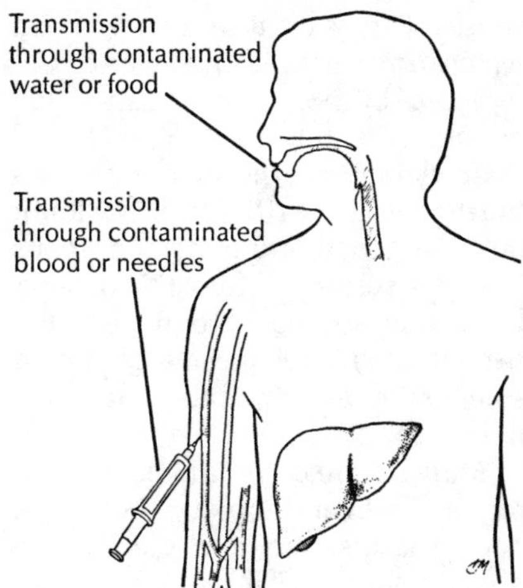

Hepatitis A can be transmitted through the digestive system by contaminated water or food. Hepatitis B is transmitted most often through contaminated blood or needles, although it is also thought to be passed by intimate person-to-person contact.

Hepatitis may also result as a complication of the viral infection called infectious mononucleosis.

Early signs of hepatitis are general fatigue, joint and muscle pain, and loss of appetite. Nausea, vomiting, and diarrhea or constipation may follow with a low-grade fever of 102°F or less. As the disease develops, the liver enlarges and becomes tender. Chills, weight loss, and distaste for smoking appear along with the characteristic jaundice. Jaundice results from an accumulation of yellow bile pigment in the blood that turns the skin and whites of the eyes yellow.

In hepatitis A, the disappearance of jaundice generally signals the beginning of recovery. However, in hepatitis B, the virus may persist for years or the duration of a lifetime.

Any sudden rise in fever, extreme drowsiness, or severe prolonged pain requires immediate medical supervision to avoid permanent liver damage. Chronic, long-term hepatitis can lead to irreversible liver failure or cirrhosis. Cirrhosis is a condition in which normal cells of the liver are replaced by fibrous scar tissue that inhibits liver function.

To determine the extent and severity of hepatitis, a physician analyzes blood and urine specimens from the suspected hepatitis patient. If the disease has progressed, the patient may have yellow skin and soreness in the upper abdomen over the liver.

More severe chronic hepatitis may require a liver biopsy, whereby a needle is inserted into the liver to obtain a sample of liver tissue. In this procedure, local anesthetic is usually injected into the upper abdomen to eliminate discomfort from the test.

A new blood test is under investigation that will speed the diagnosis of hepatitis B and identify carriers of the virus.

Because hepatitis is caused by a virus, there is no cure. Even treatment is limited, especially for acute hepatitis. Once the virus attacks, recovery is usually up to the body's regular defense system.

To encourage the healing process, physicians advise patients to avoid all strenuous activity. Strict bed rest is more important during the acute phases of hepatitis. More serious cases may require hospitalization to insure inactivity. Some of these patients may also need an exchange blood transfusion to aid recovery if the body cannot overcome contamination by itself. In addition, all hepatitis patients must avoid alcoholic beverages, because processing alcohol puts a tremendous strain on the liver.

People exposed to hepatitis can prevent or minimize the disease by obtaining an injection of gamma globulin, a disease-fighting substance in the blood. Gamma globulin usually defends against virus A and offers a modest protection against virus B. In either case, if hepatitis develops following an injection, gamma globulin seems to reduce symptoms.

Scientists are also investigating a new vaccine against hepatitis. A vaccine is a preparation of the disease-causing agent that is introduced into the body to stimulate the body to produce antibodies whose job it is to fight the disease. For now, hepatitis vaccine is only recommended for people who are in direct contact with hepatitis carriers, such as healthcare workers, but the vaccine will eventually become available for more widespread use.

See also Cirrhosis, Gamma globulin and Jaundice.

Hernia

The term hernia refers to any abnormal protrusion of part of an organ or tissue(s) through the structures that normally contain it. In this condition, a weak spot or opening in a body wall allows part of the organ to bulge through. A hernia may develop in almost any part of the body; however, the most common sites are the abdominal and groin areas.

Although a hernia is often popularly called a "rupture," this is a misleading description. Nothing is actually "torn" or ruptured in a hernia. A hernia can be congenital (present at birth) or acquired; in the latter case, it is often the result of some stress or strain on the body wall involved.

Although there are literally as many types of hernias as there are sites or locations in the body, the following are some of the most common hernias:

- Umbilical hernia, protrusion of part of the intestine at the navel or umbilicus (seen mostly in infants)

- Inguinal hernia, a protrusion of a loop of intestine into the groin where the folds of abdominal flesh meet the thighs, often the result of increased pressure in the abdomen because of lifting, coughing, straining, or accidents (accounts for about 75 percent of all common hernias)
- Scrotal hernia, an inguinal hernia that has passed into the scrotum, the bag of skin behind the penis that contains the testes
- Femoral hernia, a protrusion of a loop of intestine into the femoral canal, which is a tubular passageway that carries nerves and blood vessels from the abdomen into the thigh (this type of hernia is more common in women than in men)
- Incisional hernia, a hernia that occurs after an operation at the site of the surgical incision; often this type of hernia is due to excessive strain on the healing tissue (excessive muscular effort, lifting, coughing, or extreme obesity which puts pressure on a weakened area).

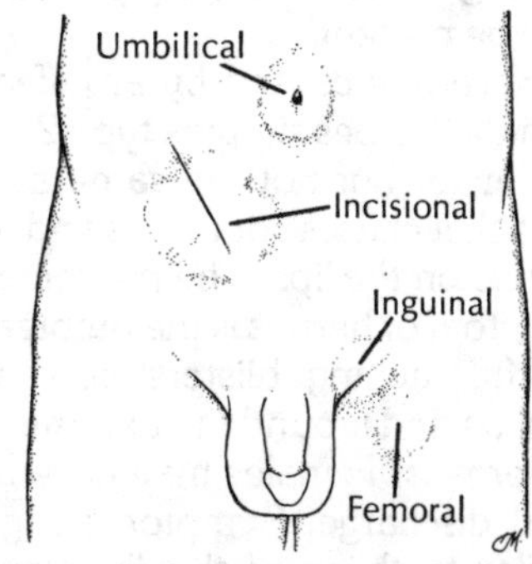

A hernia can develop in almost any part of the body, but the more common locations are shown here.

Hernias can also be classified by their condition:

- Irreducible hernia, one that cannot be restored by manipulation
- Reducible hernia, one that can be returned to "normal" by manipulation
- Incarcerated hernia, a hernia that cannot be reduced through treatment, but is not obstructed or strangulated
- Strangulated hernia, one that is tightly constricted, cutting off the blood supply of the affected tissue.

Because of the many different types of hernias, the symptoms will vary slightly depending on the cause and the body part(s) involved. However, most hernias usually begin as small breakthroughs that are hardly noticeable. At first, they may be soft lumps under the skin, a little larger than a marble, and there is usually no pain. As time goes by, the pressure of the internal contents against the weak containing wall increases, and the size of the lump increases. In the early stages, this hernia may be reducible, that is, it can be pushed gently back into its normal place. However, the hernia can easily become strangulated: as the hernia progresses and bulges out further through the weakest points in its containing wall, the opening in the wall will close behind it forming a narrow "neck." If the neck is pinched tightly enough to cut off the blood supply to the protruding tissue, the hernia will swell quickly and become strangulated—that is, the blood supply is totally cut off and unless treated, can result in gangrene (death of tissue).

Fortunately, the symptoms of this condition are usually detectable. When a hernia suddenly grows larger, becomes tense, and will not go back into place, often with accompanying pain and nausea, the hernia is strangulated. Sometimes, however, there is no pain or tenderness when this happens, especially in elderly patients.

Diagnosis of a hernia can usually be made by thorough visual examination and by studying the patient's medical history and symptoms.

For small, nonstrangulated or

nonincarcerated hernias, various supports and trusses can sometimes offer temporary, symptomatic relief. However, the best treatment is surgical closure or repair of the muscle wall through which the hernia protrudes. Surgical repair of a hernia is called herniorrhaphy. When the weakened area is very large, some strong synthetic material may be sewn over the defect to reinforce the weak area. Postoperative care is simple and involves protecting the patient from respiratory infections that would cause him/her to cough and sneeze, thus placing strain on the suture line. Recovery is usually quick and complete.

Avoiding strain or pressure on any body wall, especially those of the abdomen and groin area (in men), is the only real preventive measure against hernias.

Herpes

Herpes is a sexually transmitted disease, perhaps even more widespread than gonorrhea. A sexually transmitted disease, also known as venereal disease, is a highly contagious illness spread primarily through direct sexual contact.

Herpes can be treated but not cured. Its symptoms appear briefly, then disappear, and the disease lies dormant in the nerve cells until it is reactivated by stress or illness. It is only contagious during these active periods. Persons taking drugs that suppress the body's immune system (for instance, cancer or organ transplant patients) are at a higher risk of developing herpes because their bodies are in a weakened state. There is also some evidence that links herpes with a higher rate of cancer of the cervix in women.

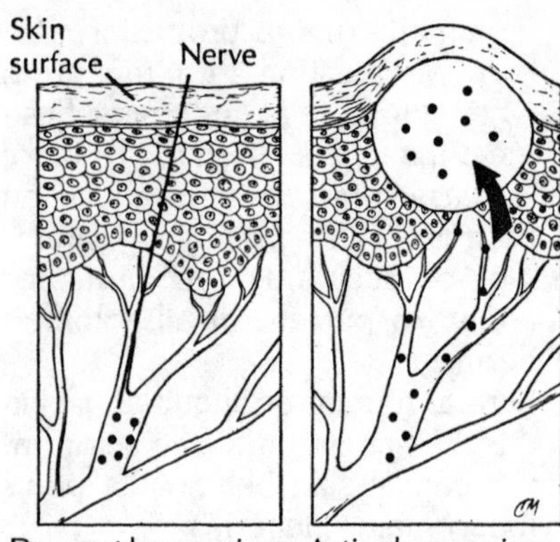

Herpes simplex type 2 virus causes painful, fluid-filled blisters in its active stage. The blisters eventually disappear, but the herpes virus lies dormant within nerve cells until stress or illness reactivate the virus triggering a new outbreak of active herpes blisters.

Although herpes is spread primarily by direct sexual contact, it can also be transmitted to an infant during childbirth, causing brain damage or death. Thus, if a woman shows signs of the active disease while in labor, the baby will be delivered by cesarean section (delivery through a surgical incision in the walls of the uterus and abdomen) rather than through the vagina where the herpes blisters may be present.

Herpes is caused by an infection with the herpes simplex type 2 virus, similar to, but not the same as, the virus that causes cold sores and fever blisters on the lips. The predominant symptom of herpes is the outbreak of painful, itching blisters filled with fluid on and around the external sexual organs. Females may have a vaginal discharge. Symptoms vaguely similar to those of the flu may accompany these outbreaks, including fever, loss of appetite, and fatigue.

The blisters will disappear without treatment in about two to ten days, but the virus will remain, lying dormant among clusters of nerve cells until another outbreak is triggered by stress, a cold, fever, or, in women, menstruation. Many patients can anticipate an outbreak by a warning sign, a tingling sensation called a "prodrome" (or premonition) of the approaching illness. Herpes is contagious only during these outbreaks, so sexual activity should be avoided while symptoms are present.

Diagnosis of herpes is accomplished by microscopic examination and culture of the blister fluid.

Herpes cannot be cured as can other sexually transmitted diseases, because any medication that will attack the virus while it lies dormant in the nerve cells will also damage the nerve cells. However, there is treatment for acute outbreaks now available that involves the use of either the antiviral drug acyclovir or laser therapy, both of which will heal blisters, reduce pain, and most importantly, kill large numbers of the herpes virus. Acyclovir has also been found to reduce the reproduction of the virus in initial outbreaks, thus possibly lessening the number of subsequent outbreaks. It should be noted, however, that to be effective, laser therapy must be started immediately after the first sores appear. In addition, herpes, as well as all forms of sexually transmitted disease, requires that every sexual partner of the infected person also be examined and treated if necessary.

Herpes can be prevented, obviously, by avoiding sexual contact with an infected person whose disease is in its active period. The chances of contracting this disease increase with the number of different sexual partners a person has. Therefore, limiting the number of partners can be somewhat beneficial in preventing herpes.

Hiatus hernia

See Diaphragmatic hernia.

High blood pressure

See Hypertension.

Hirsutism

Hirsutism is excessive hair growth in areas that are not usually hairy in women—usually the face, breasts and chest, and abdomen.

Some degree of hirsutism is present in about 30 percent of women, and it may accompany some primary disorder as a secondary symptom. Family and racial tendencies, however, account for a good percentage of hirsute women. While some hirsutism stems from a primary disorder, many cases have no known cause. It is thought, though, that hirsute women all have hair follicles that are hypersensitive to normal female androgen levels. (Androgen is a male sex hormone, but certain levels of it are normally present in women just as levels of female sex hormones are normally present in men.)

In some cases, hirsutism is only one sign of virilization (or masculination) characterized by acne, balding, and increased muscle mass, as well as by hirsutism. This condition can be caused by overactive adrenal glands (which secrete some sex hormones), ovarian tumors, adrenal tumors, steroid medications, and other causes. However, the majority of hirsute women are not masculinized. A more common cause of hirsutism is polycystic ovaries, a condition marked by numerous cysts on the ovaries (female sex glands) that leads to infrequent menstruation or absence of menstruation, absence of ovulation, obesity, and enlarged ovaries.

Hirsutism is also seen in Cushing's

syndrome, a condition that in women is characterized by excessive fat tissue in the face, neck, and trunk; absence of menstruation; convex curvature of the spine; high blood pressure; and muscular weakness. Mild hirsutism also appears in a young girl with an underactive thyroid. Absence of, or damage to, the pituitary gland, anorexia nervosa (self-inflicted starvation or excessive dieting), and some drugs such as the corticosteroids and certain birth control pills can also cause hirsutism.

The only symptom of hirsutism itself is excessive growth of hair in normally hairless areas in women: face, neck, breasts and chest, and abdomen. The hair may be soft and fine, as in anorexia nervosa patients, or coarser, depending on many factors. Diagnosis is usually confirmed through visual examination and medical history.

The treatment of hirsutism is directed at removing the cause, if it is identified. For example, adrenal hyperplasia (an abnormal increase in the number of cells in the adrenal gland) can be suppressed by corticosteroid drugs. Patients with polycystic ovaries can be treated with low-dose estrogen birth control pills or with other drugs.

In some cases, however, removing the cause does not diminish the hair growth. In these cases, hair removal is recommended for cosmetic reasons. The only safe permanent local treatment is electrolysis, destroying the individual hair follicles by an electric current. Temporary measures, such as plucking, shaving, waxing, using a depilatory wax or chemical, will temporarily mask the problem but electrolysis is the only permanent solution to hirsutism that involves considerable, permanent hair growth.

Other than prompt diagnosis and treatment of the primary cause or disorder (provided there is one), there are no known preventive measures for hirsutism.

See also Anorexia nervosa, Cushing's syndrome, and Ovarian cysts.

Histoplasmosis

Histoplasmosis is an infection following the inhalation of spores from the fungus *Histoplasma capsulatum*. The parts of the body principally affected are the lungs, the liver, and the spleen.

The *Histoplasma capsulatum* spore is found in soil and in the air. There is no practical defense against breathing the spores. Development of symptoms seems to be a matter of individual immune system response.

In most instances, histoplasmosis does not reach a point that symptoms appear. People may have the disease, but, because of the action of their immune system, never have enough damage to make the symptoms noticeable, much less create an acute condition. However, when symptoms do appear, they can be serious, especially if left unattended. The most common symptoms are as follows:

- Acute pneumonia, which is an inflammation of the lungs, accompanied by the escape of fluid and/or debris in the lungs, and severe interruption of normal lung functions
- Influenza-like illnesses, with lethargy, cough, fever, and lung involvement
- Enlargement of the liver and the spleen, with accompanying interruptions in the normal functions of those organs
- The development of fibrous scar tissue in affected organs.

Histoplasmosis can become inactive, and then be reactivated at a later date. In cases of reactivated histoplasmosis, the lungs, meninges (linings of the brain and spinal cord), heart, peritoneum (lining of the abdominal cavity), and the adrenal glands can be affected, with interruptions of the normal functioning of these organs.

Treatment for histoplasmosis begins with diagnosis. The best procedure is to cultivate growths of the *Histoplasma capsulatum* from tissue or fluid samples. Another method is by noting the rise in the body's antibody production, the protective substances produced by the body to resist the disease. Probably most affected people have histoplasmosis in a dormant form (within their bodies, but not at a stage where symptoms are evident). Fatalities occur only in cases of massive infection (which also implies massive breakdown of the body's immune system, or an immune system that is not functioning properly).

Drug therapy is the usual treatment of chronic disease. Drugs will help control the disease, but appear to have little effect on the fibrous scarring that often accompanies advanced cases of the disease.

There is no known preventive against histoplasmosis.

Hives

Hives (also called urticaria) is a reaction of the skin marked by intense itching and, most noticeably, by the rapid development of raised smooth patches or welts (also called wheals). Hives is most often a sign of an allergic reaction.

During an allergic reaction, the body overreacts to a foreign substance (called an allergen) and causes special cells called mast cells to release a powerful chemical called histamine, which is instrumental in the development of hives.

Hives is often caused by an allergy to certain foods, particularly shellfish, tomatoes, strawberries, eggs, milk, and chocolate. It can also be a reaction to drugs, food dyes, molds, bacteria, and animal skin or hair. In addition, in a susceptible person, cold, the rays of the sun, and vigorous exercise have also been known to cause hives.

Hives is characterized by an outbreak of red and white welts appearing suddenly either in small areas or all over the body and varying in size. They often appear and disappear, lasting anywhere from a few minutes to a day or two, but the outbreak can last for weeks. Accompanying symptoms are intense itching; occasionally, fatigue, fever, and nausea; and difficulty in breathing if the allergic reaction has led to a swelling in the respiratory tract.

Diagnosing the allergy and pinpointing the allergen that is causing the trouble can require extensive testing, especially when a food may be involved. Eliminating many suspected foods, then reintroducing them one at a time, sometimes helps to diagnose the cause of hives. This must be done under medical supervision and with great caution.

Hives can be treated immediately by taking antihistamines. When taken several times a day at a specific, prescribed dosage, the correct type of antihistamine will help control swelling by preventing the released histamine from triggering the hives. Drowsiness is a common side effect of antihistamines, so the type and dosage may need to be adjusted periodically. Other drug therapies such as those involving corticosteroids, which reduce inflammation, may be used to treat serious hives.

Hives can be prevented by avoiding contact with the allergen or stimulus once it is identified.

Hodgkin's disease

Hodgkin's disease is a malignant (cancerous) disease of lymph tissue. It is marked by an increase in certain cells of the lymph nodes and may be present either in a localized or generalized form in the body.

The exact cause of Hodgkin's disease is unknown. The highest incidence of the disease is found in the 15 to 35 year-old age group, and again after age 50. Studies have found no evidence that people in the immediate area of the patient will contract the disease. Recent research has suggested a number of infectious agents, including viruses, as causes of Hodgkin's disease, but this has not been confirmed.

Hodgkin's disease may be discovered accidentally on a routine chest X ray in a person without symptoms. In other cases, the first symptom for many patients is enlargement of the lymph nodes, especially in the neck, chest, throat, and underarm areas. Often there are no other complaints at this point. As the disease progresses, there may be increased swelling and prominence of lymph nodes, intense itching, fever, night sweats, weight loss, and invasion of internal lymph nodes or bone marrow. There may be a specific fever pattern, in which a few days of high fever alternate with days to weeks of normal or subnormal temperatures. One curious symptom is immediate pain in affected areas shortly after drinking any alcoholic beverage.

If bone involvement occurs, there may be pain with involvement of the backbones. The spinal cord may be compressed, resulting in paralysis in the lower legs. Other areas of paralysis may also occur, along with pain as a result of nerve root compression by tumor mass. Bile duct obstruction by tumor masses can produce jaundice (yellowing of skin and whites of eyes). Fluid buildup of the face and neck along with bluish discoloration can result from pressure on the superior vena cava (the large vein draining blood from the upper portion of the body). In addition, obstructions in the lymph nodes in the pelvis or groin area can cause fluid buildup in the leg. Lung compression can also result from enlarged lymph nodes in the chest area. Many patients show a marked decrease in immune responses and many die from other secondary infections.

Hodgkin's disease is always suspected if the patient complains of lymph node enlargement in the neck and chest/upper body area, with or without the fever, night sweats, and weight loss. Diagnosis, however, can only be made by biopsy and the study of cells. It may sometimes be difficult to differentiate Hodgkin's disease from infectious mononucleosis, leukemia, bronchial carcinoma (cancer), and tuberculosis. It is extremely important to note that lymph node enlargement, especially in a teenager and young adult, is much more frequently due to infection rather than to malignancy. Furthermore, enlarged lymph nodes do not automatically indicate that a biopsy is necessary.

It is also important for diagnostic, therapeutic, and prognostic purposes to document the extent of the disease. Hodgkin's disease conforms to four well-defined stages, and in many patients the disease—through radiotherapy, chemotherapy, or both—can be localized or arrested. Stage I is the stage in which the disease is limited to one lymph node region; Stage II, limited to two or more regions on the same side of the diaphragm (the muscle separating the chest and abdominal cavities); Stage

III, limited to the lymph nodes on both sides of the diaphragm (and perhaps the spleen); and Stage IV, extended involvement outside the lymph nodes, such as to the bone marrow, lungs, or liver.

Determining the stages of the disease requires a variety of diagnostic techniques: lymphangiography (insertion of radiographic contrast material into the lymphatic channels of the lower extremities in order to spot affected nodes by X ray), computerized tomography, and body and bone scans are commonly done. Laparotomy (surgically entering the abdominal cavity) for biopsies of the liver and abdominal lymph nodes may be done, and the spleen may be removed in special circumstances where the discovery of involved abdominal tissue would change the therapeutic plan.

Chemotherapy (drug therapy) and radiotherapy are the treatments of choice for most patients. Often, depending on the stage and cell type, the disease can be eliminated in 90 to 95 percent of the cases for an extended period of time with appropriate radiotherapy. Stage I in particular responds to radiotherapy and individuals can be rendered disease-free in about 95 percent of the cases. In Stage II, patients will respond to radiotherapy that is both generalized and directed at specific lymph nodes. Patients in Stage III benefit most from combination chemotherapy, that is, chemotherapy using a combination of four drugs. If the lymph nodes are particularly large, radiotherapy in addition may be helpful. Stage IV patients are best treated with chemotherapy.

Since Hodgkin's disease is of unknown cause, there are no specific preventive measures to be prescribed. Early detection and treatment assure a better prognosis for the Hodgkin's patient.

Hormones

Hormones are chemical substances that are secreted by organs or by cells of organs in one part of the body and are carried in the bloodstream to other organs or tissues where they control or regulate the structure or function of these distant organs. The word *hormone* (from the Greek *hormaien,* meaning "to set in motion") was once limited to the secretions of the endocrine glands, but is now applied to other chemical mediators that perform similar purposes but do not originate in the endocrine system.

Hormones can be considered chemical messengers: they are "targeted" at certain cells in the body, and their arrival in those cells causes certain activities to occur. In general, hormones have three major tasks. They regulate the activities of differing systems so that they can act together in a coordinated manner to achieve an end result. For example, the hormone adrenaline acts on the heart to increase its rate and force of contraction and on the blood vessels to increase blood flow to certain areas so that the body can cope with stress. Hormones also help control the type and rate of body growth and metabolism, and they help the body maintain a consistent internal environment.

In addition to the hormone messengers that carry their commands to various parts of the body, there are also "hormone-releasing" hormones.

These releasing hormones are secreted by the hypothalamus, a specialized part of the brain. They directly regulate the pituitary gland that secretes hormones and hormone stimulating factors. For example, if an endocrine gland is not secreting sufficient hormone, the hypothalamus signals (by secretion of a releasing factor) the pituitary which then secretes a stimulating hormone (such as ACTH) that stimulates the other gland (the adrenal gland in the case of ACTH) to produce more of its own hormone.

See also ACTH, Adrenal glands, Endocrine system, and Pituitary gland.

Huntington's chorea

Huntington's chorea is an inherited brain disease that seldom shows symptoms before early middle age. It is characterized by disorganized body movements—the word *chorea* comes from a Greek word meaning "dance" – along with mental deterioration. It is thought that Huntington's chorea is the result of a disturbance in that part of the brain that automatically regulates voluntary movements.

The condition is transmitted in a dominant gene from a parent who has the disease. There is about a 50 percent chance of a child's inheriting the disease from an affected parent. Since the symptoms of Huntington's chorea do not appear until the victim is between 30 and 50 years of age, a person with a family history of Huntington's chorea lives through the years of adolescence and early adulthood in dread of reaching the middle years when the symptoms may begin. Even more tragic, those who are unaware of a family history of the disease but do develop the disease may have children before discovering they have Huntington's chorea. In these cases, the victims have inadvertently put their children at risk of inheriting the disorder.

The first symptoms of mental deterioration are usually personality changes, in which obstinacy, moodiness, lack of interest in surroundings, and inappropriate behavior may be displayed. It should be noted that all of these types of symptoms can also be due to psychological or other disorders that have nothing to do with Huntington's chorea.

These symptoms are accompanied by irregular, jerky movements that begin in the arms, the neck, and the face. They may start as a mild form of "fidgeting," and gradually develop into facial grimaces, halting speech, irregular movements of the torso, and contractions of the neck that cause the head to rotate.

In advanced cases, the stance will become wide, in an attempt to maintain balance. The gait will become prancing, as control of the legs degenerates. As the disease progresses, the victims usually become paranoid, walking ability is lost altogether, swallowing becomes difficult, and dementia (loss of intellectual functions) increases.

No treatment has been yet found to control the symptoms or halt the disease. However, the chorea may respond somewhat to some drugs, most notably haloperidol and chlorpromazine. There is no treatment for the mental degeneration that accompanies the physical symptoms.

Short of genetic engineering (which may be the only hope for genetically transmitted conditions such as this), there is no known preventive for Huntington's chorea. Presently, genetic engineering is still in its infancy as a science. Even if it were possible to "engineer" the faulty gene away, this would not help those who presently have the disease. It would only prevent the transmission of the disease.

As of now, the best preventative for Huntington's chorea is advising affected patients not to have children.

Hyaline membrane disease

Hyaline membrane disease (HMD) is a respiratory distress syndrome, occurring in premature infants in which the newborn does not have fully functioning lungs. It is the leading cause of illness and death in premature infants in the United States today and accounts for 10,000 deaths a year.

The cause of HMD is the birth of the infant before the structures that manufacture *pulmonary surfactant* are developed. In order to begin inhaling and expanding normally, the newborn's lungs require the presence of a substance (pulmonary surfactant) that reduces the surface tension of the alveoli, the tiny air sacs at the end of bronchial tubes where oxygen and carbon dioxide waste are exchanged. Without this reduction in surface tension, the air sacs tend to collapse when the infant breathes out. This, in turn, produces incomplete expansion of the lungs. The end result is that the blood that is passing through the lungs is not fully oxygenated, at least not sufficiently to sustain life.

The symptoms of hyaline membrane disease are easily observable. There is a blue tint to the skin, from lack of oxygenation of the blood; symptoms of oxygen deprivation; irregular heartbeat; rapid, labored, and shallow breathing; flaring of the nostrils; grunting when breathing out; and swelling of tissues.

Treatment for HMD is aimed at maintaining necessary oxygen levels. The problem is lack of the ability of the lungs to oxygenate blood—until the lungs develop that ability, oxygen must be provided in such a way as to prevent damage to the infant.

Fluids, serum glucose (sugar), and electrolytes are provided by intravenous (into the vein) feedings. An oxygen face mask is used to provide warmed, moisturized oxygen with a continuous positive pressure. In more severe cases, a ventilator is necessary to breathe for the infant.

The condition will either clear up on its own as the lungs develop and begin to produce surfactant in about three to five days, or the infant will not survive.

The best preventive measure is to guard against premature labor. The mother should be carefully monitored during the last weeks of her pregnancy for any signs of premature labor. In the case of diabetic mothers, the lungs and its structures may not yet be fully formed until the fortieth week of pregnancy, so hyaline membrane disease is possible at full term in these cases.

Hydrocele

A hydrocele is a soft swelling around a testis and is noticeable as a soft mass in the scrotum, the bag of skin containing the testes. The term *hydrocele* means literally a sac of water.

There is a normal double-layered covering around each testis. Within these two layers there is usually just enough fluid for sufficient lubrication. Occasionally, however, the amount of fluid may increase, leading to the swelling around the testis. Although a hydrocele may be caused by an injury or inflammation in the scrotum among other problems (this is called secondary hydrocele), quite often there is no apparent cause (this is known as primary hydrocele). As a rule, most hydroceles in and of themselves are harmless and common, especially in older men.

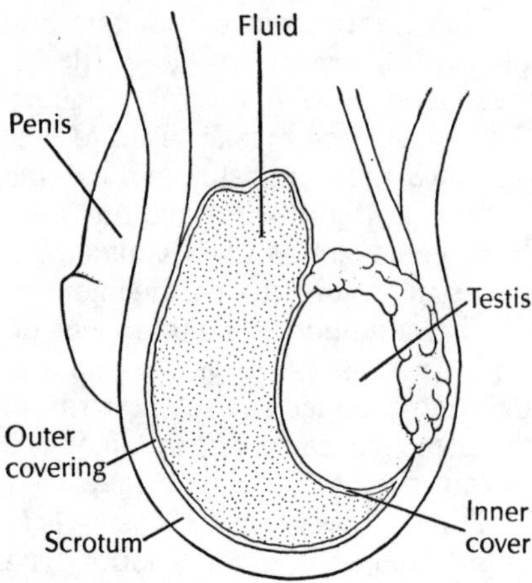

A hydrocele is the accumulation of fluid between the double-layered covering of the testis. It is usually harmless, painless, and common—especially in elderly men.

Although hydroceles are usually painless, symptoms may include pain and, of course, an obvious swelling.

A small, painless hydrocele often requires no treatment. However, if the hydrocele becomes very large or painful, treatment may be indicated. Bed rest, ice bags, and painkillers such as aspirin may afford temporary relief. Usually, however, the physician will draw off the excess fluid with a needle, a procedure done under local anesthetic. While this may bring relief, it is not always a permanent solution, since excess fluid may build up again in the area. A more permanent resolution of the problem is surgical correction.

Hydrocephalus

Hydrocephalus is an abnormal accumulation of cerebrospinal fluid within the cavities or hollow spaces of the brain. Normally, cerebrospinal fluid is secreted in the cavities of the brain and absorbed by a membrane that surrounds the cavities. If the membrane does not absorb the fluid or if the fluid is blocked, the fluid builds up in the cavities. The fluid buildup causes the head to become enlarged and the brain compressed or reduced in size. This condition has sometimes been referred to as "water on the brain" when, in reality, it is water *in* the brain.

When hydrocephalus occurs in an infant, the loosely connected bony skull plates pull apart to accommodate the swelling. As a result, the head becomes greatly enlarged. In addition to having an oversized head, the child with hydrocephalus may have an abnormally large or prominent forehead and swollen or enlarged blood vessels in the scalp. This condition can lead to paralysis, blindness, mental retardation, inability to speak, and convulsions.

Hydrocephalus is usually the result of a brain infection or malformation in the unborn baby prior to birth. While the baby's head may not appear abnormally large at birth, it expands rapidly from month to

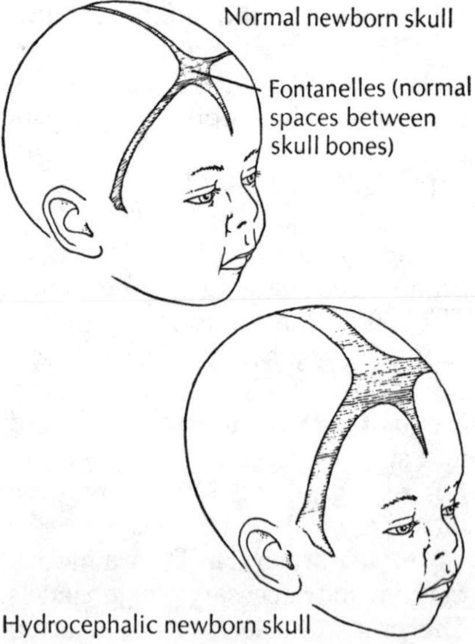

When hydrocephalus—a buildup of fluid in the brain—occurs in a newborn infant, the loosely connected skull bones spread apart to accommodate the swelling.

month, and if untreated the child usually dies by the end of the second year. If the blockage is only partial, the individual may live for a number of years, or may even live a full life.

Although hydrocephalus is usually a congenital (present at birth) condition, appearing in infants, it can occur later in childhood as a result of an infection or tumor. It can also occur in adults as a result of these same causes.

Early diagnosis, which is accomplished through the use of X rays and CAT scans, is vital to a possible cure or recovery. Surgery can make it possible, in some cases, to bypass the blockage or obstruction, causing the fluid buildup to escape through other exits. Often a small tube is shunted from a brain cavity into the abdomen or into a major blood vessel, and fluid drains from the brain into the abdomen or blood vessel. As the child grows, the tube may become blocked, again allowing pressure to build in the brain. If this happens, the tube will be replaced or the blockage removed. When surgery is successful, the probability of mental retardation is greatly reduced, and the prospects of normal development are increased.

Hyperemesis gravidarum

Hyperemesis gravidarum is a term that refers to excessive or abnormal vomiting during pregnancy. This type of vomiting is more severe than that caused by normal morning sickness, which usually clears up on its own within a few months. In hyperemesis gravidarum, the vomiting leads to starvation; dehydration, or loss of water in the body; and an imbalance in body fluids.

Symptoms of hyperemesis gravidarum include loss of weight and dehydration. The condition is most often treated in the hospital through the use of anti-vomiting drugs and of intravenous feeding to correct the possible malnutrition, dehydration, and imbalance of body fluids. A pregnant woman should not attempt to treat herself with drugs for her vomiting without consulting her doctor.

Hyperkinesis

Hyperkinesis is a nervous disorder that affects mostly children. The condition is characterized by very high levels of physical activity, consistently impulsive and immature behavior, and extremely short attention span. It is four to five times more commonly seen in boys than in girls.

Also known as minimal brain dysfunction, attention deficit disorder, and, most commonly, hyperactivity, this condition is thought to be the result of a deficiency or malfunctioning of chemicals in the brain called neurotransmitters, whose job it is to transmit impulses between the nerves.

Although hyperkinesis does no physical damage to the body, it can trigger long-lasting social, emotional, and educational problems. For example, hyperkinetic children cannot sit still and concentrate for long periods, so they may have trouble with reading, writing, and arithmetic. They often appear to be immature, uncoordinated, and boisterous and may have trouble getting along with classmates, teachers, and parents; consequently, they often suffer from a poor self-image.

The cause of hyperkinesis is not known, but several theories have surfaced in recent years. One states that the additives, preservatives, and colorings found in processed foods have a toxic or allergic effect on some children, resulting in hyperkinesis. Another theory states that a genetic defect or damage to a fetus during pregnancy causes this disorder. A third theory holds that, when deciding upon taking action, the brain has two systems—one which inspires immediate action and one which encourages hesitation and consideration—and that the neurotransmitters which control the "hesitation" response are malfunctioning in the hyperkinetic child. None of these theories has been proven or disproven.

There are no specific risk factors associated with this disorder, but it is thought that parents who were hyperkinetic tend to have children who also suffer from it.

A variety of symptoms point to a case of hyperkinesis. The hyperkinetic child is overly active, fidgety, restless, overly talkative or boisterous, impulsive, and seemingly uncoordinated. In school, this child has a very short attention span and seems to forget facts quickly, disrupts the classroom, does school work hastily and incorrectly, skips or adds words when reading, laughs too loud and hard, and prefers to play with younger children.

There are no specific tests to help diagnose hyperkinesis. These symptoms seem to be present in all children to some degree, and since hyperkinesis is rather vaguely defined, the symptoms displayed by an individual child suspected to be hyperkinetic need to be carefully observed. The quantity, intensity, and duration of these symptoms may single out hyperkinetic children from others who are merely bored with school or who are having other behavior problems.

Drug therapy has proved to be the most successful (and controversial) treatment for hyperkinesis. Several stimulant drugs appear to have a calming effect on hyperkinetic children because they affect the neurotransmitters' "contemplative" response (the one which encourages hesitation before action). However, these drugs have been shown to have unpleasant side effects such as stomach cramps, colds, nervous mannerisms, and even stunted growth. Therefore, many children on this therapy are required by their doctors to take "drug holidays" to give their bodies a break from the side effects of the medication.

Special diets which attempt to eliminate all food additives have been prescribed in keeping with the theory that additives cause hyperkinesis. Studies on this treatment have been either inconclusive or contradictory. However, many parents report dramatic changes in behavior after this treatment, although part of the change may be due to the extra attention paid to the child whose meals have to be specially prepared.

Parents can help to influence the child's actions, in addition, by praising or rewarding good behavior and ignoring or punishing bad behavior. When the child becomes too wild or uncontrollably overactive, for instance, he or she can be sent to a quiet room to settle down.

Hypertension

Hypertension, or high blood pressure, refers to persistently elevated pressure of blood within and against the walls of the arteries, which carry blood from the heart through the body. This excessive force being exerted on the artery walls may cause damage to the arteries themselves and thereby to body organs such as the heart, kidney, and brain, leading to heart attacks, kidney failure, and strokes.

Although many people believe hypertension is a condition caused by extreme activity or tension, this theory has not been proven. Actually, high blood pressure may have no known cause, or it can be associated with other diseases. When no underlying cause is discovered, the disease is called primary or essential hypertension. If another disease, such as kidney or heart disease, causes the elevated blood pressure, the condition is labeled secondary hypertension.

Contrary to popular belief, there is no typical hypertensive person. However, there are some people more susceptible to developing high blood pressure. Persons with either one or both parents who are hypertensive are at greater risk of acquiring this condition since heredity may play a role in the development of hypertension. In the past, hypertension has been attributed to aging, but current evidence shows that age is not a primary factor. Blacks, both children and adults, have at least twice the incidence of hypertension as whites.

Overweight, prolonged stress, smoking, drinking, and excessive sodium (salt) in the diet causing fluid retention may increase blood pressure, especially in people prone to hypertension. There are also indications that oral contraceptives may contribute to increased blood pressure. However, this is more likely to occur with women who are overweight, whose parents are hypertensive, or who have other hypertensive risk factors.

Hypertension has been called the "silent disease," because it often has no obvious symptoms. A person may have high blood pressure for years without noticing any symptoms. What symptoms do occur may include headache, fatigue, dizziness, flushed face, ear ringing, thumping in the chest, or possibly frequent nosebleeds. However, these symptoms may result from other conditions.

To diagnose hypertension, a simple, risk-free, painless test using a stethoscope and a sphygmomanometer, an inflatable arm cuff attached to a graduated mercury manometer (device measuring the tension of fluids) is used. Blood pressure is measured in a main artery of the arm by first shutting off and then releasing the flow of blood in the artery with the cuff and listening to the artery pulse with the stethoscope.

The blood pressure measurements are read as the systolic pressure (the first beat of the pulse after release of the cuff) over the diastolic pressure (the pressure at which the last beat is heard)—for example, 120/80 is considered normal in the average adult. The systolic pressure essentially measures the pressure of the heart during a contraction or heartbeat. The diastolic pressure is that which exists when the heart is filling between beats. Although diastolic pressure is considerably lower than systolic, there is still pressure in the body when the heart is filling. Therefore, both numbers count. An unusually high systolic pressure may mean the heart is pumping too hard or the arteries are stiff; a high diastolic pressure means that the arteries have an abnormally high tone or resistance.

Normal blood pressure is about 80/46 at birth and climbs as age increases. The normal adult pressure is around 120/80. Female hypertensives seem to do better than males; however, their risk of cardiovascular disease is still greater than that of normal females.

Fortunately, hypertension re-

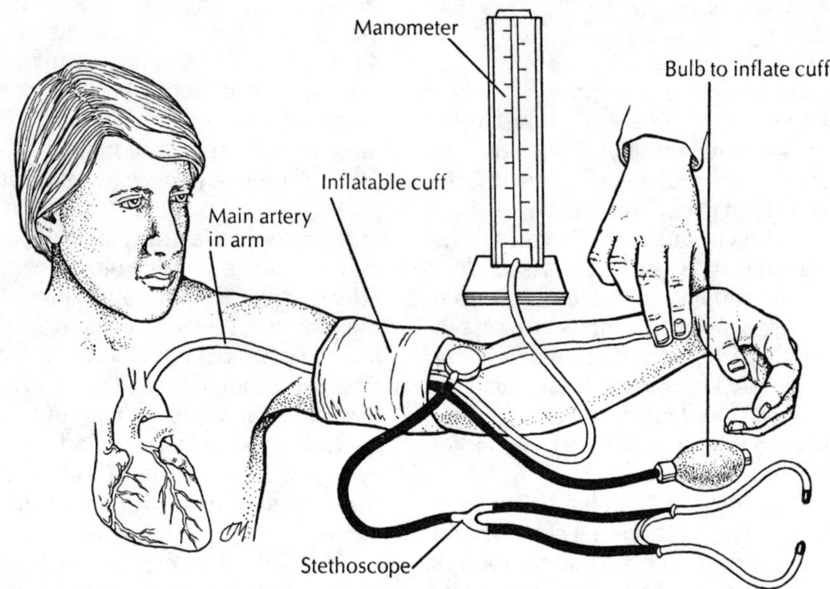

Using a sphygmomanometer—an inflatable arm cuff attached to a manometer, blood pressure is measured in a main artery of the arm by first shutting off and then releasing the flow of the blood in the artery with the cuff and listening to the artery pulse with a stethoscope.

sponds well to treatment. When the condition is mild (systolic around 140 and diastolic 90 to 94) and there is no indication of other disease, doctors may suggest lifestyle changes before prescribing medication. These changes may include weight loss for the overweight; a regular exercise program; and strict limitation of salt (sodium) intake, which affects fluid balance and volume and therefore blood pressure. Controlling salt in the diet requires restriction of table salt as well as careful scrutiny of all food and drug labels before eating.

If medication is indicated, a physician may prescribe one drug or a combination of drugs as part of a "stepped care" program. Step one may start with a diuretic, a drug that promotes water loss. Step two may be a beta blocker, a medicine that reduces the work of the heart, or a "centrally acting" drug that lowers blood pressure by affecting the blood pressure center of the brain. Step three could be a vasodilator, a drug that dilates or opens narrowed blood vessels that contribute to hypertension by increasing resistance to flow. If none of the first three steps proves effective, a combination of two or more steps may be repeated or other still more potent drugs may be used—all under the physician's close supervision.

While tension and stress do not directly cause hypertension, these factors do affect the condition. Persons with hypertension are urged to avoid high-pressure situations and learn to deal with stress. Since techniques such as biofeedback, self-hypnosis, and meditation have proven useful for reducing stress, they may help someone with hypertension. Blood pressure can be monitored at home by purchasing a special kit and learning to use the sphygmomanometer. Children of hypertensive parents especially need to have their blood pressure measured early in life on a regular basis. If three separate elevated readings (above 140/90 in adults) are detected, a trip to the doctor is in order.

Hyperthyroidism

Hyperthyroidism is a condition that results when an overactive thyroid gland produces too much thyroid hormone. The thyroid gland is a small butterfly-shaped gland located in front of the windpipe above the top of the breastbone. It affects every tissue in the body by secreting thyroid hormone which helps maintain body temperature, convert food to energy, and regulate growth and fertility. The pituitary gland, which is the control center for all endocrine glands, regulates the production of thyroid hormone by secreting thyroid stimulating hormone (TSH) when a need for thyroid hormone is present. In addition, adequate iodine is necessary for the production of thyroid hormone. Iodine in the blood is obtained either from substances taken into the body, such as food, or from the breakdown of thyroid hormone itself.

In hyperthyroidism, the thyroid gland somehow malfunctions. The pituitary gland will sense the increased levels of thyroid hormone and shut off the stimulation. However, the abnormal gland is no longer sensitive to this mechanism.

Hyperthyroidism is a descriptive term that encompasses different disorders. Grave's disease, a common form of hyperthyroidism, is probably due to the presence of an abnormal chemical stimulator of thyroid hormone production. This disease occurs most often in the young, particularly those in their 30s and 40s. It is also more common in females than in males. The occurrence of bulging eye(s) and distinctive skin problems is also a part of Grave's disease. The thyroid gland itself is frequently enlarged, smooth, and soft. Along with these unique features, patients with Grave's disease exhibit the symptoms and signs common to all forms of hyperthyroidism, including rapid heartbeat, weight loss despite increased appetite and food intake, generalized hyperactivity, tremors, increased sweating, severe nervousness and emotional instability, alterations of menstruation and fertility, and weakness.

Toxic multinodular goiter, another common form of hyperthyroidism, is a condition in which nodules (lump-like clusters of thyroid tissue) somehow form and secrete abnormally large amounts of thyroid hormone. These nodules function independent of normal regulatory mechanisms. In contrast to Grave's disease this condition is common in the middle-aged and elderly. Bulging of the eyes rarely occurs, and the gland is not uniformly enlarged, but lumpy. There has been no chemical mediator defined in this illness. Toxic multinodular goiter, of course, also produces the aforementioned symptoms and signs common to the hyperthyroid state.

The diagnosis of hyperthyroidism is made by the history and physical examination and confirmed with laboratory data. Naturally, the level of thyroid hormone in the blood must be significantly elevated, and this can be determined by a simple blood test. Further documentation and quantitation is obtained through the use of nuclear medicine scans utilizing radiolabeled iodine. Since iodine is necessary for the production of thyroid hormone, the injected, labeled iodine will gravitate to the thyroid yielding not only a picture of the gland, but a precise estimate of the degree of hyperactivity.

Treatment of hyperthyroidism depends on which condition is present.

However, treatment of the hyperthyroid state in general has several common elements. The drug propranolol, a beta-blocker, is commonly used to block the adrenaline overstimulation seen in hyperthyroidism which greatly contributes to the tremors, increased heart rate, and sweating. This drug, although it diminishes symptoms, does not get at the root of the problem: too much thyroid hormone. To decrease the amount of thyroid hormone being produced, antithyroid drugs such as propylthiouracil are used. These drugs actually interfere with the production of thyroid hormone. However, this is again usually only a temporary solution, since when the drug is stopped, the excess production may resume. The definitive therapy of hyperthyroidism is the actual destruction or removal of most or all of the gland by the use of radioactive iodine or surgery.

Grave's disease is usually first treated by blocking the adrenaline overstimulation with propranolol. Simultaneously, an antithyroid drug is started. Usually this drug is maintained for a period of one to two years and then tapered off. With this approach relapse (recurrence) is not at all uncommon. If relapse occurs or if the level of thyroid hormone is normalized, the choice then is how to reduce the amount of thyroid tissue. Whether surgery or radioactive iodine is used depends upon many complex factors and is a very controversial subject in medicine. One would be best advised to seek the opinion of a physician well-versed and experienced in the treatment of this disease before choosing. It is to be noted that both of these treatments frequently result in too little thyroid hormone in the blood, but this problem is easily remedied by supplementation with synthetic thyroid hormone.

The treatment of toxic multinodular goiter is somewhat less controversial. After blocking with a beta blocker and, frequently, normalizing hormone levels with an antithyroid drug, destruction of the gland with radioactive iodine is the treatment.

See also Hypothyroidism.

Hyperventilation

Hyperventilation is abnormally rapid and deep breathing, which serves to draw large quantities of air in along with expelling too much carbon dioxide. The diminished blood level of carbon dioxide can lead to buzzing in the ears; a tingling feeling in the fingers, toes, and lips; and lightheadedness. It may also be marked by tightness in the chest and a feeling of suffocation—that is, the inability to breathe. Hyperventilation attacks may last up to half an hour or longer and may recur several times in a 24-hour period.

Symptoms of hyperventilation may be strikingly similar to those of heart disease and other serious illnesses. The individual experiencing these symptoms should, therefore, see a doctor to rule out the possibility of any of these more serious conditions. Although hyperventilation can result from physical disease that interferes with the oxygen/carbon dioxide exchange in the lungs, most often hyperventilation is a physical response to stress, anxiety, and emotional upset. It begins slowly and builds up to a point at which symptoms appear and the person panics. The breathing then becomes even more rapid and difficult.

The symptoms of hyperventilation can often be relieved by having the person breathe into a paper bag. In this fashion, he or she immediately inhales back into the body the needed carbon dioxide he or she has just breathed out into the bag. In this way, the normal level of carbon dioxide in the blood can be restored.

Hypochondria

Hypochondria is the persistent and exaggerated worry — usually based on self-diagnosis — an individual has about his or her health, even though the person is not actually ill nor likely to become ill. It is sometimes referred to as *hypochondriasis,* which was originally thought to be the region of the stomach that was the center of melancholy or sadness.

Hypochondria reflects an often morbid concern over any unusual physical or mental sensation or feeling. For example, to the hypochondriac, a headache indicates a brain tumor; a cough has to mean tuberculosis; and a mole is sure to be cancerous. Despite test results and reassurances, this person is convinced that he or she either has a serious illness or will have one very soon.

Frequently, the hypochondriac complains of pain or discomfort in the stomach, chest, head, or neck. Symptoms common among hypochondriacs include nausea, loss of appetite, vomiting, and belching. These symptoms become worse after the person has received expressions of sympathy and concern from family members or friends. In addition, the hypochondriac often makes repeated visits to doctors and uses numerous nonprescription drug items.

Hypochondria is very difficult to treat. It has been estimated that only a small percentage of persons afflicted with this disorder recover completely. Psychotherapy is sometimes useful in such situations; however, it is often of more help if the individual can be encouraged to divert the energy spent on worrying about his or her health to more productive interests and activities.

Hypoglycemia

Hypoglycemia is the body's inability to maintain enough glucose in the blood. Glucose is a sugar released into the blood from digestion of carbohydrates (sugars and starches).

During normal digestion, increased glucose levels trigger the secretion of the hormone insulin from the pancreas located in the upper abdomen. Insulin acts to reduce the sugar level in the blood by helping certain body cells absorb the sugar for fuel.

However, if the pancreas continues to produce insulin longer than necessary or produces too much insulin relative to the level of glucose in the blood, abnormally low blood sugar levels result. This condition is called reactive hypoglycemia. Reactive hypoglycemia is a condition caused by an oversecretion of insulin and consequent rapid lowering of blood glucose levels producing symptoms of hypoglycemia in response to a glucose load. Reactive hypoglycemia is also known as post-prandial (after meals) hypoglycemia as it occurs only in response to food.

The specific causes of reactive hypoglycemia are unknown in most cases. However, certain conditions (for example, rapid emptying of the stomach with consequent absorption of a large glucose load that occurs in those patients who have had part or most of the stomach removed) commonly are associated with reactive hypoglycemia.

Another type of hypoglycemia, fasting hypoglycemia, has several known causes. Basically, fasting hypoglycemia is caused by either an insufficient production of glucose or an overutilization of the glucose present in the blood. Often, these two factors are combined to create a low fasting blood glucose level. In addition, the presence of an insulin-producing tumor on the pancreas may contribute to fasting hypoglycemia. Because alcohol disturbs the regular sugar storage and release mechanisms within the liver, heavy drinkers are at greater risk of developing the disorder. Fasting hypoglycemia can also occur in anyone who has not eaten for an unusually long interval, but this is a temporary situation. Chronic hypoglycemia is uncommon.

Hypoglycemia symptoms include fatigue, nervousness, perspiration, dizziness, headache, hunger pangs, visual impairment, and accelerated heartbeat. The condition may also bring anxiety, concentration problems, confusion, and blackouts. If sugar deprivation continues unchecked, severe hypoglycemia can produce convulsions (short-term loss of consciousness involving the nervous system and producing jerking muscle movements) and possibly deep coma (prolonged loss of consciousness).

To diagnose hypoglycemia, a doctor analyzes a blood sample to detect abnormally low sugar levels. Blood drawn during an attack of the condition provides the most accurate assessment, since symptons can then be correlated with actual blood glucose levels.

Treatment for hypoglycemia often is aimed at the underlying cause of the disease. For example, a pancreatic tumor may require surgery to remove the growth, and a hypoglycemic reaction to insulin overdose by diabetics may necessitate adjustment of insulin dosage until the body balances sugar and insulin.

With most cases of reactive hypoglycemia, however, there is no known cure for the pancreas' tendency to overproduce insulin when it is not needed. The most effective treatment involves avoiding all foods that generate attacks.

A good diet is one that is low enough in sugar and starches to moderate the body's overreaction to sugar intake and rich enough in protein to help maintain gradual elevations of blood sugar. By eating smaller meals more frequently, levels of sugar concentrated in the blood may remain more stable.

It is important to note that true hypoglycemia is an uncommon condition. Since many of the symptoms of anxiety and hypoglycemia are alike, the two diagnoses are sometimes easily confused.

See also Diabetes mellitus.

Hypotension

Hypotension is low blood pressure. Unlike chronic high blood pressure, which can be a serious health problem, low blood pressure is usually not a problem and need not be reason for concern or even treatment.

Blood pressures vary depending on such factors as age, race, sex, and environment. On rare occasions, individuals may have medical problems that, themselves, cause low blood pressure. Among such conditions are some types of heart disease, hormonal deficiencies, and malnutrition. In these cases, the hypotension will be corrected by the treatment of the medical problem.

In addition, one form of low blood pressure called postural hypotension can cause dizziness or a feeling of faintness when a person stands up abruptly from a sitting or reclining position. Normally, when an individual stands up, the blood vessels contract and otherwise act to maintain normal blood pressure in the new position. However, in those persons with postural hypotension this mechanism probably does not work properly, and upon standing these people experience a temporary reduction in the blood flow to the brain that leads to dizziness. Also, if a person stands in one position long enough, blood pools in the veins of the legs, decreasing the amount of blood returned to the heart and therefore the amount pumped to the brain.

Sometimes postural hypotension results from medication for high blood pressure; in these cases, reducing the dosage or changing the medication will correct the problem. Most often, however, postural hypotension is no cause for concern. Arising slowly from a sitting or reclining position will usually prevent the symptoms.

Hypothermia

Hypothermia is a condition in which the person's body temperature falls well below the normal temperature of 98.6°F. The lowering of the temperature can occur accidentally, or the temperature can be lowered in the course of medical treatment. When hypothermia happens accidentally, the person's condition can become serious if the symptoms or signs are ignored.

Among the causes of accidental hypothermia are the aging process, surgical procedures, certain drugs, and long periods of being exposed to the cold without having adequate clothing on. Hypothermia can occur easily in newborns and in infants, as well as in the elderly, as their heat-retaining mechanisms are respectively not fully developed and easily overtaxed.

The signs and symptoms of hypothermia include an altered level of consciousness, slow breathing, low pulse rate, listlessness, and mental confusion. The hands, feet, and abdomen of the hypothermic person will be cold to the touch.

Basic treatment for hypothermia is the gradual or slow rewarming of the cold body. The rewarming must be gradual to prevent the sudden enlargement of blood vessels at the surface of the body, which may divert too much blood from some of the body's vital internal organs. Medical help should always be obtained for a person with hypothermia. While waiting for help to arrive, the cold person should be covered with blankets and, if alert, should be offered a warm non-alcoholic beverage. Alcoholic drinks do not help because they tend to reduce body heat. Also, briskly rubbing hands or feet to restore warmth is not recommended. Any other type of treatment depends on the underlying cause of the drop in body temperature. In severe cases where body temperature is critically reduced, warm intravenous (into the vein) fluids may be given. Peritoneal dialysis (injecting and withdrawing of fluid in the abdominal cavity) with warm fluids is also an excellent way of restoring normal temperature.

The term "hypothermia" is also used to refer to a medical treatment technique. When this technique is used, the person's blood is gradually cooled, in order to lower the rate of the person's metabolism—that is, production of energy—so that the body's need for oxygen decreases. Once the need for oxygen decreases, the heart and brain can withstand a halt in the blood flow for short periods of time. Such interruptions make it possible for the patient to undergo delicate or painstaking surgery without hemorraghing or severe bleeding. Intentionally induced hypothermia has been used, for example, in open-heart surgery.

Hypothyroidism

Hypothyroidism is a disorder in which an underactive thyroid gland produces too little thyroid hormone. The thyroid gland lies in front of the windpipe above the top of the breastbone. Its job is to secrete thyroid hormone that influences every tissue in the body by participating in maintenance of body temperature, conversion of food to energy, and regulation of growth and fertility. The pituitary gland, which controls all endocrine glands, regulates the amount of thyroid hormone that is produced by raising or lowering the amount of thyroid-stimulating hormone (TSH).

The exact cause of hypothyroidism is unknown. However, the disorder may result from chronic (long-term) thyroid inflammation or deficiency of pituitary hormone. Autoimmune (destruction of the body's own tissue by its immune system) diseases of the thyroid are also a common cause of hypothyroidism. In addition, heredity may play a role in the development of thyroid imbalance. Also, women seem more prone to thyroid disorders, but the exact reason is unconfirmed. For some women, pregnancy triggers the hormone imbalance.

Hypothyroidism can also develop after suppression or partial removal of the thyroid gland as treatment for hyperthyroidism, a condition resulting from an overactive thyroid that produces too much thyroid hormone.

People with hypothyroidism may be overweight, easily exhausted, and subject to recurrent infection. They may also experience menstrual disorders, intolerance of cold, dry skin and hair, puffiness of hands and face, and mental illness.

Prolonged hypothyroidism may cause signs of reduced general body functioning. Anemia, a deficiency of red blood cells, may result from diminished function of the bone marrow, where red blood cells are formed. Heart rate may decrease, and reflexes become sluggish. In addition, an electroencephalogram, which measures brain waves, may reveal irregular patterns.

To diagnose hypothyroidism, a series of tests may be given. First, a blood test measures the amount of thyroid hormone in the blood. Pituitary thyroid-stimulating hormone is also measured. If thyroid production is too low, the level of TSH should be greatly increased (to push the thyroid to produce). If this is not the case, there may be a pituitary abnormality at the root of the problem.

Since hypothyroidism develops from a shortage of thyroid hormone, the most effective treatment is thyroid hormone supplements. Supplements are either natural hormones extracted from the thyroid glands of animals or synthetic hormones. Both types control the problem, but the natural form is usually less costly. Although treatment provides the necessary hormone control, hypothyroidism often continues throughout life. Thus, the individual may require lifelong follow-up to monitor treatment.

See also Congenital hypothyroidism and Hyperthyroidism.

Hysterectomy

Hysterectomy is the surgical removal of the uterus and its cervix. Removal

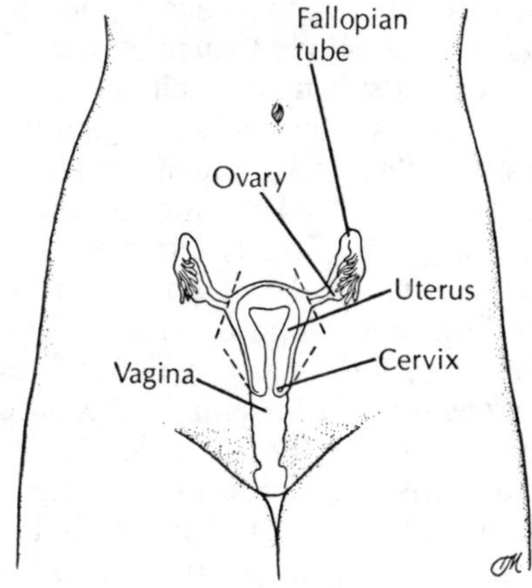

A hysterectomy is the removal of the uterus. The dotted lines outline what is usually removed, indicating that when possible the fallopian tubes and ovaries are not removed.

of the uterus may be done through an abdominal cut or incision or through the vagina (the top of the vagina is stitched together after the uterus is removed). The latter procedure requires no external incision and, therefore, leaves no external scar.

Hysterectomies may be either total or partial. The total hysterectomy involves the removal of the entire uterus. A partial hysterectomy means removal of only the body of the uterus and not the cervix.

When hysterectomy is performed, the ovaries and fallopian tubes may also be removed. Removal of the ovaries causes the patient to go through an artificial menopause—the termination of menstruation and the inability to bear children—because the ovaries produce hormones that influence menstruation and fertility. For this reason, physicians remove the ovaries only with strong indications and may need to treat the menopausal condition with the female hormone estrogen.

Hysterectomies are performed for a number of reasons. They are most commonly performed when the uterus is diseased. Symptomatic fibroid tumors, uterine prolapse, and cancer of the uterus are common reasons for a hysterectomy. Cysts and tumors of the ovaries or fallopian tubes may also require a hysterectomy.

Contrary to common belief, a hysterectomy, in and of itself, does not interfere with, or diminish the pleasure of, sexual intercourse, nor does it cause weight gain.

See also Fibroid tumors, Menopause, Ovarian cysts, and Prolapse.

I

Ileitis

See Crohn's disease.

Ileostomy

An ileostomy is the surgical opening (stoma) through the abdomen into the ileum, the lower part of the small intestine. An ileostomy is performed whenever the large intestine and rectum must be removed because of disease or abnormalities. The opening into the small intestine then becomes an artificial anus through which waste material is expelled, since waste matter can no longer travel through the normal anus.

The waste matter that is discharged through the stoma is collected in a bag that the patient wears continually. Because this waste matter does not pass through the large intestine where water is absorbed from the waste matter, the material excreted through the stoma is watery.

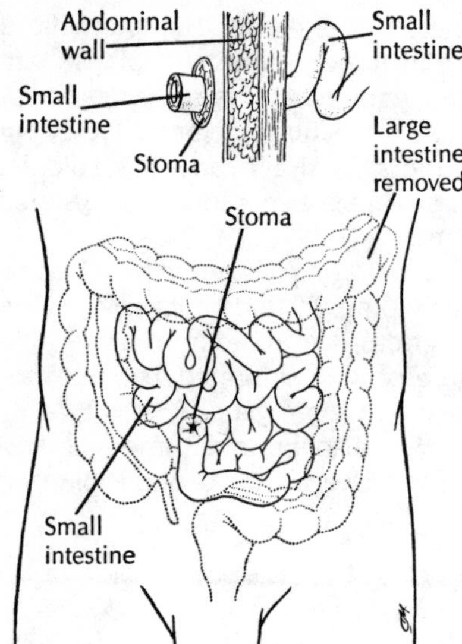

An ileostomy is a surgical opening through the abdomen into the ileum (lower part of small intestine) through which waste matter is expelled. An ileostomy is performed when the large intestine must be removed.

Eventually, the waste matter becomes firmer, but it never becomes solid.

Patients learn to care for their ileostomies in the hospital after the operation. Equipped with this knowledge, a patient can lead a normal life with an ileostomy.

See also Colostomy.

Immunity

Immunity is the body's ability to defend itself against harmful substances. Essentially, it is a resistance to infection that may be inherited or acquired naturally or artificially.

Resistance occurs when foreign organisms called antigens enter the body, causing particular specialized cells to react either by attacking the antigen directly or by producing proteins (compounds essential to living cells) that neutralize the foreign agents. The most common types of antigens are forms of bacteria (one-celled organisms that have the potential to attack body tissues or secrete poisonous substances called toxins) and viruses (the smallest organisms responsible for a variety of diseases).

The specialized cells are part of the lymph system. This system manufactures white blood cells whose job it is to destroy invading organisms. The lymph system is also a network of vessels that carries lymph, a watery fluid containing the white blood cells, to all parts of the body. Lymph drains from the blood vessels and body tissues, carrying away any waste products. The waste products, including antigens, are filtered out of the lymph by small glands called lymph nodes found throughout the body. Unwanted organisms are then trapped, attacked, and destroyed by the white blood cells.

The lymph system also manufactures antibodies. Antibodies are specialized proteins that the body produces in response to invasion of a hostile organism. The process of antibody formation begins when an antigen stimulates a lymph node into action. Antibodies then counteract invading antigens by combining with the antigen to render it harmless to the body. The antibodies coat the harmful organism so that the body's scavenger cells can destroy them more easily. Other antibodies that neutralize toxins produced by bacteria are called antitoxins.

During periods of active antibody production, lymph nodes often enlarge and become tender to the touch. A vaccination—or injection of a natural or artificial antigen to stimulate the body to produce protective antibodies — in the arm can cause swelling under the armpit, while an influenza infection can affect neck glands. Usually nodes can be felt under the skin of the armpit, groin, or neck. The spleen, an organ located in the upper left part of the abdomen is also important in the manufacture of antibodies.

Production of white blood cells and antibodies in response to an invading disease organism is called an immune reaction. This immune reaction is one of the body's primary and most efficient lines of defense. Once antibodies have been produced to fight a certain organism, that germ no longer poses a threat to the body. That is why one attack of a disease often prevents that same disease from infecting the body again. The first attack causes antibody production. In turn, these antibodies protect the body against subsequent attacks. With measles, for example, the antibodies created by having the disease or by being vaccinated with measles virus resist a second attack of the disease, thus providing immunity against its recurrence.

Sometimes, the immune system causes reactions that make the body unusually sensitive to foreign material. When the immune response is disruptive to the body, it is called an allergic reaction. What happens is that the antigens and antibodies unite on the surface of certain cells. This union triggers release of agents stored in the cells. Such powerful agents as histamine and serotonin can dilate small blood vessels and constrict smooth muscles such as those in the air passages or digestive tract. The result is an adverse reaction to the offending substance called an allergen.

Because antibodies to a particular allergen tend to increase gradually, a person rarely experiences an allergic reaction on the first encounter with a substance. However, after several exposures, allergy symptoms may appear. Offending allergens can be inhaled as with hay fever, touched as with contact dermatitis, consumed as with food or medication or injected as with drugs or insect stings.

The resulting allergic reaction can be mild enough to go unnoticed or so severe as to be life-threatening. The watery eyes and runny nose of hay fever merely annoy some people. Yet, anaphylactic shock—characterized by breathing problems; hives or itchy swellings; collapsed blood vessels; and occasionally vomiting, diarrhea, and abdominal cramps—resulting from an allergic reaction can be dangerous if not treated promptly.

Prevention of adverse immune reactions requires avoidance of the problem allergens once they have been detected. Should this not be practical, "desensitization shots" often provide relief by taking advantage of the body's ability to become immune to invading substances. Here, the doctor injects gradually increasing doses of an allergen. Over time, the body develops its own resistance to the allergen. In lieu of shots, some people find relief from antihistamines, drugs that counteract the effects of histamines.

See also Allergy, Anaphylactic shock, and Immunization.

Immunization

Immunization is the means of producing immunity, or resistance by the body to a specific disease. Doctors employ two types of immunization: *active* and *passive*.

Active immunization is accomplished by injecting a weakened or killed virus or bacteria into the body. This stimulates the body's natural defense system. Certain specialized white blood cells—which are manufactured in the bone marrow, are circulated in the blood, and are stored in lymph nodes and elsewhere–produce substances known as antibodies, carried in the bloodstream, that are tailor-made to fight the invading organisms. They remain in the body for years, sometimes a lifetime, to protect it against that particular disease.

Passive immunization involves injecting ready-made antibodies—usually extracted from the blood of animals that have been immunized solely for the purpose of producing antibodies to be used in passive immunization. Passive immunization is borrowed immunity and is only temporary but serves to protect a person who may already be infected until the body has time to create its own antibodies.

Immunization can provide protection against measles, mumps, rubella (German measles), polio, whooping cough, diphtheria, and tetanus, all of which can cripple or kill.

Children's immunizations. To be completely protected against diphtheria, tetanus, and whooping cough (pertussis), a child needs a shot of the combination diphtheria-tetanus-pertussis (DTP) vaccine at two, four, six and eighteen months and a booster shot upon entering school around age five years. When the child gets the DTP shots, he or she should also receive by mouth a drop of the oral polio vaccine (although since there are usually only four doses of polio vaccine, the child does not receive it at six months of age). At 15 months a child should have a combined shot for measles, rubella, and mumps. He or she should be tested for tuberculosis at the end of the first year and receive a tetanus-diphtheria booster shot between 14 and 16 years of age.

Parents who do not have a family physician can call their local public health department. It usually has supplies of vaccine and may give shots free.

Adult immunizations. Adults need a tetanus shot once every ten years. Otherwise, there are no routine immunizations necessary for adults in the United States, with the possible exception of influenza shots given annually (usually in the fall) to the aged and to patients with heart, lung, and other chronic diseases. (With the new purified vaccines, side effects are minor.) A vaccine for protection against 80 percent of serious pneumonias is available, to be given once every three to five years. HDCV, a new active immunization against rabies, is said to have only mild side effects for most people, with shots given on days 1, 3, 7, 14, 28, and 90 after a bite from a rabid animal (a passive vaccine is also given—once, on day 1). Immunization in advance against rabies is provided by a series of three shots of HDCV.

There are precautions to consider. Immunizations should not be given to pregnant women, nor in general to anyone whose immune system is weakened by leukemia, cancer, fever, or by prolonged X-ray or corticosteroid treatment.

Vaccination for foreign travel. Most persons traveling abroad in developed countries need no additional vaccination or medication. In general, in the United States, Canada, Australia, New Zealand, and Europe the traveler is safe without vaccinations. Travel in the less-developed countries of Africa, Asia, South America, Central America, Mexico, the South Pacific, Middle East and Far East may hold more risk, particularly in small villages or rural areas not usually visited by tourists.

In recent years no vaccination has been necessary for *direct* travel from the United States to most countries, nor to return to the United States. However, some countries require proof of vaccination from travelers who have passed through infected areas or countries, and it is best to get the shots before leaving home.

Any licensed physician can give immunizations, except that yellow-fever vaccinations must be given at an official "Yellow Fever Vaccination Center." Weeks before you plan to leave on your trip, call your local health department for latest information about vaccination requirements and recommendations for all of the countries you plan to visit. The vaccinating physician must fill out and sign an "International Certificate of Vaccination" that must be validated by a health department or by a physician with a "Uniform Stamp."

Vaccinations against cholera, which is transmitted by contaminated food and water, and against yellow fever, transmitted by certain mosquitoes, are the shots most often required for foreign travel. Because no cholera vaccine is very effective and because the risk of acquiring cholera is small, the United States Public Health Service does not recommend it for travelers unless the country visited requires it. However, yellow fever vaccinations are strongly recommended even if not required by law for travel to infected areas, usually parts of Africa and South America, and for travel outside cities in countries in "yellow fever endemic (ever-present) zones."

In no case should one be immunized for smallpox, which has been eliminated from the world. If a country still requires proof of vaccination, the United States Public Health Service recommends obtaining a written statement from a physician recommending against smallpox vaccination for health reasons (because serious complications can result for anyone). This will exempt the traveler.

Anyone not already immune to measles and mumps should receive vaccinations before traveling abroad, as should children not immune to rubella. Travelers to developing countries need diphtheria, polio, and typhoid immunizations, unless they are already immune, and a tetanus booster shot if they have not had one in the previous ten years.

Immunization cannot protect against malaria, a health threat in many developing countries. However, travelers to infected areas can take along protective medications, sleep in well-screened areas, wear protective clothing, and use chemical repellants to ward off the long-legged *Anopheles* mosquito, which transmits the disease.

Impotence

Impotence is the inability to achieve and maintain an erection of the penis, which is necessary to penetrate the female vagina during sexual intercourse. Internal spaces in the penis (called corpora cavernosa) normally fill with blood during sexual excitement and cause the penis to become rigid and erect. Impotence is a partial or total impairment of this function.

There are two types of impotence: primary impotence, in which a man is never able to have an erection adequate for sexual intercourse; and secondary impotence, in which a man quite often fails to complete intercourse to the satisfaction of both partners. Secondary impotence is the more common type.

Many men experience temporary impotence at some point in their lives, but chronic (recurring) impotence can lower a man's self-esteem and put a strain on his marriage or social relationships.

Impotence can be caused by either physical or psychological problems. It may be brought on by job-related stress, fear of causing pregnancy, unresolved conflicts about sexuality, or fear of sex after a heart attack or major surgery. Emotional problems such as these, along with drug and alcohol abuse, are some of the leading causes of impotence.

Until recently, psychological problems were thought to be the only cause of impotence; but several physical disorders are now known to trigger the problem: an imbalance in the hormonal system, which may cause a decrease in production of testosterone, the male hormone necessary for an erection; certain drugs used to treat high blood pressure, although the reason for their causing impotence is not known; diseases of the nervous system, such as multiple sclerosis; structural abnormalities of or injury to the penis; and malfunctioning of the circulatory system, which can interfere with the blood flow to the penis necessary for an erection.

The major symptom of impotence is a repeatedly limp penis that is unable to penetrate the vagina during sexual intercourse. This may be accompanied by a lack of interest in sex, but not necessarily infertility (the inability to father a child).

Several tests can help to diagnose the cause of a case of impotence. A blood test will show whether adequate levels of testosterone are present. A blood pressure cuff specially designed to wrap around the penis, coupled with ultrasound (the use of sound waves to create an image of internal structures), detects blood pressure and blood vessel problems in the penis. Another test registers the size of erections that naturally occur during sleep; if these amount to at least a 20 percent enlargement of the penis, it can usually be concluded that no physical problem is causing the impotence.

Impotence is treated with testosterone injections, surgery, penile implants, and psychological counseling. Testosterone injections may be used to relieve hormone problems, while surgery may be necessary to repair the veins and arteries that deliver blood to the penis. These procedures, however, are not always effective and therefore not recommended for everyone.

Penile implants represent a successful new treatment for impotence, with several varieties now in use. One is a silicone rod implanted in the corpora cavernosa, resulting in a penis that is semi-erect at all times. Another is a flexible silver wire surrounded by silicone, which, when implanted, allows the penis to be manipulated to an erect angle for intercourse. A third model consists of balloon-like cylinders implanted in the corpora cavernosa and attached to a container of fluid, which, when activated by a hand pump, fills them the way blood normally fills the penis during an erection.

Counseling by psychologists or trained sex therapists may be recommended for men whose impotence seems to be stemming from emotional problems; in addition, counseling may also help those with physical disorders in learning to deal with their impotence.

Avoiding the abuse of alcohol and drugs, as well as eliminating or coping with stress, should help to prevent at least some episodes of secondary impotence.

Incontinence

Incontinence is the involuntary loss of bladder and bowel control. It occurs frequently in children and in older persons.

Most often, incontinence is caused by some other underlying condition, such as a problem with the urinary tract—infection, inflammation, or pain—or with the muscles that control the bladder or bowel. It may also be caused by epileptic seizures, brain or spinal cord tumors, or a stroke. In such cases, successful treatment of those underlying causes will clear up the problem of incontinence.

Stress incontinence is the involuntary leakage of urine on coughing, sneezing, straining, or laughing. This type of incontinence is common in women whose muscles have been weakened by childbirth.

Although the first step in treating incontinence is to detect and correct any underlying problem, it is important to remember that many children have not established complete bladder and/or bowel control before they are four or five years old. Children of any age may have occasional accidents especially if they are ill or exhausted.

Persons who have problems with incontinence can help themselves by going to the bathroom often and regularly, by arranging sleeping and living quarters near bathrooms, and by wearing clothes that can be removed quickly and easily. It may also help to keep a bed pan or chamber pot next to the bed. If the problem is a urinary one, the incontinent person should drink only a small amount of water, if any, before going to bed. If the problem is bowel incontinence, the person should eat a lot of high fiber foods to establish regularity and should also keep in mind that bowels tend to move about one hour after a meal has been eaten.

While there are drugs available to aid in controlling urination, no drugs are yet available for controlling bowel movements.

Indigestion

Indigestion, also called dyspepsia, is the discomfort caused by difficulty in digesting food. It is an uncomfortable feeling of fullness, pressure, slight pain, or gassiness and is usually related to eating. (Constipation, diarrhea, heartburn, and nausea are *not* indigestion, although they may be related to the problem.)

Indigestion is usually caused by an eating problem such as eating too fast or too much; inadequate chewing; eating in an emotionally upsetting environment; eating particularly bothersome foods, such as spicy, fatty, or oily foods, or those that may cause an allergic reaction; and smoking, especially immediately before or after a meal. Indigestion can also be caused by serious disorders such as cancer, ulcers, and diseases involving the organs associated with digestion (the esophagus, intestines, gallbladder, liver, stomach, and pancreas). In addition, heart attack, tumors, and emotional problems can be accompanied by symptoms that are similar to indigestion.

Any case of indigestion that lingers for some time or that cannot be controlled in any way should be reported to a doctor for diagnosis and appropriate treatment.

The cause of indigestion is diagnosed predominantly by observing the symptoms and the conditions under which they occur. A doctor will want a description of the symptoms and of the patient's usual dietary habits; of the time, length, and location of the discomfort as well as the circumstances surrounding it and foods eaten preceding it; and of the emotional environment that usually exists during meals and snacks. X rays or stool analysis may also be used to make a diagnosis of the cause of indigestion.

Antacids often relieve indigestion (but they should not be used by people who have kidney disease, since one of their ingredients, magnesium, may interfere with kidney function). However, the best treatment consists of preventing indigestion in the first place. Eating balanced meals in a relaxed setting, eliminating foods that may be causing indigestion problems, and refraining from smoking during mealtime should be beneficial in the prevention of indigestion.

Infectious mononucleosis

Infectious mononucleosis, or mono, is a contagious viral disease that initially attacks the lymph glands in the neck and the throat. When these glands, which normally manufacture white blood cells that fight invading organisms, are weakened, sore throat, swollen glands, and fever result.

Mono is caused by a virus named Epstein-Barr virus after the scientists that first identified it in the mid-1960s. The virus enters the lymph glands and attacks the lymphocytes, the white blood cells manufactured in the lymph glands. As the white blood cells come into contact with the virus, they change shape and multiply. At first there are no symptoms, because it takes several weeks before enough of the altered cells can accumulate to generate a reaction. Gradually, however, symptoms appear. First, there is a mild sore throat, sluggishness, and fever. The symptoms worsen as the body tries to fight the infection by creating more white blood cells. Finally, symptoms diminish and disappear after about six to eight weeks.

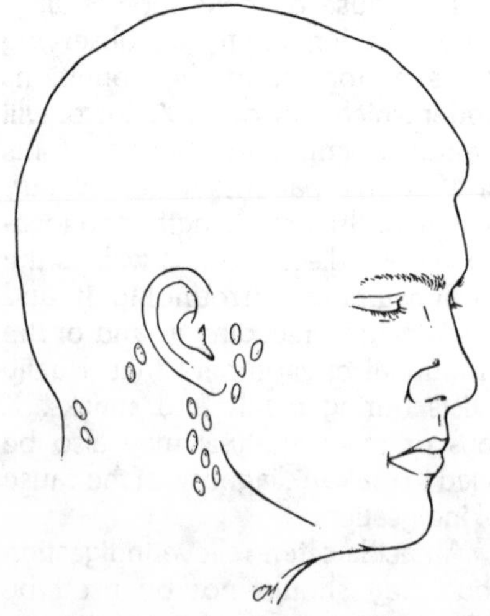
Swollen lymph glands around the throat or neck are signs of the contagious viral infection called infectious mononucleosis.

Infectious mononucleosis spreads by contact with moisture from the mouth and throat of the infected person. Kissing, sharing drinking glasses and toothbrushes, or touching anything that has been near the mouth of an infected person transmits the disease.

Teenagers and young adults seem most susceptible to mono. Sometimes, children become infected, but the disease seldom affects anyone over 35. In all cases, the infection develops so slowly with such mild symptoms that it may be initially indistinguishable from a cold or the flu. However, a sore throat that lasts two weeks or more; swollen glands around the neck, throat, armpit, and groin; a persistent fever (usually about 102°F); and tiredness indicate mono. Mono symptoms can be mild or so severe that throat pain can impede swallowing and fever may reach 105°F. Some people also experience a rash, eye pain, or discomfort in bright light (photophobia).

Most mono runs an uncomplicated course. Occasionally, however, the infection spreads to other parts of the body besides the throat and lymph glands. For example, mono may lead to hepatitis, an infection of the liver. Jaundice, a symptom of this complication, appears as a yellow discoloration of the skin and whites of the eyes. Another sign the infection has traveled is pain or tenderness in the abdomen. This discomfort may mean a swollen spleen (part of the lymph system) that could rupture or burst. Any of these symptoms should be reported to a physician for immediate attention.

When diagnosing infectious mononucleosis, a doctor takes two blood samples two weeks apart. The first sample determines if there is an excessive number of white blood cells, whether they are abnormally shaped because of the virus, and if the body is making antibodies (protective substances) to fight the Epstein-Barr virus. The second blood test shows whether the white blood cell count is still high, indicating disease is present. It is only completed if the first test shows signs of the disease.

Once mono is confirmed, standard treatment for its symptoms is prescribed. Antibiotics are ineffective since the disease is caused by a virus that does not respond to antibiotics. As long as there are no complications, the best treatment is to stay in bed, drink plenty of liquids until the temperature returns to normal, and then gradually resume normal activities as strength returns.

Antibiotics may be indicated if a bacterial infection develops in addition to mono because bacteria do respond to antibiotics. In severe cases, corticosteroid drugs that reduce swelling are prescribed. If the spleen is swollen, a doctor may recommend avoiding strenuous activities, such as lifting or pushing, that may cause sudden rupture of the spleen. Hospitalization is necessary for severe complications.

Most people recover in six to eight weeks, but some cases take as long as six months for complete recovery. A tired feeling, which may include depression, is the last symptom to disappear. Mono may return in a milder form of the initial infection within a few months. Fortunately, it almost never reappears after a year.

Infertility

Infertility is defined as a couple's failure to conceive a child after one year of regular sexual intercourse without birth control. In about 40 percent of all cases of infertility, the problem lies with the male; in 60 percent it lies with the female or with both partners.

Infertility is not sterility. The term infertility implies that the condition can be treated and reversed, that it may be a temporary problem; the term sterility is applied to a permanent, irreversible inability to have children.

Recent research has shown that a woman's fertility drops off significantly between the ages of 31 and 35 and continues to decline thereafter until menopause, when it ceases. A man's fertility also declines after the age of 40, although men can remain fertile until old age.

One of the major causes of male infertility is a low sperm count. It is measured by the number of active sperm present in a milliliter (less than one-half teaspoon) of semen (the fluid ejected from the penis during intercourse). An average "sperm count" is 90 million sperm per milliliter; a count of 40 to 60 million is thought to be necessary for conception; when the count is less than 20 million, it is highly unlikely that the man can father a child, although since only one sperm is needed to fertilize the female egg, it is still possible.

A low sperm count can be caused by low levels of testosterone, the male sex hormone; by exposure to chemicals, pesticides, and radiation;

by very frequent sexual intercourse, which depletes the sperm supply too quickly; and by heat (which slows sperm production) generated by wearing tight underwear or pants, sitting for long periods in hot cars or trucks, or working near ovens.

Infertility can also result if sperm cannot propel themselves through the female reproductive tract to reach the egg, or if sperm are irregularly shaped (only sperm with oval-shaped heads can fertilize an egg).

In addition to problems with the sperm themselves, male infertility can be caused by any obstruction in the tubes that convey the sperm from the testes to the penis. Infertility may also be caused by varicose veins in the scrotum (the pouch containing the testes), perhaps because the increased blood flow in these swollen veins brings extra heat to the area; or by a local infection or injury, although the infertility problem will probably reverse itself when the condition is corrected. In addition, surgical removal of part of the prostate gland, as well as the use of certain drugs for high blood pressure, can lead to retrograde ejaculation (a disorder in which the semen is passed backwards into the bladder, to exit with the urine, rather than out through the penis).

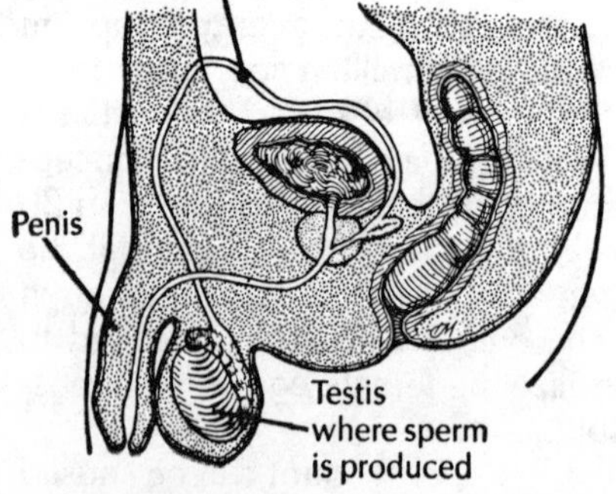

Male infertility can be caused by a blockage anywhere in the tubes that convey sperm from the testes to the penis.

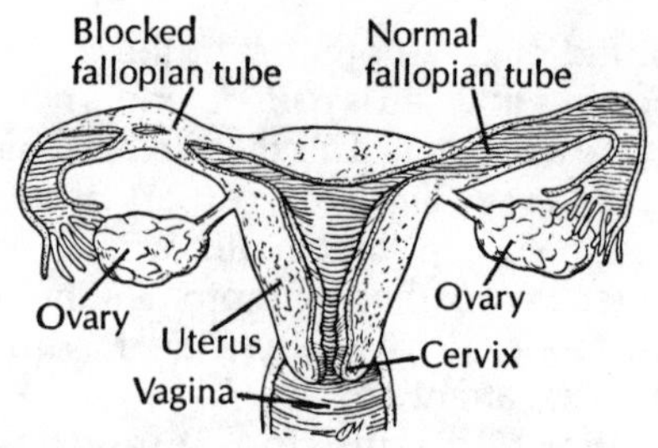

Female infertility can be caused by an obstruction in the fallopian tube through which the egg passes from the ovary to the uterus and in which the sperm and egg are united at conception.

A woman may be infertile because of a variety of conditions. It may be that she is not ovulating (releasing an egg each month); this is true in about 25 percent of all infertility cases. The fallopian tubes (through which the egg travels on its way from the ovary to the uterus) may be obstructed, often as a result of pelvic inflammatory disease (PID), which inflames the tubes and causes scar tissue to form. PID, in turn, can develop as a reaction to an IUD (intrauterine device used for birth control), a sexually transmitted disease, a ruptured appendix, or an infection of the lower reproductive tract. Endometriosis (the displacement of tissue from the lining of the uterus to outside the uterus) may also cause scar tissue to form that blocks the fallopian tubes. In addition, an imbalance of the female hormones estrogen and progesterone or of other hormones secreted from the pituitary or thyroid glands can interfere with the reproductive cycle. A weakness in the cervix (the neck of the uterus), sometimes resulting from a previous abortion or surgery, may render it unfit to hold the weight of a pregnancy; or a "hostile" cervix, one which creates an environment that in some way prevents sperm from surviving, may be the cause of the infertility.

The major "symptom" of infertility is the failure to conceive a child after regular sexual intercourse for a year. Other "symptoms" would depend on the cause of the infertility, such as a low sperm count in males or a failure to ovulate in females.

Diagnosis of the reason for the infertility problem will usually begin with physical exams and complete medical and sexual (and, in the woman's case, menstrual) histories of both partners.

A fresh sample of the male's sperm will be examined under a microscope to determine the quantity and quality of the sperm. This will provide a sperm count and will also determine whether the sperm are adequately mobile and are oval-shaped, both of which are necessary for conception.

To determine whether ovulation is taking place in the female, the basal body temperature (the body temperature upon awakening before eating or drinking) will be taken every morning for several months. If the temperature rises by 6/10 to 1 degree for a few days in the middle of the menstrual cycle, ovulation is probably taking place. An endometrial biopsy, a sample of the lining of the uterus, can also indicate whether or not ovulation is occurring.

Obstruction of the fallopian tubes can be diagnosed by injecting a dye into the reproductive tract and then taking an X ray. Another test consists of injecting carbon dioxide gas into the fallopian tubes and waiting for the patient to feel pain in the upper part of the body, indicating that the gas is passing through the fallopian tubes and that there are no obstructions.

A weakness in the cervix can be diagnosed through a physical exam and X rays; a hostile cervix can be identified by a microscopic examination of the mucus in the cervix shortly after sexual intercourse to determine the rate of sperm survival. Endometriosis is diagnosed by inserting a small, lighted, instrument into the abdomen (called a laparoscope) through which the doctor can actually see the uterus, fallopian tubes, ovaries, and any displaced endometrial tissue that may be causing the infertility. Hormone imbalances in both men and women are diagnosed with blood tests.

Treatment for a low sperm count caused by a testosterone deficiency usually consists of hormone therapy to increase testosterone levels. If the low sperm count is due to chemicals, radiation, or excess heat, these conditions need to be corrected or avoided. If the sperm count is low for some unknown reason, there is often little more that can be done.

If male infertility is caused by varicose veins, surgery may be necessary; if an obstruction exists somewhere in the tubes leading to and through the penis, microsurgery to open the blockage may correct this problem.

In females, failure to ovulate is often treated with a fertility drug called clomiphene to stimulate hormone production that regulates ovulation. About 60 percent of these patients become pregnant, and the chances of multiple births are very low. A stronger drug, which is a combination of certain pituitary gland hormones, may also be prescribed, but it carries with it a greater risk of multiple births.

Obstructed fallopian tubes may require microsurgery to open the blockage, or a new procedure in which an egg is removed and replaced beyond the point of the obstruction, where it waits to be fertilized normally. A hostile cervix can be treated with the female hormone estrogen, which stimulates the production of increased mucus necessary to transport the sperm. Sometimes sperm can be placed directly into the uterus, bypassing the cervix completely. Endometriosis can be treated with the surgical removal of displaced tissue and the scar tissue that has formed around it. Hormone imbalances can be corrected with hormone drug therapy.

Test-tube, or *in vitro,* fertilization is a new technique in which an egg is removed from the woman's ovary and is then placed in a test tube or special sterile dish containing the husband's sperm. Once the egg has been fertilized, it is then placed into the woman's uterus where it will continue to grow. This technique is primarily used in women whose blocked fallopian tubes cannot be opened by surgery.

Although recent advances in treating infertility have led to greater and greater success, about 15 percent of all female infertility problems and about 10 percent of all male problems remain undiagnosed and therefore untreatable.

See also Birth control, Conception, Endometriosis, Menstruation, Ovulation, Pelvic inflammatory disease, Prostatitis, and Reproduction.

Influenza

Influenza, more commonly called the flu, is a contagious disease that is accompanied by respiratory problems and fever. It is an uncomfortable illness that is usually not dangerous to otherwise healthy people.

Two types of viruses cause influenza: influenza A and influenza B. Each type encompasses several different strains that are named for the place where they were first identified, for example, "Hong Kong flu" and "Russian flu."

The unusual characteristic about flu virus is that once one strain spreads throughout a population, the virus strain changes in structure. Therefore, it becomes a new strain carrying a new form of influenza. The antibodies, or protective substances, produced by the body to combat the virus no longer work against recurrence of that virus because the virus has taken on different qualities. Scientists are generally able to predict what type of altered virus to expect each year, but about every ten years an entirely new strain appears.

Because influenza is thought to be transmitted by airborne particles from an infected person's respiratory system, large numbers of people in a community or even in a country can easily contract the disease in a relatively short period of time. Understandably, crowds encourage transmission of the flu. In addition, since flu spreads most easily where temperatures and humidity are low, most cases of influenza occur in fall or winter months.

Once the body is exposed to the virus, flu symptoms develop in one to three days. Some people acquire symptoms in as short a time as 18 hours. Fever, chills, headache, muscle aches, and total exhaustion can begin suddenly. Although fevers of 100°F to 104°F are more common, body temperature may rise to 106°F.

Frequently, people experience a dry cough and runny or congested nose as their initial symptoms begin to subside. These respiratory symptoms worsen and remain for three to four days. The cough, weariness, and sometimes depression may persist for two weeks or more after the other symptoms disappear.

The most common complications result from the virus settling in parts of the respiratory system. For example, adults may get pneumonia (infection of the lungs) and children may get croup (infection of the larynx). If the patient has extreme difficulty in breathing, blood in the coughed-up phlegm, bluish skin, or a bark-like cough, a physician should be consulted immediately to prevent further complications.

One life-threatening complication that affects children between the ages of two and 16 years is Reye's syndrome. It is a type of inflammation of the brain (encephalitis) that is accompanied by deteriorating changes in the liver.

Influenza cannot be cured, but usually only treated by relieving symptoms. However, there is an antiviral drug that is effective against influenza A virus symptoms and in some cases the disease itself. The drug can produce unpleasant side effects, so physicians prescribe it only when a patient is susceptible to additional complications.

In most cases, treatment for flu is the same as treatment for a bad cold or fever. Physicians recommend bed rest, extra fluids, and an aspirin substitute to reduce fever and muscle aches. Aspirin is not recommended for a child with flu. Although it has not been proven that aspirin causes or promotes Reye's syndrome, it is recommended that aspirin not be given to a child with influenza. Acetaminophen, however, has not been linked to Reye's syndrome and can be used. Nasal sprays or drops, when used sparingly so nasal tissues are not damaged, and cough medicines help relieve cold-like symptoms. A vaporizer in the patient's room that adds moisture to the air relieves congestion.

Each year, researchers prepare an influenza vaccine in an attempt to prevent spread of the virus. The vaccine is composed of several different virus strains and provides protection against influenza from these strains. Regrettably, protection is not necessarily afforded against new or different strains. Vaccines are typically between 67 and 92 percent effective.

Some people have reactions from the vaccine that range from inflammation at the site of the injection to mild flu symptoms. On rare occasions, nervous system disorders result. Children receive injections in two smaller doses four to eight weeks apart to lessen chances of any reactions.

See also Reye's syndrome.

Insect bite and sting

Insect bites and stings are minor inconveniences to most people, but to those who have an allergy to insect venom, the consequences can be serious. An allergy is an unusual reaction or oversensitivity to a foreign substance, called an allergen. Insect bites and stings are examples of injectant allergens (substances that penetrate the skin).

Reactions to insect venom show themselves in various symptoms: shortness of breath, rapid heartbeat, coughing, wheezing, and lightheadedness. The affected area swells and becomes tender or numb. In extreme cases, anaphylactic shock (a severe reaction that can be fatal, characterized by breathing problems; hives; collapse of blood vessels; and sometimes vomiting, diarrhea, and cramps) can occur. Some people experience one or more of these symptoms immediately, while others feel no discomfort for several hours after the sting.

Serious reactions to bites and stings are treated by slowing the spread of the venom throughout the body and getting emergency medical treatment as soon as possible. The venom's progress can be slowed somewhat by applying an ice pack or a tourniquet (but not so tight as to stop the blood flow) to the affected area. Emergency medical treatment will consist of an epinephrine injection, which will weaken the reaction. Many allergic people carry insect bite kits that contain epinephrine.

Prevention of recurrent allergic reactions to insect venom is accomplished with treatments of desensitization shots; starting with an initially weak solution of insect extract, doses are gradually increased with each shot. This allows the body to build its own tolerance to the insect venom.

Currently, the serum in the shots is called whole body extract, meaning that the whole body of the insect is crushed and injected into the patient. Some scientists argue, however, that to be most effective, the serum should consist of only the insect's venom rather than the whole body. However, large quantities of insect venom are not available for this purpose, so whole body extract continues to be used.

See also Allergy and Anaphylactic shock.

Insomnia

Insomnia is the inability to sleep during normal sleeping hours, when there is no apparent reason for wakefulness. The insomnia may vary from simple restlessness to wakefulness on and off throughout the night to total sleeplessness.

Although the condition is most often associated with psychological or emotional problems, it can also be related to physical disorders or even to conditions in the immediate environment.

Depression and anxiety are often the cause of insomnia. Among physical disorders that can lead to insomnia are urination problems, heart trouble, high blood pressure, infection, hardening of the arteries, spastic colon, and leg cramps. Less serious causes of insomnia can be found in the person's immediate environment —bright lights, noise, overheated or underheated bedroom, lack of ventilation. Insomnia may also be caused by too many or too few bed clothes; constipation; hunger; and too much coffee, tea, cola, or other beverages containing caffeine which is a stimulant.

Strangely, drugs to promote sleep can cause insomnia. The careless or inappropriate use of tranquilizers and sedatives can disrupt sleep patterns. If high doses of tranquilizers or sedatives are taken, the wake-sleep rhythm or pattern can be reversed and sleep can become irregular. The person may doze throughout the day and then be unable to sleep at night.

A person who has chronic or persistent insomnia should consult a physician so that the underlying cause of the insomnia—emotional or physical—can be diagnosed and treated.

Ways of preventing or coping with simple insomnia include taking a ten or 15 minute walk before bedtime, taking a warm bath, drinking warm milk (milk contains a substance called tryptophan that naturally promotes drowsiness), reading, or watching TV. Taking sleep-promoting medications should be discussed with a doctor.

Interferon

Interferon is a substance—a complex protein—produced by body cells in response to an invasion of a virus. Once produced, interferon moves to other cells, making them resistant to the virus and preventing the growth and reproduction of the virus. Interferon, which is detectable two hours after the body becomes infected, is effective not only against the virus that caused it to be produced, but also against other viruses that invade the system.

The release of interferon is part of the body's attempt to protect itself against viral infection. Much research is being conducted in an attempt to develop a means of using interferon to prevent disease. Unfortunately, studies have shown that interferon is effective only in the species that produces it. In other words, it is not possible to extract interferon from animals to use against human infections. However, work is being done to discover a way of artificially stimulating the human body to produce more interferon.

Intestinal bypass

See Bypass surgery.

Irritable bowel syndrome

Irritable bowel syndrome, also called spastic colon or mucous colitis, is a collection of symptoms caused by irritability and irregularity in the movement of both small and large intestines. The syndrome is usually influenced by emotions. Feelings of nervousness, anxiety, guilt, depression, or anger may bring on this very common disorder. Coffee, raw fruits and vegetables, hormones, drugs, and overuse of laxatives can promote it, as can an inability of the body to digest the natural sugar in milk. Women are affected three times as often as men.

Not a disease, irritable bowel syndrome is a collection of symptoms that includes both constipation and diarrhea, often alternating and sometimes accompanied by straining and abdominal cramps. Stools may be loose or compacted and may include mucus, which has been manufactured as a lubricant by the irritated bowel lining. Gas, bloating, nausea, headache, or fatigue often accompany the other symptoms.

There are two main types of irritable bowel syndrome. The first is spastic colon, which often begins at mealtime and is marked by cramps or a dull aching pain in the abdomen, usually the lower part. The pain may disappear after a bowel movement. The second type of irritable bowel syndrome is painless diarrhea, which is characterized by an urgent need for a bowel movement upon awakening or during or right after a meal. Incontinence (involuntary loss of bowel control) can occur.

For anyone who appears to have irritable bowel syndrome, the doctor will first want to rule out diseases with similar symptoms. The patient may be asked to bring in a stool specimen to be cultured and examined for traces of blood and parasites. The colon may be x-rayed, following a barium enema. The doctor may insert a sigmoidoscope (a lighted tube) into the colon through the anus, the opening at the end of the intestine, to check for serious disorders such as ulcers that can lead to ulcerative colitis.

If no organic disease is found, the doctor will reassure the patient and discuss ways in which the symptoms can be relieved. There may be methods by which the patient can reduce the anxiety or depression that may be causing the syndrome. The doctor may prescribe a tranquilizer, sedative, mood elevator, or antispasm medicine — but only on a short-term basis, so that the individual does not become dependent on a drug. Long walks, bike rides, or other exercise may help to relax the person while promoting better bowel action. If constipation is a problem, the doctor will advise the patient to add bulk such as whole bran to the diet; to stop depending on laxatives; and to take pills that absorb water, add bulk, and help to stabilize the large bowel. If diarrhea is present, avoiding laxative foods, such as beans, may help. Patients bothered by gas will be warned against foods such as cabbage. Milk may even be barred from the diet. Most people, except many of northwest European origin, lose the ability to digest the natural sugar (lactose) in milk by the time they are 20 years old. A test for this is an oral dose of lactose. If it results in diarrhea and bloating, it is a tip-off that the symptoms could have been caused entirely or in part by drinking milk.

If irritable bowel syndrome continues despite the treatment, it is important to remember that it is not dangerous. However, to be on the safe side, a regular physical checkup should be scheduled with your doctor—every year—especially if you are over 40.

Ischemia

Ischemia is an inadequate flow of blood to a specific part of the body caused by an obstruction of the blood vessels supplying that part of the body. The obstruction is the result of the narrowing, compression, or destruction of arteries and is due to such factors or conditions as a blood clot or hardening of the arteries (atherosclerosis). In the latter condition, the hardened arteries gradually narrow to a point where not enough blood can pass through them.

An ischemic attack in the brain

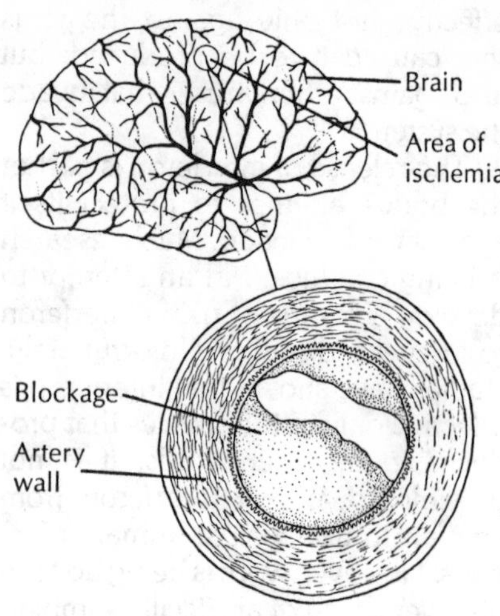

Ischemia is an inadequate flow of blood to a part of the body because of a blockage in the blood vessel nourishing that part of the body.

occurs when the supply of blood to the brain is reduced. This type of attack resembles a stroke. If the brain is deprived of blood, and thereby life-giving oxygen, for more than four minutes, the result is irreversible brain damage and often death.

When the blood supply to the heart is reduced, angina pectoris results. When the blood supply to the heart is cut off, a heart attack occurs. The less blood that gets through to the heart, the greater the severity of the attack. If a weakened heart is unable to pump an adequate supply of blood to other parts of the body, the other organs will work at less than capacity, and the whole system may break down.

Occasionally, ischemic attacks can be controlled by medications called vasodilators that dilate or enlarge blood vessels. Angina pectoris is often managed in this way. For more serious cases, surgery to remove or to bypass the obstruction is recommended.

See also Angina pectoris, Bypass surgery, Heart attack, Stroke, and Transient ischemic attack.

Itching

Itching is an uncomfortable or irritating sensation felt by the nerve endings located on the surface of the skin, accompanied by the urge to scratch. It has been described as a pricking, stinging, burning, or crawling feeling, and may be a symptom of a variety of disorders.

The biological reactions that lead to itching are not clearly understood, but it is known that this stimulation of the nerve endings can be caused by both physical and psychological factors.

Itching can be caused by insect bites; small cuts or scrapes; hives and other allergic reactions; a fungus infection; the rash that often accompanies infectious diseases such as chicken pox; dry skin, often stemming from bathing or showering too frequently or using harsh soaps; reactions to drugs; and psychological stress.

Itching is characterized by an uneasy discomfort on the skin, the urge to scratch, and possibly redness, peeling, and other irritations of the skin as a result of scratching. Itching of just the scalp and forearms with no obvious cause may be triggered by psychological stress.

Treatment of itching depends on its cause. Itching from dry skin is usually treated by applying skin lotions or creams to small areas and using body lotions or bath oils for larger areas; reducing showers and baths to only twice weekly, as water tends to dry the skin; and trying new brands of soap or shampoo.

If itching seems to be a reaction to a drug, the doctor should be consulted before making any changes in medication. (A patient should *never* stop taking a drug without the consultation of a doctor.) The doctor will either lower the dosage to relieve the itching or give advice on treatment of the itching while maintaining the original dosage.

If no visible symptoms or outside substances seem to be triggering itching, psychological stress may be the cause, and the best treatment will involve removing the stress or learning how to deal with it.

If itching persists for more than a week after attempts at self-treatment, a doctor should be consulted because persistent itching with no visible cause may be a symptom of diabetes, thyroid disease, kidney failure, liver disease, or cancer.

Some itching can be prevented. Limiting bathing to twice weekly and using humidifiers to keep the air moist should help prevent the itching caused by dry skin.

Jaundice

Jaundice is a yellowish discoloration of the skin, whites of the eyes, mucous membranes, and other tissues of the body, and is caused by the abnormal accumulation of bile pigment (or bilirubin) in the blood.

Bilirubin consists primarily of the hemoglobin of used red blood cells and is found in bile, a bitter, yellow-green fluid that aids in digestion by breaking down fat. Bile is secreted by the liver, stored in the gallbladder, and discharged into the intestine when it is needed for digestion.

In many cases, jaundice occurs when bile is prevented by obstruction from being discharged into the intestine. The obstruction may be caused by gallstones, by tumors or, uncommonly, by parasites in the bile ducts. Jaundice may also be an accompanying sign of hepatitis, a disorder in which the inflamed or damaged liver cannot process the bilirubin it receives. Occasionally, jaundice appears if too many red blood cells are too rapidly destroyed, sometimes as a result of an anemic condition, and the liver cannot accommodate the excess. In addition, jaundice is associated with, or symptomatic of, many other diseases in which the normal functioning of the liver is disrupted. These diseases include certain cancers and certain viral and parasitic infections. Over 50 percent of full-term and 80 percent of premature newborns show signs of jaundice by the second or third day after birth. In most of these cases, however, the condition is nothing to worry about and disappears in a week or so.

When jaundice occurs, the liver usually has become enlarged and functions less effectively. Bowel movements may be clay-colored, and urine can vary in hue from light yellow to a brownish green. Jaundiced skin ranges in color from lemony yellow to dark olive green.

Routine blood testing will determine the origin of most cases of jaundice, but occasionally it may be necessary to observe the bile ducts, by means of an X ray. Certain dyes injected into the blood will collect in the liver and bile ducts to show the point of obstruction on an X ray. Other alternatives include ultrasound, in which sound waves bounce off internal body structures and form an image of them, and a CAT scan, a special technique that provides a cross-sectional picture of the area.

If a backup of bile is observed, surgery to eliminate the obstruction may be indicated. Otherwise, treatment will be determined by the nature of the cause of the jaundice.

See also Gallstones and Hepatitis.

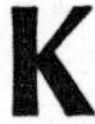

Keratitis

Keratitis is an inflammation of the cornea—the transparent covering over the iris and pupil of the eye—which commonly produces redness, tearing, tenderness, sensitivity to light, and blurred vision.

The most common type of keratitis is caused by herpes simplex virus, the same virus that produces cold sores. Although herpes simplex keratitis is not painful, at first there is a sensation that foreign matter may be present. If left untreated, all feeling in the cornea is eventually lost. Like cold sores, the infection tends to come and go, but it should be taken care of when the first sign—a whitish lesion on the cornea—appears. Treatment usually consists of eyedrops or ointment, but some specialists prefer to scrape the cornea and cover the eye temporarily.

Traumatic keratitis occurs when a corneal injury leaves scar tissue after the injury itself has healed. If the scar tissue covering the pupil is considerable, blindness may result. This condition can be cured by corrective surgery.

Interstitial keratitis is most often caused by congenital (present at birth) syphilis in children or by tuberculosis. This type of keratitis produces deep deposits of scar tissue, which cause the cornea to become hazy and give it a ground-glass appearance. There is little that can be done for this condition, although the inflammation and redness usually diminish after a month or two. Vision may or may not be impaired thereafter.

Ketosis

Ketosis, also known as ketoacidosis, is an abnormal condition that occurs when the body burns fat instead of glucose (a sugar that is the body's chief source of energy) and, as it does so, emits more poisonous by-products called ketones than the body can tolerate. Under normal circumstances, ketones are broken down into carbon dioxide and water by the liver and other organs.

Ketosis occurs most often in those people with insulin-dependent diabetes mellitus, a disorder in which the pancreas produces little or no insulin, a hormone secreted into the bloodsteam to regulate glucose levels. This imbalance, in turn, prevents the body from absorbing enough glucose and forces it to obtain its energy by burning fat. Ketosis is also a consequence of starvation, another condition in which the body must rely excessively on stores of fat for energy.

The most common symptoms are a vinegar-like breath odor, increased thirst and urination, weakness, abdominal pains and generalized aches, nausea, and vomiting. If allowed to continue unchecked, ketosis can lead to breathlessness and possible coma. Ketosis is diagnosed by testing the glucose and ketone levels of blood or urine (the urine test is less reliable).

An injection of insulin ends diabetic ketosis. Diabetics are especially susceptible to ketosis before their condition is diagnosed, while they are fighting an infection, or when they neglect their diet or medication. Treatment of ketosis caused by starvation consists of feeding the individual sugar-containing substances by mouth or administering glucose solution intravenously (into the vein).

See also Diabetes mellitus.

Kidney failure

The kidneys are two bean-shaped organs located in the back of the upper abdomen. Their functions are to filter chemical wastes from the blood, excrete these wastes in the form of urine, and regulate body concentrations of water and nutrients. When kidney failure occurs, certain abnormalities within the kidneys prevent them from functioning normally, leading to chemical imbalances and the buildup of toxic (poisonous) substances and fluid within the body. This may eventually lead to organ damage and possibly death.

There are two forms of kidney failure. In the acute form, there is a sudden malfunction of the kidneys leading to a rapid buildup of toxins and fluid within the body, often within several hours. In the chronic form of kidney failure, there is a slow, progressive malfunction of the kidneys leading to a slow buildup of toxins and fluid, often occurring over several months to years.

Numerous conditions can cause kidney failure. Untreated high blood pressure, kidney stones or other urinary tract blockage, adverse reactions to chemicals or drugs, serious injury, infectious disease, shock following surgery, heart attack, blood transfusion with incompatible blood, severe dehydration (loss of body fluid), complications during pregnancy, immunologic disease, or congenital (existing from birth) kidney defects may all lead to kidney failure.

The most characteristic symptoms of kidney failure are a reduction in urine volume and edema, a condition in which fluid accumulates in the tissues. As a result, feet and hands and the area around the eyes may swell and become puffy. Urine color may change indicating kidney disease. In kidney failure, the urine may be bloody, wine-colored, or cloudy.

More generalized signs of kidney failure include drowsiness and fatigue, loss of appetite, diarrhea, nausea, dry skin, and difficulty in breathing. Delirium, coma, and death will eventually occur in untreated cases.

Analysis of blood and urine samples is used to diagnose kidney failure. Urine tests may reveal substances such as white blood cells, sugars, or protein that have slipped through the normally efficient filtering system of the kidneys. Similarly, when the kidneys are not filtering waste materials from the blood, blood analysis identifies the waste products that remain in the blood. X rays or ultrasound scans of the kidneys may determine any structural abnormalities or blockage.

In the case of acute kidney failure, treatment begins with diagnosing and correcting the cause of the kidney damage, and restoring normal kidney function as rapidly as possible. For example, shock may be treated with blood transfusions or kidney stones may be surgically removed.

Complete bed rest is essential as the kidneys recover. In addition, limited fluid intake, except in cases of unusual fluid loss from diarrhea or vomiting, relieves the strain on the sensitive kidneys. Physicians often recommend a low-protein diet to reduce the extra strain that is required to process the waste products of protein metabolism in the kidneys.

Should these measures prove ineffective, the patient may be helped by dialysis. Dialysis is a process that cleans and filters toxic substances from the blood by an artificial kidney machine. Most dialysis patients receive treatment by traveling to the hospital three times a week. However, a newer portable technique allows more freedom for dialysis patients.

In the case of chronic kidney failure, destruction of the kidney has progressed to the point where treatment cannot bring kidney function back to normal. Treatment of these patients involves a diet low in salt and protein and dialysis at least three times a week. Dialysis will offer a chance to prolong life, but it is not a cure for the kidney failure. Only surgically replacing the damaged kidneys will cure the kidney failure. In recent years, methods of matching kidney donors with recipients have improved, thereby limiting transplant rejection and serious complications. Today, kidney transplants are a highly successful treatment for chronic kidney failure.

See also Dialysis and Kidney stones.

Kidney stones

Kidney stones are deposits of mineral or organic substances that form in the kidney. Their size may vary from that of tiny pebbles to walnut-like formations.

The formation of kidney stones depends upon what types and amounts of excess substances are found in the urine, the fluid mixture of water and waste products produced in the kidney and excreted from the body. When abnormally high levels of minerals, such as calcium, are in the urine, they may condense into hard masses, forming stones in the kidney. Increased levels of calcium in urine may come from drinking large quantities of milk. Eating foods rich in Vitamin D, which helps the body absorb calcium, can also contribute to an overaccumulation of calcium. In addition, fractured bones can release extra calcium that may condense into stones in the kidney.

Certain disorders encourage building of mineral deposits in the kidney. Gout is a joint disease that results from high blood levels of uric acid (a waste product from breakdown of protein) that crystallizes into stones in the urine. Urinary infections that impede bladder function can also cause retention of urine that then harbors higher concentrations of elements that can solidify into stones. In addition, overactive parathyroids (endocrine glands that regulate calcium absorption) permit increased mineral absorption into the body, and this may lead to the development of kidney stones.

Middle-aged men and people with gout or chronic urinary tract infections are more susceptible to kidney stones. However, in many cases, no one can pinpoint the cause of the kidney stones.

Kidney stones may remain inactive for years and never produce any symptoms. On the other hand, some stones can cause problems as they pass out of the kidneys, including severe pain and tenderness over the affected kidney, frequent and painful urination, nausea, blood in the urine, fever, chills, and extreme exhaustion.

A more serious condition develops as the stone enters the ureter (the tube that carries urine from the kidney to the bladder) where it lodges and produces excruciating pain across the back, abdomen, and reproductive organs. If blockage occurs in the urethra, the tube that conveys urine from the bladder to the outside of the body, urine output decreases. The trapped urine may back up, distending and injuring the urinary tract. This situation requires immediate medical treatment to prevent loss of consciousness, shock, and possible kidney damage.

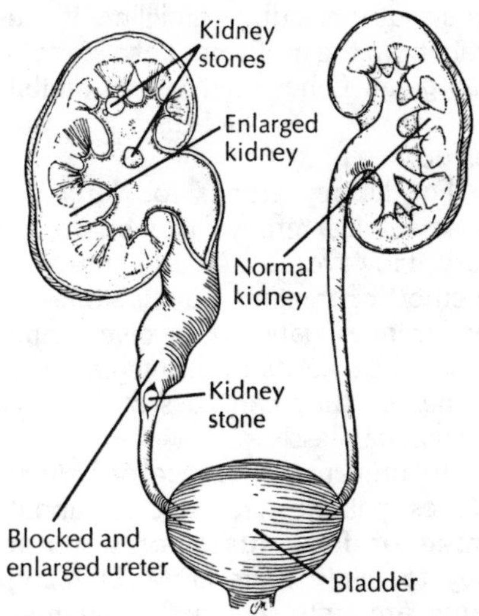

Kidney stones are formed in the kidney but may migrate to the ureter, creating an obstruction with swelling and damage above the blockage.

Kidney stones that are too small to be noticed may still cause damage to delicate tissues as they move through the urinary tract, scraping organ linings and leaving internal scars.

To determine the type of kidney stone formation, a physician analyzes the blood and urine samples. X rays or an ultrasound scan, in which high-frequency sound waves bounce off internal body structures and outline their image, reveal the location and nature of the stones.

The recurrence of kidney stones may often be controlled by diet. Reducing or eliminating intake of foods with high levels of stone-producing minerals can prevent worsening of the condition and the formation of new stones.

Since calcium contributes to kidney stones in most cases, the diet should be low in milk products and Vitamin D foods. Gout patients should decrease their protein consumption, since uric acid is a by-product of protein digestion.

As yet, there are no drugs available to dissolve kidney stones. Doctors may prescribe painkillers if the pain from the movement of a stone is too great. Other medications inhibit absorption of calcium from the blood.

For kidney stones too large to pass, surgical removal may be necessary. However, a new less intrusive method of treating kidney stones is under investigation. It involves using tiny shock waves to disintegrate the stones so they can pass out of the system painlessly.

To prevent recurrence of kidney stones, patients need to drink about three or four quarts of water a day to dilute their urine. Drinking large amounts of fluid, sometimes throughout the night, reduces urine concentration so stones cannot form. Surplus water can also flush the system of any small stones.

See also Cystitis and Gout.

Laryngitis

Laryngitis is an inflammation of the mucous membrane (or lining) of the voice box (larynx), located in the upper part of the respiratory tract. It causes hoarseness and even possibly a temporary loss of speech.

Laryngitis may result from a bacterial or viral infection, such as a cold or flu, from an irritation of the mucous membrane of the larynx, such as that caused by smoking, or from overuse of the voice.

Symptoms of this condition—other than hoarseness or loss of voice—include dryness and scratchiness of the throat, coughing, and pain from speaking.

Chronic or persistent laryngitis is

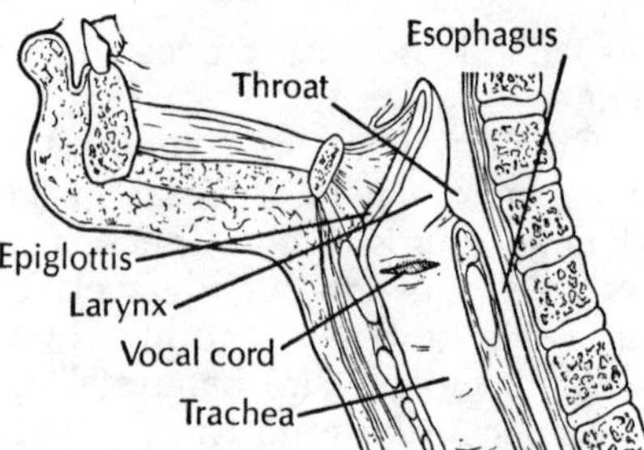

The larynx, or voice box, is located in the upper part of the respiratory tract.

most often caused by smoking, air pollution, dust, or smoke. It may also stem from tonsillitis, tuberculosis, early cancer, or paralysis of the vocal cords. Because laryngitis may be a symptom of a more serious condition, persons who consistently suffer from it should consult a physician.

Laryngitis is best treated by totally resting the vocal cords. Pain may be eased with throat sprays, steam inhalations, and mild pain relievers such as aspirin or acetaminophen.

Legionnaires' disease

Legionnaires' disease is a severe respiratory infection caused by an uncommon form of bacteria. There has been no person-to-person transmission of this disease documented as yet.

Legionnaires' disease, which usually presents itself as pneumonia, has symptoms similar to many other respiratory diseases (including influenza), making it difficult to differentiate and diagnose. Symptoms include dry coughing, high fever, chills, diarrhea, shortness of breath, chest pains, headaches, sweats, nausea, vomiting, and abdominal pain. Occasionally, bloody sputum (phlegm) is produced. Lethargy and confusion may also be accompanying symptoms in progressive, serious cases.

The elderly, cigarette smokers, and individuals taking drugs that diminish the power of the immune system are more likely to contract Legionnaires' disease than other people. Persons who have some other medical problem—heart trouble, cancer, respiratory illness, or kidney disease—are also believed to be particularly susceptible.

The first identifiable outbreak of Legionnaires' disease occurred in 1976 in the city of Philadelphia. Over 180 people attending or visiting the state convention of the American Legion became afflicted with the disease. Among them, there were 29 fatalities. Other outbreaks have occurred since in the United States and Europe. Studies have also shown that outbreaks of respiratory diseases, later identified as Legionnaires' disease, occurred as early as 1947.

Subsequent investigations have indicated that contaminated water droplets from air conditioners or other water-based coolant units may be harboring the agent of the illness.

Although Legionnaire's disease is uncommon, it should be considered in anyone (particularly the elderly and the chronically ill) who has a respiratory infection that worsens over about four days. The disease can be mild and appear to be an episode of flu. The diagnosis is made by the history and physical examination, chest X rays, and special tests of the blood and sputum (phlegm) that determine the presence and changing amount of antibodies (protective substances to fight off the infection) present.

As of now, there is no preventive vaccine against Legionnaires' disease. If an outbreak is suspected, public health officials may search for and attempt to eliminate the potential offending source. Common sources that may harbor the bacteria are air-conditioning vents, bodies of water, and areas of excavation.

If the victim of Legionnaires' disease is diagnosed and given the correct antibiotic (erythromycin) early in the course of the illness, the outlook for recovery is good.

Leukoplakia

Leukoplakia is a tough, fibrous lesion—most often in the form of a white patch—appearing on the lips, tongue, gums, and on other areas where there are mucous membranes (linings) such as the female genital organs.

The oral condition can be caused by badly fitted dentures, excessive smoking, overconsumption of alcohol, and a diet of highly spiced foods. Leukoplakia is often referred to as smoker's patches or smoker's tongue. Although these lesions are generally not painful, they may cause difficulty and discomfort when the person talks or swallows, especially if the patches are on the lips, gums, or tongue. In addition, leukoplakia may develop into a cancerous growth and may also be a symptom of syphilis.

If a person notices these persistent white patches, a physician should be seen immediately. A biopsy is often taken since the presence of cancer cannot be determined by merely looking at the lesion. These patches should be examined by a physician frequently, since a cancer may develop in the future. In most cases, however, the physician will probably advise that the lesion be entirely removed.

After the physician examines the lesion, he or she may advise having dentures refitted or cutting down on smoking and the consumption of alcohol and spicy foods.

If an unusual white patch appears on any skin surface, a physician should be seen immediately. One should never attempt to self-treat such a condition.

Leukorrhea

Leukorrhea is an abnormal discharge from the vagina. All women will have some normal discharge, and this results from a secretion of mucus by the cervix (neck of the uterus) and the vagina. This normal discharge helps to lubricate the vagina and to some extent prevent infection. At the time of ovulation, when an egg is released from the ovary, this discharge is most noticeable, but it is generally present during the entire menstrual cycle.

An abnormal vaginal discharge usually has the following characteristics: it may be heavy, it may be associated with itching of the genital organs and anal area, and it may have a disagreeable odor. This discharge is usually caused by an infection of the vagina, but it may also be caused by an infection of the cervix, a tumor or other abnormal growths, the presence of foreign matter in the vagina such as a tampon, or, less commonly, an inflammation of the vagina caused by chemicals in douches or contraceptive creams or jellies.

Vaginal infections are usually caused by one of three different organisms: yeast (a fungus), trichomonad (a parasite), or by a variety of bacteria.

To diagnose the cause of the discharge, the doctor will perform a pelvic examination and will often take a sample of the discharge and look at it under the microscope. Sometimes a culture of the discharge may also be taken so that the organism causing the problem can be grown in the laboratory and identified.

Once the cause of the abnormal discharge has been identified, specific steps will be taken to treat it. If the discharge is caused by bacteria, oral antibiotics or antibiotic vaginal creams may be prescribed. Specific oral drugs or vaginal creams will be prescribed if the discharge is caused by either yeast or trichomonad. In some cases, a biopsy of the cervix or vagina may be required if the doctor suspects that a tumor may be causing the discharge.

Douching with vinegar and water or other solutions available at the drugstore generally will not cure the discharge even though symptoms may improve for a few days. A woman with an abnormal vaginal discharge should consult her doctor before attempting to treat herself.

See also Vaginitis.

Loss of appetite

Loss of appetite (also known as anorexia) is a disinterest in and lack of desire for food. Loss of appetite should not be confused with the willful suppression of the urge to eat (called anorexia nervosa), which often occurs in young women. Rather, loss of appetite is a common symptom that accompanies many illnesses.

Appetite is controlled by two areas of the brain—the "feeding" center and the "fullness" center—that work to regulate feelings of hunger depending on the body's need for food. Appetite loss can, very rarely, be caused by damage to these areas of the brain, but more commonly it results from fatigue, the common cold, and psychological problems such as anxiety and depression. Serious disorders that may lead to longer periods of appetite loss include certain types of cancers as well as glandular and intestinal diseases.

Loss of appetite is indicated by a general disinterest in food or eating, reduced food intake, and, in severe cases, weakness and a decrease in the body's natural resistance to disease.

A doctor's advice should be sought if appetite loss stems from emotional or psychological problems, if it lasts for long periods, or if it seems to have no obvious cause. Counseling may be beneficial for those who have emotional problems connected to this disorder.

See also Anorexia nervosa.

Lumpectomy

A lumpectomy is the surgical removal of a malignant lump in the breast. This procedure is currently being evaluated as an alternative to mastectomy when the surgeon believes that the cancer is confined to the lump and no spread has occurred. After a lumpectomy is performed, the patient must be closely followed to be certain that the cancer does not recur.

See also Mastectomy.

Lungs

The lungs are part of the respiratory system whose function is to supply the blood with necessary oxygen and relieve the blood of the waste product carbon dioxide. This exchange of oxygen and carbon dioxide occurs in the lungs. Air from the outside enters through the nose where it is warmed, moistened, and filtered before it passes through the throat into the trachea (windpipe). The trachea divides into two bronchi, passageways leading into each lung. Within each lung the bronchi divide and subdivide until the smallest bronchial tubes end in small cup-shaped sacs called alveoli. It is in the alveoli that the oxygen/carbon dioxide exchange takes place. Each alveolus is served by numerous tiny blood vessels called capillaries. Oxygen in the alveolus crosses the alveolar and capillary walls to enter the blood while carbon dioxide passes from the blood through the capillary wall into the alveolus. The oxygen is then carried by the blood to the body's cells and the carbon dioxide is released by the alveolus into the outside environment on exhalation.

During inhalation and exhalation the lungs expand and contract. However, they have no muscle tissue and are expanded and contracted by the ribs and the diaphragm, the large muscle separating the chest and abdominal cavities. During inhala-

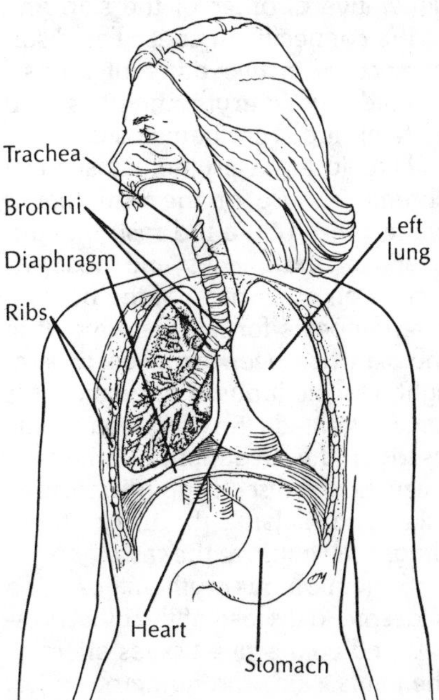

The lungs are part of the respiratory system whose function is to supply the blood with oxygen and relieve the blood of carbon dioxide.

tion the diaphragm contracts which causes it to descend and the chest cavity to expand. At this point the air pressure inside the chest cavity is less than that of the air outside the body; consequently, air from the outside rushes into the lungs. During exhalation, the diaphragm relaxes and moves up, reducing the chest capacity and pushing air out of the lungs.

The expansion and contraction of the lungs is eased by the pleura, a thin, moist membrane that covers the lungs and lines the chest cavity. The pleura permits the various surfaces of the lungs and chest cavity to slide and glide past each other as the lungs expand and contract.

Lupus erythematosus

Lupus erythematosus is a degenerative disorder of the skin and of the connective tissues. The disorder occurs in two different forms—discoid lupus erythematosus and systemic lupus erythematosus.

Discoid lupus erythematosus is a chronic disease of the skin that is characterized by a red rash that appears on the cheeks and nose, as well as on other parts of the body. It often appears for the first time after the skin has been exposed to sunlight. Discoid lupus erythematosus is usually treated with drugs commonly used in the treatment of malaria. Even though discoid lupus is not at all related to malaria, the use of these drugs may improve the rash.

Systemic lupus erythematosus is a widespread disease of the blood vessels and connective tissues affecting the joints, skin, and numerous other organs in the body including the heart, lungs, liver, intestine, and kidneys. Red patches appear on the cheeks and nose that resemble an open-winged butterfly. Symptoms may also include severe pain in the joints, an intermittent fever, and unusual fatigue. The inflammation may involve many other parts of the body and cause severe and irreversible damage to the blood vessels and to the kidneys.

Cortisone and other steroids are used to control the inflammation in the joints and in other parts of the body; aspirin and other analgesics are used to control the pain. As with discoid lupus, antimalarial drugs are used to treat the rash.

This disease may be mild or it may progress rapidly to affect many organs seriously. Death may result in severe cases.

Lymphocytes

Lymphocytes are a type of white blood cell produced in the bone marrow and lymph nodes and stored in the thymus gland, spleen, and lymph nodes (which are found throughout the body; the most easily felt lymph nodes are found in the neck, armpits, and groin).

Lymphocytes play an important role in the body's immunity. Divided into T and B cells, lymphocytes make their way through the lymph channels into the bloodstream, where they identify and "memorize" the characteristics of foreign elements called antigens. B cells manufacture antibodies, which are protein-based substances whose job is to destroy the antigens—also essentially proteins—by combining with them. T cells, which are 70 percent of the lymphocyte total, regulate antibody production and oversee immune responses.

Lymphocytes normally constitute between 22 and 28 percent of the cells in an adult's circulating blood. In cases of infection, specifically those caused by viruses, the percentage of lymphocytes in the blood may increase to above 50 percent.

Lymphocytes are normally the second most numerous type of white blood cells in the body. The most common white blood cells are called polymorphonuclear leukocytes. These white blood cells act by engulfing bacteria and killing them.

See also Antibody/antigen and Immunity.

M

Macular degeneration

Macular degeneration is the deterioration of the macula, a yellowish depression in the back of the retina of the eye. The retina, which is sensitive to light, is the innermost of the three coatings of the eyeball. The other coatings are the choroid, which encircles the retina, and the sclera (white of the eye), which covers the choroid layer. These coatings surround the inner globe of the eye, called the vitreous cavity.

The macula is located on the retina near the optic nerve at the very back of the eye. The function of the macula is distinguishing fine detail in the central vision field. Thus, the macula is that part of the eye with the sharpest vision. As light enters the eye, any image that is focused on the macula is the one that is most accurately perceived in the brain. Consequently, degeneration of the macula leads to blurring of central vision.

Macular degeneration is often secondary—that is, a result of—other conditions of the eye and is usually hereditary. However, one form is not hereditary and occurs primarily in persons over 60 years of age. In many of these cases, the blood vessels of the eye narrow, possibly as a result of atherosclerosis, and the macula's blood supply is diminished. Since the macula requires a plentiful blood supply, any deficiency causes degeneration of the macula.

Macular degeneration develops slowly and painlessly. Therefore, the blurring of central vision is gradual. If both eyes are affected—as is almost always the case—activities requiring sharp vision, such as reading or driving, usually have to be curtailed. Eventually, all central vision disappears, although peripheral vision is unaffected.

There has been no treatment for macular degeneration until recently. It has now been found that about 5 percent of affected individuals may be helped by treatment with laser beams. Early in the course of the condition, vision may be improved by special powerful eyeglasses.

See also Eye.

Mania

Mania is a term that refers to an abnormal elevation of mood, characterized by wild excitement, talkativeness, overactivity, and lack of concentration. It is also characterized by excessive irritability, hostility, and sometimes violence.

Mania is the opposite of depression in the manic-depressive disorder, in which periods of elevation alternate with periods of depression, with periods of normalcy in between. Persons in the manic stage are likely to go on spending sprees; start, but not finish, new projects; become sexually promiscuous; exhibit restlessness and distractibility; and chatter rapidly and often incoherently. In addition, their judgment is often impaired. Because persons in the manic state think they are functioning at their very best, manic individuals overestimate personal capacity for activity. As a result, many overextend themselves, becoming involved in many activities without considering the physical, mental, or social consequences.

Mania, and manic-depressive disorder as well, are usually treated by medication and/or psychotherapy. The medication most commonly used is lithium carbonate. Lithium is most useful in preventing manic episodes. However, it may require several weeks for lithium to be effective and blood tests to monitor blood levels are essential since excessive lithium levels can cause serious side effects. It is not known exactly how lithium works to combat mania, although it has been shown that lithium affects chemical transmitters in the central nervous system.

See also Depression.

Marijuana

Marijuana, or cannabis, is the dried flower clusters, stems, and leaves of the Indian hemp plant (also known as *Cannabis sativa*), which look like coarse tobacco. It is also known as "weed," "pot," "grass," "tea," and "Mary Jane," as well as a number of other slang equivalents.

Marijuana has been eaten, drunk, smoked, or sniffed throughout recorded history. When marijuana is rolled into a cigarette, it is called a "joint" or a "reefer." When it is smoked, it smells like burning rope.

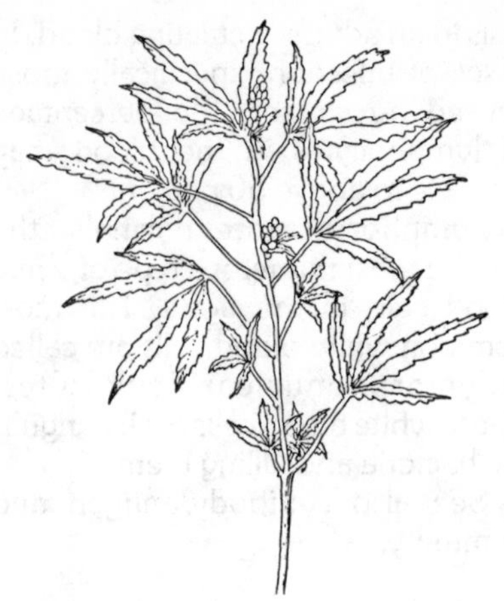

Marijuana (cannabis) is obtained from the flowering tips and shoots of the *Cannabis sativa* plant which grows wild or is cultivated all over the world.

Marijuana relaxes the body and the mind. It gives a feeling of exhilaration, inner joy, and euphoria. However, it also produces mood swings. In addition, marijuana heightens perceptions. Colors are brighter, music is more intense, and time is extended. These effects can be accompanied or followed by panic, depression, hallucinations, and fear of death, particularly if marijuana is being used in combination with other drugs. Marijuana does not, however, increase intellectual functioning or creative capacity.

Visible symptoms of marijuana use include red eyes, dilated pupils, and lack of physical coordination. Sometimes, users feel lethargic and nauseous. Reactions to use of the drug differ. The person may be happy, talkative, and silly, or may become withdrawn.

Users of marijuana often become psychologically dependent upon the drug because it represents a way for not facing the problems and stresses in individual lives. Marijuana users do not, however, become physically addicted to it and do not suffer serious withdrawal reactions when they abstain from its use. Most users of marijuana do not progress to use of hard drugs, such as heroin or cocaine, although that risk does exist.

It is believed that use of marijuana may cause long-term physical effects, including damage to the brain, heart, lung, and reproductive system. It may also cause a general decrease in motivation. Marijuana impairs judgment, and driving a car while under the influence of marijuana is especially dangerous.

Mastectomy

Mastectomy is the surgical removal of a breast or part of a breast, usually as a treatment for cancer.

There are several types of mastectomy, each characterized by the muscles, glands, tissues, or skin removed.

- Lumpectomy—removal of the tumor along with some of the surrounding breast tissue
- Partial mastectomy—removal of the tumor along with approximately one half of the breast
- Simple mastectomy—removal of the entire breast and possibly some of the lymph nodes in the armpit
- Modified radical mastectomy—removal of the entire breast plus more of the armpit lymph nodes than in the simple mastectomy
- Radical mastectomy—removal of the entire breast, all the lymph nodes in the armpit, and the chest muscles
- Extended radical—removal of

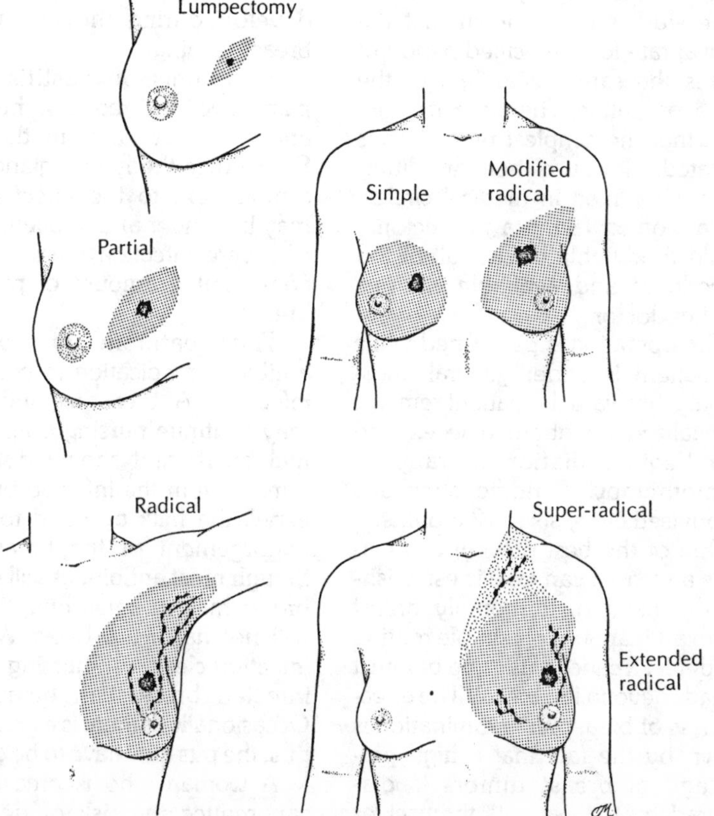

The shaded portions show the area affected by each type of mastectomy.

breast plus additional tissue in the chest as well as the armpit lymph nodes and chest muscles

- Super radical mastectomy—removal of the same tissues and muscles as in the extended radical but in addition tissues and lymph nodes up into the neck.

The type of mastectomy is determined by whether the cancer is still localized in the original site or whether the cancer has spread into neighboring lymph nodes. The lymph nodes in the armpit will have a biopsy done on them—a biopsy is the removal of a small tissue sample to examine it for malignant cells. In addition, other tests may be done to determine if the cancer has spread to other areas of the body.

There is some question about how extensive the surgery needs to be. Some studies have shown that the survival rate for a specified period of time is the same regardless of the type of operation. Therefore, it would seem that the simplest procedure is indicated. However, there are differences of opinion in medical circles, and a woman facing a mastectomy should thoroughly discuss all of the procedures and available options with her doctor.

The operation is performed while the patient is under general anesthesia. Afterward the patient remains hospitalized for about a week and may begin radiation therapy or chemotherapy. Periodic checkups are advised every six to 12 months.

One of the best preventive measures a woman can take is establishing the habit of a monthly breast self-examination. This simple routine can detect a cancerous lump before it spreads beyond the breast. The effectiveness of breast self-examination is shown by the fact that a high percentage of breast tumors is discovered by the patients themselves during a monthly breast self-examination.

See also Cancer for instructions for a breast self-examination.

Mastitis

Mastitis is inflammation of the breast caused by bacterial invasion and infection.

This condition occurs most frequently in nursing mothers and comes from bacteria normally found on the skin and nipples that enter the breast through the nipple and infect the milk glands and ducts. In many cases, it occurs in the third to fifth day after the birth of the baby, because cracked nipples through which the bacteria enter the breast may develop during the first week of breast-feeding.

Symptoms of mastitis include pain, swelling, redness, high fever and a tender lump in the breast. Sometimes the lymph glands in the armpit next to the affected breast may be tender and swollen. In cases of severe infection there may be a considerable amount of pus in the breast.

The treatment for mastitis is antibiotic medication to combat the infection. A breast-feeding mother may continue nursing from the normal breast and should discontinue nursing from the infected breast but expell the milk by hand to prevent engorgement of the breast. Even though most antibiotics will enter the breast milk in small quantities, this will not harm the baby. When the infection clears up, nursing from the infected breast can be resumed. Occasionally, if there is a great deal of pus, the pus may have to be drained.

A woman who is breast-feeding can reduce the risk of developing mastitis by keeping the nipples clean and dry between feedings and by wearing clothing that does not rub or irritate the nipples.

Another more common form of mastitis is not infectious and is called chronic fibrocystic mastitis. In this condition breasts contain small cysts and nodules and are usually very painful. This condition is readily treated by a physician, who will check to be sure that the cysts and nodules are not cancerous.

See also Fibrocystic disease of the breast.

Mastoid infection

A mastoid infection is a bacterial invasion of the mastoid air cells, small air-filled cavities located in the mastoid bone. The mastoid bone is the bulge in the skull behind the ear.

A mastoid infection is most often a complication of a middle ear infection. This infection can lead to mastoiditis, which is characterized by ringing in the ear, a discharge of pus from the ear canal, and, very often, fever. Other indications include

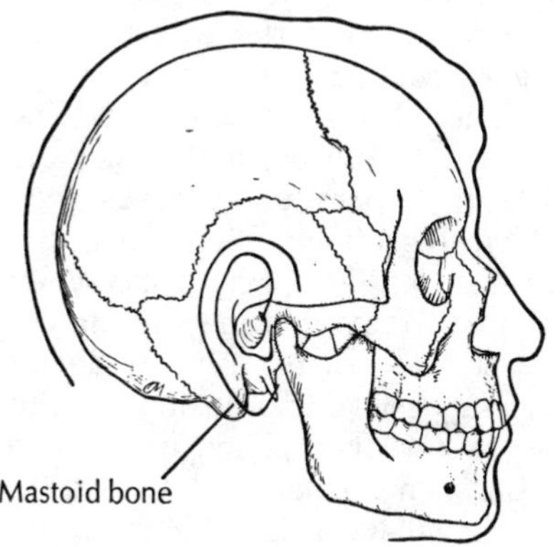

A mastoid infection is an infection of the air cells—air-filled cavities—in the mastoid bone, which is the protrusion of the skull immediately behind the ear.

swelling and tenderness of the mastoid bone. In severe cases, an abscess (pus-filled cavity) may develop in the mastoid bone. This is a serious complication because it carries the risk of spreading to the interior of the skull and infecting the meninges, membranes that cover the brain. This is called meningitis.

Since antibiotics are so effective against ear infections and mastoid infections, mastoiditis is fortunately now rare. Sometimes, however, surgery is required to remove the infected cells if antibiotic treatment is started too late or is not effective. This procedure is called a mastoidectomy.

See also Ear infections.

Measles

Measles is a contagious disease that mainly affects the respiratory system, skin, and eyes. It was once considered one of the more dangerous childhood diseases because the threat of serious complications was so great. Fortunately, development of a vaccine to prevent measles has drastically reduced its occurrence.

Another name for measles is rubeola. Rubeola is caused by a virus that invades the body and infects living cells. The virus comes from the respiratory system of an infected person and is spread via airborne droplets of moisture. Some researchers contend that the virus enters the body through the eyes.

Incubation period for measles—the time between being exposed to the illness and actually showing symptoms—is eight to 12 days. During this time, the infected person is contagious up to four days before symptoms begin and up to six days after the rash develops.

Measles usually begins much like a cold with runny nose, nasal congestion, sneezing, a dry cough, and fever between 102°F and 104°F. After three or four days, eyes may become sensitive to bright light as they grow red and swollen. Then the fever drops. At this time, red spots with tiny white centers appear in the mouth. These are called Koplik's spots after the man who first diagnosed them.

By the fourth or fifth day, the fever increases again, and a rash appears. The rash usually starts on the face, neck, and behind the ears before spreading to the rest of the body. As the spots multiply, they grow larger, become raised, and sometimes blend together. Their color turns dark red and then brown before the skin begins to fall off in small flakes. This process takes about one week after the rash first emerges, although skin discoloration can last as long as two weeks. Other symptoms usually disappear within seven to ten days from the start of the disease.

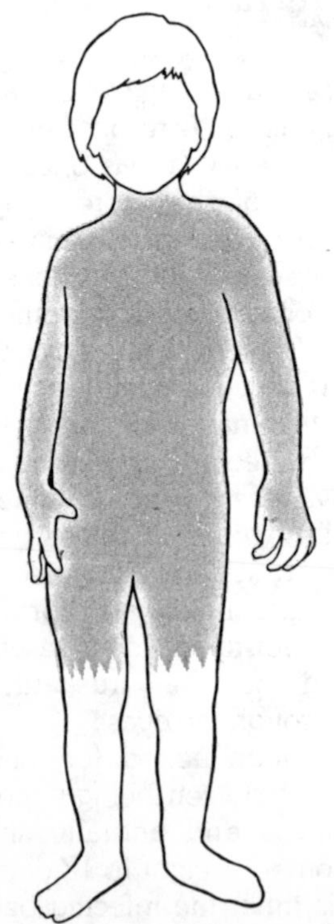

The measles rash—dark red spots that blend together as they spread—usually begins on the face, neck, and behind the ears and then spreads over the body as far as the knees.

Breathing problems, increased coughing, earache, or extreme drowsiness may indicate complications that warrant consulting a doctor immediately. The more serious complications are pneumonia (infection of the lungs) and encephalitis (inflammation of the brain). Additionally, subacute sclerosing panencephalitis (SSPE), a rare but often fatal disease of the brain, has been linked to measles. Severe ear infections can also result, particularly in young children. In addition, bronchitis, laryngitis, and swollen neck glands can complicate measles and make the course of the illness last longer or even return after apparent recovery.

Generally, physicians diagnose measles by the initial symptoms. To confirm diagnosis, nasal discharge, blood, or urine can be tested for signs of the virus.

Measles, being caused by a virus, does not respond to antibiotics. For this reason, treatment focuses upon relieving uncomfortable symptoms. A vaporizer in the patient's room eases cold-like symptoms by adding moisture to the air. If the eyes are irritated, warm compresses may relieve the inflammation. Also, dim lights are easier on the eyes. When washing, soaps that may irritate the skin should not be used. A doctor may suggest adding baking soda to bath water or applying a soothing lotion, such as calamine lotion, to the rash to relieve itching. Most physicians recommend an aspirin substitute to reduce fever.

Today, measles has been almost eliminated because of a vaccine given to children as an injection around 15 months of age. The vaccine, which is prepared from measles virus, stimulates antibody (protective substance in cells) action within the body to produce immunity or resistance to the disease. A low vaccine effectiveness rate in very young children is the reason that babies are not vaccinated before 15 months of age. Most babies under six months of age already have immunity that they acquired from their mothers before birth. Should a baby be exposed to measles, however, a doctor should be consulted. Measles is dangerous for anyone under three years of age or for anyone with chronic long-term disease.

Meniere's disease

Meniere's disease is the result of an increase in pressure in the inner ear because of a buildup of fluid in the labyrinth—the part of the inner ear that controls body balance and equilibrium. This buildup of pressure distorts and sometimes ruptures the membrane or lining of the labyrinth wall.

Meniere's disease is an uncommon disease, and its cause is unknown. However, it is thought that the pressure changes may be brought on by an infection, a small hemorrhage in the ear, or an allergic response. It occurs most commonly in men aged 40 to 60.

Symptoms of Meniere's disease include recurring and violent attacks of vertigo or dizziness, ringing in the ears, noises that sound muffled or distorted, and nausea that is sometimes accompanied by vomiting. Deafness in one or both ears may eventually develop.

Mild attacks of Meniere's disease may last from a half hour to several days before fading away naturally. They may recur regularly at intervals of weeks, months, or years. Severe attacks may last for several weeks, requiring the person to be confined to bed. In such cases, almost any movement of the head will result in bizarre and disturbing sensations that the floor and the furniture in the room are spinning around. Severe cases may also be accompanied by anxiety attacks and migraine headaches.

The use of certain drugs such as diuretics and antihistamines may help to relieve severe and recurrent attacks. In severe cases, surgical destruction of certain nerves in the ear may be necessary.

See also Dizziness.

Meningitis

Meningitis occurs when bacteria or viruses enter the spinal fluid and infect the meninges, the three layers of membrane that surround the brain and spinal cord. Meningitis can be fatal, although this is becoming less and less common because of the increased use of effective antibiotics.

Meningitis seems to strike males more often than females and is most commonly seen in children up to the age of four years and in adults over the age of 60. Swelling of the brain, as well as epilepsy, blindness, amnesia, and deafness, can result when meningitis is not properly and promptly treated.

The three layers of meninges are called the dura mater (the outermost layer), the arachnoid (the middle layer), and the pia mater (the innermost layer). A space between the inner two layers (called the subarachnoid space) is filled with clear fluid (called cerebrospinal fluid), which is produced in the brain. When bacteria or viruses invade this fluid

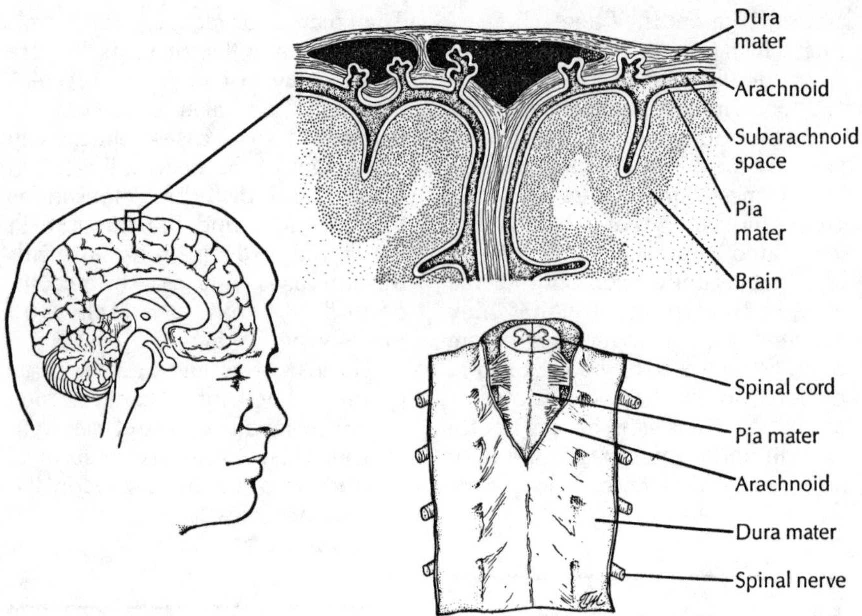

Meningitis is an infection of the meninges, the membranes that cover the brain and spinal cord. The three membranes are the dura mater, the arachnoid, and the pia mater. Between the two inner layers is the subarachnoid space filled with cerebrospinal fluid. When an infection invades the spinal fluid and then infects the meninges, meningitis results.

and form pus, the surrounding membranes soon become infected, resulting in meningitis.

Meningitis is caused by an infection that enters the system through a serious head wound or through the bloodstream from a source of infection in another part of the body. The bacteria may also reach the meninges from an abscess (localized infection) of the brain itself, but this is quite rare.

A deficiency in the body's immune system, which can be either inherited or acquired over time, may lead to a greater chance of contracting this disease. Also, newborns may be at a greater risk if the mother had a genital infection such as herpes during the last week of pregnancy, if the membranes of the uterus ruptured prematurely, or if labor was prolonged.

The symptoms of meningitis are a "bursting" headache, high fever, rising pulse rate, irregular breathing, vomiting, and sensitivity to light. Pain extends down the neck, into the back and lower limbs; the neck may be stiff, and it will be difficult for the patient to bend forward. As the disease progresses, convulsions or coma may occur.

If the doctor does not think there is increased pressure in the brain, meningitis may be diagnosed using a test called a lumbar puncture in which a sample of the cerebrospinal fluid is withdrawn and examined to see if it is clear (normal) or cloudy (pus-filled) and to identify the bacteria causing the infection. A physical exam, blood cultures, and cultures from the secretions of the respiratory tract may also be taken to determine the type of bacteria present. A viral infection, however, is much harder to diagnose; it may not show up on any tests although meningitis symptoms are clearly observed.

Immediate treatment is very

important, so the doctor may prescribe medication for the meningitis patient even before the specific infecting agent is identified; once the cause is determined, an appropriate medication, most often an antibiotic, can be administered. The patient will be hospitalized where measures can be taken to reduce fever and control brain swelling.

Viral infections, again, are much harder to treat. There is no medication that will kill a virus that has entered the central nervous system. Treatment in this case is limited to hospitalization, where supportive therapy will be administered until the disease has run its course.

Prevention of meningitis may be possible with some vaccines now available, which combat certain bacteria strains that cause meningitis. Research is still being done on vaccines for other bacteria strains.

Menopause

Menopause is the normal, natural stage in a woman's life when her menstruation and ovulation cycles stop, ending her reproductive years. Also called climacteric or the change of life, it occurs around age 50 but can start anywhere between the ages of 40 to 60. During the years immediately preceding its onset, menstrual periods may become scant and irregular.

Scientists do not fully understand what causes menopause but they believe that it is triggered when the female sex glands, the ovaries, stop responding to the gonadotropic (sex gland) hormones that are secreted by the pituitary gland to control normal function of the ovaries. The ovaries' subsequent decline in the production of the female hormone estrogen sets off the bodily changes.

Physical symptoms may include hot flashes (a warm and flushed feeling that comes over the face, neck, and chest and lasts a few minutes at a time but recurs throughout the day), excessive perspiring, dryness in the vagina (which can lead to painful or difficult intercourse), pounding heartbeat, joint pains, headaches, itching skin, increased facial hair, and decreased armpit and pubic hair.

Nonphysical symptoms are depression, anxiety, irritability, apprehension, decreased ability to concentrate, lack of confidence, and insomnia.

Symptoms may last from a few weeks to more than five years. Not every woman experiences the same changes, other than an end to menstruation; about 25 percent notice no other changes, 50 percent discern some physical and/or psychological symptoms, and the other 25 percent note very uncomfortable or distressing symptoms.

During this time, it can also be difficult for a woman to face the aging process and its physical ramifications, the end of the childbearing years, and a sense of uselessness because of a possible decrease in family responsibilities.

It is important not to attribute all physical changes to menopause to the point of overlooking the symptoms of disease. This is a good time to schedule an examination and discuss the bodily changes with a doctor. A woman should see a doctor immediately if she starts to bleed in between menstrual periods, bleeds excessively, or has another period six months or more after they had apparently stopped.

Fertility and the need to practice birth control at this stage depend upon a woman's age at the time of her last period. Under age 50, a woman can still conceive for up to 24 months after the date of her last period; over

50, conception is possible for up to one year.

Treatment for the physical symptoms of menopause includes replacement of the female sex hormones, commonly estrogen or a combination of estrogen and progesterone in tablet or vaginal cream. The lowest effective dose is administered (because of possible side effects) for the first few months and then tapered off (unless symptoms reappear) until the changes in the ovaries are completed.

Artificial estrogen can help a woman's psyche, bones, joints, and skin but it does harbor potential side effects, including coronary or cerebral thrombosis and cancer of the uterus. Estrogen is not given to women with circulatory or liver disorders and is carefully controlled when prescribed to those with diabetes, epilepsy, and heart or kidney disease. Progesterone is not prescribed for women with liver disease and is carefully controlled in those with asthma, epilepsy, and heart or kidney disease. The benefits and hazards can be discussed with a doctor; other medication is available to treat certain menopausal symptoms in women who cannot take hormones.

Treatment for the psychological or emotional symptoms may include tranquilizers, antidepressants, sleeping pills, or psychotherapy.

It is important to remember that any treatment merely lessens the discomfort of menopause; it cannot stop or slow down menopause or the aging process.

After menopause, a woman may be more prone to osteoporosis (a disease that makes bones porous and brittle) and high blood pressure. Both of these conditions can be controlled under medical supervision.

See also Hypertension and Osteoporosis.

Menorrhagia

Menorrhagia is a term referring to an abnormally long—more than seven days—or heavy menstrual flow, frequently accompanied by the passing of large blood clots.

It is a common problem, one that is often caused by a disturbance in the hormones controlling the menstrual cycle. It can also be caused by fibroid tumors in the uterus, inflammation of the pelvis, and hypothyroidism (underactive thyroid gland).

The condition, which is especially common in women nearing the late 30s and 40s, seldom indicates the existence of a serious disorder. However, it may result in iron deficiency anemia because of excessive blood loss.

If this abnormal menstrual flow continues over a long period of time, a physician should be consulted. The physician may perform a number of tests to determine whether there is a serious underlying cause as well as do a Pap test, a cervical biopsy (tissue sample from the cervix), or a biopsy of the uterine lining to check for cancer. The physician may also do a blood test to check for anemia.

It is suggested that persons having this disorder reduce the level of their activities during menstruation and be sure to get enough iron so that they will not become anemic.

Menstruation

Menstruation is the monthly breakdown and discharge of the endometrial tissue that lines the uterus. The endometrial tissue thickens during each menstrual cycle to prepare the uterus for possible pregnancy. Approximately midway through the cycle, ovulation occurs. Ovulation is the process in which an ovary—one of two glands near the top of the uterus that secrete female sex hormones—releases an egg. Extending from either side of the uterus are the fallopian tubes, which are four to five inches long with finger-like projections at their ends. When the ovary releases an egg, the projections on the nearby tube sweep the egg into the tube where it slowly inches toward the uterus.

If during that time, the egg is fertilized by a sperm, the male reproductive cell, it moves to the uterus and implants itself into the rich uterine lining where it grows for the next nine months. If the egg does not become fertilized, the uterine lining breaks down and passes, along with the unfertilized egg, out of the cervix (neck of the uterus) on through the vagina and out of the body. This discharge is known as menstruation, and this monthly cycle is controlled by the female hormones, estrogen and progesterone, secreted by the ovaries.

Young women start menstruating and ovulating at puberty, which occurs between the ages of nine and 14, and normally do so every month (except while pregnant) until they reach menopause around age 50 or so.

Menstruation may be accompanied by complications of varying degrees of seriousness in many women at some point in their reproductive lives. The most common

Stages of menstrual cycle

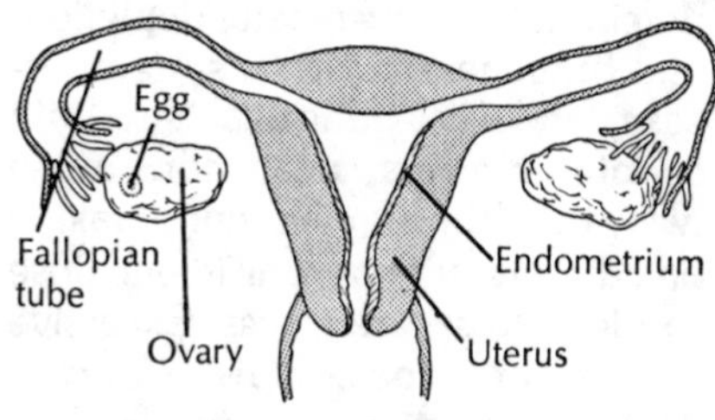

In the first stage while the egg is still inside the ovary the endometrium (lining of the uterus) is fairly thin.

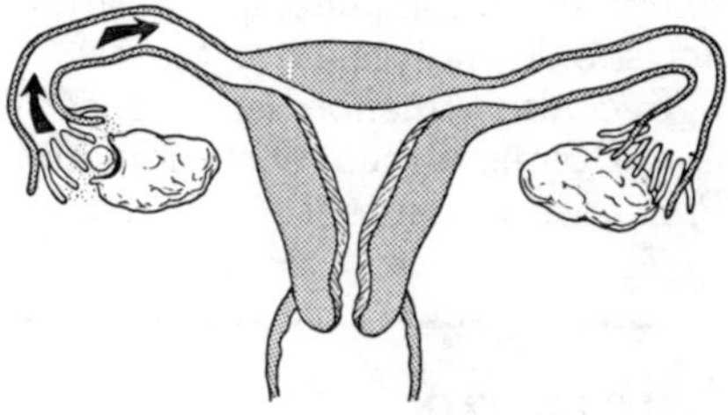

When the egg is released and begins to move into the fallopian tube, the endometrium begins to thicken in preparation for a possible pregnancy.

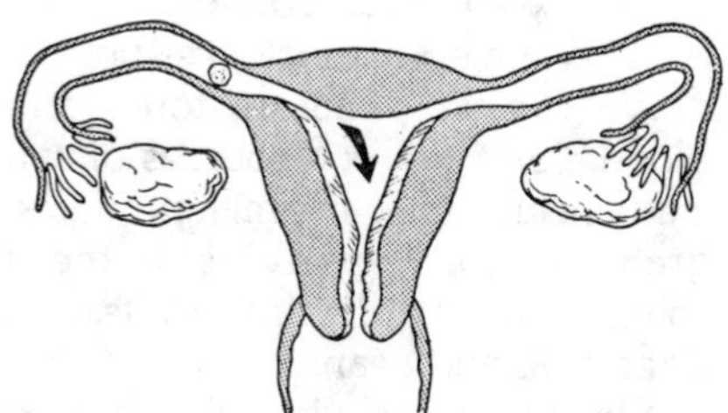

The egg moves through the tube toward the uterus. This is the point at which conception may occur. The egg is met by the male sperm cell in the fallopian tube, and the fertilized egg moves on to the uterus. During this time the endometrium continues to grow.

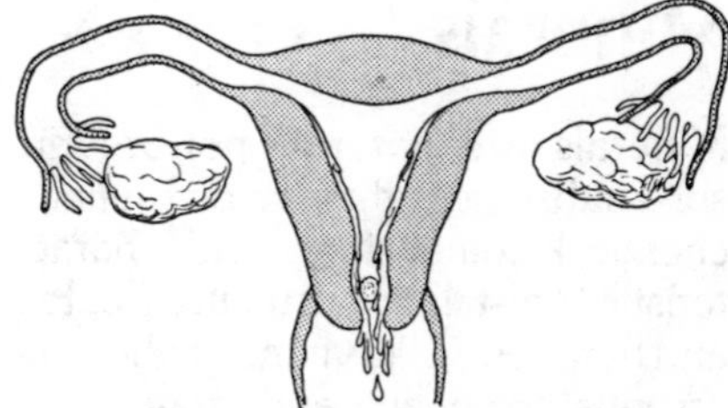

If conception does not occur, the endometrium ceases to grow and thicken. At this stage, the endometrium breaks down and is discharged, along with the unfertilized egg, from the uterus. This is menstruation. (In this drawing the egg has been enlarged for the sake of illustration; normally the egg is only visible under a microscope.)

problems are dysmenorrhea, painful menstruation; amenorrhea, the absence entirely of a menstrual period or the missing of several periods; and premenstrual tension (PMT), distinct feelings of irritability and discomfort in the days before the period begins.

For many years the symptoms of these disorders have been attributed to emotional factors. Research, however, has shown that most are caused by very real physical changes, and many new methods of treatment have been developed.

Although the disorders themselves are generally not dangerous, they can be physically and emotionally incapacitating. Furthermore, they may be symptoms of a disease in the reproductive organs. Therefore, medical treatment for annoying symptoms accompanying menstruation should always be sought.

See also Amenorrhea, Conception, Dysmenorrhea, Ovulation, and Premenstrual tension.

Migraine

See Headaches.

Minerals

Minerals are natural, nonorganic solid substances that have a definite chemical composition and characteristic crystalline structure, color, and hardness. Like vitamins, they are essential for health and growth and perform two functions in the body: minerals build (bones and soft tissues) and regulate (the cardiovascular system, the internal pressure of body fluids, nerve responses, and oxygen conduction).

The body requires some minerals in relatively large amounts; these macrominerals are calcium, phosphorus, sodium chloride, potassium, magnesium, and sulfur. Others are called trace minerals because they are needed only in minute (tiny) quantities: iron, manganese, copper, iodine, zinc, cobalt, fluorine, and selenium. Still other minerals are harmful: lead, mercury, and cadmium.

Although minerals are necessary, they are essential only in certain small amounts and can be harmful if taken in excess. Those who use mineral supplements should take care not to surpass the daily requirement. An overload can upset the balance of other minerals and block their performance; can result in decreased physical ability; and can contribute to such conditions as anemia, bone demineralization (mineral depletion) and brittleness, nervous system disease, and fetal abnormalities. With certain minerals, even consuming twice the daily requirement or taking one day's requirement all in one dose can lead to severe illness. Excessive minerals are especially risky for children, pregnant or nursing women, and the elderly.

Calcium is the most prevalent mineral in the body; in fact, bones and teeth together contain an average of two to three pounds. It regulates certain body processes—normal nerve function, muscle tone, and blood clotting. Good sources of calcium include milk and milk products, green leafy vegetables (except spinach and chard), citrus fruits, and dried peas and beans.

Phosphorus coexists with calcium in the bones and teeth but is also present in most body tissues. Phosphorus is present in so many foods that a deficiency is rare; it is most abundant in meat, poultry, fish, eggs, and whole-grain foods.

Sodium and chloride combine to

form sodium chloride (table salt) yet each element functions separately. Sodium maintains regular water balance both inside and outside the cells and is found in blood plasma and fluids outside the cells. Foods rich in sodium include meat, fish, poultry, eggs, milk, and processed foods like bacon, ham, bread, and crackers. Chloride, part of hydrochloric acid which is basic to the digestive system, is concentrated in gastric (stomach) juices. People who perspire heavily may have to add salt to their diet, but generally most people eat too much salt because of their high consumption of processed food and added table salt. Surplus salt increases the body's water retention (edema) and is associated with high blood pressure, kidney disease, cirrhosis of the liver, and congestive heart disease.

Potassium, mainly present in the fluid in cells, regulates the balance and volume of body fluids in tandem with sodium. Most foods, both plant and animal, are rich in potassium so a deficiency is very rare, although it may show up in conjunction with prolonged diarrhea, use of diuretics (medication that removes water from the body), or a diet that lacks protein.

Magnesium is contained mostly in bones although it is present in all body tissues. It is vital to the special chemicals called enzymes that help convert food into energy. Magnesium deficiencies usually occur only in post-surgical patients, alcoholics, and others who do not eat a well-balanced diet. Magnesium-rich foods include bananas, whole-grain cereals, dry beans, milk, nuts, peanuts, peanut butter, and most dark green vegetables.

Sulfur, found in all tissues, is a part of several important amino acids and of the vitamins thiamine and biotin. It is not yet understood how it works in the body.

Most trace elements rely on organic compounds for transport, storage, and function.

Iron is apparent throughout most of the body, chiefly in the blood, liver, spleen, and bone marrow. It is an integral part of the compounds that are necessary to transport oxygen to the cells and to regulate its use there. These foods provide significant amounts of iron: liver, meat products, egg yolks, fish, green leafy vegetables, peas, beans, dried fruit, whole-grain cereal, and food made from iron-rich cereal.

Manganese is fundamental for the normal building of tendons and bones and is part of some enzymes. Food rich in this mineral include bran, coffee, tea, nuts, peas, and beans. Manganese deficiency in humans is virtually unknown.

Copper, an element involved with the storage and release of iron to form the oxygen-carrying hemoglobin for red blood cells, is most vital in the early months of life. If a pregnant woman's intake is sufficient, her baby will be born with enough copper. It is most available in processed food as well as in organ meats, shellfish, nuts, and dried peas or beans.

Iodine is only necessary in minute amounts but is indispensable for the normal working of the thyroid gland. A shortage can result in thyroid enlargement (goiter). Before the introduction of iodized salt in the United States in 1924, iodine-deficiency goiter was common in inland areas. Food harvested from the sea is abundant in iodine.

Zinc is a fundamental part of the enzymes that move carbon dixode in the red blood cells from the tissues to the lungs for exhalation. A deficiency of zinc may show up as a loss of the sense of taste or delayed healing of wounds. Associated with protein, zinc is found in meat, poultry, cheese, dry beans, nuts, cocoa, fish, egg yolks, and milk. Although it is available in whole-grain cereal, it is not likely to be absorbed because of the presence of other substances.

Cobalt, not needed in the body by itself, is part of the nutrient Vitamin B_{12}, available in meat, eggs, and dairy products.

Chromium acts with insulin in the use of glucose (sugar). A shortage produces a diabetic-like condition. It is present in dried brewer's yeast, whole-grain cereals, and liver.

Selenium works in conjunction with Vitamin E. Not much is known about selenium, except that it is important in the body and that it is found in animals and plants where it is accessible in the earth.

Fluorine is important to the formation of teeth and resistance to dental caries (cavities), especially in children, and helps maintain calcium in the bones of the elderly. It is available in small and varying amounts in water, soil, vegetables, and meat.

See also Fluorides and Vitamins.

Miscarriage

A miscarriage, in medical terms a spontaneous abortion, is the end of a pregnancy, brought on by the premature delivery of the fetus (unborn baby) before the beginning of the twentieth week of pregnancy. At that point, the fetus is not developed enough to survive outside the uterus on its own. (After the twentieth week of pregnancy, a spontaneous abortion is considered a premature delivery or, if the baby is born dead, a stillbirth. A pregnancy that is ended artificially is commonly known as an abortion, although the medical term is termination of pregnancy.) Most miscarriages occur within the first 14 weeks of pregnancy.

It is impossible to know the number of miscarriages that happen during the first month of pregnancy before a woman realizes she is pregnant; the only indication is a slightly late menstrual period with a heavier than normal flow. However, about 10 to 15 percent of the known pregnancies end in miscarriage.

There are different categories of miscarriages. A "threatened" miscarriage is experienced by about one out of every five pregnant women when they bleed vaginally during the first three months; although it may indicate a spontaneous abortion, with proper care it is rarely more than a threat and the pregnancy will continue normally. An "inevitable" miscarriage refers to a situation in which bleeding occurs and the cervix begins to dilate (open). A "missed" miscarriage occurs when the fetus dies in the uterus but is not naturally expelled, and the woman has no bleeding or pain to signify that the pregnancy is not progressing; the physician usually notices when the uterus stops growing.

The reason that a miscarriage occurs is not always understood, but it is believed that a fetus usually aborts because it is not developing normally. Several factors can contribute to a miscarriage including abnormalities in the father's sperm; disease in the mother, most notably an acute infection, glandular disorder, high blood pressure, kidney or heart disease, diabetes, or thyroid problems; abnormalities in the uterus; the mother's poor nutrition and use of cigarettes, alcohol or drugs; environmental pollutants; or the mother's involvement in a severe accident or trauma.

The expulsion of the fetus because of an abnormality is thought to be a chance event, not due to a problem or defect in either parent. Of women who miscarry once, most (80 percent) have a successful subsequent pregnancy. Women who miscarry two or three times, whether or not they deliver successfully in between, are known as "habitual aborters."

The symptoms of miscarriage are vaginal bleeding (from a few drops to a heavy flow) and cramps (either dull and constant or sharp and intermittent) in the lower abdomen or back. The bleeding can start suddenly or follow a brownish discharge. A solid clot of material or tissue may pass from the vagina. If possible, this should be saved for the doctor who may be able to examine it and determine a reason for the expulsion. A miscarriage can be complete–the uterus expels all the tissue–or incomplete–tissue remains inside the uterus.

A pregnant woman who starts bleeding or experiences pain should contact her physician immediately.

There is no medical treatment to stop or avert an inevitable miscarriage. (The drug diethylstilbestrol, DES, was prescribed to deter miscarriages until it was discovered that it had little effect and could cause abnormalities in babies.) The physician generally directs the woman with symptoms to rest in bed and abstain from sexual intercourse.

After an inevitable, incomplete, or missed miscarriage, any remaining fetus or placenta must be removed by a surgical procedure known as dilatation and curettage (D and C) in which the physician expands the cervix and gently scrapes residual material from inside the uterus. Without this precaution a woman is more likely to be susceptible to infections caused by the retained tissue.

It is normal for a woman to feel depressed by the loss of the expected child, but it is usually safe for her to attempt to conceive soon afterward—six to eight weeks later — on the advice of her physician.

More and more information is becoming available about the use of drugs and about the nutritional and environmental factors that can affect a pregnancy. It is advisable for a woman, at the beginning of her pregnancy, to seek counseling or educate herself so she is aware of the most up-to-date information on the substances and practices that may contribute to a miscarriage.

See also DES and Dilatation and curettage.

Mole

A mole is a cluster of cells, usually pigmented (colored), that appears on the skin. Moles are sometimes present at birth, but more often they appear during childhood, adolescence, or pregnancy. Although moles, which are commonplace, can become cancerous, they seldom do.

Moles vary in size, shape, and color. They may be large or small, flat or raised, or smooth or warty. They may be skin-tone or their color may vary from yellow-brown to black. Some moles have one or more hairs.

The most common type of mole is the intradermal nevus, which forms in the lower layer of skin. It is a raised cluster of cells that ranges in color from skin-tone to black. Other types of moles include the (1) lentigo nevus, a flat, uniformly pigmented brown or black spot, (2) junctional nevus, a flat or slightly raised blemish that ranges in color from light brown to nearly black, (3) compound nevus, which is raised and is usually dark in color, and (4) halo nevus, a pigmented mole in the middle of a ring of depigmented skin.

Moles are often removed for cosmetic reasons. However, any mole that enlarges suddenly, becomes darker, begins to bleed, or changes in any other unexplained way should be removed and the cells examined.

Mono

See Infectious mononucleosis.

Mucous colon

See Irritable bowel syndrome.

Multiple sclerosis

Multiple sclerosis is a chronic disease of the central nervous system, consisting of the brain and spinal cord. Damage to the nerves results after the myelin sheath degenerates. The myelin sheath is the fatty substance insulating the nerve fibers of the nervous system. Once this protection disappears, body functions may become impaired. Ultimately, the patient may be wheelchair-bound or even die.

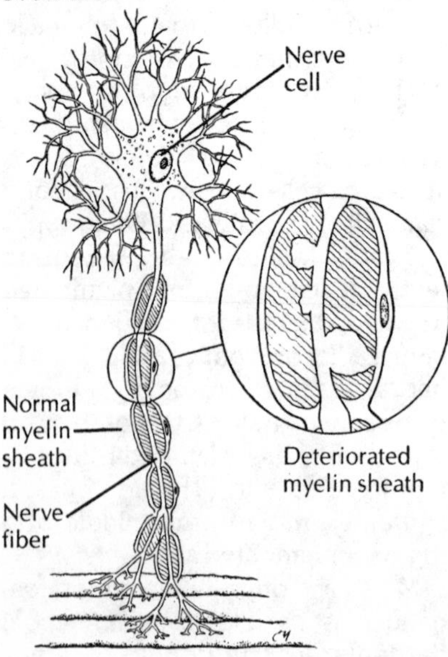

Multiple sclerosis results when the myelin sheath, the fatty substance that insulates the nerve fibers, deteriorates.

As yet, researchers have not determined the exact cause of multiple sclerosis. Some studies indicate that the disease follows exposure to a virus (contagious microorganisms attacking living cells). The virus may lie dormant (inactive) for some time before certain environmental factors, such as a second exposure to the virus or stress, trigger the disease.

Another theory suggests that multiple sclerosis affects people who have some defect in their immune system (the response of the body that attacks and inactivates disease-causing agents) that makes them more susceptible to the disease after exposure to the virus.

Initial attacks of multiple sclerosis are most common in people in their late 20s and early 30s. The disease begins with tingling and numbness in the arms and legs, muscle spasms, partial loss of vision, difficulty in walking, and impaired bladder control. After the first attack, there is usually a period of remission (a time without symptoms) for as long as two to three years.

Subsequent attacks occur at irregular intervals and cause gradually increasing disability. Frequent episodes cause weakness, general incoordination, impaired speech, and a burning sensation in the affected areas. Sexual function lessens, and mood swings are common.

More extensive nerve damage may result in loss of muscle control and require the patient to use a wheelchair. Usually the earlier the onset of disease the more slowly it progresses. Ten years after onset, less than half of these patients can continue regular daily activity. After 20 years, less than one quarter are able to function normally.

Physicians diagnose multiple sclerosis through physical examination and observation of symptoms. Often, diagnosis remains unconfirmed until a second attack occurs years later.

Since there is no prevention or cure for multiple sclerosis, treatment concentrates on relieving the symptoms. Doctors prescribe muscle relaxants to help ease muscle spasms. Some patients find that corticosteroid drugs shorten acute attacks of the disease by reducing inflammation of the nerve tissue. However, steroid drugs should be used cautiously because they may have adverse side effects.

Besides drugs, many patients are more comfortable if they are well rested. Afternoon naps and adequate sleep at night offer some relief. In addition, cold temperatures sometimes improve symptoms, whereas heat makes them worse.

Mumps

Mumps is a highly contagious viral disease that is usually contracted during childhood. More than 85 percent of the cases occurs before age 15, especially between six and ten years of age.

Mumps is caused by a virus that attacks cells of the parotid (saliva) glands. This invasion results in painful swelling of the face beneath the ear along the jawline. Mumps virus spreads by contact with airborne moisture from the infected person's nose or throat. Sometimes, the infection comes from someone who either has the disease without symptoms, or who is not yet aware of the symptoms. The disease occurs most often during spring months, though it can happen any time of year.

Symptoms can be so mild that they are nonexistent or they can be very severe. Fever (101°F to 103°F), headache, and loss of appetite usually develop first, followed by earache. Then the characteristic swelling of the saliva glands appears. Swelling may start on one side of the face and then appear on the other side within a few days. Sometimes, however, only one side swells. The inflammation may cause soreness and difficulty in eating or swallowing.

Other glands, such as the sex glands, may become swollen as well. Boys who have one or both testes inflamed may be in considerable pain. The affected testicle may shrink somewhat, but it always returns to normal size within time. Medically, this condition is known as orchitis. Contrary to popular belief, mumps

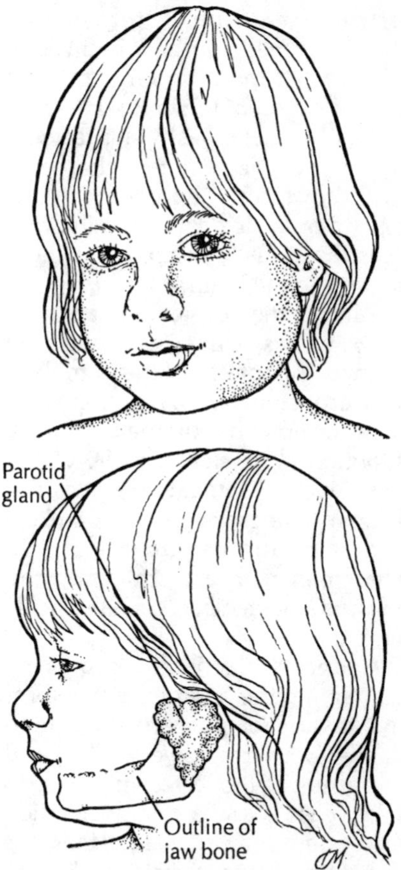

Mumps is caused by a virus that infects the salivary glands, especially the parotid gland. The infection causes a painful swelling of the face in front of the ear.

uncommonly leads to sterility in males. Girls may have swelling in the ovaries (female sex organs), but there is seldom any severe discomfort. In addition, swelling may occur in other glands and organs including the breasts, other saliva glands, liver, and the brain.

Although mumps can be unpleasant, it rarely has long-term complications. If they occur, encephalitis or inflammation of the brain is the most dangerous complication of mumps because it carries the risk of death. Another possible result of mumps encephalitis is hearing loss or even deafness. However, hearing may return to normal after several months. A milder form of brain complication is meningoencephalitis (inflammation of the brain or its covering, the meninges). This disease causes stiff neck, headache, high fever, drowsiness, bright light sensitivity, and possible delirium—all symptoms that usually disappear without damage to the brain.

Pancreatitis, or inflammation of the pancreas, can also result from mumps. Symptoms of this complication are stomach pain, vomiting, chills, fever, and extreme weakness. Although these signs usually vanish and leave no damage, diabetes can result in rare cases. Other complications of mumps include nerve inflammation, heart problems, and nervous system disorders—all usually temporary.

A doctor diagnoses mumps by examining the characteristic form and texture of the swollen parotid glands. Boys may have swelling and tenderness in the testes. Exposure to the disease is also a clue. Incubation—time between exposure to the virus and signs of symptoms—is 14 to 21 days. If mumps is suspected, secretions from the saliva glands can be tested for mumps virus.

Treatment for mumps involves relieving discomfort of the symptoms, since there is no cure for the disease. Bed rest is usually not necessary. Soft foods and liquids may be easier to swallow. However, fruit juices with high acid content, like orange or grapefruit, may sting.

If glands are severely swollen, a physician may prescribe painkilling drugs. Steroid drugs may be recommended for men or boys with extremely swollen testes, but these drugs may prove ineffective. Warm or cold compresses including an ice pack may relieve some pain. Most mumps symptoms disappear within about ten days.

There is a vaccine that is 95 percent effective in preventing mumps. The vaccine encourages antibodies (protective substances) to be produced by the body to resist the disease. Mumps vaccine is usually combined with measles and rubella (German measles) vaccines and given to children as a shot during their second year.

Muscles

Muscles are connective tissues that have the ability to contract. Body movement is affected by three different types of muscle: striated, smooth, and cardiac. Striated, or striped, muscle consists of layers of connective tissue divided into bundles of interwoven fibers running parallel to each other. These layers are attached to the skeleton (bony framework of the body), and they aid the body in voluntary movement. As muscles shorten, they pull on adjacent tendons (fibrous tissue connecting muscles and bones) and bones. This interaction of connecting body parts causes movement.

Smooth, or organic, muscle lines most of the internal organs of the body, including the intestines, bladder, and blood vessels. Therefore, this type of muscle assists all functions controlled by the autonomic nervous system which governs functions under involuntary control. For example, smooth muscle helps circulate blood and gland secretions throughout the body, move material through the digestive tract, and regulate breathing in the lungs. Smooth muscle contains elongated spindly cells arranged parallel to one another that are often grouped into irregular size bundles. Under a microscope, this muscle appears smooth in comparison to the rougher surface of the striated muscle.

Cardiac muscle is the muscle of the heart, and its job is to pump blood within and from the heart. The unique characteristic of this muscle is that its fibers are striated, but they are controlled by the autonomic system.

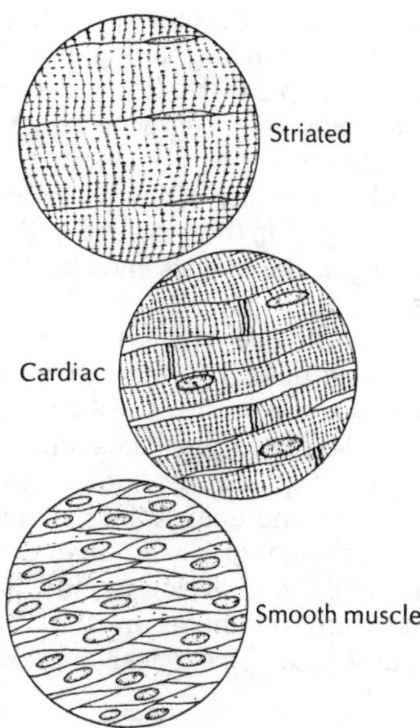

Muscles are connective tissues that have the ability to contract. There are three types of muscles: striated that aid in voluntary movement, smooth that assist functions under involuntary control, and cardiac that is the muscle of the heart.

Muscular dystrophy

Muscular dystrophy is the general term for a group of diseases in which the body's muscles weaken and waste away. Muscular dystrophy almost always strikes in childhood and is usually inherited. Duchenne muscular dystrophy, which is usually inherited through the mother, is probably the most common form of the disease, but all forms—including that one—are fortunately rare.

Boys under the age of three are most apt to develop Duchenne muscular dystrophy. Girls are rarely affected. The disease is progressive, that is, it becomes worse rapidly once it takes hold. In severe forms of muscular dystrophy, the child must use a wheelchair to get around by the age of eleven or twelve. Scoliosis, or curvature of the spine, may also result from the disease.

Severe cases may be fatal, often when the patient is a young adult. Pneumonia is sometimes a fatal complication for the muscular dystrophy patient because of weakening of the chest and diaphragm muscles associated with breathing.

Muscular dystrophy is sometimes confused with multiple sclerosis. The latter is a disease of the nervous system that can ultimately result in crippling. However, there is no deterioration of the nervous system in muscular dystrophy.

Symptoms of muscular dystrophy may vary. Muscles usually begin to weaken first in the hips, legs, and shoulders. A child of four or five who waddles from side to side, who has difficulty standing up properly, or who falls frequently should be checked by a family physician or pediatrician. Sometimes the child even has difficulty standing up straight or raising an arm high above the head.

Parents should not be overly concerned about the natural awkwardness that occasionally overtakes the older toddler. However, a child near five years of age who consistently has problems with muscular coordination should be checked.

The physician may want a muscle biopsy, (a small tissue sample) to confirm a diagnosis of muscular dystrophy.

Traditionally there has been no treatment for severe cases. An exercise program designed by a physical therapist may be helpful in mild cases. In such cases, the prescribed exercises should be performed faithfully to help slow down or hinder the weakening of the muscles.

In any case, physicians advise the parents of the patient to regulate the diet so that the child does not become overweight. The patient is not as active as other children and thus cannot eat as much. Overweight taxes the child's weakening muscles and makes life more difficult.

Because muscular dystrophy is an inherited disease, women in the family should be tested to see if they are carriers—which means they could pass on the disease to their children. Such women should receive genetic counseling regarding any pregnancy.

Myasthenia gravis

Myasthenia gravis is an uncommon disease of the nerves and muscles characterized by great fatigue and weakness in the muscular system, most notably in the face and throat, with slow and progressive paralysis, although the muscles do not atrophy (wither or waste away). It is most likely to strike adults, especially women between the ages of 18 and 25 and men older than 40, but it can affect any individual of any age.

Myasthenia gravis is sometimes associated with hyperthyroidism (overactive thyroid gland), excessive tissue in the thymus (a gland in the chest that is essential to the immune system), or tumors in the thymus.

The condition is a neuromuscular disorder; the muscles fail to receive messages from the nerves because of a lack of the important neurotransmitting chemical, acetylcholine. Experts believe the problem originates in the autoimmune system, making the body fight against tissues instead of protecting them.

The muscular weakness first shows up in the face: eyelids droop, often causing squinting and double vision; there is an inability to move the mouth and lips with subsequent difficulty in talking, chewing, and swallowing; cheeks generally droop or sag, resulting in a characteristic smile or stoical expression. Sometimes the arms and legs are afflicted, affecting basic motor movements like walking, standing, lifting a cup, and other simple tasks. It can also impair breathing. The degree of paralysis or weakness varies from hour to hour and day to day, although it tends to be mininal in the morning and worse at night. Blood tests and chest X rays aid in the diagnosis.

Myasthenia gravis is usually not curable but drugs are available that restore nerve transmission to the muscles. The drugs neostigmine and pyridostigmine reestablish muscle strength and enable the patient with myasthenia gravis to live a more normal life. If it is determined that the problem originates in the thymus gland, it can be surgically removed.

Myopia

Myopia, also called nearsightedness, is a very common optical defect in which the eyes can see close objects clearly but faraway objects look blurred. About one in every five people is myopic; it tends to be hereditary, developing around age 12 and progressing until about age 20.

The defect is caused by an eyeball that is too long from front to back. Normally, the eye's cornea (the curved transparent tissue that covers the front of the eye) and lens (elongated fibers just behind the front of the eye responsible for focus) refract or bend light coming from the viewed distant object so that the image focuses on the retina (a layer of light-sensitive nerve cells that line the back of the eyeball). In myopia, the focused image falls short of the retina because of the greater length of the eyeball, resulting in a fuzzy image.

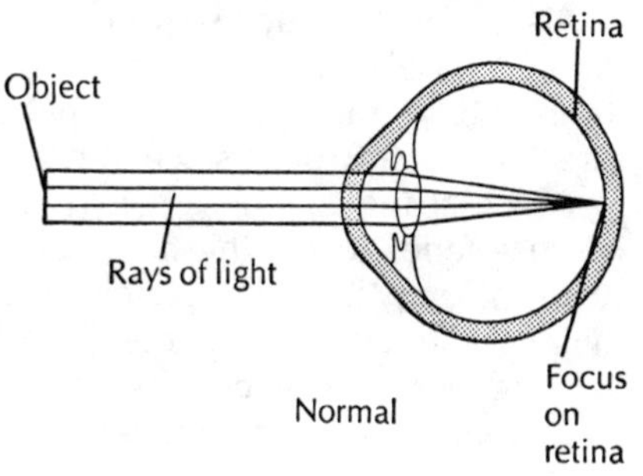

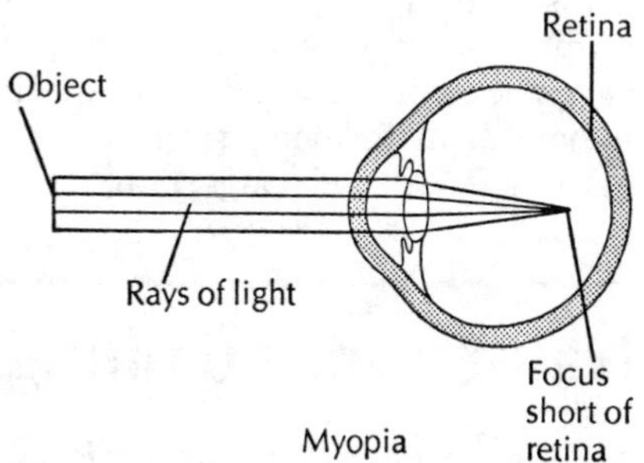

Myopia—nearsightedness—is a vision defect in which the eye can clearly see close objects but distant objects appear blurred. It is caused by an eyeball that is too long front to back causing incoming light to fall short of the light sensitive retina. This results in a fuzzy image.

There are several kinds of myopia. Curvature myopia refers to an excess curve of the refractive surfaces of the eye causing light to enter the eye in an abnormal path. The curvature is either in the front surface of the cornea or the lens. In index myopia, there is an increase in the light-refracting properties of the lens. It is sometimes associated with future development of cataracts or iritis (inflammation of the iris). Progressive myopia is an uncommon form in which the eyeball continues to elongate throughout a person's life, eventually leading to degeneration of the retina or a detached retina.

Blurred or fuzzy vision should be examined by an ophthalmologist (physician who is an eye specialist) who will look inside the eyes with a special instrument (ophthalmoscope), diagnose any disorders, and test the acuity (sharpness) of vision. Nearsightedness is easily corrected with a concave (inwardly curved) lens that pushes the images back to the retina and focuses them clearly.

A surgical procedure known as radial keratotomy corrects myopia but is considered controversial. It involves cutting 16 "spokes" in the cornea coming out from the center; as the cornea heals, it flattens and counteracts the problem.

Myopia rarely progresses after age 30. In fact, the onset of middle age sometimes lessens the condition.

N

Narcolepsy

Narcolepsy is a disorder in which the afflicted person is subject to a recurring, irresistible, uncontrollable desire to sleep, accompanied by muscular weakness and intense emotional reactions. The desire occurs during waking hours and often at inopportune times—during a business meeting, while driving a car, in the middle of a conversation. Although the person falls into a deep sleep, it lasts only a few minutes. The person wakes up feeling refreshed but is likely to fall asleep again soon.

Narcolepsy is not necessarily related to a disease or condition, although it may be associated with cataplexy, a condition in which a person suddenly collapses to the floor at times of stress or unexpected emotional stimulus like laughter. It is thought that narcolepsy may be related to lesions or disturbances in the hypothalmus, a part of the brain, that cause a disorder in the endocrine system.

Amphetamines, which are stimulants, are prescribed to treat narcolepsy.

Nasal congestion

Nasal congestion occurs when the blood vessels in the nose enlarge, thus taking up more space in the nasal cavity and allowing less air to pass through with each breath. These enlarged blood vessels also leak fluid into the surrounding tissues, which fills the nasal cavity and further impairs breathing.

Nasal congestion is not a serious problem in itself, although it may be bothersome enough to interfere with daily activities and sleep. Persistent cases should be reported to a doctor, as nasal congestion may be a symptom of mild infections or more serious disorders.

The common cold, influenza, allergy, and bronchitis are the most frequent causes of nasal congestion. Persistent cases may be caused by structural abnormalities in the nose or by the daily use of certain drugs, particularly those often prescribed for high blood pressure, which act to enlarge all blood vessels, including those in the nose.

Occasional nasal congestion is often treated with nonprescription decongestants such as nasal sprays, nose drops, and nasal inhalers, all of which act to shrink swollen blood vessels in the nose and stop fluid secretion. However, they also may shrink blood vessels elsewhere in the body, resulting in increased blood pressure and heart rate, as well as in nervousness and insomnia. For this reason, over-the-counter decongestants should not be used by those with high blood pressure, heart disease, diabetes, or thyroid disorders.

Also, those who do use decongestants for nasal congestion should use them only for brief periods, perhaps three days at the most; since they act to constrict the blood vessels, their overuse tends to tire the blood vessels, relaxing them completely and making the nose more congested than it was before decongestants were used. This is called rebound congestion.

In addition, specific medicine that is inserted in the nose may be prescribed by a doctor. Also, the use of vaporizers or humidifiers is often beneficial in relieving some of the discomfort of nasal congestion.

Nausea and vomiting

Nausea is an extremely uncomfortable or queasy feeling in the stomach area, often accompanied by an urge to vomit. Vomiting is the forceful ejection of the contents of the stomach through the mouth.

Both nausea and vomiting can be

symptoms of relatively mild upsets in the body chemistry such as motion sickness or of very serious disorders such as peptic ulcer.

Nausea and vomiting originate in an area of the brain called, interestingly, the vomiting center. The vomiting center receives impulses from the network of nerves extending throughout the body. When nerves which supply information from both the digestive system and the inner ear (part of which controls balance) deliver the message that vomiting is necessary, the person will vomit.

Nausea and vomiting are usually temporary conditions and are sometimes beneficial, because they result in the expulsion of something potentially harmful to the body. However, persistent or recurring vomiting can lead to a dangerous loss of fluids and salts (called dehydration) and of nutrients, as well as to damage to the esophagus (the passageway from the mouth to the stomach) or upper stomach.

Several relatively mild conditions and disorders may cause nausea and vomiting, including motion sickness, the morning sickness of pregnancy, excessive alcohol intake, emotional upset, drug side effects, eating too much, eating especially bothersome foods such as oily or greasy foods, and eating spoiled food. More serious conditions that may be accompanied by nausea and vomiting are severe injury or pain, serious disorders of the digestive system (such as peptic ulcer or gastritis), heart disease, and gland disorders. Additionally, vomiting without the feeling of nausea preceding it may be a symptom of brain injury or brain tumor.

The symptoms that accompany nausea include a "sour" or queasy stomach, chills, perspiration, drowsiness, headache, rapid heartbeat and breathing rates, and salivation (excess saliva).

Most nausea and vomiting will require little or no treatment, as these symptoms will subside when the factor causing them is removed or corrected. However, if vomiting occurs regularly or frequently without an obvious cause, or if blood or red or dark brown spots appear in the vomitus, medical treatment should be sought immediately and a sample of the vomitus may be examined.

Home remedies will often help to relieve the discomfort of occasional bouts of nausea and vomiting. Drinking tea, non-cola beverages, especially ginger ale, and soup or broth is often suggested because liquids need to be replaced because of the fluid loss experienced during vomiting. Solid food usually is not recommended, but when vomiting subsides, toast or crackers may be tried before returning to a normal diet.

Several medications can successfully control the urge to vomit, but they need to be prescribed by a doctor and should only be used with caution. In addition, any woman who is pregnant or thinks she may be pregnant should consult with her doctor before taking this or any other type of medication.

See also Dehydration and Hyperemesis gravidarum.

Necrosis

Necrosis is the death of individual cells, group of cells, or localized areas of tissue or bone while the surrounding tissue remains alive and healthy.

The tissue or bone dies because it has not survived the ravages of an infection or because it has been cut off from its blood supply by any one of several diseases or conditions. Necrosis can occur in tumors that outgrow their blood supply; in any area of the body where the nurturing blood vessels have been blocked by fatty deposits (atherosclerosis), clots, or emboli; in small areas of the heart following a heart attack; or in bones where osteomyelitis (inflammation of the bone due to infection) chokes off the arteries supplying the bone.

The symptoms and management of necrosis vary widely depending upon the underlying infection or blockage.

See also Gangrene.

Nephritis

See Glomerulonephritis and Pyelonephritis.

Nephrotic syndrome

Nephrotic syndrome is a disorder most commonly affecting children in which the glomeruli, tiny clumps of blood vessels in the kidneys that filter urine, do not work properly. The defective glomeruli allow proteins, most notably albumin, to escape from the bloodstream and seep into the urine while letting fluid that should be eliminated as waste accumulate under the skin.

As a result, the child's body gradually swells up (edema), becoming especially bloated around the face, abdomen, and ankles. In addition, the child urinates very little, about one fifth the normal amount. The syndrome usually affects children between the ages of one and six years, more often boys than girls. If initial blood and urine tests point to nephrotic syndrome, the doctor will order more tests and possibly a kidney biopsy (tissue sample) to confirm the diagnosis.

Nephrotic syndrome is caused by other diseases that affect the kidneys and although it is a relatively rare disorder, it is a serious one that requires careful treatment for children who are afflicted by it. The syndrome causes a vulnerability to other infections, including peritonitis (inflammation of the lining of the abdominal cavity), and the risk that the condition may persist and develop into chronic glomerulonephritis and eventually kidney failure.

With proper medical care, however, usually in a hospital where medication (diuretics to eliminate excess fluid and steroids to control inflammation) and diet (high in protein and low in salt) can be carefully supervised, the condition can be controlled. Symptoms are likely to clear up after a few weeks and the child can finish recuperating at home, sometimes with no aftereffects, other times with a relapse after several weeks or months.

To prevent complications, a doctor should be consulted as soon as a child either urinates less often or has unusual swelling in the face, abdomen, or ankles.

Nervous system

The nervous system is a complex network of specialized tissue that regulates thoughts, emotions, actions, sensations, and basic body functions. The basic element of the nervous system is the neuron, or nerve cell. In combination, these neurons form nerve fibers that transmit impulses throughout the body. To protect neural function, myelin, a fatty substance, provides insulation for fibers of the nervous system.

There are two major divisions of the nervous system, the central nervous system and the peripheral nervous system. Distinctions between

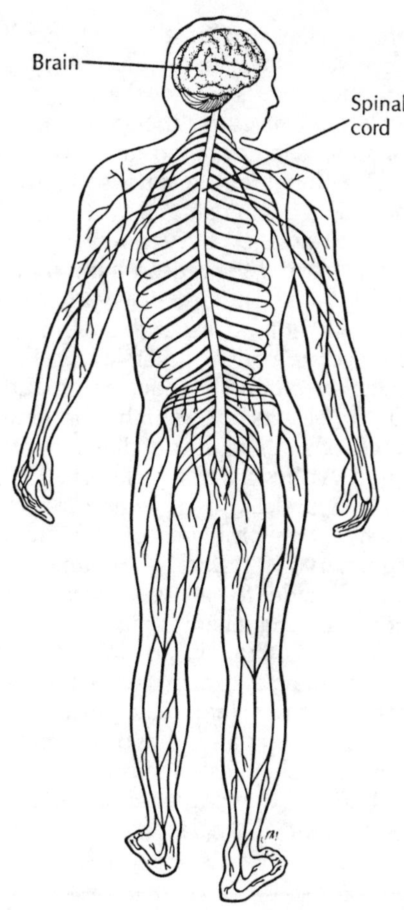

The nervous system has two major divisions: the central nervous system and the peripheral nervous system. This illustration shows the central nervous system (brain and spinal cord) and the peripheral nervous system (nerves that branch out from brain and spinal cord).

them depend upon function and location. The *central nervous system* consists of the brain and spinal cord. The brain is the control center of the body that lies within the skull (bony formation of the head). It governs body functions by sending and receiving messages through the spinal cord. Protecting the brain and spinal cord are bones, layers of tissue, and spinal fluid.

Once messages leave the central nervous system, they are carried by the *peripheral nervous system*. The peripheral system includes the cranial nerves (nerves branching from the brain) and spinal nerves (nerves branching from the spinal cord). These nerves convey sensory messages from receptor cells in the body to the central nervous system. They also transport motor impulses from the central system back to the body where muscles and glands can respond to the impulses.

The *autonomic nervous system,* which is part of the peripheral nervous system, regulates all activity that is involuntary but necessary for life, including activity of the internal organs and glands.

Working together, the entire system coordinates adjustment and reaction of the body to internal and external environmental conditions.

See also Brain.

Neuralgia

Neuralgia is pain that runs along the course of a damaged nerve. The condition ranges from mild and temporary to severe and chronic, but the pain itself is characteristically sharp and extreme, lasting only a few seconds at a time but tending to recur.

The source of the injury to the nerve depends upon the type of neuralgia. Tic douloureux or trigeminal neuralgia, the most common form, affects the faces of people over age 50 (except in cases of multiple sclerosis) and more commonly over age 70. The trigeminal nerve controls sensation in the face, teeth, mouth, and nasal cavity and triggers the muscles that move the jaw. The pain, usually excruciating, covers one side of the face and can be set off by eating, washing, or even by a gust of air. Eventually the stabbing pains occur closer together until they are constant. The cause is unknown, and, although not serious, it can become very disabling.

Sciatica pain is initiated by pressure on the body's largest nerve (sciatic) which runs from the spinal cord through the lower body and legs. The pressure is usually caused by a slipped disk between the vertebrae (backbones). The pain burns through the buttocks and along the back of the thighs and worsens if the patient coughs, sneezes, or bends.

In peripheral neuropathy, impairment of the peripheral nerves, those outside the brain and spinal cord, occurs as a complication of other disorders—diabetes mellitus, alcoholism, a vitamin deficiency, anemia, tumors, or overexposure to certain chemicals and drugs (typical of farm and industrial workers). Symptoms begin as a tingling sensation in the hands and feet that slowly spreads up the limbs to the trunk; numbness follows in the same pattern, the skin becomes sensitive, and neuralgic pain ensues. Numbness in the hands leads to a loss of dexterity and susceptibility to accidents. A special risk is that a numbed part of the body can sustain an injury without the patient's awareness until it becomes infected or ulcerated. The muscles gradually atrophy (wither away), and paralysis may set in.

Carpal tunnel syndrome is compression of the large nerve that passes through the "tunnel" created by the wrist bones. It is fairly common, especially in pregnant women. Numbness, tingling, and a burning pain in the hand at first wake the patient at night and then begin occurring during the day.

Shingles or herpes zoster is a viral infection characterized by intense pain and skin rash along the course of a nerve. Red blisters appear in a band usually along one side of the chest, trunk, or abdomen and can attack a nerve across the forehead. It occurs in adults during times of stress or after exposure to chicken pox which is caused by the same virus. Shingles can be diagnosed by sight.

Treatment for the various types of neuralgia depends upon the location of the damaged nerves, severity of the pain, and the reason behind the impairment. Therapy may vary from cold or hot packs and aspirin to stronger prescription painkillers. For shingles, ointments may soothe and dry up blisters but, as with most viral infections, there is no direct treatment. A physician may refer a patient with neuralgia to a neurologist, a specialist in problems of the brain and nervous system. A neurologist may decide to sever a damaged nerve to eliminate the pain.

There is virtually no way to prevent neuralgia, except to treat underlying diseases that may precipitate nerve damage and to avoid overexposure to chemicals and drugs.

See also Carpal tunnel syndrome, Sciatica, and Shingles.

Neurotransmitters

Neurotransmitters are chemicals that transmit nerve impulses from one nerve cell to another. The basic units of nerves are neurons, and their action is both electrical and chemical. At the ends of threadlike fibers extending outward from the core of each neuron are tiny sacs containing neurotransmitter chemical. After an electrical nerve impulse has traveled across a neuron, it reaches the nerve ending and stimulates the release of neurotransmitters from their sacs. The neurotransmitters travel across the gap (synapse) to the nerve ending of the next neuron and stimulate the production of an electrical charge that carries the nerve impulse forward. The process is then repeated until a muscle is moved or relaxed or a sensory impression is noted by the brain or a lower part of the central nervous system.

Night blindness

Night blindness—or nyctalopia—is a condition whereby a person can see well in good light but not in dim or fading light.

Photoreceptors (nerve-end organs sensitive to light) in the retina make the adjustments that govern the eyes' ability to adapt to varying degrees of light. The retina is a layer of light-sensitive nerve cells that lines the interior of the eyeball; it acts as the film for images the eye sees. The nerve cells are either cones or rods. Cones, concentrated in the center of the retina, distinguish fine detail and color while rods, which are around the edges of the retina, are sensitive to the intensity of light and do most of the work of seeing in dim light. Rods contain the pigment rhodopsin or visual purple that becomes temporarily bleached out by bright light. The speed at which rhodopsin adjusts to darkness depends upon a sufficient supply of Vitamin A in the body.

Night blindness is caused by either a severe deficiency of Vitamin A or by retinitis pigmentosa, an inherited degenerative disorder of the retina. In cases of extreme Vitamin A shortage, the cornea may soften or start to dissolve (keratomalacia) or the eyes may become excessively dry (xerophthalmia). The Vitamin A deficiency can be treated with doses of the vitamin but there is no cure for retinitis pigmentosa.

The only way to prevent night blindness is to include enough Vitamin A in the diet.

See also Retinitis.

Nongonococcal urethritis

Nongonococcal urethritis (NGU), also known as nonspecific urethritis, is a sexually transmitted disease that causes an inflammation of the urethra. A sexually transmitted disease, also known as venereal disease, is a highly contagious illness spread primarily through direct sexual contact.

NGU, left untreated, can lead to arthritis, prostatitis (inflammation of the prostate), and epididymitis (inflammation of the ducts leading from the testes) in men, and pelvic inflammatory disease (an inflammation of the fallopian tubes) in women. It can be transmitted from a mother to her baby during childbirth, resulting in ear infections and pneumonia; it has also been linked to an increased risk of stillbirths and sudden infant death syndrome.

NGU is transmitted by direct sexual contact with an infected person. It displays symptoms similar to gonorrhea, although it is not caused by the gonorrhea bacterium but by several others including one called chlamydia.

Sometimes no symptoms are evident when NGU is present; in other cases there is a discharge from the penis or vagina, painful and burning urination, and other symptoms similar to those of gonorrhea. In fact, NGU can occur at the same time that gonorrhea is present, so if symptoms persist after treatment for gonorrhea, it may be that NGU also exists.

Diagnosis of NGU is often difficult because there is no one simple test for it; a sample of secretions from the penis or vagina may be taken to determine if chlamydia is present, but many labs do not do this test and those that do may charge a very high fee. Therefore, NGU is often diagnosed by ruling out other disorders that may display similar symptoms, such as gonorrhea or cystitis (bladder infection).

Penicillin has no effect on NGU, so this disease is treated with other antibiotics, such as tetracycline. This is the reason that treatment for gonorrhea, usually penicillin, will not affect NGU.

A person who has NGU or any other sexually transmitted disease should abstain from sexual activity until all tests have indicated that the disease is no longer present. This disease requires that every sexual partner of the infected person also be examined and treated if necessary.

NGU can be prevented by avoiding sexual contact with someone who has the disease. Since this is not always possible, it should be remembered that the chances of contracting NGU or any other sexually transmitted disease increase with the number of different sexual partners a person has.

See also Cystitis, Gonorrhea, Pelvic inflammatory disease, and Prostatitis.

Nose

See Ear, nose and throat.

Nosebleeds

A nosebleed occurs when there is a break in the blood vessels in the inner lining of the nose, causing bleeding from the nose. Nosebleeds seldom require medical attention, but it is possible, although quite rare, for nosebleeds to be symptoms of serious illnesses.

Nosebleeds can be caused by an injury to the nose; breathing dry air for long periods; repeated blowing or picking of the nose; tumors in the nose; or high blood pressure or other blood diseases.

Very persistent or frequently occurring nosebleeds will require the attention of a doctor who may cauterize (use heat or the application of the chemical silver nitrate to seal off) the blood vessels in the back of the nose.

However, occasional nosebleeds can be treated by simply sitting up and leaning forward, so as not to swallow the blood, and pinching the entire soft portion of the nose between the thumb and forefinger for ten minutes. If the bleeding does not stop, cold packs can be applied to the bridge of the nose for 15 to 20 minutes. If bleeding still persists, a doctor should be notified.

Frequent nosebleeds from dry air may be relieved by the use of a humidifier. Also, those who have frequent nosebleeds should not blow the nose too harshly or blow through one nostril.

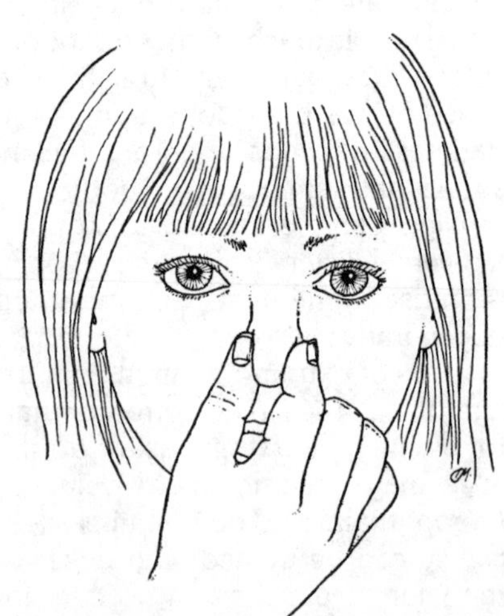

An occasional nosebleed can be treated by sitting up and pinching the entire soft portion of the nose between the thumb and forefinger for ten minutes.

When nosebleeds occur along with colds or other respiratory infections, a nasal decongestant may help to shrink the blood vessels in the nose. However, these decongestants should not be used by anyone with high blood pressure, heart disease, diabetes, or thyroid disorders, because decongestants also shrink blood vessels in parts of the body other than the nose, which can lead to complications for these patients.

Nystagmus

Nystagmus is the involuntary, rhythmic, and rapid movement of the eyeballs in a horizontal, vertical, or rotary direction. A person who sits in a moving vehicle and watches the scenery flashing by demonstrates normal nystagmus.

Abnormal nystagmus is brought on by one of three problems: defective vison in which the eye does not receive enough stimulation for it to concentrate on one object; disturbances in the elaborate mechanisms in the ear responsible for balance; and diseases of the nervous system especially those parts of the brain responsible for eye movement and coordination. Generally, the only symptoms are double vision or vertigo and dizziness. Treatment depends on the underlying cause.

O

Obesity

Obesity is a term commonly applied to body weight that is 20 percent or more above normal weight. It has been linked statistically to high blood pressure, diabetes, cardiovascular disease, and chronic back and joint pains, among other ailments, and it is a potentially serious condition that shortens life span.

The risk of disease and death among the obese is greater for men than for women, but for both it increases in direct proportion to the degree of overweight. For example, among those who are 20 percent overweight there are 25 percent more deaths for men and 21 percent more for women than among those of normal weight in a given age group; and for those 30 percent overweight, there are 42 percent more deaths for men and 30 percent more for women.

Obesity tends to occur more frequently in some families than in others. This may indicate a hereditary tendency, or it may be due to family food patterns and attitudes toward food. Women tend to gain weight after the menopause and men gain in middle age. Overweight chil-

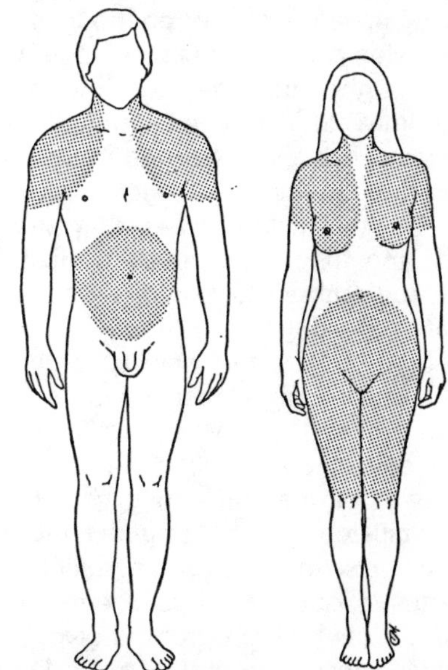

The shaded areas show where fat buildup most commonly occurs in men and women.

dren often grow up to be overweight adults. This is particularly true when food is used as a reward for a child or is withheld as a punishment. Food may then come to represent security and love—an attitude toward food that often continues into adult life.

The cause of obesity is virtually always the direct result of taking in more food than is "burned off" in activity. (Certain glandular disturbances can affect the appetite or the distribution of fat on the body, but these conditions are uncommon.) The appetite for food is influenced by habit as well as by emotional factors, and it is not always prompted by hunger. The appetite center, or feeding center, is the area in the brain that controls the appetite. It is thought to be located in the brain area called the hypothalamus. The coined term "appestat," suggested by the word "thermostat," has been used for the mechanism of appetite control.

The connection between smoking, appetite, and weight gain is unclear. Smoking has been said to inhibit, or decrease, appetite, so that giving up smoking is often thought to be followed by increased appetite and weight gain. The gain in weight that may follow when smoking is stopped has also been attributed to the dependence of some smokers on oral satisfaction; when they stop smoking, they are impelled to substitute the oral satisfaction of eating for that of smoking.

The treatment of obesity is twofold: eat less and exercise more. A low-calorie diet that is nutritionally well-balanced and that can form the basis of permanent eating habits is the first step. Combined with a regular exercise program, such a diet can eliminate obesity. Anyone embarking on such a program, however, should consult a doctor for a checkup and for guidance.

Appetite-decreasing drugs can be harmful and should be taken only under medical supervision. Even physicians who use them in selected cases recognize that these drugs are at best only a temporary prop and not an answer to the problem of overweight over a period of time.

Crash diets and fad diets can lead to vitamin and nutritional deficiencies; if they are effective at all, it is basically only because they furnish fewer total calories. The quick weight loss that many such diets promise is often merely a loss of fluid from the body tissues, and the weight lost will quickly be regained as the fluid is replaced.

Massage is not effective in removing or redistributing local fat deposits. Hot baths and sweating serve only to remove water from the tissues, which will soon be replaced.

In extreme cases surgery is sometimes resorted to to remove excessive layers of fatty tissue, such as pendulous breasts; but the expense of the operation and the inherent dangers of any surgery make this a treatment of last resort. The same caution should be exercised with stomach-stapling surgery or bypass surgery.

It is particularly important for parents to teach children good eating habits and to control any tendency to overweight before it has become a serious problem. The old notions that children should have food urged on them and that a fat child is a healthy child should be recognized as not only false but harmful. Older people, too, need to take special care to avoid overweight. They tend to be less active than in their younger days, yet may continue to follow their established eating patterns. Reduced activity may make it necessary for the elderly to seek out means of regular exercise — whether it be calisthenics or sports such as swimming, bicycling, bowling, or hiking—that are suited to their capacities and tastes.

One safeguard for those of all ages is to control overweight strictly, at an early stage, by weighing daily and embarking on a diet-and-exercise plan as soon as the weight is three to five pounds above the norm for the individual's height and body type. It is far easier to take off a few pounds than to wait until massive obesity requires a protracted and difficult struggle. Increased life span and improved health and vigor will be a satisfying reward.

See also Bypass surgery.

Occult blood

Occult blood is a term referring to amounts of blood so minute (small) that they cannot be seen by the naked eye and are only detectable with a chemical test or a microscopic examination. The term is generally used in reference to blood in the stools, or feces, that indicates bleeding along the gastrointestinal tract.

Often, the only symptom of occult bleeding is the fatigue caused by the loss of oxygen-carrying red blood cells. Between 50 and 200 milliliters (three to 15 tablespoons) of blood can be passed in one stool with no visible indication that it is present.

Such bleeding is not always constant, so tests are typically run on three samples of stools if a problem is suspected. The patient must not eat red meat for three days before taking the samples because even cooked blood from meat can test as positive for occult blood.

Occult blood may also be present in the urine, indicating bleeding at some point in the urinary system.

Onychogryphosis

Onychogryphosis (or onychogryposis) refers to unusual nail growth, to the extent that the nail begins to resemble a claw or horn. The nail becomes thick, long, horny or raised, and green or black in color with an opaque surface. It happens most often in toenails.

Injury caused by going barefoot or wearing tight shoes is the usual cause of onychogryphosis, but the condition can also be hereditary or connected to congestive heart failure, in which there may be a shortage of blood circulation to the feet; peripheral neuritis which affects nerves in the legs causing decreased sensation in the feet and therefore increasing the chance that the foot will be injured; ichtyosis (dry, scaly skin); hormonal disorders; syphilis; and stroke.

Properly-fitting shoes, hot baths, massage with warm oil or hydrogen peroxide, or treatment of the underlying disease should clear up the condition.

Onychomycosis

The most common of inflammatory nail disorders, onychomycosis is a fungal infection of the nails that is prevalent among those with a low resistance to infection (diabetics or patients taking corticosteroid, or hormonal, drugs), those who work with their hands in water and are prone to paronychia (inflammation of the skin around the nail), or those with ingrown toenails.

Onychomycosis is caused by a number of fungi and is most often a result of paronychia. Chronic but painless, the affected nails look dull, opaque, and brittle; are marked with grooves or ridges; and appear flaky. The surrounding cuticle may become red, tender, and swollen, and ooze pus if a bacterial infection accompanies the disorder. The fungi can be identified by examining nail scrapings in the laboratory.

The condition is treated with griseofulvin, an antifungal drug that can be taken orally or applied topically. However, it may take months to cure. Furthermore, the condition may never clear up at all, especially if the toenails are affected. Cutting the nails short or removing the entire nail can help the healing process.

To prevent onychomycosis, fingernails and toenails should be dried thoroughly after bathing; footwear should be changed often if feet tend to perspire. Thorough drying eliminates the moisture that fungi thrive in.

Oophorectomy

Oophorectomy is surgical removal of an ovary, either one of the two female sex glands situated above and on either side of the uterus. The ovaries are almond-shaped organs, about an inch and one-half long, that produce an egg for fertilization each month and also secrete the female sex hormones. An oophorectomy is a major operation, usually performed through either a vertical or horizontal incision in the abdominal area but occasionally through an incision in the vagina.

Removal of one ovary (unilateral oophorectomy) may include a salpingectomy—removal of all or part of the nearby fallopian tube that transports eggs to the uterus. Removal of both ovaries is a bilateral oophorectomy. A bilateral salpingo-oophorectomy – removal of both ovaries and both fallopian tubes – ends a woman's ability to conceive children. A hysterectomy (removal of the uterus) is generally performed in conjunction with a bilateral oophorectomy because the uterus has no purpose without either ovary and, if left, can harbor tumors later on.

Oophorectomies correct a number of conditions in which the ovaries are the site of the trouble, including an ectopic pregnancy, in which the embryo is lodged in the ovary, and benign (noncancerous) and malignant (cancerous) ovarian cysts and tumors. In women with recurrent cancer or endometriosis (a condition in which parts of the uterine lining are displaced outside the uterus), physicians do oophorectomies intentionally to stop hormone production, which tends to aggravate the problem. Breast cancer, as well, may be dependent on hormones to grow; about one third of the women with breast cancer show a decrease in breast cancer growth after removal of their ovaries.

For a woman in her childbearing years, doctors make every effort to save any healthy ovarian tissue. Because the ovaries are fed by an excellent blood supply, they heal quickly and even a small bit of preserved ovarian tissue will function, secrete hormones, and discharge eggs. The woman remains fertile and avoids an early menopause.

Some physicians recommend a bilateral oophorectomy when the uterus must be taken out. There are pros and cons to removing healthy ovaries. Arguments for their removal are: it eliminates the possibility of ovarian cancer, since the hysterectomy may interfere with blood supply to the ovaries; a small number of women will develop cystic ovaries and pain, requiring a second operation anyway; and, if a woman is in her 40s, the ovaries will naturally stop functioning within a few years. Arguments against a routine oophorectomy are: it causes the onset of premature menopause, which brings with it greater risks of high blood pressure and osteoporosis (loss of bone mass); the abrupt end of hormone production is less natural than the gradual tapering off of a natural menopause, provoking severe menopausal symptoms, such as hot flashes and vaginal shrinkage; and estrogen, the hormone usually prescribed after a bilateral oophorectomy, may increase the risk of breast cancer.

In women past menopause, for whom fertility is no longer an issue and in whom the ovaries are no longer producing estrogen anyway, both ovaries and uterus are commonly removed even if only one ovary is abnormal.

See also Hysterectomy and Ovarian cysts.

Osteitis deformans

See Paget's disease of the bone.

Osteoarthritis

See Arthritis.

Osteomyelitis

Osteomyelitis is inflammation of the bone and bone marrow due to a pus-producing bacterial infection. It is considered a childhood disease, occurring most often in boys between the ages of five and 14, but also occurs among adults. Since the introduction of antibiotics, osteomyelitis is rare in the United States, but still common in countries lacking good medical care and proper nutrition.

Although bone is fed essential oxygen and nutrients by blood vessels, blood may also carry bacteria, which tend to settle in the capillaries of the long (arm and leg) bones. Germs can also reach the bones directly from adjacent infected tissue or through an open wound or fracture. Usually osteomyelitis affects only one area of the bone or bone marrow, but can attack more than one bone at a time.

Symptoms include: pain and excruciating tenderness near a joint or at the affected area; fever in the 102 and 104°F range; redness and swelling. Although a physician can often diagnose osteomyelitis from the visible symptoms, X rays and blood tests confirm its presence.

Complications may prolong treatment. The child with the condition is often hospitalized and given antibiotics in liquid, tablet, or intravenous (into the vein) form. Doctors may drain the pus and clean the area in a minor surgical procedure and then immobilize the limb in a splint. The child is released from the hospital once the healing begins, but may have to take antibiotics for six more weeks.

Possible complications are blood poisoning (septicemia); destruction of the bone; spread of the infection to a nearby joint, possibly resulting in a permanent deformity or stiffness; transference of the infection to the surface of the skin where it erupts as an abscess (collection of pus in a cavity); damage to the bone cartilage (elastic connective tissue) that retards bone growth; and suppurative (infectious) arthritis.

Chronic (long-term) osteomyelitis is a possible delayed complication of acute (sudden) osteomyelitis, especially if it results from a fracture or the presence of a foreign body in a wound such as a bullet or metal surgical piece. The major signs of chronic osteomyelitis are a flare-up or reopening of an abscessed wound with a fluctuating discharge of pus and pain, and bone that feels thickened and is covered over by scars. X rays show irregular bone and pieces of dead bone. Chronic osteomyelitis can be prevented by immediate antibiotic treatment of the acute variety.

Treatment for chronic osteomyelitis may be extensive. It may take several successive operations to remove all the dead bone and tissue, completely drain the abscess, and repair bone when possible. Large doses of antibiotics may be required.

To prevent osteomyelitis, clean and disinfect all wounds thoroughly and, especially in children, apply a bandage to keep the area clean until it has healed.

Osteoporosis

Osteoporosis is a common disorder characterized by a decrease in the calcium content of bone tissue that leaves the skeletal system thin and susceptible to fracture.

To date, the cause of osteoporosis is unknown. However, chances of acquiring the disease seem to increase dramatically with age, especially for women. One prevailing theory maintains that osteoporosis results from a loss of the female hormone estrogen, which affects the calcium content of the bones. Menopause (cessation of menstruation or periods) often leads to osteoporosis because the body's production of estrogen is reduced at this time. Almost one third of all women over 60 years of age have the disease to some extent.

For reasons not entirely known, white and Oriental women are likelier to develop osteoporosis than black women. In addition slender females, especially those with fair skin, run a higher risk than stouter, thicker-skinned women.

Besides developing spontaneously, osteoporosis can also appear as a result of other conditions. Surgical removal of both ovaries (the female sex glands that produce estrogen), chronic arthritis (inflammation of the joints), or Paget's disease (a disorder of unknown origin that results in bone destruction) may lead to osteoporosis. People who are inactive, either by choice or because of confinement from illness, seem more susceptible to the disorder. In addition, a diet without various nutrients, especially calcium, that promote bone development may also contribute to osteoporosis.

Depending upon the strength of the bones, osteoporosis may initially show either no symptoms or extreme pain, commonly in the lower back. The disease is not life-threatening, but it may lead to serious fractures which, for the elderly, can result in serious complications. Initially, sudden back pain may follow fracture of the vertebrae, bones in the spine. Pain from the fracture itself may subside but discomfort from osteoporosis may continue. This pain may lead to further inactivity which may weaken additional vertebrae. Hence, a vicious cycle develops whereby pain leading to inactivity encourages osteoporosis which, in turn, increases bone fragility.

As the disease progresses, the spinal column may become reduced in length or may become curved due to the pressure of body weight—hence, the term "widow's hump" or "dowager's hump." As osteoporosis progresses, the individual may actually lose several inches in height.

Often, osteoporosis progresses undetected until a fractured bone develops and an X ray is taken. At this time, a physician may notice that bone thinning has become a generalized condition throughout the body.

Physicians urge patients with osteoporosis to follow and exercise program that will strengthen the mus-

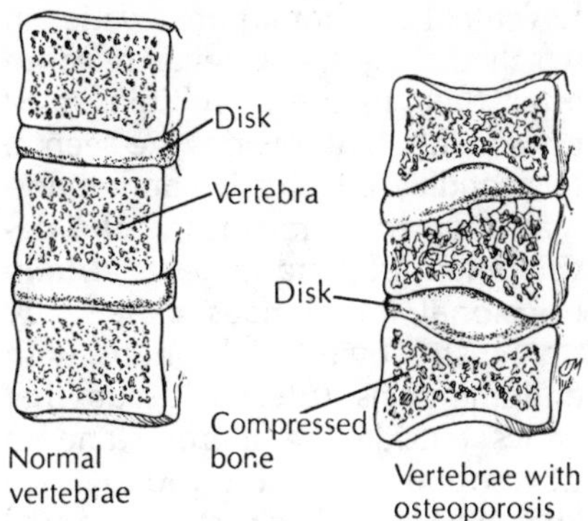

Osteoporosis, a condition in which the bones weaken and break easily, may lead to compression of the vertebrae (backbones) because of the pressure of the body's weight on the weakened vertebrae.

cles supporting weakened bones. To protect bones in the spinal column, however, lifting heavy objects should be avoided. For advanced cases, a back brace may be necessary to support body weight while sitting or standing. Crutches, walkers, or a cane may assist walking.

Sometimes, physicians prescribe the female hormone estrogen to women to decrease bone loss. Women taking these medications need careful supervision as the hormones may cause adverse side effects. Anyone receiving estrogen therapy should have a physical examination and a Pap test (examination of cells scraped from the vagina and cervix to detect cancer) every six months because of a suspected link between estrogen supplements and uterine and breast cancer. Men may be given the male hormone testosterone, which stimulates growth of body tissues, to treat osteoporosis.

For people prone to injury from osteoporosis, a balanced diet is an important factor in preventing or controlling the disease. Foods rich in vitamins and minerals, particularly calcium and Vitamin D, encourage bone formation. When the diet is deficient in these ingredients, vitamin and mineral supplements may be prescribed.

Otitis media

See Ear infections.

Otosclerosis

Otosclerosis is an abnormal spongy overgrowth of bone in the middle ear that leads to totally or partially muffled hearing or deafness. The excess bone grows at the entrance to the middle ear where it immobilizes the base of the stapes, a tiny stirrup-shaped bone that is one of three interconnected bones transmitting sound waves to the inner ear. As a result, sound-conducting vibrations are diminished and impaired hearing results. In most cases, both ears are affected. The cause of otosclerosis is unknown, but the condition tends to be hereditary.

Hearing loss generally begins in the late teens or early 20s; the rate of deafness may accelerate and stabilize several times, but ordinarily the loss is complete within ten to 15 years, sometimes sooner in children. In some cases, the hearing loss stops just short of deafness and the affected person still can hear loud sounds. Otosclerosis usually affects one ear before the other and is preceded by tinnitus (ringing in the ear). Special hearing tests aid in diagnosis.

The only way to halt or reverse otosclerosis is surgery—treatment that is successful about 70 percent of the time. Although a hearing aid can help, most doctors prefer to operate. In a procedure called a stapedectomy, a surgeon folds back the eardrum, removes the affected stapes and replaces it with a synthetic or wire substitute that restores the conductive vibrations of the inner ear. Because the bones involved are the tiniest in the body, the surgery is very delicate and carries a 2 to 5 percent risk of failure. However, in most cases the operation is only done on one ear at a time, thereby reducing the risk.

After surgery, the hearing of most patients is greatly improved within two to three weeks. Sometimes a residual blood clot at the site of the surgery temporarily blocks hearing until it dissolves. Patients with advanced otosclerosis in both ears are usually advised to undergo the stapedectomy as soon as possible.

See also Deafness.

Ovarian cysts

Ovarian cysts are abnormal swellings or sac-like growths on an ovary, either one of the two female sex glands situated above and on either side of the uterus that produce eggs and female sex hormones. Ovarian cysts may be liquid-filled or semifluid.

Most cysts are small but can vary in size from less than an inch in diameter to as big as 15 to 20 inches in diameter and, depending on their size, type, and location, can be symptom-free or can cause severe pain and complications. They are common among women between the ages of 20 and 50 and can grow alone or in groups, on one ovary or both. Approximately 85 percent are benign (noncancerous).

The origin of most ovarian cysts is unknown. In some instances, they develop from an abnormal egg. Others originate as eggs that stay in the ovary instead of leaving after they ripen. Still others are related to abnormalities in the ovary.

Polycystic ovaries (the Stein-Leventhal syndrome) are ovaries in which the eggs are never released after they mature. Multiple small cysts within both ovaries are seen in this condition. Excessive and abnormal body hair growth and the development of acne may result from hormonal imbalances caused by polycystic ovaries. Women with endometriosis (uterine tissue that grows outside the uterus) tend to develop growths on the ovaries known as chocolate cysts, so named because their fluid resembles chocolate. Dermoid cysts are most commonly found in women under age 30; they arise from the ovarian cells that produce the eggs, and the cysts may contain fragments of hair, teeth, bone, and sweat and oil glands.

Symptoms of ovarian cysts vary with the type of growth. Some bear no symptoms and are only discovered during a routine pelvic examination. Others cause firm, painless swelling in the lower abdomen; pain during sexual intercourse; frequent urination (if they press against the bladder); irregular vaginal bleeding; an increase in body hair (if they affect the hormone-producing capabilities of the ovaries); or pain, nausea, and fever (if the cysts rupture or grow on stalks that get twisted).

Cysts can rupture during sexual intercourse, a fall, childbirth, surgery, or for no apparent reason. The resulting effect depends upon how irritating the cystic fluid is to the surrounding tissues, which immediately emit a fibrous material, or adhesions, to defend themselves against the contents of the cyst. The situation can be dangerous if the fluid is infected, cancerous, or extremely irritating.

Ovarian cysts are diagnosed by pelvic, or vaginal, examination or laparoscopy (a surgical procedure in which a telescopic-like instrument is inserted through the abdominal wall to view the pelvic organs). Sometimes they are difficult to diagnose accurately because symptoms can resemble acute appendicitis or other abdominal problems. In addition, it can be hard to determine if a cyst is malignant or not and if it is actually on the ovary or some other pelvic organ without performing either laparoscopy or a laparotomy (examination through an incision in the abdomen). Ovarian cysts that develop during pregnancy are also difficult to diagnose.

Some cysts require no treatment if they are small, not creating any problems, or are likely to disappear on their own. If treatment is necessary, cysts may be drained with a laparoscope, but most are removed surgically. Removal involves either taking out the entire ovary (oophorectomy) or taking out only the cyst (cystectomy).

If the ovarian cyst proves to be cancerous, it is necessary to remove both ovaries, both fallopian tubes, and the uterus since the cancer may have spread from the ovarian cyst to these other structures. If an ovarian cyst is found in a woman after menopause, it must always be removed since these cysts often prove to be cancerous. Removal of both ovaries, tubes, and the uterus is also performed in this case.

See also Cyst, Hysterectomy, and Oophorectomy.

Ovulation

Ovulation is the process in which an ovary—one of two glands near the top of the uterus that secrete female sex hormones—releases an egg. The egg develops in a small fluid-filled sac called a follicle. When ovulation occurs, this sac ruptures, releasing an egg from the ovary.

Extending from either side of the

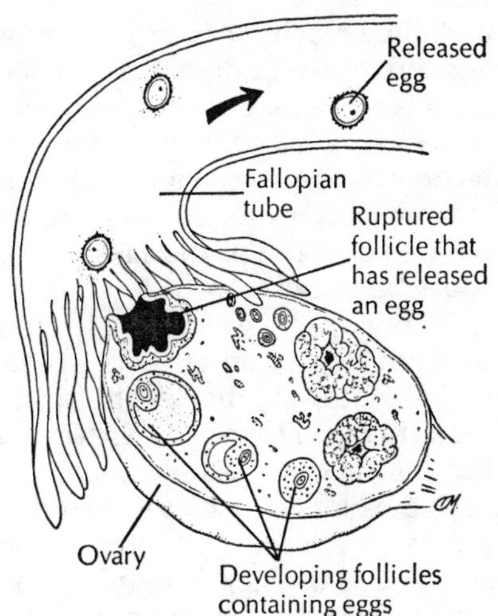

During ovulation the ovary releases the ripe egg which moves up the fallopian tube toward the uterus.

uterus are the fallopian tubes, which are four to five inches long with finger-like projections at their ends. When the ovary releases an egg, the projections on the nearby tube sweep the egg into the tube where it slowly inches toward the uterus.

If during that time, the egg is fertilized by a sperm, the male reproductive cell, it moves to the uterus and implants itself into the rich uterine lining where it grows for the next nine months. If the egg does not become fertilized, the uterine lining breaks down and passes, along with the unfertilized egg, out of the cervix (neck of the uterus) on through the vagina and out of the body. This discharge is known as menstruation.

Ovulation is regulated by a complex system of hormonal and chemical secretions from the ovaries, the hypothalamus (part of the brain), and the adjacent pituitary gland (the master gland of hormones).

Young women start ovulating — and menstruating — during puberty, which occurs between the ages of nine and 14, and normally do so every month (except while pregnant) until they reach menopause around age 50 or so. Some women feel cramps in the lower abdomen during ovulation. The only other ways to recognize when ovulation is happening are to take body temperature before rising in the morning with a special thermometer or to count 14 days from the first day of the last menstruation in an average 28-day cycle. However, the length of the menstrual cycle can vary. Sperm that has been ejaculated inside a woman's vagina as long as two to three days before the release of the ripe egg can still fertilize it. Therefore, there is an almost seven- to ten-day period during which a woman can become pregnant during each cycle.

See also Birth control, Conception, and Reproduction.

P

Paget's disease of the bone

Paget's disease (osteitis deformans) is a disorder in which the normal turnover (breaking down and reforming) of bone is greatly accelerated. The disease develops in three stages. In the first stage (destructive), bone tissue breaks down but is replaced with blood vessels and dense fibrous tissue making the bones very vascular (having a great deal of blood flowing through them). During the following stage (mixed), new bone formation takes place at a rate geared to the breakdown process. In the third stage (sclerotic), the breakdown process slows, allowing for the hardening of new bone which becomes quite dense.

Although any bone can be affected, Paget's disease most commonly invades the pelvis, skull, thighbone, shin, vertebrae (backbones), collarbone, and the ribs.

The condition normally affects 1 to 3 percent of the elderly, especially males. Its incidence is higher in some European countries than in others and rare in Asia, Africa, and South America. The cause is unknown.

Bone pain is one of the most prevalent symptoms. Sometimes complications develop. The thickened, enlarged bones are susceptible to fracture, particularly during the destructive phase of the disease. When the disease attacks the skull bone, it can compress the auditory nerve that relays signals from the ear to the brain and cause deafness. Heart failure can result from stress of the increased blood flow through the bones. Malignant bone tumors are another complication, but fortunately are uncommon. The disease can affect appearance if it enlarges the head, bends the back, or bows the legs. In some severe cases particularly if the person is immobile, calcium levels in the blood and urine increase and may lead to formation of urinary stones.

A history and physical examination, blood tests, and particularly X rays confirm the diagnosis.

Although there is no cure, analgesics (painkillers) like aspirin offer some relief. Severe pain or other complications are sometimes managed with chemotherapy (drug therapy), or corticosteroids (cortisone). Injections of calcitonin, a hormone normally produced in the thyroid gland that promotes calcification of bone, may help block bone breakdown.

Pain

Pain is an unpleasant or uncomfortable sensation that can range from mild irritation to excruciating agony. It is probably the most commonly reported symptom and is linked to innumerable disorders and diseases. (A symptom is an abnormal physical or psychological condition that accompanies or results from a disease or disorder, and that often serves as a clue in diagnosis.)

Pain occurs when specialized nerve endings are stimulated; within a fraction of a second this pain "signal" travels through a network of nerves to the brain. Pain can be a warning sign, indicating impending damage to the body, or it can be a protective mechanism, causing the person feeling pain to remove the cause or reflexively draw away from the source. Most healthy people have occasional, brief twinges of pain that have no specific cause and are usually harmless. However, bothersome, recurring, or persistent pain can be caused by thousands of factors. Most commonly, pain is a symptom of disease, injury, or abnormal changes in the body.

There are many types of pain. Pain can be dull and constant, sharp and sudden, crushing, burning, piercing, or aching. When it is felt in areas other than the location of the disorder (for example, when the pain of heart attack is felt in the arm), it is called "referred pain." Unexplainable pain should be reported promptly to a doctor for investigation and possible treatment.

Diagnosing the cause of a pain may be difficult. It is best to observe any accompanying symptoms and to keep in mind the answers to two questions that a doctor may ask in trying to diagnose the pain: "What brings on the pain?" and "What brings relief?"

The ideal treatment for pain consists of finding and correcting its source. In some cases, however, such as in widespread cancer, this would be impossible, so the pain itself needs to be treated, most commonly with analgesic drugs (painkilling medications). Aspirin and acetaminophen are probably the most common painkillers that can be obtained without a prescription. Other more potent painkillers, such as narcotics, must be prescribed by a doctor. Other drugs, both prescription and nonprescription, are designed to treat and relieve the pain of a specific disorder (for example, antacids treat the discomfort of heartburn and/or ulcers).

If the pain comes from the muscles such as in overexertion or from injury to soft tissues such as a bruise, adequate rest of the affected area may bring relief. Also, surface treatment of this type of pain can be very beneficial; this consists of massage or application of heat or cold (depending on the injury and the time elapsed since incurring it) to the painful area.

Pancreatitis

Pancreatitis is an inflammation of the pancreas, an organ located behind the stomach, close to the liver and gallbladder.

The pancreas has many functions. The exocrine pancreas secretes digestive enzymes (proteins that help chemical reactions along), for example, amylase which aids in the breakdown of starches and lipase for the breakdown of fats. The endocrine pancreas secretes hormones directly into the bloodstream, such as insulin and glucagon which are critical to the body's processing of glucose (sugar).

The existence and degree of inflammation in the pancreas may be hard to determine not only because of the gland's hidden position and dual purpose, but also because symptoms are easily confused with other abdominal disorders.

Pancreatitis commonly results from an obstruction of the pancreatic ducts. Why these blockages occur is often hard to determine. It has been observed that the majority of pancreatitis cases are related to gallbladder disease and alcoholism. Acute attacks are frequently associated with gallstones or alcoholic binges. If hereditary factors are involved, the disease may begin in childhood, as early as eight or ten years of age. Direct blows to the abdomen or injury during an operation may also lead to pancreatitis, sometimes a year or more after the event. Mumps and other viral infections; drugs including steroids (cortisone), diuretics, and oral contraceptives; and tumors have all been connected with pancreatitis.

The disease is characterized by the sudden onset of steady, severe, boring upper abdominal pain (frequently radiating to the mid-back) accompanied by nausea and persistent vomiting. Eating, or even the sight of food, may seem to bring on the pain or to make it worse. Vomiting provides no relief, a feature which can distinguish it from some stomach or intestinal disorders. Fever, shock, jaundice (yellowish discoloration of the skin), dehydration, bleeding, and infection may occur in severe attacks. After an acute episode of pancreatitis, tissue debris, blood, and pancreatic enzymes may form a "pseudocyst," that is, an organized collection of material without its own true sac. Rupture or enlargement of a pseudocyst can be a very serious or even fatal event. If a pseudocyst is formed and is not resolving on its own, surgery is necessary to drain it.

Blood and urine tests as well as microscopic tissue examination may be inconclusive, but can at least be helpful in excluding other abdominal disorders. A newer test, endoscopic retrograde cholangiopancreatography, enables visual inspection of the pancreatic ducts through an X ray. The technique is performed by inserting a gastroscope (a lighted tube) through the mouth and stomach into the duodenum (beginning of the small intestine). In the duodenum is the opening to the common bile and main pancreatic ducts. A special device is inserted through this opening and X-ray contrast material is injected. From the films taken, obstructions, tumors, or characteristic ductal patterns associated with chronic pancreatitis can be seen. This test is usually not performed within several weeks of an attack of pancreatitis.

The patient is usually hospitalized from three to 14 days for a mild to severe acute attack. Correction of an underlying problem, such as removal of stones, improves the chances for complete recovery.

Initial treatment is aimed at relieving the pain and reducing stomach secretions which can stimulate the pancreas. Pancreatic function is diminished by eliminating eating and drinking and by suctioning out stomach acids to allow the pancreas to rest. Large pseudocysts which do not dissolve on their own may require surgical drainage to prevent rupture. During convalescence, a low-fat, high-protein diet should be followed and antacids may be prescribed. If the disease is chronic, it may be necessary to use pancreatic extracts to supplement insufficient volume of enzymes secreted by the diseased pancreas. This helps to normalize digestion thereby maintaining reasonable nutritional status.

Chronic pancreatitis is an indication of continued degenerating tissue damage which may impair pancreatic function. In some cases of recurrence, surgical exploration might be considered to locate a previously unidentified blockage or to remove diseased tissue; however, surgery is unlikely to help the patient who continues to drink alcohol to excess.

Paralysis

Paralysis is the loss of the ability to move a part of the body, usually brought on by damage to either the muscles or to the nervous system. Paralysis can vary in severity and degree from one small muscle to almost the entire body. Irreversible and permanent paralysis results when a nerve is completely severed and destroyed, whereas paralysis caused by some diseases that cause inflammation without actual destruction of nerve tissue may diminish partially or totally as the condition is treated and the body recuperates.

There are numerous causes of paralysis. Brain damage resulting from disease or a stroke can lead to partial or total paralysis of various parts of the body. Such damage interferes with the transmission of nerve impulses from the brain to the muscles. Other diseases such as myasthenia gravis (a severe muscular weakness due to imbalances in the neurochemical transmission system) and poisons such as botulism or nerve gas sometimes also prevent nerve impulses from making contact with muscles, but do not necessarily cause complete loss of movement.

A spinal cord damaged or cut at mid to lower back can paralyze the legs and the lower part of the body, including the bladder and rectum; this condition is called paraplegia. A spinal cord that is injured around the neck affects both arms and legs; this is known as quadriplegia.

Diabetes, cancer, alcoholism, vitamin deficiency, or drug reaction among others can injure peripheral nerves (those outside the brain and spinal cord) which then either weaken or totally immobilize the muscles they control, as well as cause loss of sensation in the areas they serve.

Well-being and survival depend on the cause and extent of the paralysis. Obviously, paralysis that affects muscles involved in breathing is vitally significant because the very job of breathing has to be taken over by machines. However, artificial breathing may enable a patient to survive until the paralysis improves or disappears.

Patients whose paralysis does not require artificial measures for survival may benefit from physical or occupational therapy. These patients can learn to reuse a muscle or to develop other muscles to compensate for a disabled muscle. All patients with disabled muscles require special attention to prevent muscle atrophy (withering away), and ulcers (skin sores).

Paranoia

Paranoia is a mental disorder or personality disorder characterized by delusions of grandeur and suspicion of persecution.

Paranoid personalities display unreasonable distrust and constant unfounded suspicion that others are out to do them harm; interpret innocent comments as personal attacks; develop grandiose or exaggerated estimations of their own worth, yet feel that others do not recognize their value; believe they are the center of attention because everyone else openly criticizes them; and strenuously defend their fears with reason and logic.

Occasionally, paranoia shows itself as unwarranted and extreme sexual jealousy.

An internal conflict between the need for recognition and the compulsion to guard certain aspects of emotional life may be the root of paranoia. Often, unconscious sexual conflicts play a role in the development of paranoia.

Paranoia differs from paranoid schizophrenia, a much more serious problem in which the individual not only has delusions of grandeur and a persecution complex, but also demonstrates deranged thought processes, hallucinations, and other signs of disturbed personality.

True paranoia can generally be helped with psychotherapy and medication, if necessary.

It is important to remember that almost everyone exhibits some harmless, short-lived paranoia from time to time, usually from excess worry over an embarrassment or from disappointment.

Parkinson's disease

Parkinson's disease is a progressive disorder characterized primarily by uncontrollable tremors in the limbs, a shuffling gait, and generalized muscular rigidity. It most often strikes people over the age of 60.

Parkinson's disease is usually not fatal, but it leads to changes in the entire body, making the patient more susceptible to other diseases. It can be present in a mild form for 20 or 30 years, but a severe case can lead to a serious disability within five to ten years.

The cause of Parkinson's disease is unknown, thus it is also not known why it strikes certain people. No inherited, medical, or environmental factors have been found definitely to cause the disease. The one exception to this is an epidemic of encephalitis (brain inflammation) that occurred some years ago following World War I. This disease produced a collection of symptoms and signs indistinguishable from true Parkinson's disease. However, since this is not true Parkinson's disease, the syndrome is referred to as "Parkinsonism."

It is known, however, that Parkinson's disease may be a reflection of a chemical imbalance in the brain. Those with the disease have been shown to have low levels of a neurotransmitter called dopamine. (Neurotransmitters are chemicals in the brain that transmit impulses across junctions between nerves; the balance of neurotransmitters in the brain is thought to be responsible for muscle control.) To date, no cause for this chemical deficiency has been found.

The symptoms of Parkinson's disease are uncontrollable shaking of the limbs, stiff muscles, drooling, reduced blinking, an expressionless face, stooping posture, and a shuffling walk. Tremors may worsen during rest periods and times of increased anxiety. Interestingly, the tremor may decrease when the patient reaches for an object or when he or she must act quickly under a great deal of stress.

As the disease progresses, speech slurs and sentences trail off into unintelligible muttering. Small muscle movement becomes increasingly difficult—reducing the ability to write, eat, chew, and swallow—and all movements seem overly stiff and slow. The term "cogwheel rigidity" is often used to describe the typical arm motion these patients may display; when pulled from a flexed position, the arm seems to jerk up and down as if controlled by a ratchet like that found in a cogwheel.

Excitement and tension can cause these symptoms to worsen, as can depression. Depression is common among Parkinson's disease victims, who are understandably upset by their loss of muscle control.

Diagnosis involves a simple history, physical examination, and observation of the symptoms. If

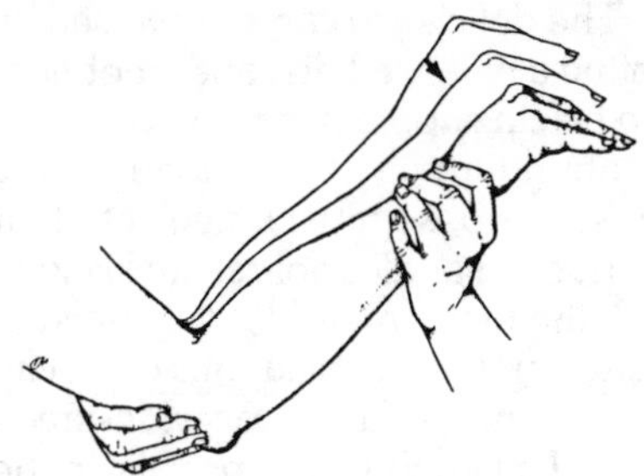

"Cogwheel rigidity" in a Parkinson's disease patient occurs when the arm is pulled straight and moves in a jerky fashion as if controlled by a rachet such as is found in a cogwheel.

tremors are the only symptom displayed, the examination tests may be done to rule out the possibility that other disorders are causing the tremors, such as liver disease, multiple sclerosis (a debilitating muscular disorder), chronic alcoholism, or overactive thyroid gland.

Treatment of Parkinson's disease consists of correcting the chemical imbalance caused by the dopamine deficiency. Dopamine itself cannot be absorbed directly into the brain from the bloodstream, so a substance called levodopa is prescribed to help the brain manufacture more of its own dopamine.

Levodopa has several undesirable side effects, among them nausea (which is decreased if the drug is taken with meals), an uneven "on-off" effect (causing symptoms to disappear and then reappear), and a loss of effectiveness over time. For these reasons and others, levodopa often is not prescribed or is given in smaller doses in combination with other types of drugs known as anticholinergics. These drugs decrease nerve to muscle transmission, thereby reducing tremor and rigidity. They also decrease drooling. Bromocriptine, a drug that enhances dopamine's effects, has also been successful, as have other drugs.

Physical therapy and exercise are also important in a treatment program for Parkinson's disease. In addition, emotional support and understanding are critical.

Patent ductus arteriosus

Patent ductus arteriosus is a congenital (present at birth) heart disorder in which the ductus arteriosus, an extra blood vessel present in the fetus (unborn child) which allows the blood to pass from the pulmonary artery to the aorta (two of the main blood vessels leading directly from the heart), fails to close after birth. It is most common in premature babies.

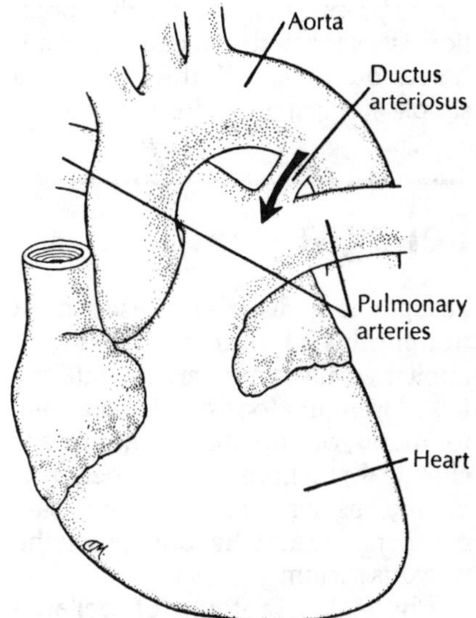

If the ductus arteriosus fails to close after birth, incorrect flow of blood will put a strain on the baby's heart.

During the gestation period (the nine months of fetal growth and development in the uterus), the fetus is immersed in amniotic fluid and, thus, the lungs are not used. Therefore, the blood bypasses the lungs and the fetus receives oxygen from the placenta (which nourishes the unborn child) through this extra vessel.

If the ductus arteriosus remains open after birth, blood continues to flow through it; any excess blood passes through the lungs. Congestive heart failure can develop.

Although the cause of the defect is unknown, the heart of a fetus is completely formed by the third month of pregnancy and any disorder may originate during that time.

Although obvious symptoms are rare, the affected infant may display shortness of breath or develop congestive heart failure.

Patent ductus arteriosus can be treated with medication if diagnosed early (various prenatal—before birth—tests have become available in recent years for diagnosis if the condition is suspected) or can be eliminated by tying off the duct in a simple surgical procedure.

Pellagra

Pellagra is a disorder caused by a deficiency of niacin (otherwise known as nicotinic acid), a vitamin found in many foods . Niacin is vital to many of the body's important chemical reactions used to generate energy, as well as to healthy skin maintenance and the functions of the nervous system.

Physical symptoms of pellagra include weakness; loss of appetite; sore, red, cracked skin with symmetrical spots that turn brown and scaly; a painful scarlet mouth, tongue and gums; a burning sensation throughout the digestive tract; diarrhea; and headaches. Psychological symptoms are anxiety; forgetfulness; insomnia (inability to sleep); irritability; and dementia (loss of intellectual abilities).

The deficiency can be reversed by eating a balanced diet and/or obtaining niacin supplements. Since niacin is abundant in many foods, only those who seriously neglect their diets, such as alcoholics, are likely to lack the recommended daily need of between 9 to 12 milligrams of niacin. At one time pellagra was widespread in the United States, especially in the South, but today it occurs far less frequently.

Pelvic inflammatory disease

Pelvic inflammatory disease (PID), or salpingitis, is an infection of a woman's fallopian tubes, two four- to five-inch long ducts that conduct egg cells from the ovaries to the uterus. Although the term is widely used to refer to infections of all the parts of the pelvic cavity above the vagina, PID is properly restricted to the fallopian tubes.

The causes of PID are not always fully known, but it is usually caused by certain bacteria transmitted during sexual intercourse, an intrauterine device (IUD) that has become infected, or certain vaginal infections. One of the commonest agents causing PID is gonorrhea, a widespread sexually transmitted disease.

It is suspected that a woman is more vulnerable to PID if her cervical canal (the opening from the vagina into the uterus) has been dilated at some point by either recent surgery or recent childbirth or miscarriage. Under normal circumstances, the cervix prevents bacteria from the vagina from entering the uterus.

PID symptoms include severe pain and tenderness in the lower abdomen, fever, a foul-smelling vaginal discharge, early menstrual bleeding, pain during sexual intercourse, nausea, vomiting, fatigue, and pain during urination or defecation.

If it is not diagnosed early, the infection can cause abscesses (pus-filled cavities) to form in the fallopian tubes or around the ovaries (the female sex glands, which secrete female sex hormones and discharge eggs). PID can also damage and irreversibly scar pelvic tissue and, if the tubes are blocked, PID can prevent conception. The infection can also result in bacteria entering the bloodstream and spreading to other parts of the body and in peritonitis (inflammation of the membrane lining the pelvic and abdominal cavities).

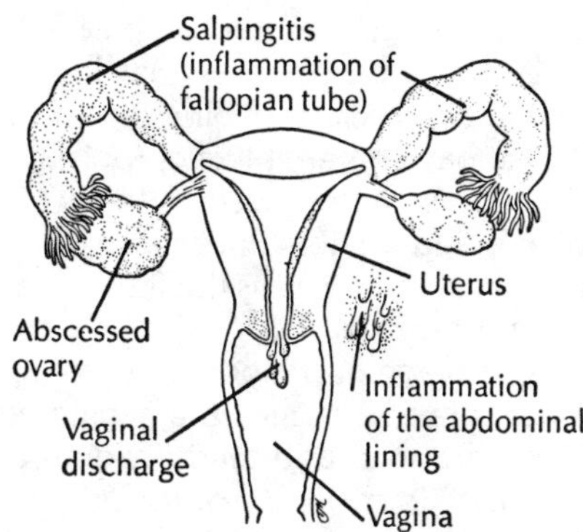

Pelvic inflammatory disease is an inflammation of the fallopian tubes (salpingitis) that can lead to an abscessed ovary, an inflammation of the abdominal lining, and perhaps blocked fallopian tubes.

It is important to seek medical attention as soon as symptoms occur so the infection can be treated before it worsens and spreads. The physician will take a sample of fluid from the cervix to identify the infecting organism.

The doctor will prescribe antibiotics to fight the infection and aspirin or other painkillers for pain relief. The woman may be advised to rest in bed, abstain from sexual intercourse, and apply heat to the lower abdominal area. These measures generally succeed in curing the infection; if not, the woman may have to enter the hospital to receive antibiotics intravenously (in the vein). In some cases, a laparoscopy (a view of the internal organs through a special tube), or possibly surgery to drain blocked tubes or abscessed tissue may be required. Sometimes, the damage is too extensive and the fallopian tubes, the uterus, and the ovaries may have to be removed. This will cure the infection; however, conception will then be impossible.

A woman can minimize her chances of contracting PID by taking precautions any time her cervix is dilated; for example, by avoiding tampons, sexual intercourse, douches, and tub baths for at least several weeks after childbirth, an abortion, D and C (dilatation and curettage, surgical scraping of the interior lining of the uterus), or miscarriage. She should check with her doctor regarding when these activities may be safely resumed. Also, if a woman suspects she may have gonorrhea, she should have this treated immediately before PID develops.

Peptic ulcer

See Ulcer.

Pericarditis

Pericarditis is an inflammation of the membranous bag surrounding the heart, known as the pericardium. Often with pericarditis, a great deal of fluid collects between the membrane and the heart (a condition called pericardial effusion), which may lead to complications.

The inflammation commonly stems from an infection, such as pneumonia or tuberculosis. Viral infections are also common causes of pericarditis. Pericarditis can also be seen in noninfectious diseases such as diseases of the connective tissues and chronic kidney failure. Occasionally, pericarditis can occur after a heart attack or chest injury.

Although mild pericarditis occurs commonly in conjunction with a viral infection, serious pericarditis is unusual. Pain in the center of the chest (and possibly the shoulders, neck and upper arms) that worsens with coughing, lying flat, or breathing may signify pericarditis. Since this type of pain is a symptom of several serious illnesses, a doctor should be consulted about any severe chest pain that lasts more than a few minutes. A chest X ray, electrocardiogram (ECG) and blood tests, along with the history and physical examination, will usually identify pericarditis and, quite often, its cause.

When a large effusion exists, the motion of the heart may be restricted, thereby preventing it from filling and pumping effectively. This can be life-threatening and must be corrected as soon as possible. The fluid may be drained by inserting a needle through the chest into the pericardial sac. This is done either to diagnose the condition or to relieve the effusion. Once the cause is diagnosed, the doctor will treat the underlying cause (such as using dialysis in kidney failure or antibiotics for bacterial infection) in order to eliminate the pericarditis and/or effusion.

Occasionally, long-term pericarditis arises from a chronic condition, most notably tuberculosis, but also from many other causes of pericarditis. The chronic inflammation causes thickening and contraction of the pericardium to the point that it restricts the heartbeat. Called constrictive pericarditis, this condition is not quite as common anymore because of the decrease in reported tuberculosis cases, but it is a severe condition calling for immediate attention.

With constrictive pericarditis, the legs and abdomen swell and, without surgery, this cannot be corrected. In this case, a pericardectomy to remove the scarred pericardium is the appropriate surgical procedure.

Periodontal disease

Periodontal disease, or periodontitis, is a progressive deterioration of the gums and bones around the teeth.

One theory is that the condition begins with an accumulation of bacteria and food particles that lodges within tissues surrounding the teeth. These bacteria emit toxins (poisons) that cause gum tissues to swell, bleed, and erode. Gingivitis, inflammation of the gums, is the first stage.

Pyorrhea (running of pus), the second stage of periodontitis, results when the soft tissues are separated from the bone and teeth leading to "pocket" formation. Pockets of bacteria and pus accumulate around the teeth leading to weakening of the fibers holding the teeth in their sockets as well as to destruction of the bone supporting teeth. As the disease advances, teeth become loose and fall out. They may also move out of alignment with one another and cause problems with chewing.

In the early stage of periodontal disease, gums become sore, red, and slightly swollen. They may be sensitive to the touch and bleed when brushed or flossed. Pus in the gums around the teeth signals the beginning of the second disease stage. If pus remains in the gum tissue without draining, extreme pain and swelling can result.

A dentist diagnoses the beginning of periodontal disease by examining

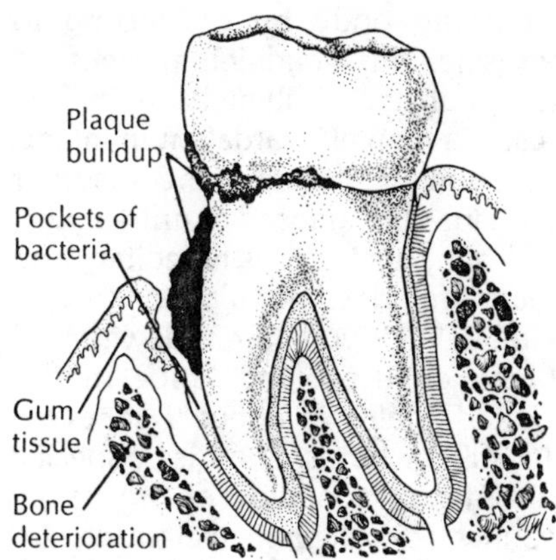

The left side shows what periodontal disease can do; the right side shows a healthy tooth, bones, and gums.

the swollen gums and the deposits of bacteria and plaque around the teeth. Once detected, continued care of the mouth at home can help prevent extensive periodontal disease and reduce gum problems.

Oral hygiene to prevent gum disease is the same as treatment to prevent tooth decay. Ideally, the mouth needs to be cleaned after every meal. More realistically, a thorough cleansing before bed may minimize the chances of gum disease. Dentists suggest brushing teeth with a soft-bristled brush. Gentle movements within the crevices dislodge decay-causing material, while firm strokes over the teeth remove plaque.

Flossing is recommended to clear plaque from between teeth. After brushing and flossing, vigorously rinsing the mouth with mouthwash containing antimicrobials (substances that kill bacteria) can also help eliminate bacteria formation; but mouthwash alone cannot prevent plaque.

For self-checking, a dental mirror provides a view of the teeth and gums in the back of the mouth. Disclosing wafers, which when chewed discolor plaque, reveal any invisible film to be removed.

For advanced cases, a dentist may scrape the affected tissue pockets and apply antiseptics (germ-killers) every few months in an effort to kill the bacteria. Should this procedure fail to check the spread of the disease, surgery by a periodontist (gum specialist) may be needed to remove deep pockets in the gum. Once the bacteria are eliminated, good oral hygiene practices should keep the disease under control.

See also Tooth decay.

Peritonitis

Peritonitis is a term used to describe an inflammation and/or infection of the thin double-layered membrane (peritoneum) covering the abdominal organs. The condition occurs when the peritoneum is invaded by bacteria, toxins (poisons), bile (a substance produced by the liver and stored in the gallbladder), blood, or urine. Because the peritoneum is well-sealed, the only way it can be infiltrated is when one of the hollow organs of the abdomen ruptures; when a solid organ is somehow damaged, causing it to leak; or when there is a penetrating injury from the outside. For example, if the bladder is ruptured in an accident, sterile urine is discharged into the peritoneal cavity. Although germ-free, the urine is quite irritating, thereby causing a "chemical peritonitis." If, however, the colon is perforated, fecal contents, containing loads of bacteria and toxins, are discharged. This creates a bacterial peritonitis. Both of these conditions are extremely serious and must be immediately remedied.

A main symptom of peritonitis is severe pain that intensifies with any movement and often forces the person to lie very still with legs drawn up.

The abdominal area is very tender and grows rigid; commonly there is vomiting, fever, and dehydration (loss of body fluids). When the peritoneum is inflamed, fluid begins to leak out of the blood vessels into the peritoneum. If not corrected, this may lead to shock (failure of the circulatory system because of loss of blood volume). After some time, the abdomen may swell. This is a danger sign that the intestines have become paralyzed and bloated with air. These symptoms and signs signify a need for immediate medical care, including intravenous (injected through the veins) antibiotics to fight infection. Intravenous fluids are also given to restore lost volume. In addition, usually a tube is inserted through the nose and into the stomach to relieve the bloating and remove pooled fluids. After the patient is stabilized with these procedures, surgery to remove or repair the cause of peritonitis is done. Chances for recovery are usually excellent.

Pharyngitis

See Sore throat.

Phenylketonuria

Phenylketonuria (PKU) is a congenital (present at birth) disorder characterized by the presence of increased amounts of amino acids in the blood and urine. (Amino acids are the chemical building blocks of protein.) The condition is marked by the inability to convert phenylalanine, a naturally occurring amino acid essential for optimal growth in infants and for nitrogen balance in adults, into tyrosine, another amino acid. Since excess phenylalanine is eliminated from the body by converting to tyrosine, this condition permits an accumulation of phenylalanine. The result is mental retardation in infants or young children if the disorder remains undiagnosed or untreated.

Phenylketonuria is hereditary and found in most population groups, although it is very rare in Jewish and black children. Incidence in the United States is about 1 in every 16,000 live births. There is no specific disorder or condition of pregnancy connected with phenylketonuria.

Early diagnosis of phenylketonuria is vital since symptoms are usually not obvious in a newborn infant. Therefore, screening tests are mandatory for babies born in most hospitals in the United States. Sometimes infants with PKU will show neurologic (nervous system) disorders, very light skin coloring, eczema (a skin disorder), and a "mousy" odor about the body; older children may be extremely hyperactive. Often the light hair and skin coloring is an early clue to the disease; the infant will have lighter skin, hair, and even eyes than other members of the family.

Treatment of this disorder within the first few days after birth is vital if the mental retardation that is PKU's most dreaded effect is to be prevented. Treatment consists of limiting the child's phenylalanine intake so that the essential amino acid requirement is satisifed without any excess. This can be done by feeding the infant special formulas with little or no phenylalanine. Regular milk is a protein food and thus rich in phenylalanine. When the infant is started on solid foods, low-protein natural foods, such as fruits, vegetables, and certain cereals, are also permitted.

If PKU is not diagnosed in the first few days of life, the later results are usually extreme hyperactivity, seizures, and mental retardation. Some physicians think that treatment and special diet must be continued throughout the child's life. Others say it can be ended when brain development is virtually complete, around five years of age.

It is important to remember that, although untreated PKU can lead to retardation and other problems, early diagnosis and treatment can enable the child to develop normally and to lead a normal life.

Phimosis

Phimosis is a constriction of the foreskin (skin fold over the head of the penis) that prevents the foreskin from being drawn back over the head (glans).

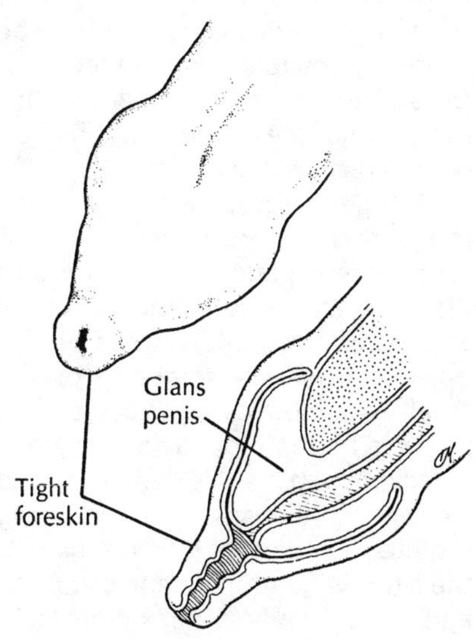

Phimosis occurs when the foreskin cannot be pulled back over the penis.

The cause of phimosis is either congenital (present at birth) or acquired. The acquired form is usually due to an infection involving the penis that leaves adhesions—growths of tissue that adhere both to the inner aspect of the foreskin and to the glans itself. Phimosis also prevents debris (common dirt, dead cells, and normal fluid secretions) from escaping, thereby causing the debris to stagnate between the foreskin and glans providing an excellent place for bacteria to grow. Once infection is established, ulceration of the glans and swelling of the lymph nodes in the groin can occur.

The definitive treatment for this condition is circumcision—the surgical removal of the foreskin. If, for some reason, this must be delayed, there must be careful attention to keeping the area clean and dry and free from infection until the situation is corrected.

See also Circumcision.

Phobia

Phobia is a psychological disorder characterized by persistent, abnormal, and unfounded dread and fear of something that is not inherently dangerous or threatening to most people. It is also a suffix or word ending, which denotes unreasonable fear or abhorrence of a specific element as in claustrophobia, an intense fear of being closed in.

A phobia resembles acute or chronic anxiety but, unlike "free-floating" anxiety, it is linked to specific environmental stimuli: heights, open places, the state of being alone, travel, even blushing. True phobia affects fewer than 1 percent of the total population.

Phobia, like anxiety, seems to occur more often in some families. The anxiety itself is a fearful reaction to the emergence of forbidden or unconscious drives. In most cases, a set of psychological mechanisms called *projection* and *displacement* focuses the anxiety on specific external objects, persons, or situations that then come to stand for or represent the original cause of the anxiety. In shifting attention to the secondary symbol, the patient learns to use avoidance of the object or situation (spiders, heights, open places, and so on) to prevent rearousal of the painful anxiety. The "choice" of the phobic object is often at random; it may be the first object or situation at hand when the original anxiety first appears.

Often, the very thought or mention of the phobic object induces anxiety in the patient. The closer he or she comes to the reality of the situation, the more the anxiety mounts towards panic. As a result, the patient spends more time avoiding the phobic stimulus and this very avoidance often begins to restrict his or her daily activities. Examples include the man or woman who cannot travel because of fear of flying or the victim of agoraphobia who avoids all open places in order to remain secluded at home where he or she feels "safe."

The symptoms of the phobias depend, of course, on the phobic object. *Agoraphobia* (a fear of open, public places, such as stores, malls, parks, theatres, or stadiums, or of crowds and crowded situations) is the most common phobia, accounting for about 60 percent of all such cases. Often, the agoraphobic person experiences the phobia selectively—he or she can face the phobic situation fairly well in the company of someone close or trusted.

Other phobias, called simple phobias, involve objects. Some are childhood phobias, such as fear of the dark or of animals, and disappear with age. But adults, too, experience phobias of specific objects or situations: spiders, heights *(acrophobia)*, or being alone *(monophobia)*. If the objects are easily avoided, as with spiders, or snakes, there is usually no great problem. However, fear of flying may cause great inconvenience for a person whose work or social life involves constant air travel, and monophobia may handicap a worker whose job requires long periods of isolation to complete a project.

The phobias of function, or social phobias, are those in which the presence of others causes the anxiety. Among the most common are *erythrophobia* (a fear of blushing) or the fear of eating, which makes the patient incapable of eating in the presence of others or in a public place such as a restaurant or cafeteria.

Phobias usually begin in early adulthood and follow a long course of alternate improvement and worsening of symptoms. Agoraphobia, the severest of the phobias as well as the most common, is the least likely to show significant improvement. The longer the patient has phobic symptoms (any time period over a year), the less likely he or she is to achieve a complete recovery.

A type of psychotherapy called insight therapy may be helpful in less severe cases; patients learn to recognize the real, underlying object of anxiety and come to see the phobic object as merely symbolic of the "real" fear. More extreme cases often respond better to behavioral therapy in which the patient is deconditioned to the phobic stimulus by being required to confront the stimulus. At the same time, the patient is encouraged to try various relaxation techniques to combat anxiety. In the most severe cases a technique called flooding is used in which the patient is forced to experience prolonged phobic anxiety with a constant exposure to the dreaded object or situation.

Although drug therapy alone generally is less effective than when it is combined with psychotherapy, minor tranquilizers and antidepressants often can help delay or dull the onset of panic attacks.

See also Agoraphobia and Claustrophobia.

Photosensitivity

Photosensitivity is an abnormally increased sensitivity of the skin to the rays of the sun.

The causes of this condition are not fully understood, although it is known that certain substances when combined with ultraviolet light produce the reaction. Among those substances are: contraceptive pills; hexachlorophene, a skin antiseptic; sandalwood oil; coal tar; certain perfumes; and a variety of orally taken drugs. In these reactions, it appears to be the combination of ultraviolet rays with the agent that triggers the response.

The symptoms of photosensitivity range from burning reactions, similar to those ordinarily suffered after prolonged exposure to the sun, all the way to rashes; scaling; welts (raised areas) on the skin; and excessive burning, dizziness, nausea, and vomiting. The most common symptom is a rash.

The most effective treatment is to discover the basic cause of the heightened sensitivity and to eliminate it. If, for example, photosensitivity is a reaction to a contraceptive pill, a different kind of pill or form of contraception could be prescribed. Treatment of photosensitivity symptoms duplicates that used for sunburn: ointments, topical anesthetics, and creams. It should be remembered that these treatments are standard topical therapy for the skin but do not eliminate the underlying causes of photosensitivity.

If it is impossible to isolate the cause of photosensitivity, the next best step to take is to avoid exposure to light by wearing light-colored clothing, white gloves, and broad-brimmed hats. Commercial sunscreen products are also helpful. Obviously, contact with the substances already listed should be avoided.

Pica

Pica is an abnormal craving to eat objects and materials not ordinarily considered to be foods.

The causes of pica are not completely understood. In the case of a pregnant woman who eats laundry starch, pica may be an almost instinctive effort to make up for deficiencies in the diet. In the case of lead poisoning in children, as a result of the consumption of lead-based paint, the causes are less clear: it could be a teething impulse, or it could be the result of unconscious drives not fully understood.

Although lead poisoning is the most serious pica problem with children, the effects of pica are as varied as the poisonous substances that are consumed. The most common poisons eaten as a result of pica are those that are used as ingredients in manufacturing processes. They include: inorganic metals and nonmetals, used in paints, matches, and the like; volatile organic poisons, used in paints, soaps, and cleaners; and pesticides.

While all pica sufferers do not eat non-foods indiscriminately, any person (especially a child) suffering from pica may consume one or more inedible substance as part of a general tendency to eat non-foods. Some doctors also include consumption of a variety of growing plants, such as mushrooms, century plants, and toxic (poisonous) plants (poison ivy), as evidence of pica.

The treatment for pica is not simple, since medical science has not as yet pinned down the root of the compulsion. Obviously, if the craving is induced by a deficiency of an element such as iron, the treatment is to remedy the deficiency. Medical treatment for the effects of pica-ingested non-foods depends on the nature of the substance consumed. If a child is the pica sufferer, the first line of defense is to remove the toxic material from his or her reach, and to search the immediate area for other toxic substances.

Prevention of pica may be as simple as the maintenance of a balanced diet. When the causes cannot be found and pica activity persists, the first practical move is to remove toxic sources.

Pinworms

Pinworms is a term that refers to a condition in which the gastrointestinal tract and occasionally other sites such as the female reproductive tract are infested by any of a variety of worms, called *oxyurids*. These worms are tiny (about 3 to 10 millimeters in length).

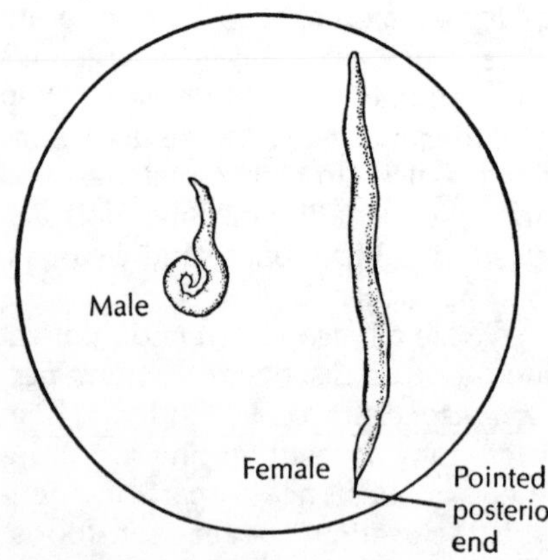

Pinworms is the common name of small worms called oxyurids.

The usual cause of the infestation is the ingestion (consumption) of the worm's fertilized eggs by eating food contaminated with the eggs. Contamination results from contact with fingers that have been in contact with feces. Eggs can also survive on bedclothing and linens for two or three weeks.

Many children who have pinworms do not have obvious symptoms. Such symptoms that may occur are itching around the anus (the opening from the large intestine to outside the body), accompanied by inflammation of the anal tissues. After being ingested, the eggs hatch and release their larvae into the upper portion of the small intestine. The larvae mature as they pass up through the first part of the large intestine. After mating, the adult male worms die and the females migrate on down the large intestine to the anal region, where they lay their eggs around the anus. The eggs are transferred from the anus to the mouth on the child's hands, and the cycle continues. Pinworms can be transmitted to other children and adults in the same manner. Also, the hatched larvae can migrate back through the anus and into the bowel. This is called retroinfection and occurs primarily in adults.

Worms can also cause irritation, inflammation, and obstruction in the appendix. In addition, pinworms can work their way into a female's vagina and urethra (the passageway from the bladder to the outside) and cause inflammation and/or infection in the vagina, the reproductive system, and bladder.

Aside from noting the symptom of itching, the diagnosis is made by identifying the eggs or worms under a microscope. An easy and inexpensive way to accomplish this is to wrap a piece of cellophane tape—sticky side out—around a tongue depressor. This swab is then placed against the anal area. The contents from the swab are then transferred to a slide for microscopic examination. This procedure should be done in the morning before bathing and on several consecutive days.

Treatment of pinworms is not difficult. Usually one dose of the drug pyrantel pamoate is sufficient. Other medications are also available. In addition, in group infestations, all members should be treated simultaneously, and their bedclothes, linens, and underwear laundered at the same time. Also, the eggs around the anus should be removed by cleaning the anal area thoroughly at the time of treatment. Reinfestation is common, and when symptoms develop, another course of treatment is necessary.

It is important to teach children clean eating habits, to encourage them to wash their hands frequently, and to keep an eye open for other children who may be infected (as evidenced by scratching around the anus).

Pituitary gland

The pituitary (also called the *hypophysis cerebri*) is a small gland located just beneath the base of the brain, between its two frontal lobes, and directly above a cavity called the phenoid sinus.

The pituitary gland has two lobes or parts, each with its own function. The front, or anterior, lobe secretes the following hormones: *somatotrophin* (also known as growth hormone that affects the body's general growth); *thryotropic hormone* (also known as thyroid-stimulating hormone that acts on the thyroid gland to stimulate production of thyroid hormone); *adrenocorticotrophic hormone* (ACTH—which stimulates the adrenal cortex); two gonadotrophic hormones (follicle-stimulating hormone and luteinizing hormone that are concerned with maturation and release of egg and sperm cells); and *prolactin* (which acts on the mammary glands to promote the secretion of milk).

The posterior lobe of the pituitary secretes the following hormones: *oxytocin* (which stimulates smooth muscle tissue to contract and is critical in labor of childbirth) and *vasopressin* (which regulates the kidney's function of taking or releasing water in the system).

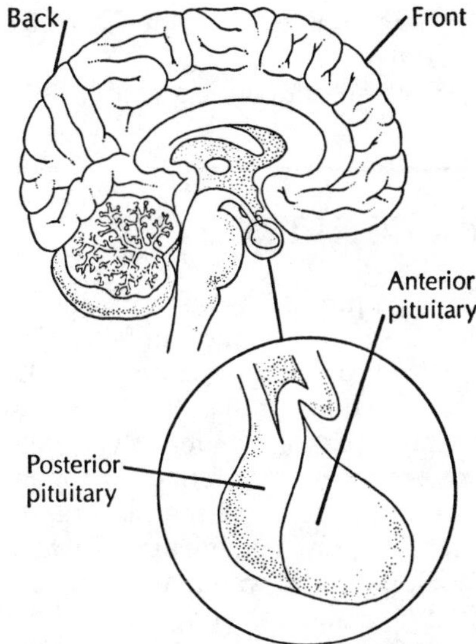

The small pituitary gland is one of the most important glands in the body.

Despite its relatively small size, the pituitary gland is so important to bodily functions that it is sometimes called the "master gland." Disorders of this gland, often the result of tumors, can result in disastrous abnormalities in growth and body maintenance. Excessive secretions of growth hormone by the anterior lobe produces giants, while deficient secretion produces dwarfs (if disorders in secretions occur during the years in which the skeleton would be growing naturally). If oversecretion occurs after a person has become an adult, a condition called *acromegaly* results, in which the victim's hands, feet, jaws, and facial bones grow disproportionately large.

A condition known as diabetes insipidus (which is unrelated to the more common diabetes mellitus, or high blood sugar levels) is one of the malfunctions of the posterior lobe. With this disorder, there is a deficiency of vasopressin, resulting in abnormally high urinary output of water. Control can be regained with the administration of synthetic vasopressin that will inhibit excessive water release.

See also Endocrine system.

Placenta previa

Placenta previa is an abnormal condition after conception in which the fertilized egg, or zygote, travels to the lower portion of the uterus, to attach itself to a part of the uterine wall near or even over the uterine *os* (opening). In these cases, the placenta (a temporary organ in the uterus, which develops during pregnancy to conduct nourishment and oxygen from mother to unborn child) forms in such a way as to cover all or part of the uterine opening and thus interfere with normal delivery. There are three types of placenta previa: (1) partial, in which only a portion of the cervix (or uterine mouth) is covered; (2) complete, in which the cervix is completely covered; and (3) low-lying (or marginal), in which the placenta does not cover the cervix, but is close enough to it possibly to interfere with normal delivery. There is one placenta previa in every 100 to 500 pregnancies. They are more prevalent among women who have had two or more children than among those for whom it is the first pregnancy.

Placenta previa is not the result of a disease or necessarily inadequate precautions on the part of the mother. The cause of this condition is unknown. Some authorities feel that a placenta will never implant on the same part of the uterine wall twice. If a woman has several pregnancies, only the lower part of the uterus may be left on which the placenta can implant.

The major symptom of placenta previa is painless vaginal bleeding. Profuse bleeding may begin as early as the 24th to 26th week of pregnancy, with no apparent cause. The blood will be bright red, indicating that it is fresh blood. Bleeding occurs as the placenta separates from the wall of the uterus near the uterine opening. This bleeding occurs without any injury (from a fall, for example). In some cases, the blood flow is light (spotting).

Any vaginal bleeding during pregnancy is abnormal and should be reported to the doctor immediately. An ultrasound scan of the mother's abdomen will then be performed. If a placenta previa is present, this will be seen with the ultrasound scan.

There are two types of treatment: delayed and active. The purpose of delayed treatment is to give the fetus time to mature so that it can survive a cesarean delivery (through an incision in the abdomen) and be mature enough to survive a premature birth. In the case of active treatment, the fetus is delivered by cesarean section as soon as possible.

The degree of vaginal bleeding will usually dictate the type of treatment. If vaginal bleeding is slight, delayed treatment is chosen. If vaginal bleeding is heavy, active treatment, that is, a cesarean section, will be performed immediately.

Bleeding from placenta previa may be extremely heavy, leading to severe blood loss from the mother. This bleeding stops only after the fetus and placenta have been delivered by cesarean section. Unless treatment is rapid in this case, death of both the mother and fetus may occur.

Platelets

Blood platelets (also called thrombocytes) are tiny disk-shaped cells that play a critical role in the process of blood coagulation, or clotting. They are manufactured in the bone marrow, and usually live for about ten days.

The number of platelets per unit volume of blood plays an important role in proper platelet function. The normal number ranges between 200,000 and 500,000 platelets per cubic millimeter of blood. Platelets initiate the coagulation process by aggregating (or clumping) together,

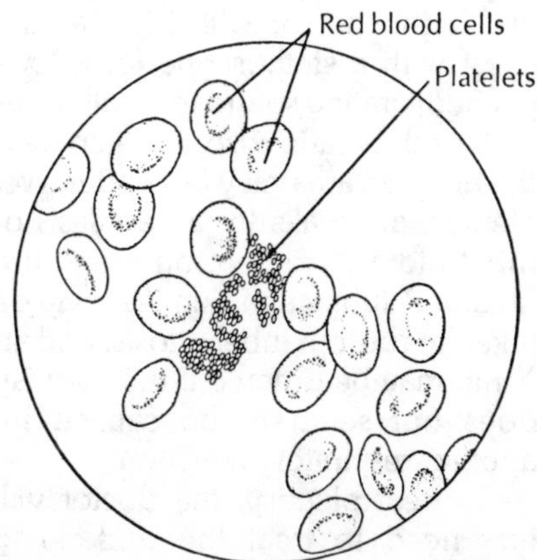

Blood platelets, compared to red blood cells, are tiny, yet they are vital for coagulation.

and the usual amount of time for adequate coagulation is five minutes or less.

Blood coagulation is a complex process requiring the presence of many substances in the blood besides platelets. However, without platelets, coagulation would be impossible.

A low platelet count may be seen with many different diseases including certain liver diseases, uncommon forms of anemia caused by vitamin deficiencies, and certain cancers (such as leukemia) of the blood-forming organs.

The most common cause of a low platelet count is destruction of platelets by the body's immune system. For an unknown reason, the bodies of some individuals may recognize platelets as foreign, and these platelets will be destroyed by antibodies.

When a lack of platelets prolongs bleeding time, several types of treatment may be attempted, depending on the cause of the low platelet count. If the platelet count is too low, prolonged bleeding results. If the platelet count is too high, emboli (clots or clumps of blood materials that obstruct vessels) may develop. Neither condition is desirable, so increasing platelet counts must be done with care.

The usual method to increase the number of platelets in the blood is by transfusion. These transfusions are normally reserved for patients with severe platelet deficiencies.

Care should be taken by any patient whose platelet count is low, since bleeding will be prolonged and coagulation will not occur within normal time limits. For this reason many physicians recommend that, until normal platelet counts are attained, patients should (in severe cases) avoid anything that may cause bleeding such as toothbrushes, abrasive foods, and enemas. They should also avoid any kind of contact sports and accidental hard contact with objects such as furniture, or automobile doors.

Pleurisy

The term pleurisy is another name for pleuritis and refers to any inflammation of the pleura, the membrane that covers the outside of the lungs and lines the chest cavity. It is a complication that generally develops from other upper respiratory tract infections such as pneumonia or tuberculosis.

There are two types of pleurisy: dry pleurisy, the more common inflammation; and wet pleurisy, a similar condition except that fluid oozes from the inflamed tissue into the space between the lungs and the chest wall. Compression of the lungs by this fluid may occur, making breathing difficult.

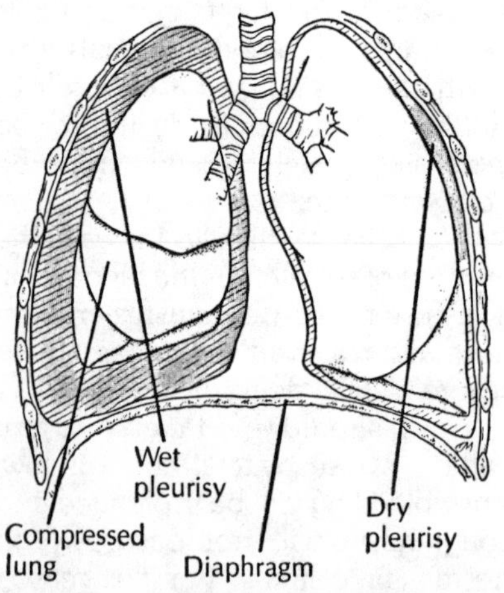

Pleurisy is an inflammation of the pleura, the membrane covering the lungs and lining the chest cavity. A simple inflammation is called dry pleurisy; if fluid is produced by the inflamed pleura, the condition is called wet pleurisy. This fluid may compress the lung.

Dry pleurisy is caused by an infection already in the lungs, often viral or bacterial pneumonia or acute bronchitis (inflammation of the air passages). It can arise as a complication of tuberculosis or because of a tumor. Wet pleurisy can also develop from an infection, tuberculosis, or a tumor, as well as from an injury or a liver disease. Certain liver diseases can inflame the diaphragm (the muscle separating the organs of the chest region from those of the abdomen) and also the part of the pleura that covers the diaphragm. People highly susceptible to respiratory infections are more likely to develop pleurisy.

The major symptom of dry pleurisy is a sharp, stabbing pain toward the side and lower part of the chest. The pain also may be felt along the shoulders, neck, and abdomen. Any action in the chest, such as breathing or coughing, will aggravate the pain, which will be accompanied by shortness of breath, dry cough, and sometimes fever.

Wet pleurisy is characterized by similar symptoms, but there may also be difficult breathing, chills, and often a blood-tinged mucus discharged with the cough, indicating pneumonia.

A diagnosis of pleurisy usually requires a physical exam during which the doctor will listen to the chest with a stethoscope for a low-pitched, grating sound that will occur with each breath. Also, the skin near the affected area may be tender. Wet pleurisy also calls for an analysis of the fluid that is oozing from the pleura. A tuberculin skin test may be taken to rule out tuberculosis, and an X ray may be ordered if the pleurisy does not seem to be caused by another respiratory infection.

To treat pleurisy, the doctor will first need to treat the underlying infection or disease that has triggered it, often with antibiotics. The symptoms of pleurisy can be relieved somewhat by bed rest, by use of a humidifier or vaporizer to add moisture to the air, or by strapping the chest with a tight binder. The latter is not always recommended, however, as it may prevent deep breathing and coughing up of mucus, both of which are necessary to clear the respiratory system of mucus. Painkillers may help to relieve chest discomfort at least enough so that the patient will not need to stifle the painful coughing that is necessary to loosen the mucus.

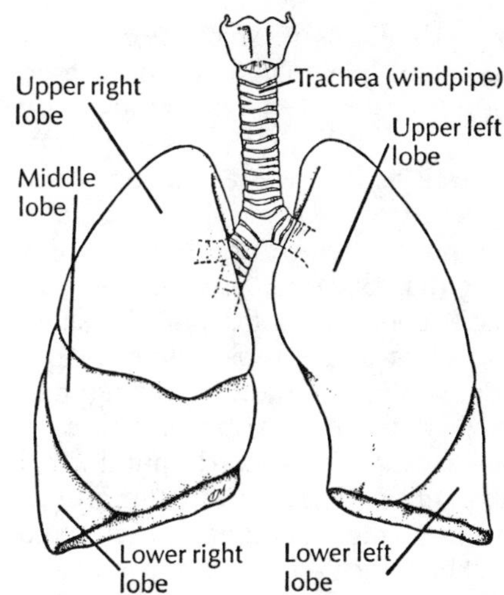

Pneumonia

Pneumonia is an infection of the lungs in which tiny air sacs in one or more sections of the lungs become inflamed and filled with fluid and white blood cells, which try to fight off the infection. It can be fatal, usually for the very young and very old.

There are several types of pneumonia, distinguished by the part of the lung that is infected. Lobar pneumonia is an infection in only one section, or lobe, of the lungs. Double pneumonia is an infection in a lobe or lobes of both lungs. Bronchial pneumonia, a complication of acute bronchitis, is the term used to describe an infection in the section of the lungs near the bronchi (the airways connecting the windpipe and lungs). Walking pneumonia is a general term people often use to describe the condition of someone who has pneumonia but is not aware of it and has not sought treatment.

Pneumonia most often strikes the person whose resistance is lowered, often by another upper respiratory tract infection or a systemic (bodywide) disease. It is often a secondary disease stemming from inadequate defense mechanisms, from cold or flu, or from long-term diseases, such as chronic bronchitis, emphysema, asthma, diabetes, cancer, or sickle-cell anemia.

Viruses, bacteria, fungi, or other microorganisms may cause pneumonia. Also, it may develop if a person inhales certain chemicals or if food, vomit, or a foreign object passes through the trachea (the windpipe) instead of the esophagus (the passageway from the mouth to the stomach) and settles in a lung. Smoking, excessive drinking, a prolonged period in bed, anesthesia, sedatives, and immune-suppressing drugs may make an individual more likely to develop pneumonia if exposed to an infectious organism. Pneumonia is most common during flu and cold epidemics and during the winter months when people are indoors where bacteria and viruses are easily spread.

All types of pneumonia are characterized by four major symptoms: chest pain, a sudden rise in temperature, coughing, and difficult breathing. Viral pneumonia, more common and generally less serious than other varieties, is recognized by coughing and other cold symptoms, as well as by general fatigue. Also, fever, chest pain, and difficult breathing may signal the presence of this disorder. Bacterial pneumonia generally comes on suddenly with shaking chills and a rapid, steep rise in temperature; shallow breathing; and a cough that brings up a bloody, dark yellow, or rust-colored sputum. An oxygen shortage that sometimes accompanies bacterial pneumonia will be indicated by other symptoms such as headache; nausea; vomiting; and cyanosis, a blue discoloration of the lips and fingertips.

Pneumonia is diagnosed by listening to the chest with a stethoscope in order to detect the presence of fluid in the lungs; X rays and an analysis of the discharge that is coughed up may also help to identify pneumonia.

Viral pneumonia is usually treated with commonsense remedies: staying in bed; drinking lots of fluids; maintaining a light diet; and using pain relievers to combat discomfort and, sometimes, oxygen to ease breathing difficulties.

The more serious bacterial pneumonia, however, requires antibiotics such as penicillin. Patients also need to stay in bed, or, if the case is serious enough, enter the hospital for care and supervision. If breathing difficulty worsens, oxygen may be administered.

There are vaccines that may help in preventing some types of pneumonia. Bacterial pneumonia caused by certain bacteria can possibly be prevented with a vaccine and it is especially recommended for the elderly or for those with chronic diseases that may weaken the respiratory system. Viral pneumonia caused by certain flu viruses may be prevented with a vaccination against influenza A, a virus which often leads to pneumonia.

The very young, the very old, and the chronically ill are the most likely to contract pneumonia, so care must be taken to protect those who fall into these categories from respiratory infections.

Poisoning

See Emergency first aid section at the end of this book.

Polycythemia

Polycythemia is a chronic disorder characterized by an increase in red blood cell mass and in concentration of hemoglobin (the substance in red blood cells that carries oxygen). Polycythemia literally means "many blood cells."

The condition is classified as a myeloproliferative disease, a disease characterized by overproduction by the bone marrow and its components of blood cells.

The exact cause of polycythemia remains unknown. The average age of the patient at onset of the disease is 60 years, but 5 percent are under 40 when the ailment first appears. It is more often seen in males and people of Jewish descent, but others are also affected. Its occurrence is rare; about seven per one million persons.

The initial symptoms include fatigue, difficulty in concentration, headache, drowsiness, forgetfulness, and dizziness. Half of its victims complain of itching, especially after a hot bath. Reddish skin color, or flushing, may be observed. On the other hand, patients may have completely normal skin color, with redness only of the mucous membranes, especially the inner lids of the eyes. Patients may complain of blurred vision, ringing in the ears, and circulatory disturbances.

Later symptoms include abnormal increase in all bone marrow material, abnormal increase in the body's blood volume, strain on the heart, and impaired blood flow.

Phlebotomy–incision of a vein and withdrawal of blood to counterbalance the overproduction of red blood cells–is probably the safest treatment since it does not interfere with the functions of bone marrow. Usually, three to six separate phlebotomies are needed for red blood cell and hemoglobin levels to return to normal. Iron-deficiency anemia often develops after a phlebotomy is performed. However, supplemental iron must not be given and foods with very high iron content should be avoided since they will raise the hemoglobin to abnormal levels. Phlebotomy followed by radiation therapy to suppress bone marrow activity produces positive results in most patients.

Pregnancy

Pregnancy is a condition in which an embryo or fetus (the embryo is an early stage and the fetus a later stage of an unborn child) is developing within the mother's uterus as a result of fertilization of her monthly egg cell by one of the father's spermatazoa (a male reproductive cell).

Fertilization, or conception, occurs in the fallopian tubes (two tubes linking the uterus to the ovaries, the female sex glands) after the egg has been ejected from the surface of one of the ovaries. The fertilized egg, also called a zygote, then travels down the fallopian tubes into the uterus, where it attaches itself to the uterine wall. It will remain there to grow and develop until birth, in most cases, nine months later.

The first symptom usually noticed by the mother is a missed menstrual period. Nausea and vomiting ("morning sickness") are also common symptoms of pregnancy. During normal pregnancy, many changes will take place in the mother's body. The abdomen will stretch and the breasts will enlarge, grow sensitive, and prepare to produce milk for the baby. In some cases, the skin will develop brown spots or splotches; blood volume will increase up to 30 percent; and breathing will stem more from the chest and less from the abdomen (because of the increased abdominal space taken up by the expanding uterus and the developing fetus). The amount of blood flowing through the kidneys will increase 25 percent to 40 percent and the bladder will pull up higher into the abdomen. There will be a slight increase in the acidity of the saliva (this may be one of the causes of nausea and vomiting). A hormone called "relaxin" will cause the bones of the pelvic area to widen during the tenth or twelfth week of pregnancy. Many of the mother's glands will expand in size; calcium and phosphorus, two essential minerals in food, requirements will almost double and there will be an increase in the demand for iron and many other elements.

Most women wait until they have missed a second period before consulting their doctor. Once the doctor confirms the pregnancy, he or she will begin a program of prenatal (before birth) care. Prenatal care consists chiefly of making sure that nothing is wrong, in other words, that there are no complications. A healthful diet is recommended and gradual caloric increases are not only allowed but advisable, provided the additional food does not come from emp-

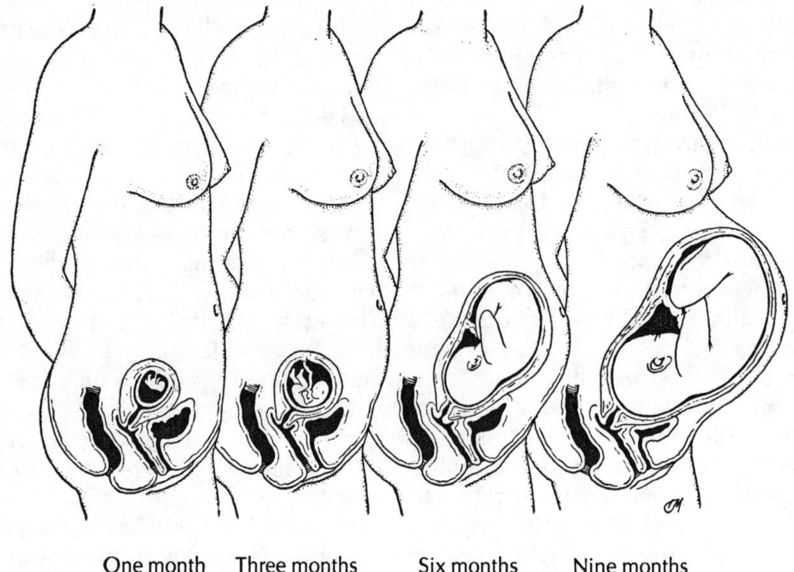

As the unborn baby grows within the uterus, the mother's body changes both internally and externally.

ty calories such as excess starches and sugars. Generally, if the woman was consuming 2,000 calories before pregnancy—with no weight gain—she should raise her intake to 2,200 or 2,400 calories in the early pregnancy period and she may be advised to increase that figure to 2,600 calories by the later stages. If the baby's weight is included, most women should gain approximately 23 to 26 extra pounds by the ninth month. It should be emphasized that this additional weight puts more stress on the back and on the legs, sometimes resulting in problems such as swayback or varicose veins (swollen veins close to the skin surface in the legs). These conditions can be eased by proper rest, exercise, and, for varicose veins, special hosiery.

Proper rest and exercise are important throughout the pregnancy. In general, a woman can participate in most, if not all, of the activities and sports she was taking part in before her pregnancy. Her doctor can help advise her about any limitations.

One of the most important aspects of prenatal care is safety in the use of medications. A pregnant woman, or one who even suspects she is pregnant, should never take a medication without her doctor's recommendation or approval. This caution includes over-the-counter preparations—even aspirin—as well as prescription drugs. In addition, a woman should not smoke during pregnancy, and she should limit, if not eliminate, alcoholic beverages. Smoking has been linked to miscarriage (the expulsion of the fetus before it is capable of surviving on its own), low birth weights, and prematurity. Alcohol, too, has been linked to miscarriage, and studies have shown that alcohol can affect the brain of the fetus. The best guideline to remember is that no drug or substance can be assumed to be harmless during pregnancy.

Once the initial nausea and vomiting period is over (usually after two or three months), many women increase their calorie intake, sometimes in a mistaken attempt to "make up for what the baby is taking." As a consequence, they show drastic gains in weight, with all of the complications, such as swollen ankles, that such gains bring. At the other extreme are those mothers who cannot eat normally because the nausea symptoms persist throughout pregnancy. In each of these cases, both the mother and the fetus may suffer. If any sudden weight gain or loss is experienced, the physician should be informed.

Either through rapid weight gain or inadequate kidney function, some women tend to swell significantly in the ankles and lower legs and, to a lesser extent, in the hands and fingers. Under no circumstances should nonprescription diuretics (drugs causing increased urinary output) be taken for this condition. The doctor should be consulted.

A normal pregnancy that runs its full time span is called a "full term pregnancy." Here, the baby is born after a full gestation (or developmental) period of 40 weeks or thereabouts. Sometimes the baby will come earlier, an event known as prematurity. During labor, the mother will begin to experience light or mild contractions of the uterus. As they become more frequent and more powerful, the amniotic sac in which the baby is growing may break (this is commonly called "breaking the water").

When delivery, or birth, is imminent, the contractions will continue to grow in frequency and strength until the baby's head (in a normal delivery) or buttocks (in a breech delivery) begins to travel through the cervix and down the vagina. When the baby's head appears at the vaginal opening, the event is called "crowning." Today, in one out of six pregnancies, the delivery is performed by cesarean section.

After delivery, milk production and breast-feeding will begin in earnest and will continue for several months until the baby is capable of taking other nourishment, unless, of course, the mother prefers to start the baby on artificial formula. In this case, she will be treated with medication and icepacks to curtail milk production. Most doctors advise that breast-feeding is best for the baby's growth and future health.

After breast-feeding ends, the breasts will return to normal size. Exercises will restore the abdominal muscles to their normal tone.

See also Conception, Ovulation, and Zygote.

Premenstrual tension

Premenstrual tension is the nervousness and irritability experienced by some women during the week before their menstrual period begins. Menstruation is the process in which the endometrium, or inner lining of the uterus, sloughs off the buildup of tissues triggered each month by hormonal releases to prepare the womb for the fertilized egg cell. If the egg is not fertilized, menstruation, in the form of a slow, bloody discharge over four or five days, ensues. In the past, this and other menstrual problems were thought to be caused by emotional instability or hysteria, but modern research has shown that there are physical reasons for menstrual disorders.

Premenstrual tension is thought to be caused by fluctuations in the production of female hormones in the course of the menstrual cycle. These hormonal changes apparently increase the amounts of salt and fluid retained in the body (called edema) during the week before the period begins. Neither the exact cause for this fluid and salt retention nor the reason for its effect on certain women is fully understood.

The symptoms of premenstrual tension appear during the week preceding menstruation and usually disappear as soon as the menstrual flow begins. In addition to nervousness and irritability, this disorder is characterized by a bloated or puffy feeling that results from fluid retention. Other symptoms include depression, headache, fatigue, tenderness in the breasts, and acne.

Premenstrual tension is often treated by reducing salt intake or taking medications (called diuretics) which help to eliminate excess fluid from the tissues. Tranquilizers as well as psychological counseling may be recommended for cases in which emotional problems are an underlying cause. A balanced diet, moderate exercise, and adequate rest may also be beneficial in treating the condition.

A reduction of salt intake in general may also help to prevent the initial edema which accompanies premenstrual tension.

Prolapse

Prolapse involves the collapse, falling, or change in position of tissue or an organ so that it turns outward, falls down, or reverses its position in reference to surrounding tissue. Prolapse is caused by injury, disease (with internal swelling), parasitic infestation, such as worms, or other inflammation.

Symptoms of prolapse vary, depending on the structure that is involved. There are four common types of prolapse.

- *Prolapse of the umbilical cord* occurs when the umbilical cord (the connection between the fetus, or unborn child, and the mother) bulges ahead of the fetus as it emerges during birth.
- *Prolapse of the iris* is a condition in which the iris (the colored portion of the eye) protrudes through the cornea (the clear covering over the iris and the pupil).
- *Rectal prolapse or prolapse of the rectum* (the lower part of the large intestine) results when the rectal tissues protrude through the anus, the opening from the rectum to the outside. (This can be caused by parasitic infestations.)
- *Prolapse of the uterus* may be one of three types, depending on severity: (1) first degree prolapse, in which the uterus sags downward to cause the cervix (the womb's open-

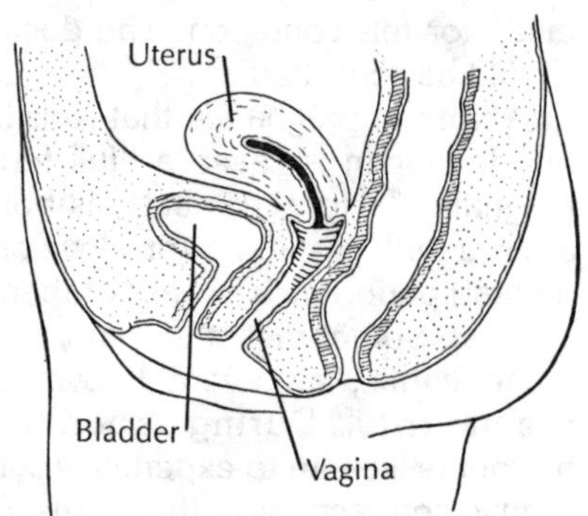

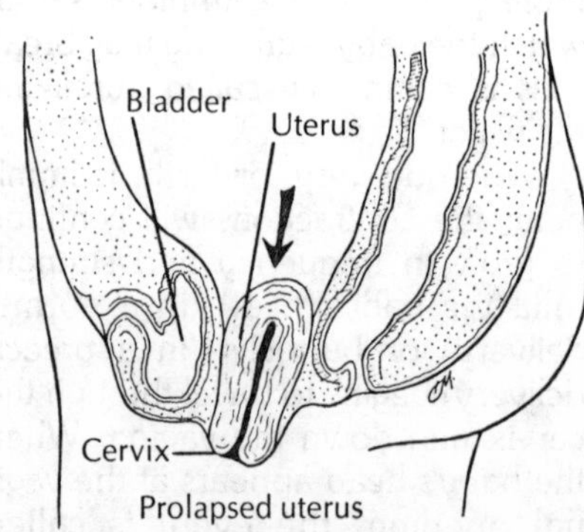

In this second degree prolapse of the uterus, the organ has fallen to a point where the cervix is outside the vagina.

ing) to fall to a point where it is flush with the entrance to the vagina; (2) second degree prolapse, in which the cervix is outside the vagina; and (3) third degree prolapse, in which the entire uterus is outside the vagina.

If the prolapse is the result of injury or stress, a surgical repair may be indicated, in which the prolapsed organ is returned to its proper place and sewn or stapled into position. If the prolapse is the result of disease or swelling, the cause of the prolapse must first be controlled and then eliminated. Afterward, the organ or tissue is returned to its original position and secured there. In mild cases of prolapse, the structure may return to its proper place without surgery.

It is especially important to monitor and prevent prolapses of the iris, the rectum, and the uterus. Iris prolapses can permanently affect the vision by damaging the cornea through which the iris protrudes. This kind of prolapse signals severe eye infection, with probable destructive internal damage. Changes in the visual field should warn about prolapse of the iris before it actually occurs. A corneal transplant may be necessary to restore vision in the affected eye, given that the infection causing the prolapse has not destroyed the internal parts of the eye. Prolapse of the rectum can lead to other serious problems such as necrosis, or tissue death, if the blood supply is cut off to affected areas. A prolapsed uterus can make future childbirth difficult, and may damage other organs, which in turn necessitates other repairs.

See also Cystocele and Rectocele.

Prostaglandins

Prostaglandins are fatty acid substances similar in chemical structure to hormones that occur naturally in the human body. Like hormones, prostaglandins appear to regulate or trigger activity in various tissues and organs. The first prostaglandin was isolated in the human prostate gland, which is how the substances got their name. More than 16 prostaglandins in six groups have now been identified. They stimulate smooth muscle, affect heart rate, influence blood pressure, and contract the uterus. Prostaglandins affect the cardiovascular (heart and blood vessel) system, the central nervous system, the gastrointestinal (digestive) system, the endocrine (hormonal) system, and the urinary tract. In the endocrine system, for example, a prostaglandin triggers the release of the vital growth hormone by the pituitary gland.

Medical researchers have been experimenting with various preparations of synthetic prostaglandins as drugs, for both diagnosis and treatment of disease. One prostaglandin stimulates contractions of the uterus in childbirth, so a prostaglandin preparation can help speed up some cases of difficult labor. Another prostaglandin has been used to reduce blood pressure in research subjects, but is not yet available as a prescription drug. Prostaglandins are also being studied in the treatment of asthma, emphysema (a serious respiratory disease), shock (a sudden, dangerous slowing down of blood circulation), and even the common cold. Researchers have successfully used a prostaglandin to halt the growth of leukemia and melanoma, two types of cancer, in cells in the laboratory.

Prostate gland

The prostate gland is a small doughnut-shaped organ located in the male genital area and positioned so that it completely surrounds the urethra (the urinary tube that leads from the bladder to the outside). The prostate gland secretes an alkaline (basic) substance that makes up the major portion of seminal fluid, which carries sperm outside the body.

The sperm, or male reproductive cells, are protected from acid (present both in the vagina and in the male urethra) by this alkalinity of the prostate's secretions. Sperm are also capable of the greatest mobility (ability to move) when in a slightly alkaline medium. Proper prostate secretion is thus essential to proper sperm action.

See also Prostatitis.

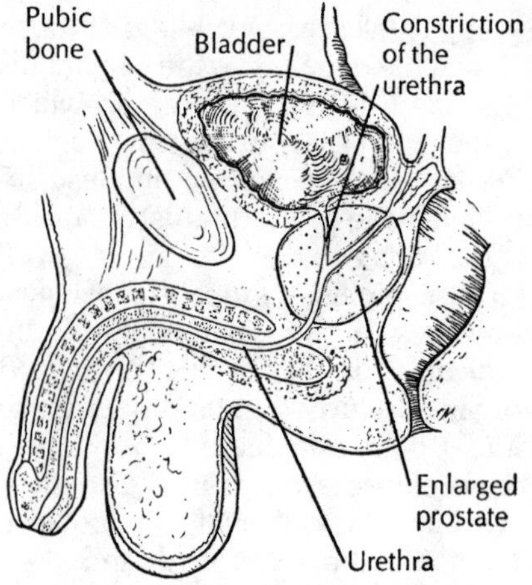

An enlarged prostate, caused by inflammation of the prostate gland, may constrict the urethra passing through and interfere with urination.

Prostatitis

Prostatitis is an infection or inflammation of the male gland called the prostate. It predominantly affects older men, usually in the form of chronic (recurring) flare-ups. Though not a serious disorder, prostatitis can be irritating and uncomfortable because it disrupts normal urination; in advanced stages, it can cause bladder or kidney damage.

Located just below the bladder, the prostrate is a small, doughnut-shaped gland that surrounds both the neck of the bladder and the urethra (the narrow tube which carries urine, from the bladder through the penis, to be expelled). As men get older, they sometimes develop an enlarged prostate, which may constrict the urethra and eventually trigger a condition called prostatism, which is a disruption of normal urination marked by prolonged effort or repeated attempts to start the flow, decreased force, and dribbling toward the end of the flow. Some urine is almost always left in the bladder, forming a fertile breeding ground for bacteria and subsequent infection common in prostatitis. Advanced cases of prostatism may cause a sudden, total blockage of urine flow, requiring emergency treatment because the backup of urine can lead to kidney and bladder damage.

An isolated bout of prostatitis can result from a sexually transmitted disease or a urinary tract infection when the bacteria from these disorders also infect the prostate gland. However, chronic prostatitis, the more common form, seldom results from an infection; in fact, its cause is unknown. It has been theorized that too much or not enough sexual activity may cause a chronic disorder, because the prostate secretes a substance during ejaculation which helps to transport sperm cells.

The most common symptoms to look for, if prostatitis is suspected, are trouble in starting the urine flow, reduced force, and dribbling as it ends; increased frequency of urination; and increased feelings of urgency, even during sleep. An infected prostate may be marked by discomfort in the lower back and genital area, a burning sensation while urinating, fever, and chills.

Prostatitis is diagnosed by an examination of the prostate to check its size, shape, and firmness. An infected prostate will be tender to the touch and, when it is massaged by the doctor, pus cells will be forced out and will then appear in the urine. A culture of the urine specimen will be examined for bacteria, although very often no bacteria are identified in a case of chronic prostatitis. However, a urinalysis may show some evidence of infection, and if a trace of blood is present, the urine will be additionally tested for the presence of malignant cells.

An enlarged prostate is diagnosed by means of a procedure called intravenous pyelogram (IVP), in which dye is injected into a vein in the arm, allowed to travel through the bloodstream to the kidneys, urinary bladder, and out through the penis. The dye will show any enlargement or obstruction in the ureters. Then the patient will be required to urinate; if the IVP shows a large quantity of urine left in the bladder, a partial obstruction caused by an enlarged prostate generally can be diagnosed.

Most prostate infections can be treated quite successfully with antibiotics. Chronic nonbacterial prostatitis, however, is not treated with antibiotics. Instead, drinking large quantities of water and nonalcoholic fluids, as well as taking hot baths, is often recommended.

An enlarged prostate that causes symptoms is normally treated by surgical removal of the excess tissue through one of two procedures: transurethral surgery (performed through the urethra), in which the center of the prostate gland is scraped out by an instrument that has been inserted into the penis; or prostatectomy, a more complicated procedure requiring an incision in the lower abdomen or between the legs. There is little danger of impotency resulting from either of these surgical procedures, but they may lead to retrograde ejaculation, a harmless condition in which semen is passed back into the bladder to be expelled with the urine, rather than out through the penis during intercourse.

Proteinuria

Proteinuria is a symptom of kidney problems marked by an excess of proteins in the urine.

Proteinuria can be caused by, among other conditions, kidney malfunctions, heart disease, the consumption of certain foods, pregnancy and adolescent changes, and overexertion from certain sports such as jogging, marathon running, and boxing.

In most adult cases of proteinuria, the disorder is first diagnosed as an unexpected finding in a routine physical examination. Usually, the person will experience no symptoms and will be essentially healthy, with no evidence of kidney disease. The total protein excretion in the urine in these early-diagnosed cases is usually less than 1000 mg per day (the norm is less than 150 mg per day). Nevertheless, the majority of patients do not show any deterioration of kidney function.

In about half of the diagnosed cases, proteinuria ceases spontaneously within a year to several years. However, there are instances in which the patient continues to lose greater and greater amounts of protein in the urine. Eventually, high blood pressure and kidney failure may develop.

When proteinuria is constant, measures of protein excretion should be made on a regular basis. In these tests, the total protein excreted in the urine in a 24-hour period is measured.

Treatment of proteinuria depends on its cause and its severity. As mentioned earlier, many cases disappear spontaneously. However, the patient should be carefully monitored and tested regularly in order to note any change in the condition. Any change in the protein level should be followed with other appropriate diagnostic testing of kidney function.

Psittacosis

Psittacosis (parrot fever or ornithosis) is a rare form of pneumonia caused by bacteria that are transmitted to humans by certain birds. The disease was first observed in parrots and later in other birds and domestic fowl. It is often accompanied by fever, coughing, and enlargement of the spleen (an abdominal organ that performs a number of blood-related functions).

Psittacosis is found principally in such birds as parrots, parakeets, lovebirds, and less often in poultry, pigeons, and canaries (in which the disease is often called ornithosis). Human infection usually takes place when a person inhales dust from feathers or excrement of infected birds. It can also be transmitted directly to a person by a bite from an infected bird or, rarely, by cough droplets of infected persons. Person-to-person transmission is rare.

After a one- to two-week incubation period (the time between exposure to the illness and the appearance of symptoms), the disease usually begins with fever, chills, headache, muscle aches, and loss of appetite. The patient's temperature continues to rise and a dry cough develops that brings up mucus and pus in the later stages. Chest X rays made during the first week of noticeable symptoms will show inflammation of the lungs. During the second week, the typical symptoms of pneumonia develop. The patient's temperature will remain above normal for at least two to three weeks and then slowly will begin to fall. A steady increase in pulse and respiratory (breathing) rates may be potentially serious. About 30 percent of untreated cases end in death. Recovery in those people who receive treatment may be gradual.

The most common drug to treat psittacosis is tetracycline, an oral antibiotic. Strict bed rest is necessary in most cases. Cough preparations with codeine are also advised. In severe cases, tetracycline may be given intravenously (through the vein).

Infected flocks of pigeons or other birds, dust from feathers, bird cage contents, and any sick domestic birds or fowl should be avoided. Specially treated feed is often used to prevent the spread of infection among imported parrots, parakeets, and lovebirds, as well as among turkeys raised for market.

Psoriasis

Psoriasis is a persistent skin disease producing thick red eruptions—often covered by silvery scales — either in small patches or over large areas of the body. Although it is not contagious, psoriasis is fairly common, affecting 1 to 2 percent of the population. The condition often first appears between the ages of 15 and 30 years and usually requires lifelong treatment.

The cause of psoriasis is unknown, but researchers believe the disease may be related to skin growth and regeneration (cell replacement). With normal skin, the epidermis, or outer layer, continually sheds old cells and replaces them with new ones formed in the skin's deeper layers. Cells live for about one month before they die and flake off. With psoriasis, the rate of cell growth accelerates. Skin cells may move to the surface and die in as short a time as four or five days. Increased cell growth causes buildup that can be extremely dry and irritating. While the normal shedding process is usually unnoticeable, psoriasis can produce very obvious blemishes.

Psoriasis seems to show a strong hereditary factor, although only one third of its victims can recall a relative who had the disease. There seems to be some relationship between the condition and arthritis, as well.

Once psoriasis develops, outbreaks of the disorder can be triggered in several ways. Injury to the skin, such as a cut or burn, may provoke a flare-up, usually eight to 18 days after the trauma. Seasonal changes may also affect psoriasis, with the disease worsening during winter months. Many patients have greater problems during periods of physical and emotional stress. Infections, too, such as upper respiratory or throat infections, seem to aggravate psoriasis.

Psoriasis is characterized by reddened, raised patches of skin with silvery scales called plaques. These clearly defined plaques appear more on the elbows, knees, trunk, or scalp, although underarm and genital areas may also be involved. Patches on the scalp shed large silver-white scales at the hairline that resemble severe dandruff. Those patches found in moist areas, such as underarms, are usually less scaly and red. All patches may itch. If fingernails are involved, the nails may be pitted or discolored. More advanced cases may show the nails separated from the nail bed.

Usually, psoriasis produces no general health problems. Sometimes, however, the disease becomes so severe that chills, painful redden-

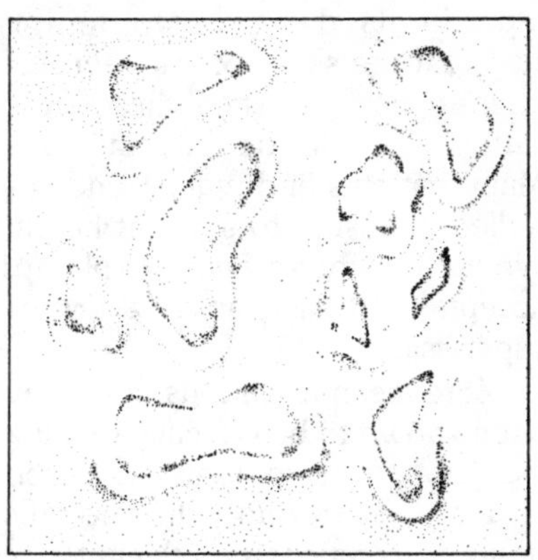

Psoriasis eruptions are clearly defined reddish, raised patches of skin with a silvery covering called plaques.

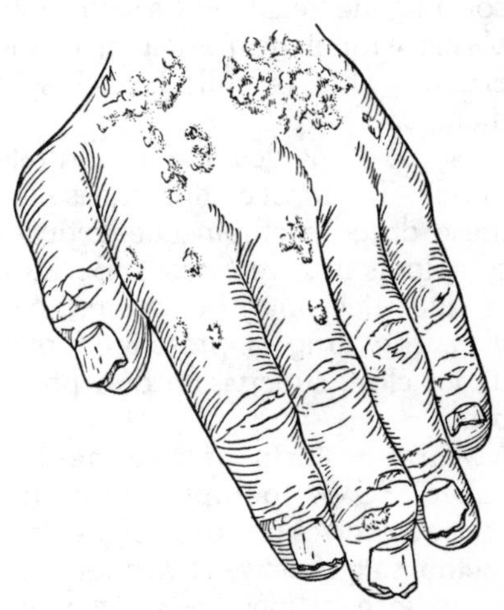

Psoriasis that has spread to the fingernails may cause pitting and discoloration of the nails.

ing of the skin, cracking of the skin around joints, and shedding of large areas of scaled skin result. This condition is exfoliative psoriasis, and patients often require hospitalization for intensive therapy.

As yet, there is no known cure for psoriasis, and treatment offers only temporary relief from symptoms. Cleaning the skin is important to prevent infection. Over-the-counter lotions and creams can cleanse irritated skin and reduce itching, as well. These preparations often contain small amounts of coal tar and other ingredients designed to remove scales. If the skin becomes sensitive after application, use of these preparations should be discontinued. Many patients find regular and controlled exposure to sunlight helpful. Where sunlight is scarce, a sunlamp is acceptable if used under a doctor's supervision.

More recently, various drugs have been shown to be effective in relieving psoriasis symptoms. Cortisone and newer steroids (hormonally-based medications) can clear plaques in about 50 percent of the cases when applied directly to the affected skin. Many physicians recommend covering the treated areas with a thin plastic wrapping in addition to the cream. This is called occlusive therapy.

Some drugs slow the growth rate of cells. The most commonly used of these drugs, methotrexate, reduces symptoms in severe cases. Because its side effects may be severe, however, the drug is prescribed only under close supervision of a physician.

Another form of treatment is called PUVA therapy. Here, the patient receives one dose of the drug methoxsalen followed two hours later by a dose of long-wave ultraviolet light. This procedure is repeated twice weekly until the psoriasis clears up (usually 20 to 25 treatments). More than 80 percent of the patients given this therapy report at least partial relief. However, these benefits need careful weighing against the premature skin aging and skin cancer that PUVA therapy may cause.

Psychosomatic illness

Psychosomatic (or psychophysiological) illnesses are a broad, loosely-defined group of disorders in which physical symptoms are of mental, emotional, or psychological origin. They are not specific "diseases" or "disorders," as these terms are commonly used, but instead symptoms that are at least partly psychological in origin.

There are many ways in which psychosomatic illness can be fully defined. In some cases, psychological factors can contribute directly or indirectly to the cause of some physical disorders, as with heart disease and Type A (heart attack-prone) personalities, who show aggressiveness, competitive drive, preoccupation with deadlines, a chronic sense of impatience, and a feeling of time urgency. On the one hand, a Type A patient's heart attack is not psychosomatic in that the illness itself is of physical and not psychological origins, but on the other hand, the personality type can be linked rather definitively with this set of physical symptoms.

There are other cases in which psychiatric symptoms are direct expressions or symptoms of disease, as in disorders involving the nervous system or endocrine (hormone-producing) organs. In other cases, psychological symptoms occur as reactions to the physical illness, especially if the illness is recurring or chronically disabling.

Thus, the term "psychosomatic symptoms" or "psychosomatic illness" covers all these cases, but common usage confines the term "psychosomatic" to conditions in which psychological factors appear actually to cause the illness.

Current thinking on psychosomatic illness suggests that social stress may appear disguised in somatic form—that is, in the form of physical symptoms. Often the patient overlooks or denies the underlying emotional disturbance. Subsequent testing fails to reveal the source of the problem in many cases and diagnosis is vague.

Almost any type of symptom that can be imagined by a patient can be psychosomatic in origin. In fact, it is estimated that one third of all patient complaints to a doctor may be at least partially psychosomatic in cause. Sometimes, the patient may have previously experienced the symptom as a real condition, and at a time of social stress the symptom "reappears." Or the patient has a real illness or injury, is treated and cured, but still insists the symptoms are persisting. Occasionally, the patient may "borrow" the symptoms from another person (for example, he or she complains of chest pains while caring for a relative with a heart attack).

While almost any sort of symptom may be psychosomatic, the most typical complaint is pain—facial pain, headaches, generalized abdominal pain, backache, painful menstrual cycles in women, and so on.

There is also a psychological disorder called Munchausen's syndrome, which is the technical name for pathological malingering or chronic fictitious illness. This syndrome involves repeated fabrications of illness, usually acute, dramatic, and generally convincing, by a patient who goes from doctor to doctor, hospital to hospital, clinic to clinic, for treatment. Many of the "patients" have studied medical textbooks closely and have learned to mimic the symptoms of unusual or dramatic diseases. Sometimes they even practice self-mutilation and give themselves abscesses, scars, rashes, even infestations of pinworms and other organisms. In some bizarre variations, a child or other relative is used as a surrogate patient and the parent or other relative will falsify medical history, injure the other person with drugs, add blood or bacteria to urine and blood samples, all in order to simulate a disease of his or her choice.

Diagnosis of psychosomatic disorders is often difficult since the patient may be quite skilled at manipulation and deception or may be unaware of his or her own motivations.

For patients with true psychosomatic disorders, such as those with Munchausen's syndrome, successful treatment is rare. Often, complying with the patient's wishes for treatment or testing relieves the symptoms temporarily, but usually the demands grow, and if the doctor refuses additional or more dramatic treatment methods, the patient often becomes angry and moves on to another doctor, clinic, or hospital. Psychiatric treatment is often refused or circumvented. Therefore, treatment is usually limited to early recognition of the true nature of the disorder, avoidance of risky or expensive procedures and testing, and refusal to administer unwarranted medication. If the patient can accept any kind of counseling or psychiatric help, that will, of course, become the treatment of preference.

Pulmonary embolism

A pulmonary embolism is a clump of matter that blocks a blood vessel in the lungs. Emboli are composed of a variety of materials, and when they travel, they eventually come to vessels too tiny for them to pass. When this happens in the lungs, these clumps are called pulmonary emboli.

Emboli develop from a variety of causes. They may break off venous thrombi (blood clots that originate chiefly in the lower extremities, especially the thigh), which may be

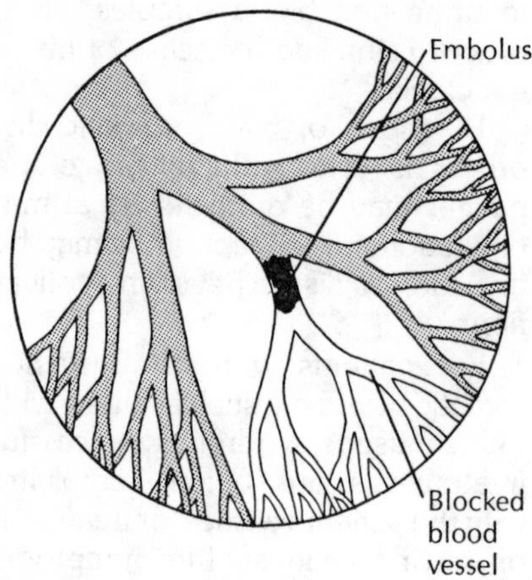

Pulmonary embolism occurs when the blood vessels of the lungs are blocked by a clump of matter. The blood supply in the area behind the blockage is thus cut off.

caused by an increase in number and clumping of platelets (the blood elements that help in clotting), as the result of injury, surgery, and peripheral vascular diseases. Also, venous thrombi are sometimes the result of an increase in the thickness of the blood (as would occur in polycythemia—an increase in the total number of red blood cells in the blood).

Other types of emboli may consist of either pieces of matter that have broken loose from their points of origin (as in pieces of tumors or whole tumors) or the clumping of blood cells around a foreign body such as a catheter particle or a foreign protein (for example, venom or other poisonous substances).

Emboli may be classified as solid (detached blood clots, clumps of tumor cells, or bits of foreign objects); liquid (globules of fat); or gaseous (air). Emboli may also be either bland (nonpoisonous) or septic (poisonous or infectious). Any one or more of these types of emboli may find its way into the lungs and become a pulmonary embolus.

The sudden development of the following symptoms may indicate the presence of a pulmonary embolus: wheezing; dyspnea (labored or difficult breathing); chest pains; hemoptysis (spitting up blood); unexplained low oxygen levels in arterial blood; and right heart strain, as indicated on an ECG (electrocardiogram).

Diagnostic procedures for detection of pulmonary embolism may include a test of arterial blood (blood pumped out of the heart), an ECG, and a lung scan with X rays. The definitive diagnostic procedure is pulmonary angiography, which consists of an X-ray scan of the lungs after the introduction of a dye into the bloodstream. This will show the embolus in relief against the contrast dye and can pinpoint its location. As serious as pulmonary emboli potentially are, only a small number are lethal.

In the event of pulmonary embolism, oxygen is adminstered and blood pressure, as well as heart functions, are supported by medication or manual resuscitation, if necessary. Anticoagulant medication (to slow blood clotting) is administered, in order to prevent the development of additional emboli. The drugs usually given are heparin and warfarin.

In about 20 percent of pulmonary embolism cases in which a venous thrombus is determined to be the origin, the inferior vena cava (the main vein for the lower limbs and the pelvis) may be deliberately blocked by an "umbrella filter" or a clip in order to keep a venous thrombus from traveling farther.

Sometimes the embolism must be removed surgically. This is done only when the patient demonstrates low blood pressure as a side effect of the embolus, and when surgery can be done only a few hours after the embolism has occurred.

The best prevention of pulmonary emboli is early detection and treatment of venous thrombosis.

See also Embolism.

Purpura

The term purpura refers to a group of bleeding disorders that are all characterized by purplish or brownish-red discolorations, easily visible through the skin's outer layer, caused by hemorrhages (internal bleeding) into the tissues.

Common purpura is the most widespread of such disorders and is marked by easy bruising and increased blood vessel fragility. It is an inherited condition occurring mostly in women, particularly following menopause. The result is simple, or senile, purpura, which often affects thigh tissue and produces large bruises rather than hemorrhages. The bleeding pattern is usually under the skin and may be intensified by surgery or injury.

Allergic purpura and anaphylactoid purpura are also known as Henoch-Schonlein purpura. This is a condition that is most often seen in children and can be associated with arthritis, gastrointestinal disorders, kidney failure, and erythema (skin inflammation). Purpura fulminans, a similar problem, is also seen in children, mainly after an infectious disease. It is marked by fever, shock (a dangerous, sudden lowering of blood pressure), anemia, rapidly spreading symmetrical skin hemorrhages in the lower limbs, as well as by intravascular thrombosis (blocking of a blood vessel by a solid mass) and gangrene (tissue death).

Thrombocytopenic purpura is any form of purpura in which the platelet (the tiny elements in the blood that are vital to clotting) count is decreased, whether as a primary disease or as a consequence of another blood disorder. This form of purpura is characterized by anemia, side effects in the nervous system, and minor blood clots in tiny blood vessels.

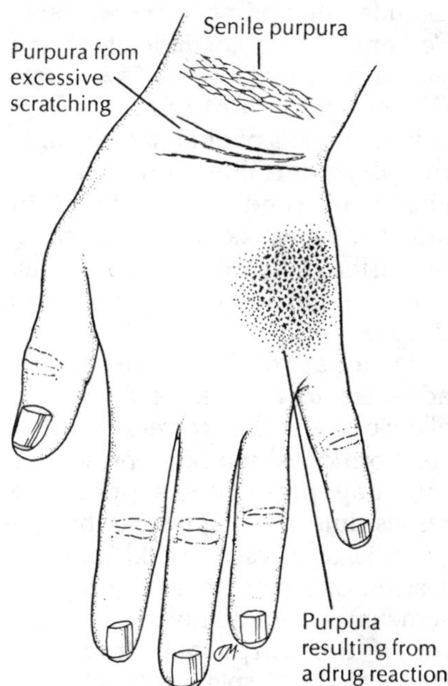

Purpura, or bleeding of the smaller blood vessels beneath the skin's surface, may have many causes.

Causes vary with the type of purpura. For example, common purpura, when it occurs in postmenopausal women, appears to result from decreased estrogen (female hormone) levels and thinning deep-layered skin tissues. Allergic purpura may result from the development of immunities that often follows an infection or allergic reaction. The secondary purpuras always accompany other diseases or disorders, and purpura sometimes is seen in the elderly because of the skin's fragility. There are also temporary forms of purpura in which vascular bleeding occurs as a result of fever, hypothyroidism (low output of thyroid hormone), generalized illness, defects in the small vessels, or a drug reaction to certain medications such as aspirin. Finally, purpura can sometimes stem from overly tight clothing or from injuries, such as a black eye.

Laboratory testing is essential in the case of all the purpuras in order to exclude other primary causes if any. Perhaps the most difficult of the purpuras to diagnose is allergic (Henoch-Schonlein) purpura. Joint pain and bouts of abdominal pain in this disorder may mimic acute abdominal conditions or forms of arthritis. Later, kidney involvement during the course of this purpura may cause a misdiagnosis of kidney disease.

In the case of allergic purpura it is advisable to eliminate the possible allergic cause. Corticosteroids (artificial hormones) are often prescribed but may produce disappointing results. Immunosuppressive therapy (artificial suppression of the immune system, often by means of drugs) is sometimes, though not always, useful. If the purpura is thrombocytopenic, the spleen, an abdominal organ tied into the circulatory system, may be removed if it is hoarding too many platelets. Milder cases of any form of purpura often improve spontaneously.

Estrogen therapy has proved helpful in preventing or relieving common purpura in postmenopausal women. Other than preventive measures to avoid infections or allergic reactions, there is little that can be done to prevent purpura.

Pyelonephritis

Pyelonephritis is a bacteria-caused inflammation of the kidney, affecting both the kidney tissue and the renal pelvis (the funnel-shaped expansion of the upper end of the ureter where it joins the kidney).

There are two types of pyelonephritis, *descending* and *ascending*. In the descending type, bacteria reach the kidney through the bloodstream, infecting first the kidney tissues themselves, and then "descending" or moving downward to infect the renal pelvis of the kidney. In the more common ascending type, the bladder is infected first, and the infection then spreads by moving upward from the bladder to infect the kidney tissues.

Causes of pyelonephritis may include scars from previous infections, urinary tract infections, abnormal growth of the prostate (a male gland secreting fluids), kidney stone and tumors, stagnation of urine due to backflow from the bladder, diabetes mellitus (a condition of excess sugar in the bloodstream), and pregnancy.

Symptoms of pyelonephritis are low back pain, difficulty in urinating, burning sensation upon urination, edema (swelling, including puffiness under the eyes), mental confusion, nausea, vomiting, and—in extreme cases—loss of consciousness. Although some cases of chronic (recurring) pyelonephritis can be traced to an acute onset or initial attack, with persistent, recurrent bacterial infections following, there are many cases in which there is no such acute phase. Often patients will have no real evidence of past or current infections.

Acute pyelonephritis is treated with antibiotics given orally or intravenously (through the vein). Recurrent episodes should be treated with any of a number of appropriate antibiotics. Chronic pyelonephritis requires careful management and frequent reevaluation. Patients should be treated with an antibiotic even during periods when they feel no symptoms and receive long-term therapy after that.

Pyloric stenosis

Pyloric stenosis is a narrowing of the passage between the stomach and the small intestine. The stomach has two openings: at the top, where it joins with the esophagus, which is the food passage between the throat and the stomach, and at the bottom, where it joins with the small intestine. The lower opening is called the pylorus.

Pyloric stenosis (stenosis means narrowing or constriction) can be caused by many conditions including cancer, spasm, a nearby ulcer in the part of the intestine directly below the pyloric opening, gastritis (inflammation of the stomach, or enlargement of the pyloric sphincter muscle (the muscle that rings the pyloric opening and controls its movement).

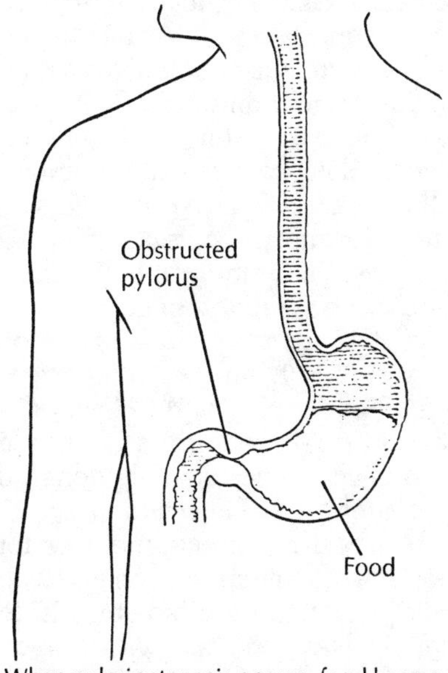

When pyloric stenosis occurs, food has no way of entering into the intestines from the stomach.

In the case of congenital (present at birth) pyloric stenosis, ten days to three weeks after birth the infant will experience regurgitation (weak "spitting up" of part of the stomach's contents), projectile vomiting (vomiting with great force), weight loss, and dehydration (loss of body fluids) without appetite loss. Adults with pyloric stenosis experience discomfort in the upper and middle portion of the abdomen, pain, bloating of the abdominal area, nausea and vomiting, and weight loss.

In mild cases of pyloric stenosis, the condition can be treated by taking small feedings or meals, restoring normal fluid levels, and administering anticholinergic drugs (drugs that block the strength of the nerve impulses that are making the pyloric muscle contract).

In severe cases, a pyloromyotomy (a lengthwise incision into the pyloric muscle) may be indicated. Also, a portion of the pyloric sphincter muscle may be removed.

Pyorrhea

See Periodontal disease.

R

Rabies

Rabies (hydrophobia) is an acute infectious viral disease of the central nervous system of mammals, especially carnivores (meat eaters), which is characterized by central nervous system (CNS) irritation, followed by paralysis and, in some cases, death. Human infection usually follows the bite of a rabid animal (dogs, skunks, cats, foxes, coyotes, and so forth). In the later stages of the disease, it is marked by paralysis of the swallowing muscles and by throat spasms, which are set off by drinking or even the sight of liquids (hence, hydrophobia or "fear of water"). Convulsions, tetanus and respiratory (breathing) paralysis are other symptoms of the last stages. Fortunately, because of animal immunization programs, there are now no more than about five reported cases of rabies per year in the United States.

Rabies is caused by a virus that is present in the saliva of rabid animals. Rabid animals transmit the infection by biting other animals or human beings. Rabies can also be acquired by exposure of a mucous membrane or of an open skin wound to infected animal saliva.

The rabies virus travels from the site of entry to the spinal cord and brain, where it multiplies. It then spreads to the salivary glands and into the saliva itself. In human beings the incubation period (the time between exposure to the virus and development of symptoms) may extend from ten days to one year, but the average incubation period is 30 to 50 days. The incubation period is shortest in persons who have been bitten on the head or trunk or those who have multiple bites.

The first symptom is a short period of mental depression, restlessness, and fever. In the next stage of the disease, the restlessness increases to an uncontrollable excitement and hyperactivity. There is excessive salivation ("foaming at the mouth") and painful spasms of the throat muscles. The spasms can be easily initiated—by a breath of air, a slight breeze, an attempt to drink water. Generally, the patient experiences overwhelming thirst, but cannot drink. In untreated cases, death occurs within three to ten days. However, patients often survive the disease if diagnosis and treatment are prompt.

In human patients, diagnosis of rabies is usually suspected by a report of an animal bite or exposure to the saliva of a rabid animal. The diagnosis is confirmed by testing for the virus once the symptoms appear. A domestic animal with no symptoms, such as a cat or dog, that suddenly bites a human should be confined and observed by a veterinarian for ten days. If the animal still shows no symptoms, it was not infectious at the time of the bite and is usually released. However, if the animal is apparently rabid or is a wild animal, it should be captured. Local police or health departments should be notified so that they can capture and examine the animal.

As soon as the bite or exposure of an open wound to animal saliva occurs, the contaminated area should be cleansed immediately and thoroughly with a 20 percent solution of medicinal soap. Deep puncture wounds should be flushed out with soapy water. It is not advisable to cauterize (seal by heat) or sew up the wound.

The next step is antirabies serum for passive immunization. This is followed by vaccine for active immunization. HDCV, a new active immunization, is said to have only mild side effects for most people. Both active and passive immunizing products should be used at once.

HDCV injections are given on days 3, 7, 14, and 28 after exposure. The WHO (World Health Organization) recommends that a sixth injection be routinely done 90 days after the first injection.

The best preventive measure for rabies is to minimize contact with rabid or suspected rabid animals. In many cases, persons with a high occupational risk of animal bites receive "preexposure" injections. This is especially helpful for zoo personnel and persons whose work or hobbies take them into areas where they are likely to encounter rabid animals.

As for domestic animals, restraining dogs and cats and impounding stray animals is the best preventive measure. Immunizing 70 percent or more of the dog population of major cities has helped to restrict transmission of rabies, even in areas where wild animals have the disease.

Controlling rabies in wildlife areas is more difficult, although rabies as a disease is self-limiting because it tends to kill off susceptible hosts in an area. Expensive control efforts are generally limited to areas where humans are apt to be exposed to wildlife—in campgrounds, parks, wildlife preserves, and so on.

Radioactive isotopes

Radioactive isotopes, or radioisotopes, are used primarily as a diagnostic tool to detect tumors, blood clots or malfunctioning organs in the body.

A radioisotope is a variation of a normal chemical element that contains a different number of neutrons in its unstable nucleus (which is the center of the atom, the element's smallest part). Because it is unstable, the nucleus disintegrates and gives off electrically charged energy (ionizing radiation).

Certain elements are attracted to, or are used by, particular organs. For example, iodine, when given by mouth or injected, will travel to and is used by the thyroid gland. Radioactive iodine, when administered to a patient, will also travel to the thyroid gland, but, because of its special properties, it will show up on X rays. A machine, called a scanner, is placed near the patient and picks up the radiation emitted by the radioactive isotope as it travels to the organ being studied. The scanner converts the radiation into flashes of light and then into an image, which is put on an X ray film or projected onto a screen.

Using this technique, a physician can determine the position, shape, and size of an organ or the presence of a tumor. By looking at the rate at which the radioisotope is absorbed and eliminated, the doctor can also see how the organ is functioning.

Radioisotopes are mainly used to study the "soft tissues" (thyroid gland, brain, liver, spleen, and kidney), which do not show well on regular X rays. The most recent advance in radioisotope diagnosis has allowed doctors to observe the heart muscle. Although the procedure is still quite costly, it holds out much promise for victims of heart attack or other abnormalities. Some conditions that can be detected by using radioisotopes are over- or underfunctioning organs, tumors, blood clots, injuries, bone marrow disease, red blood cell irregularities, cirrhosis of the liver (a condition in which the internal tissues of the liver are scarred and otherwise damaged), hepatitis (inflammation of the liver), nonabsorption of Vitamin B_{12}, and certain anemias.

Radiation poisoning poses no danger to the individual being tested. Because very small amounts of radiation can be detected and measured, only a minute amount of a radioisotope is required.

Rash

A rash is an eruption on the surface of the skin, covering either small areas of the body or extensive areas, in the form of red spots, patches, or blisters. Often, a rash causes itching, but this is not always the case. A rash is usually a temporary condition, appearing and disappearing within a few days if not sooner. If so, there is little need for worry; however, a rash can also be a symptom of infectious diseases or other disorders.

Rashes may be caused by exposure to the sun, heat and cold, the chemicals in household cleansers or detergents, fabrics, or certain foods (these are called allergic rashes). A rash can appear as a visually distinctive and major symptom of certain diseases, including allergies, measles, rubella (German measles), chicken pox, shingles, and some sexually transmitted diseases.

Rashes that appear regularly with no other symptoms may indicate the presence of an allergy; if a rash is accompanied by other symptoms, it is more likely that the cause is an infectious disease.

Any rash that lasts for more than a few days should be examined by a doctor. A rash will usually disappear when its underlying cause is treated. In the case of allergy, perhaps the only possible treatment will be something to relieve minor itching and irritation, but a diagnosis and allergy testing may at least indicate which irritant (allergen) to avoid in the future.

Raynaud's phenomenon and disease

Raynaud's phenomenon and disease involve a spasm or spasms of the arterioles (small artery branches), especially in the fingers and hands and occasionally in other parts, such as the nose and tongue. It is often accompanied by intermittent paleness or cyanosis (bluish discoloration) of the skin.

Raynaud's phenomenon may be of unknown cause, in which case it is called Raynaud's disease, or it may be a secondary symptom of conditions such as connective tissue disorders (scleroderma), nerve disorders, drug reactions, pulmonary hypertension, and myxedema (a dry, waxy swelling of the skin sometimes called "non-pitting edema"). If it is caused by another condition, it is called Raynaud's phenomenon.

For whatever reason, Raynaud's disease is most common in young women. Often, the attacks are precipitated by exposure to cold or by emotional upsets or stress. The color changes may come in three stages—pallor (extreme paleness), cyanosis, and then extreme redness, called reactive hyperemia. On the other hand, the color changes may go through only two cycles: cyanosis and then redness. Normal color and sensation are restored when the hands are warmed. Color changes in the hands do not affect the joints and seldom affect the thumb. Pain is usually not present, but numbness, tingling, or burning are common complaints.

Raynaud's disease differs from secondary Raynaud's phenomenon in that both sides of the body are involved. Raynaud's disease also tends to continue for at least two years with no progression of symptoms.

If Raynaud's phenomenon is associated with diseases such as scleroderma, there can also be tightness and thickening of the skin of the hands, arms, and face; difficulty in swallowing; painful open sores on the fingertips; blood vessel lesions on the hands, wrist, and lips; and sometimes blockage of the artery nearest the wrist.

Therapy for secondary Raynaud's phenomenon depends chiefly on diagnosing correctly and then treating the underlying disturbance.

Mild cases of Raynaud's disease can be helped substantially by protecting the body and extremities from extreme cold. Also mild sedatives, taken orally, can be of help. The patient is always advised to stop smoking, since nicotine acts as a constrictor of blood vessels. Reserpine, an antihypertensive and tranquilizer, may be useful but there are side effects, such as depression.

A more extreme measure is regional sympathectomy (an interruption of some part of the nerve pathways). This operation is reserved for patients with progressive disability; while it abolishes the symptoms, the relief may last for only a year or two. Results of the surgery are usually better in patients with Raynaud's disease than in those with the secondary phenomenon.

Rectocele

Rectocele is a condition in which a portion of the rectum, the tubular-shaped organ at the end of the intestinal tract, protrudes into the vagina. The usual cause of this condition is a weakening of the back wall of the vagina due to the stretching caused by childbirth.

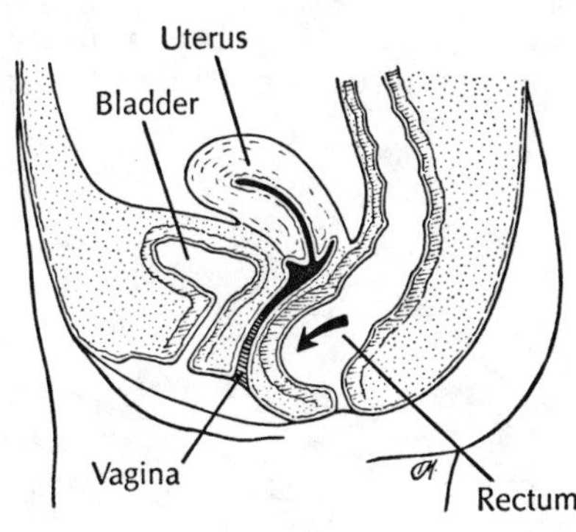

Rectocele occurs when the rectum protrudes onto the back wall of the vagina.

A minimal protrusion may produce no symptoms or a mild pressure sensation during bowel movements. More severe protrusion of the rectum may lead to chronic constipation and painful bowel movements.

A rectocele is easily diagnosed by the doctor during a pelvic examination. After straining or coughing, the rectum may be seen bulging into the vagina.

Rectocele is not a dangerous condition and generally requires no treatment. If severe constipation or painful bowel movements develop, surgical repair is often curative. Mild symptoms may be relieved by avoiding straining and heavy lifting and by drugs and diet that will ensure a soft bowel movement.

Reiter's syndrome

Reiter's syndrome is a simultaneous occurrence of *urethritis* (an inflammation of the urethra, the tube from the bladder to the outside of the body), *conjunctivitis* (an inflammation of the conjunctiva, which is the membrane that covers the front of the eyeball and the insides of the eyelids), and *arthritis* (an inflammation of the joints). Diarrhea occurs in some cases. It is a condition that affects males more often than females.

The syndrome develops from sexual transmission, but is not caused by the gonorrhea microbe. Instead, it is thought that Reiter's syndrome is caused by a virus-like organism called chlamydia.

Reiter's syndrome exhibits multiple symptoms, any one of which might be mistaken for another disease. The conjunctiva becomes inflamed, with corresponding discomfort around the eyes. The intestinal tract exhibits the symptoms of diarrhea, with a corresponding loss of water (which should be replaced immediately). Urethritis causes discomfort during urination. Arthritic symptoms appear, with swelling and pain in the joints. Furthermore, most victims develop fever, lesions (on the palms of the hands, the soles of the feet, trunk, and mouth), watery growths on the skin, and iritis (an inflammation of the iris, the part of the eye that gives it color).

Treatment for Reiter's syndrome is similar to that for rheumatoid arthritis: aspirin or, if aspirin is ineffective, anti-inflammatory drugs such as indomethacin or phenylbutazone. The antibiotic tetracycline may help control the urethritis. Conjunctivitis may be treated with cortisone eyedrops.

Reproduction

The reproductive system includes those organs in the male and female body that function to create new life and, in the female, to nourish it during the developmental stage until birth. Some doctors include breasts as reproductive parts, because they may nourish the new life after birth.

Female reproductive system. The female reproductive system consists of those structures within the female body designed to create and nourish new life. The system includes the ovaries, fallopian tubes, uterus, cervix, and vagina.

Breasts, or mammary glands, are often considered organs of reproduction, but they are actually a type of sweat gland. However, their development is regulated by the reproductive system. For example, hormones manufactured by the ovaries control breast growth during puberty (the time of life around 11 or 12 years when sex organs begin to mature) and milk production after childbirth.

The reproductive process begins in the ovaries. Ovaries are small, egg-shaped glands located in the lower abdomen. These glands monitor the cyclic functions of the reproductive system based on ovulation. Ovulation is the monthly production and release of a mature egg (occasionally two or more eggs). This action and other reproductive functions result from stimulation of

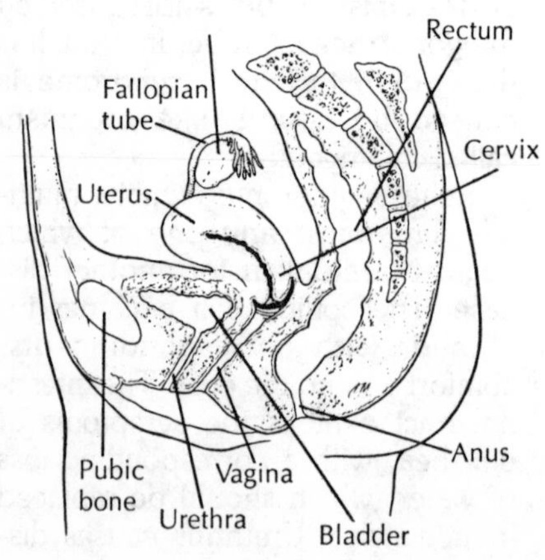

A side view of the female reproductive organs.

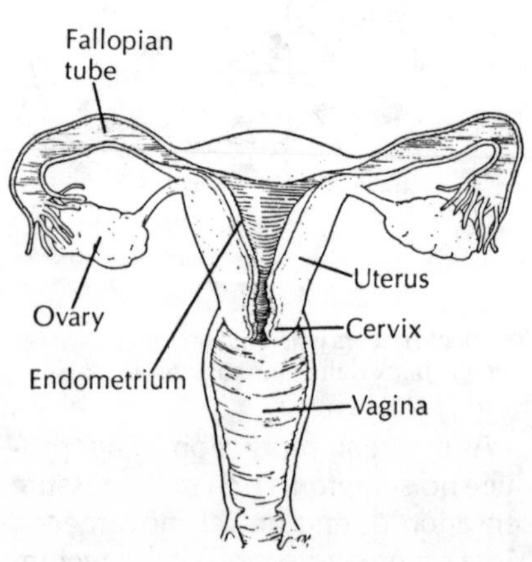

A front view of the female reproductive organs.

hormones—estrogen and progesterone—secreted by the ovaries. Estrogen regulates the secondary sex traits of body hair growth, breast development, ovulation, and menstruation. Progesterone contributes to reproduction, as well as to enlargement of the breasts during pregnancy and milk production after childbirth. The two hormones coordinate to control the menstrual cycle. When either hormone level increases or decreases, menstrual irregularities result.

Once an egg is released, it travels through the fallopian tubes. There are two fallopian tubes and they extend from each ovary into the uterus. Their reproductive function is to contain the egg until fertilization (union between the egg and sperm, or male sex cell) takes place. Fallopian tubes direct the sperm to the egg and then propel the fertilized egg into the uterus.

The uterus is a pear-shaped hollow organ normally about the size of a lemon. Its muscular walls are lined with rich, soft tissue called the endometrium. Each month the lining adds layers in anticipation of receiving and nourishing a fertilized egg. Should conception (union of sperm and egg) occur, the lining nourishes the fertilized egg in the uterus until birth. However, if the egg remains unfertilized, the uterus sheds the endometrium and the unfertilized egg, which leaves the body as menstrual discharge.

The cervix is a narrow opening to an inch-long canal. The canal connects the lower end of the uterus to the upper portion of the vagina. This canal transports sperm on their way to fertilize an egg and is the passageway for menstrual discharge and babies leaving the uterus.

The vagina, or birth canal, is a passageway leading from the uterus to the outside of the body. In the average adult woman, it measures four to five inches in length. Although vaginal walls are normally close together, they separate to accommodate a descending baby during childbirth and the erect male penis during sexual intercourse.

The vagina produces natural secretions that provide continual lubrication and cleansing of the organ. The amount of secretion may vary with the menstrual cycle and emotional state.

Male reproductive system. The male reproductive system consists of those structures in the male body designed to create life. The system includes the two testes, a network of ducts, a set of glands, and the penis.

Testes are two oval-shaped glands located in the scrotum, a pouch of skin hanging behind the penis. Their job is to produce male sex hormones (called androgens and testosterone) and sperm (sex) cells. Sex hormones control secondary male sex characteristics from puberty on, including penis growth, body hair growth, voice change, and increased muscle mass.

Testes discharge sperm cells into the epididymis, the first structure in the duct system. Other passageways include the vas deferens, the ejaculatory duct, and the urethra. The entire duct system transports sperm from the testes to the outside of the body.

The epididymis runs along the top and side of each testis. Inside the epididymis are several ducts which direct sperm from the testes into the vas deferens. The vas deferens, or continuation of the epididymis, loops up into the body before descending into a duct in the seminal vesicle gland. This duct from the seminal vesicle becomes the ejaculatory duct. From here, the duct stretches through the prostate gland and enters the upper segment of the urethra, the

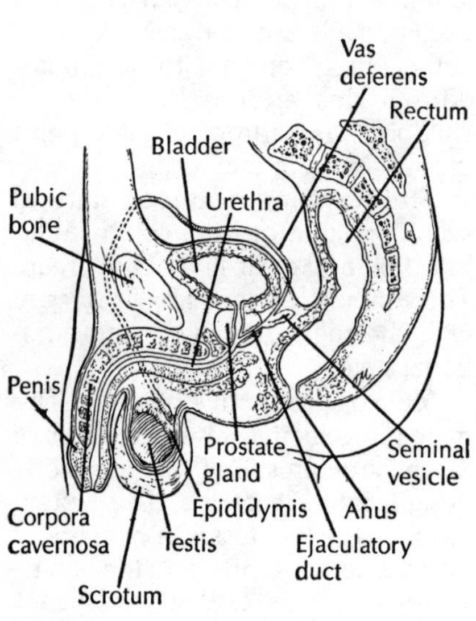

A side view of the male reproductive organs.

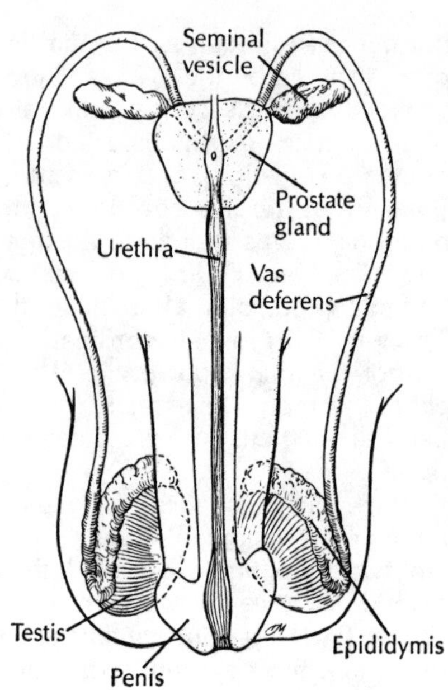

A front view of the male reproductive organs.

tube from the bladder to the outside of the body. At different times the urethra functions as an exit tube for urine as well as for sperm.

As sperm travel through the duct system, they combine with fluids from the male glands. The two main types of male glands are the seminal vesicles and the prostate gland. Seminal vesicles each lie near the underside of the bladder (storage depot for urine before elimination from the body). They discharge a sticky, thick fluid that unites with the sperm cells emerging from the testes.

The prostate gland surrounds the upper portion of the urethra as it leaves the bladder. This gland secretes a thin fluid which combines with the sperm cells and seminal vesicle fluid. Prostate fluid helps activate the sperm.

Sperm mixed with glandular fluids is called semen. Semen forms in the urethra and travels out of the penis during sexual excitement, or ejaculation.

The penis is the external organ that propels sperm into the female during sexual intercourse. When sexually excited, the large internal spaces, or corpora cavernosa, within the penis fill with blood. As the penis engorges, it becomes rigid enough to enter the female vagina, or entryway to the female reproductive system.

Respiration

See Lungs.

Restless legs syndrome

"Restless legs" syndrome (also called Ekbom syndrome, "jimmy legs," or "jitter legs") is a feeling of uneasiness, shakiness, twitching, and restlessness that affects the legs after a patient has gone to bed for the night. Insomnia (inability to sleep) is almost invariably a result of the syndrome.

Precise cause of the syndrome is not known, although some authorities consider it to be brought about, or intensified, by poor blood circulation. It is most common in neurotic (mildly psychologically disturbed) individuals, but is also seen in normal persons. Some physicians claim that it is more common in hyperactive patients; others say that it can be brought about by intense activity, especially physical activity, just before bedtime.

Since the syndrome has been connected with circulatory disorders, drugs that increase the circulation to the lower extremities may prove helpful. A mild sedative at bedtime is also useful in preventing insomnia and assuring the patient a restful night of sleep.

Retinitis

Retinitis is an inflammation of the retina, the innermost layer of the eye that is sensitive to light. There are several types of retinitis, each one dependent on the cause.

Toxoplasmic retinitis, which is either acquired or present at birth, is caused by a microbe from outside the body. (If it is present at birth, the microbe was passed to the unborn baby through the placenta, the temporary organ in the uterus that nourishes the unborn baby.) A similar retinitis is caused by blood infection that settles in the eye. Exudative retinitis stems from unknown causes, but results in detachment of the retina from the eyeball.

The most common form of retinitis, however, is retinitis pigmentosa. It is an inherited disorder in which excess amounts of a substance called phytanic acid accumulate in the system and cause extensive damage to the retina. Phytanic acid is a form of phytol, a compound found in green vegetables.

The symptoms of retinitis pigmentosa are night blindness, inflammation of the retina, pronounced limitation of the field of vision (tunnel vision), loss of kinesthetic sense (sense of where the body is), shrinkage of the retina, clumping of retinal pigment (the element giving it its color), and dislodgement of the retina's blood vessels.

Many of the same symptoms are found in the other forms of retinitis. Sometimes, they are accompanied by a cloudiness in the liquid filling the eyeball (called vitreous fluid). This can be seen by a physician examining the interior of the eye.

In the case of retinitis pigmentosa, there is little that can be done except to avoid foods containing phytols. If the retina is detached, a condition often caused when a hole in the retina allows the eye's fluid to seep in and create a pocket, surgery is usually the treatment. The pocket is eliminated either by freezing or by heat, sometimes with a laser. If the retinitis is the result of blood infection, the obvious course to follow is removal of the underlying problem.

There are no clearcut preventive measures against retinitis.

See also Detached retina.

Retinopathy

Retinopathy is a condition in which deterioration of the retina—the light-sensitive, image-receiving innermost lining of the eye—is caused by damage to or overproduction of its blood vessels.

The vast majority of retinopathy

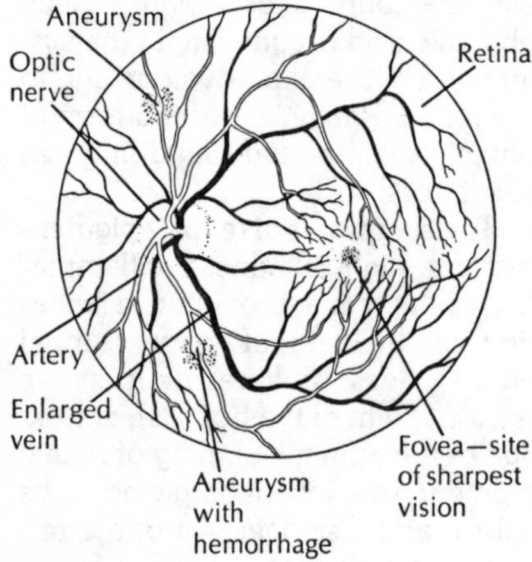

Retinopathy is a condition in which the light-sensitive innermost lining of the eye, the retina, deteriorates because of damage to or overproduction of its blood vessels.

cases stems from diabetes. Although fewer than 5 percent of all diabetics completely lose their sight because of retinopathy, that figure still means diabetes is one of the leading causes of irreversible blindness today. Other conditions that increase susceptibility to retinopathy include high blood pressure (in which the retinal veins and arteries are either constricted or entirely blocked); hemorrhaging resulting from the sudden appearance of a blood clot, fat globule, or cholesterol plaque; and chronic kidney failure.

If retinopathy is triggered by sudden hemorrhage, total blindness in the eye can strike swiftly, so the victim is advised to seek immediate medical attention. In cases of high blood pressure or diabetic retinopathy, vision usually worsens over time.

Controlling diabetic or high blood pressure retinopathy is best achieved by strict control over glucose (blood sugar) levels or blood pressure, either through diet or medication depending on the severity of the condition. If diabetics chronically allow their glucose levels to exceed normal bounds, retinal damage can be extensive and may require laser treatments to burn and seal off leaking blood vessels. In cases where these excess or weakened veins and arteries have clouded the eye's normally clear vitreous liquid, doctors can siphon off the fluid and simultaneously replace it with a harmless salt water solution.

Reye's syndrome

Reye's syndrome is a type of encephalitis (inflammation of the brain) that also affects the liver. It is a somewhat rare, noncontagious disease that strikes children under the age of 18, often after they are recovering from a viral infection such as influenza or chicken pox. It is most commonly seen in children between the ages of five and 11 years and most often between the months of December and March.

Reye's syndrome is a serious disease that requires immediate treatment. It is fatal in 25 percent of all cases.

This disorder is different from other types of encephalitis because it not only causes the brain to swell but also causes fatty deposits to collect in the liver, thereby resulting in malfunctions in both organs. Brain damage, coma, or death can result if it is not diagnosed and treated quickly.

The exact cause of Reye's syndrome is not known, but since it almost always follows a viral infection, it has been theorized that the virus combines with another unknown substance in the body and produces a damaging poison.

The symptoms of Reye's syndrome are sudden vomiting, abnormal sleepiness or hyperactivity, and confusion. Convulsions and coma (complete loss of consciousness) may occur as the disease progresses.

Early diagnosis is crucial. Reye's syndrome is diagnosed by careful observation of the symptoms; testing of a sample of cerebrospinal fluid (the clear fluid of the central nervous system, produced in the brain) but only if there is no suspicion that there is increased pressure in the brain; blood tests to determine the presence of liver damage; and tests of the blood sugar level because it is often low in young children who develop this disease.

There is no known cure for Reye's syndrome. Treatment usually consists of helping the child to weather the first few days of the illness, maintaining normal blood sugar levels and reducing pressure on the swollen brain. Usually, if the child survives for three or four days, the symptoms will subside and recovery will follow.

If blood sugar is low, normal levels should be restored with the injection of glucose, a form of sugar, into the veins. Increased pressure on the brain from the swelling is also reduced with medication.

There are no specific steps to prevent Reye's syndrome. However, although it has not been proven that aspirin causes or promotes Reye's syndrome, it is recommended that aspirin not be given to children with a viral infection, especially chicken pox and influenza.

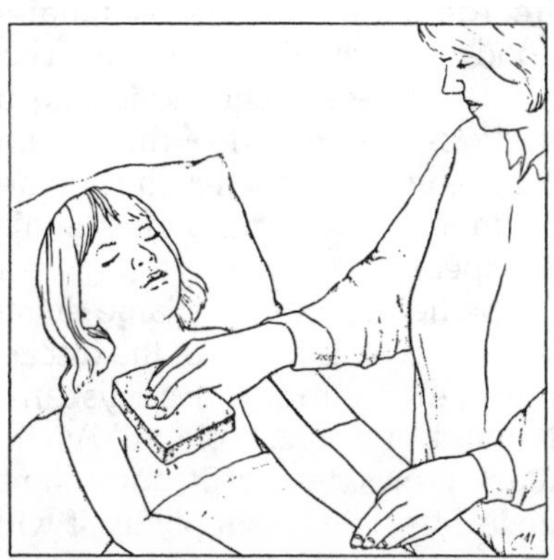

Sponge baths can be used instead of aspirin to reduce fever in children with viral illnesses, especially chicken pox and influenza.

Rheumatic fever

Rheumatic fever is the result of a bacterial disease characterized by inflammation, swelling, and soreness of the joints—especially the ankles, knees, and wrists—and inflammation of the heart. Commonly occurring in children and adolescents, it is a serious illness that can result in permanent damage to the heart. The attacks of fever may recur over a period of years and last from a few weeks to several months.

The disease is considered to be a late stage of a streptococcal infection such as a "strep throat," even though in some cases the earlier infection may have been so minor that it cannot be recalled. The body's immune system, by which antibodies are formed to attack infecting bacteria, apparently becomes disordered and the antibodies turn on healthy tissues such as that of the joints and the heart. The disease is more prevalent in some families than in others; but whether this indicates a hereditary factor or is due simply to sharing the same environment and living habits is not clear. Only 1 percent of all cases of streptococcal infection in children and adolescents are followed by rheumatic fever, so it is believed that a special susceptibility may be involved.

Rheumatic fever should immediately be suspected when a child or teenager develops an unexplained fever with joint inflammation a few weeks after an untreated (or unrecognized) throat infection or tonsillitis (inflammation of the tonsils). Other joints then become inflamed one after another, and a peculiar skin rash develops, lasting a day or two. Chorea, a spasmodic jerking and twitching of the limbs and facial features, may be among the symptoms if the infection spreads to involve the brain. Fortunately, it leaves no lasting brain damage and passes off after some weeks or months even without specific treatment. If the heart becomes involved, nodules may emerge over the elbows, kneecaps, and other bony prominences.

The acute stage of joint involvement leaves no permanent deformity or crippling, but damage to the heart is permanent when it involves destruction of heart valve tissue. Scar tissue is then eventually formed on the valves, so that they cannot open and close properly. The heart, unable to carry out efficiently its function of pumping blood through the circulatory system, must work harder and becomes enlarged. Blood clots may form on its inner lining and be carried in the blood throughout the body, often lodging in a blood vessel and blocking it.

The chief treatment for rheumatic fever is the use of antibiotics over an extended period of time—long enough to eliminate all bacteria. Aspirin is commonly used to bring down fever and relieve inflammation and pain. Hormones such as cortisone are usually given if there are signs of heart involvement, and sedatives may be prescribed if chorea becomes severe. The long periods of immobilization in bed once recommended are now believed to be unnecesssry, although bed rest during acute attacks may be prescribed. Seriously damaged heart valves can often be repaired surgically or even replaced by artificial valves.

The only form of prevention of rheumatic fever is prompt diagnosis and adequate treatment of all streptococcal infections in children and young people, especially those involving the throat and ears. It has been suggested that special precautions, such as the administration of antibiotics, be taken during dental treatment of rheumatic fever patients to prevent the spread of bacteria to the heart.

See also Rheumatic heart disease.

Rheumatic heart disease

Rheumatic heart disease consists of a variety of abnormal cardiac conditions, including heart valve scarring and endocarditis (inflammation of the lining of the heart).

This disease is a potential aftermath of rheumatic fever, once one of the prime killers of children. Rheumatic fever is an inflammatory disease that primarily affects the heart, tendons, joints, and arteries. Rheumatic fever may cause an inflammation of the heart valves that reduces their ability to close. This allows oxygenated blood that should be pumped out to the body from the heart's left ventricle (lower chamber) to seep back into the left atrium (upper chamber), thereby reducing the total amount of oxygenated blood in the circulatory system. This, in turn, causes a chronic feeling of tiredness on the part of the patient, which is unrelieved when the primary rheumatic fever symptoms finally disappear.

The heart tends to enlarge drastically during this phase of the disease in order to meet the system's demands for fresh blood. As the heart grows larger, it sometimes grows less able to supply itself with blood. As a result, a point of diminishing returns is reached, and the patient's activities sometimes become permanently restricted, leading to a completely sedentary life.

Among the chronic effects of rheumatic heart disease are: heart "murmur," caused by the backflow of blood from the left ventricle into the left atrium; the formation of microscopic blood clots in the heart, which can break loose, enter the bloodstream, and find their way into the vessels of the retina (the light sensitive tissue lining the back of the eye), causing hemorrhaging (internal bleeding) and possible impairment of vision; kidney dysfunction in middle or later life; shrinkage of muscular tissue from underactivity; irregular pulse, shortness of breath and fainting spells; and lack of muscular or cardiovascular endurance.

Presently, rheumatic fever is treatable by a number of antibiotics. Penicillin has been used for 30 years as a preventive against recurrences. Many victims of rheumatic heart disease, even those who contracted it in the late 1930s, have gone on to live extremely active lives, despite heart murmurs, heart enlargements, and damaged valves. Although rheumatic heart disease is a serious matter, regular exercise, a sensible diet, and quiet determination can mean the difference between a sedentary and an active life.

Supervision by a physician is a must for anyone who suffers from rheumatic heart disease and wants to embark on a regular exercise program. In some cases, however, it may be impossible for a patient to participate in vigorous physical activity, especially if the heart damage is advanced or severe. For some of these individuals, surgery, in which an artificial valve may be implanted, can offer relief.

See also Rheumatic fever.

Rheumatoid arthritis

See Arthritis.

Rh factor

Rh factor refers to a characteristic of blood in which it can be classified as either Rh positive or Rh negative. Rh positive blood has the Rh (named for the Rhesus monkey, in whom it was first discovered) antigen on its red cells; Rh negative blood does not. An antigen is a substance that can provoke an immune, or protective, response to the presence of foreign bodies. An estimated 85 percent of the population has Rh positive blood, that is to say, they possess the Rh antigens.

Blood consists of several components: plasma (the liquid portion), erythrocytes (red blood cells, which contain hemoglobin, their oxygen-carrying element), platelets (tiny cells which play a critical role in the coagulation process), white blood cells, and various other elements. Yet is is the antigens that induce the production of antibodies whose action is crucial to the functioning of the body's immune system.

Each antigen causes the manufacture of antibodies that will interact only with that antigen. These antibodies will treat blood not of its type as a foreign substance. Transfusions of blood of different blood groups (Types A, B, AB, or O) will not be successful: the blood of the person receiving the transfusion will reject the blood being transfused.

Each of the lettered blood groups have different antigens, hence different antibodies. They are as distinctive as fingerprints. Within this classification, Type A has antigen A on its red cells, Type B has antigen B on its red cells, and Type O has neither antigen A nor antigen B on its red cells.

Blood of different types and different Rh factors literally do not mix. Type A blood plasma, for example, does not contain any anti-A antibodies. It does, however, contain anti-B antibodies. If Type B blood is transfused, the anti-B antibodies in the plasma will destroy the type B red cells that have type B antigens on them.

Blood normally has no anti-Rh antibodies. But these anti-Rh antibodies can develop in the Rh negative blood if Rh positive blood is introduced into the bloodstream. This can come about in two ways: if a person with Rh negative blood receives a transfusion of Rh positive blood, or if a woman with Rh negative blood conceives a baby with Rh positive blood (inherited from the father) and some of the Rh positive substance from the unborn baby finds its way into the bloodstream of the mother.

In either of these cases, the Rh positive red cells will stimulate the person's body to form anti-Rh antibodies. If this happens, the blood will form clumps and a potentially lethal situation will develop: the clumps may block the blood vessels, leading to death.

If difficulties do not appear with the formation of these antibodies during the first transfusion or the first pregnancy, they will surely appear if any Rh positive blood is ever again introduced into the person's bloodstream. The antibodies are already present, and the introduction of additional Rh positive blood will result in a mobilization of existing antibodies and the production of even more. In addition to clumping of blood, other problems will arise. For example, hemolysis (the liberation of hemoglobin from the red blood cells) will make it impossible for the red cells to carry oxygen, thus producing the symptoms of anemia and lack of oxygen.

There are potential dangers to an unborn baby if the mother's blood contains anti-Rh antibodies. If the unborn baby has Rh positive cells, anti-Rh antibodies may pass through the placenta from the mother's bloodstream to cause hemolysis of the baby's blood cells. Once born, the baby may have to have massive, possibly total, transfusions of Rh negative blood to prevent clumping, as well as hemolytic anemia. Nowadays, this situation is relatively rare following the introduction of injections given to the Rh negative mother after the birth of her first Rh positive baby. These injections inhibit the formation of the potentially dangerous antibodies.

Rubella

Rubella, or German measles, is a relatively mild viral infection with cold-like symptoms and a short-lived rash. The disease is contagious, but it is usually not dangerous. One exception is when rubella infects pregnant women. In this instance, the virus can also affect the unborn child, causing serious long-term problems. However, rubella outbreaks are infrequent since the development of a vaccine to prevent the illness.

Rubella results from a virus that invades the cells of the body. The virus spreads from one person to another by contact with airborne moisture from the infected person's respiratory system. An infected person can spread the virus as early as one week before the rash appears and as late as five days after the rash fades. A baby with congenital rubella syndrome can transfer the virus until the child is about 12 to 18 months old. Although instances of second infections have been reported, rubella seldom occurs twice in the same person.

Although rubella is generally a mild infection, some complications can arise. Encephalitis, or inflammation of the brain, occurs in one in 5000 cases. Thrombocytopenic purpura, a blood disease, can prove fatal when it accompanies rubella. High or prolonged fever and extreme fatigue should be reported to a physician to prevent further complications.

Another serious complication of rubella is congenital rubella syndrome, or rubella infection that is present at birth. Here the pregnant woman transmits the disease to the fetus (unborn child) during pregnancy. Rubella virus may cause one or more serious organic and growth disorders, particularly if contracted during the first three months of pregnancy when the fetus is forming. The most common problems include congenital heart defects, hearing and vision problems, blood disorders, and mental retardation and other brain disorders.

The first symptoms of rubella are runny nose, swollen neck glands, and low fever (up to 101° F). About two days after these signs, a rash with very small red or pink spots appear on the face and neck. The spots are flat initially. Then they become slightly raised and fade within a day or two. As the first spots fade, more spots develop until the rash gradually spreads over most of the body. The rash lasts only two to three days, but swollen glands may persist for as long as a week. All other symptoms usually disappear by then. When there is joint pain, as is common with older women, discomfort may last another week.

Under normal circumstances, rubella is difficult to diagnose because the symptoms are so mild and variable. Sometimes a rash is absent and the disease resembles a cold. Other cases may be so severe that the infection may be confused with measles. A doctor identifies the virus by taking a blood test and tracing any history of exposure to the disease. Incubation, or time between contact with the virus and beginning of symptoms, is 14 to 21 days.

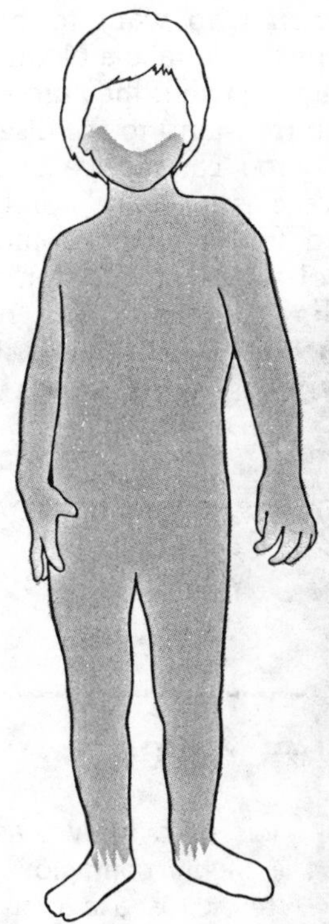

The light pink rubella rash first appears on the face and the neck and then gradually spreads over most of the body.

Most patients require little or no treatment for rubella because the symptoms are so mild. Aspirin or an aspirin substitute may afford relief for any joint pain. Otherwise, drugs are not needed. Some patients may want bed rest, but most people feel well enough to be somewhat active.

Rubella rarely occurs now because children routinely receive rubella vaccine at about 15 months of age. The vaccine is combined with measles or mumps vaccine in one injection. Rubella vaccine works in the body to stimulate antibodies (protective substances) that fight the disease.

Women who want to become pregnant should take a blood test to determine whether they are already immune (resistant) to the disease. If not, they too, can receive a vaccination. Vaccinations are not recommended for pregnant women because of a risk of infection to the fetus. For this reason also, doctors caution women to wait at least three months after vaccination before becoming pregnant.

S

Scarlet fever

Scarlet fever (also known as *scarlatina*) is a highly contagious childhood bacterial disease caused by Group A hemolytic streptococci.

The symptoms of scarlet fever include fever; sore throat; widespread scarlet rash beginning in the armpits and groin and spreading to the neck, chest, back, extremities, and even the tongue; and peeling and scaling of the skin, even on the palms and soles. The incubation period—the time between exposure to the disease and appearance of symptoms—is two to four days.

Scarlet fever in the past was an often fatal disease, but today it is easily treated with penicillin and complications are rare. In addition to the penicillin, bed rest and a nourishing diet with plenty of fluids help speed recuperation.

Schizophrenia

Schizophrenia is not a single mental disorder, but rather a group of mental disorders that impair functioning and that are characterized by psychotic symptoms involving disturbances of thinking, feeling, and behaving. Among the characteristics common to most types of schizophrenia are withdrawal from reality, delusions, hallucinations, ambivalence, inappropriate emotional responses, and bizarre behavior.

Most cases of schizophrenia are considered to be "caused" by a complex interaction between inherited and environmental factors. Approximately 10 percent of close relatives of schizophrenics are diagnosed as schizophrenic themselves sometime in their lives. A genetic susceptibility appears to be an important factor in schizophrenia, but it should be stressed that schizophrenia is not "inherited." Even if the susceptibility is there, the obvious signs of the illness are connected to stressful life events and the individual's ways of coping with them.

Schizophrenia is not confined to any single age, race, sex, socioeconomic, or racial/ethnic group. It has a worldwide distribution, affects persons of all ages (although it commonly starts in later adolescence or early adult life), and seems to be a bit more prevalent in lower socioeconomic groups (however, some authorities guess that this is misleading; the diagnosed schizophrenic's inability to focus on career, profession, education, and related matters allows him/her to drift farther and farther down the socioeconomic scale). One interesting side note: most of those who develop schizophrenia in later life are widowed, unmarried, or handicapped.

There is no specific personality type that can be singled out as "preschizophrenic." Many schizophrenics do show such traits as extreme sensitivity, shyness, lack of emotion, anti-social behavior, and paranoid attitudes early in life, but an equal number of people with the same symptoms continue to lead normal lives.

The onset of schizophrenia may be sudden or gradual. However, even in cases with an acute or abrupt onset, there will be definite stages: a prodromal period of increasing withdrawal and disintegration of previous levels of functioning; then a residual phase, with the onset of persistent delusional beliefs and emotional withdrawal. In the full-fledged schizophrenic state that follows, some or all of these symptoms may occur:

- *Thought disorders.* Clear, goal-directed thinking becomes increasingly difficult and thought/speech grow more diffuse. Sudden, incomprehensible changes of subject, fringe associations, a private symbolism, and obvious flaws in reasoning occur. Some patients report a thought block while others claim their thoughts are broadcast and shared with others.
- *Emotional changes.* Lack of emotion and inappropriate emotion are the most common symptoms, but mood disturbances (depression, excitement, anxiety, elation, perplexity) are also common.
- *Perceptual disorders.* "Hearing voices" is the most common, but all the other senses may be affected as well. The "voices" often are giving a running commentary on the patient's behavior or seem to be talking about him or her.
- *Delusions.* Delusions may involve persecution, illness (hypochondria), religious ideas, jealousy, sexual problems, grandeur, thought blockage or broadcasting, telepathy, or special significance (such as the belief that one is the Messiah or is the victim of a conspiracy).
- *Catatonic symptoms.* These can range from hyperactivity and excitement to stupor and immobility. Assuming odd positions for long periods of time can occur, and affected mannerisms (exaggerated gait, grimacing) are common.
- *Violent behavior.* Self-mutilation and petty crimes, as well as suicide, are common especially when committed at the command of the "voices." Violent schizophrenics often commit a crime in the quest for recognition or acclaim and may seek out someone in an authoritative position, such as a parent or teacher, or a popular "authority figure," such as a movie star, rock star, or political figure.
- *Nonspecific symptoms.* These include withdrawal from reality, abnormal activity (rocking, pacing), eccentric dress or grooming or dishevelment, perplexity, ritualistic behavior and "magical" thinking, depression, anxiety, anger, and hypochondria.

The *diagnosis* of schizophrenia normally requires that the patient and his/her illness meet at least these specific criteria: (1) presence of certain psychotic symptoms, delusions, hallucinations, and formal thought disorders; (2) deterioration from an earlier level of functioning; (3) continuous symptoms for a period of at least six months; (4) onset before age 45; (5) symptoms not traceable to other emotional disorders; and (6) symptoms not due to organic mental disorders or mental retardation. Diagnosis must also rule out "mimicking" conditions, such as drug dependence, infectious disorders, and other mental disorders such as simple paranoia or manic-depressive syndrome.

The diagnosis of schizoaffective disorder is often made when the physician cannot draw a clear line between true schizophrenia and other emotional disorders. It often covers cases of an isolated incident (or incidents) of schizophrenic behavior with no recurrence.

The chief treatment measures for schizophrenia include drug therapy, psychotherapy, counseling including social support, and gradual rehabilitation and retraining. For a first illness or acute relapse, hospitalization is usually indicated in order to stabilize the patient's condition. However, hospitalization for more than a few months may be inadvisable; if the patient is able to function outside of an institution, leading some semblance of a normal life may actually be therapeutic.

The drugs usually prescribed are antipsychotic medications. When patients refuse to continue oral doses of antipsychotic drugs, long-acting injections are often preferable to reduce the risk of relapse. Patients who display remission of symptoms should be given a "drug holiday" at intervals to test functioning without drugs, but careful observation and monitoring of symptoms should continue. Antidepressants may be substituted in some cases.

Electroconvulsive therapy is used only for catatonic patients or for those with the severest, most immobilizing depressions.

The cornerstone of most treatment programs is psychotherapy. Occupational therapy and gradual social involvement should also be arranged, as should a structured rehabilitation program. Careful control of environmental pressures is important. Both overstimulation and understimulation should be avoided.

It should be remembered that schizophrenia is not necessarily a chronic disorder. About 30 percent of patients recover completely and most of the remaining ones show marked improvement, although impaired emotional response and lowered drive usually persist. With treatment, even active cases can be controlled within four to eight weeks.

No specific preventive measures are known at this time.

See also Depression, Electroconvulsive therapy, and Paranoia.

Sciatica

Sciatica is a condition characterized by pain that extends along the entire length of the sciatic nerve (which runs down the lower back and outer side of the thigh, leg, and foot), radiating across the back of the pelvis through the buttocks and into the leg.

Sciatica is most commonly associated with injury to or the rupture of a lumbar disk, one of the disks located between the lumbar (lower back) vertebrae. When the injured disk moves against the sciatic nerve, pain radiates down the nerve.

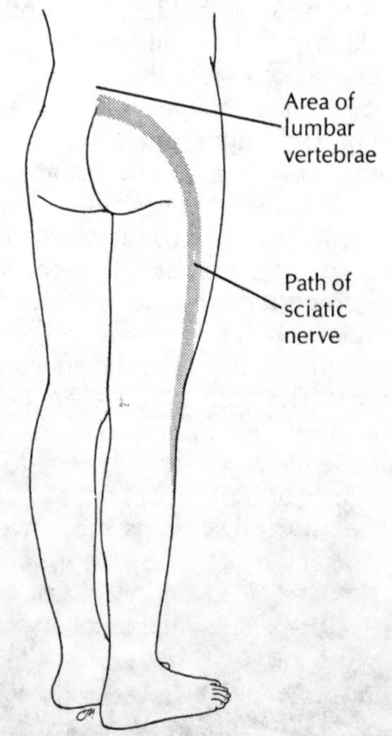

Sciatica is a condition in which pressure on the sciatic nerve causes pain to radiate along the path of the sciatic nerve as shown here.

The symptoms of sciatica vary in intensity depending on the extent to which the injured disk presses on the sciatic nerve and according to the individual's susceptibility to pain. In mild cases, the pain may be a slight discomfort in the lower back and along the leg. In severe cases, the pain is excruciating in the same areas and often completely immobilizes the victim. Furthermore, since the cause is usually a ruptured or "slipped" disk, it is difficult to know when an attack will begin. A sudden cough may cause the disk to move and press on the sciatic nerve, resulting in the pain that such pressure causes.

It is commonplace for sciatica patients to be free from pain one moment and in agony the next moment, depending on the position of the offending disk. Also, repeated problems with movements of the ruptured disk can cause a general inflammation of the sciatic nerve. In these cases, it is not a matter of the pain existing one time and disappearing another time. Instead, it is a matter of having less pain at one time than at another.

In treating sciatica, the first line of attack is to make certain that the involved disk no longer presses on the sciatic nerve. Treatment to accomplish this may require placing the patient in traction, so that the spine is pulled from opposite directions, in the hope that the disk will slip back into place.

Physical therapy (under a doctor's supervision or according to a doctor's prescription) is also used to relieve the pain of sciatica. This treatment includes hydrotherapy, in which a stream of water is directed to the affected area, including the area of the ruptured disk. Also, many therapists advise their patients to overcome the effects of the ruptured disk by developing the core muscles—the four muscle groups that form the waist—in order to provide a supportive column of muscle that will help keep the disk in place.

In extreme cases, surgery is indicated. In this instance, the spine is fused in the area of the ruptured disk, and the possibility of further pressure against the sciatic nerve is eliminated.

See also Neuralgia and Slipped disk.

Scoliosis

Scoliosis is sideways curvature of the spine. There is usually a main curve in one direction and an upper and/or lower curve to compensate for it in the opposite direction.

Scoliosis can result from unequal leg lengths, or it may be due to defective development of the vertebrae (backbones) while an unborn baby is growing in the uterus. Paralysis of trunk muscles on one side of the body caused by polio, cerebral palsy, or muscular dystrophy; tilting of the pelvis in hip disease; or deformities of the spine caused by rickets or rheumatism can also lead to scoliosis.

There is no known cause, however, for the most common kind of scoliosis, known as idiopathic (cause unknown) scoliosis. It occurs during childhood and results in the curvature of a previously straight spine. Before the age of three years, mostly boys are affected, with an upper curve to the left and a lower curve to the right. Between the ages of four and ten years, both boys and girls are affected in equal numbers, and the curves are varied. Most prevalent is the adolescent form, usually affecting girls between age ten and the time their skeletons mature. Most often, the upper spinal area (behind the chest) curves to the right, with compensating curves to the left in the lower neck area and in the small of the back. If untreated, scoliosis can produce diminished lung capacity, back pain, spinal arthritis, and disk disease.

Parents should be alert for the signs of scoliosis, which may be noticed first as an apparently uneven hemline, unequal pant legs, or one hip higher than the other. To inspect your child, ask the child to stand up straight with shirt off while you observe from the rear. Notice if one shoulder is higher than the other or if one shoulder blade sticks out. With the arms hanging loosely at the sides, notice if one arm hangs away from the body farther than does the other. See if one hip appears higher or more prominent than the other. See if the child seems to tilt to one side. Finally, ask your child to bend forward, arms hanging in front and palms together at the level of the knees. A hump on the back at the ribs or near the waist may be a sign of scoliosis, as may be any "one-sidedness" noticed in the tests above. If you have any suspicions, report them to your child's doctor, who will give the child a similar checkup and if necessary take X rays or call in an orthopedic surgeon (bone specialist) to confirm the diagnosis.

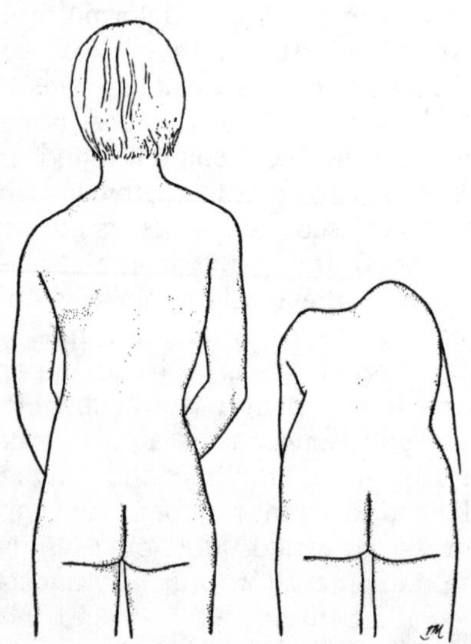

Severe scoliosis can be seen when viewing a child from the back, and even mild scoliosis can be noticed when the child bends at the waist. Bending forward rotates the chest making one side of the back more prominent.

Treatment of scoliosis may involve only exercises if the curvature is mild. Sit-ups, exercises to stretch the spine, and breathing exercises may strengthen the muscles of the trunk enough so that they will correct the situation. Frequent X rays and physical examinations are needed to determine if the exercises are working.

More severe scoliosis may require a special brace, which is constructed of a leather or plastic pelvic girdle holding one vertical brace in front and two in back, connected to a ring around the neck. This often must be worn 24 hours a day, except when the patient is bathing or exercising, until the child's skeleton has matured. It is adjustable for growth.

The most severe scoliosis requires spinal-fusion surgery, in which certain vertebrae (backbones) are fused together, with stabilization provided by metal rods, cable, and/or staples. Before the operation, the patient needs to be placed either in a body cast for three to six months or in dynamic traction (with weights and pulleys) for seven to ten days. Frequent checkups are needed after surgery to make sure that the correction is being maintained.

Scurvy

Scurvy is a disease caused by Vitamin C deficiency, and it is characterized by anemia (deficiency of red blood cells), spongy gums, a tendency to bleed, and abnormal bone and tooth formations. The disease may be either acute or chronic.

Vitamin C is essential for the formation and maintenance of connective tissue, bone tissue, and teeth. It is also essential for the healing of wounds and burns.

There are two forms of scurvy, infantile and adult.

A primary Vitamin C deficiency in infants is due simply to lack of supplementary Vitamin C. In adults, scurvy is usually due to unusual food habits or to improper diet; often adult scurvy results from an "ulcer diet" for gastrointestinal disorders that limits citrus fruits and juices because of their acid content. Pregnancy and breast-feeding increase the Vitamin C requirement; pregnant women and nursing mothers must make sure to include adequate Vitamin C in the diet. In addition, diarrhea, inflammatory disease, burns, surgery, and exposure to intense cold all increase the Vitamin C requirement in adults.

Infantile scurvy usually appears between ages six months and one year. The earliest symptoms include irritability, loss of appetite, and failure to gain weight. Often the child screams or cries whenever he/she is moved and may hold the legs motionless because of internal bleeding of the bone surface. There may be abnormal enlargements or hardening of the joints or long bones (especially in the thigh) and a tendency toward gum hemorrhage as the teeth erupt. Fever, anemia, and increased pulse and respiration rates are also common symptoms.

Adult scurvy usually remains inactive for a period of three to 12 months following severe Vitamin C deficiency. Lassitude; weakness; irritability; weight loss and/or loss of appetite; multiple splinter hemorrhages at the nails; swollen, purplish and spongy gums; loosening of teeth; and failure of wounds to heal are among the earliest symptoms. Secondary infections, gangrene (death of tissue), breaks in old scars, spontaneous hemorrhaging, muscle pains and pains in the joints, and small hemorrhagic spots on the skin of the legs are all symptoms of a more advanced stage. In some cases there is edema (fluid retention) of the lower extremities and an arthritis resembling rheumatoid arthritis. There may even be bleeding in the conjunctiva, the membrane that covers the front of the eye and lines the eyelids.

Diagnosis of a case of infantile scurvy will include an X ray of the ends of the long bones of the leg, which will show a crosswise thickening and increased density, the so-called white line. It is often difficult to differentiate infantile scurvy from rickets, polio, osteomyelitis, rheumatic fever, and certain hemorrhagic disorders such as allergic purpuras. In cases where diagnosis is doubtful, a therapeutic dose of Vitamin C given orally will stop the pain of infantile scurvy almost immediately and reduce the swelling and bleeding of the gums within 72 hours.

In adults, scurvy can mimic arthritis, hemorrhagic disease, and gingivitis (inflammation of the gums). The blood level of Vitamin C is usually low, but this is not always an accurate diagnostic tool. Vitamin C in the urine will be low, and there may be anemia not caused by blood loss.

Fortunately, scurvy is easy to treat. Vitamin C given orally for one week, supplemented with orange and tomato juice, is the remedy for infantile scurvy. If diarrhea or vomiting is present, half the recommended oral dose can be given intravenously.

For adult scurvy, Vitamin C is taken orally until symptoms have disappeared; then the patient can go on maintenance doses. Vitamin C in divided doses is given for several months in chronic scurvy that appears in connection with gingivitis, hemorrhaging, or joint symptoms.

A balanced diet with plenty of Vitamin C is the best preventive measure for scurvy. Fortunately, natural sources of Vitamin C are plentiful—besides citrus fruits and tomatoes, many green vegetables such as green peppers are rich in Vitamin C. In the case of patients on bland diets or "ulcer diets," a physician should be consulted as to how to prevent Vitamin C deficiency.

See also Vitamins.

Senility

Senility is the term applied to the mental and physical deterioration associated with old age. While the term covers both physical and mental problems, most people think of mental deterioration when they hear the word.

The causes of senility are many: arteriosclerosis (hardening of the arteries); heart disease (with an accompanying loss of oxygen to the brain and other body tissues); lung disease (with a decrease in the lungs' ability to oxygenate blood); blood vessel diseases; and diseases of the liver, the kidneys, and other organs. Senility is not linked to a single disease, nor is it thought to be inevitable (some people are mentally alert at ages past 100). However, the years take their toll, and chronic disorders hasten senility. Life-long harmful habits are also a cause of early senility, alcohol, tobacco, and drug use being among the worst offenders.

Gradual loss of physical and mental vigor is the most common symptom of oncoming senility. A lack of interest in the surroundings or in activities once enjoyed is another symptom. Victims experience a loss of complex skills, such as the ability to do puzzles, math problems, logic problems, or even their personal checkbook balances. If the onset of senility is sudden, as it is with a condition called Alzheimer's disease, the victim will often be in a panic, as he or she feels mental powers deteriorating more and more each day. Short-term memory is one of the first faculties to go, and many victims are completely aware of the fact that their minds are deteriorating: they can remember everything except the events of only moments ago.

Physical senility is gradual, unless a chronic illness accelerates the process. The skin becomes dry and loses its resilience (often also becoming mottled in appearance), the muscles lose their tone and become weak, the bones lose their strength and become brittle, and the organs gradually fail in their functions.

While there is no way to stop the clock, there are many ways that one can continue leading a vigorous, active life all the way into the 60s, 70s, and 80s. Regular exercise; balanced diets; avoidance of toxic substances such as tobacco, alcohol, drugs, carbon monoxide, and other pollutants; and proper amounts of vitamins and minerals seem to have a positive effect on people at any age. Protection from debilitating disease and avoidance of injury (falls, broken bones) can also add years of activity to the lives of the elderly.

Much of mental senility could be avoided by simply not "turning off" the mind upon retirement. To stay mentally active takes an act of will. The mind begins to deteriorate quickly if it is not used—in some ways similar to the shrinking that unused muscles experience.

See also Alzheimer's disease, Atherosclerosis, and Osteoporosis.

Septicemia

Septicemia, often called blood poisoning, is a form of bacteremia, or invasion of the blood circulation by bacteria. Specifically, septicemia occurs in those situations in which bacteremia is associated with symptoms and signs of infection.

The causes of septicemia usually are traceable to some surgical procedure, to the use of intravenous devices or catheters, and to childbirth injury complicated by streptococcus infection or other infections. Septicemia is also a common side effect of intravenous drug injections, particularly in drug abusers. Other diseases and disorders often associated with septicemia include endocarditis (inflammation of the lining of the heart); genito-urinary tract infections; and sometimes diseases of the skin, bones, and joints.

Few symptoms are unique to septicemia, so it is often confused with other illnesses. However, fever, often variable and intermittent, is generally present. Chills may occur at the outset of the disease. Skin eruptions are common and may be petechial (small red dots or splotches), purpuric (purple and bruise-like), or may take any of several other forms. Often septicemia begins abruptly with chills, fever, nausea, vomiting, diarrhea, and general collapse.

Complications may include secondary infections of the body's organs and bones.

The diagnosis of septicemia is established by blood cultures, which test for various kinds of bacteria. Normally, there should be no bacteria in the blood. A single negative culture does not exclude septicemia; in some patients who have had prior antibiotic therapy, there is never a single positive blood culture. Bone marrow culture is actually the most sensitive diagnostic tool.

Treatment of septicemia relies heavily on antibiotics. Therapy should continue until the patient has been free of symptoms for at least one week.

Sexually transmitted diseases

See Genital warts, Gonorrhea, Herpes, Nongonococcal urethritis, and Syphilis.

Shingles

Shingles, or herpes zoster, is a painful viral infection of one or more nerves. The infection produces a blistery, itchy skin rash above the affected nerve.

Shingles rash looks identical to the rash of the chicken pox virus. Shingles and chicken pox are caused by the same virus called varicella zoster. Moreover, previous infection with chicken pox is necessary in order to develop shingles. Why shingles occurs in certain people and not others at any given time is unknown. Scientists believe that after recovery from chicken pox the varicella zoster virus lies dormant in the body. One theory contends that the virus is reactivated after injury to the affected area or other emotional or physical upset to the body. Sixty-five percent of the cases studied confirm this assumption.

Another theory proposes that with shingles the number and strength of antibodies (protective substances) produced by the body to fight the varicella zoster virus may diminish after a bout of chicken pox. This reduction in force makes some individuals susceptible to another attack of the virus. Because some antibodies endure, the person gets shingles rather than chicken pox. Yet, if someone is exposed to the virus as an adult and has not had chicken pox, he or she will get chicken pox, not shingles.

Incidence of the disease increases

with age. Shingles rarely occurs in people under age 15. More than 50 percent of those who get shingles are over 45 years of age.

Shingles begins with a prickling or tenderness in the skin over the infected nerve. Burning or shooting pain in the same area is also an early symptom. Within two to four days a rash with small, red spots appears over the affected part of the body. As the spots enlarge, they blister and sometimes blend together. Eventually they fill with pus, burst, and crust over much the same as with chicken pox rash. With shingles, however, the process takes longer and is confined to the skin area above the affected nerve.

Shingles rash is very itchy. In addition, pain increases as the area beneath the rash becomes more red and swollen. Shingles attacks nerves on the chest, back, neck, arm, or leg most often. However, facial nerves are involved frequently. The rash appears in a band or strip following the path of the nerve, usually on one side of the body. The rash persists

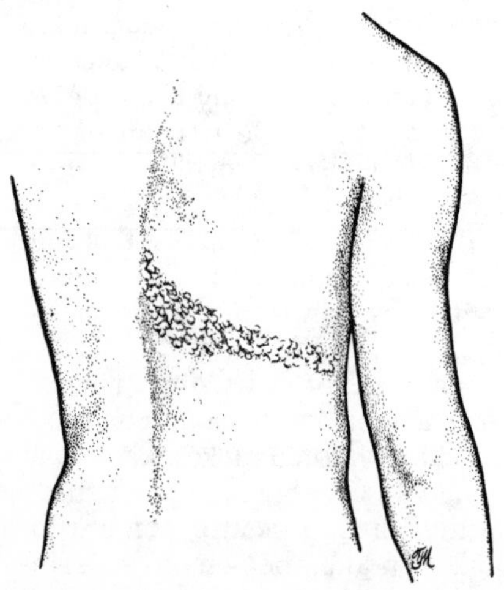

Shingles is an infection of a nerve characterized by a blistering skin rash following the path of the affected underlying nerve. The rash itself is identical to the rash of chicken pox, since both diseases are caused by the same virus.

two to three weeks before clearing, while the pain continues for three or four weeks. Sometimes, pain may linger for a month or more. In people over 60, pain may persist for several months after the rash disappears.

Occasionally, shingles rash becomes generalized and spreads over the entire body. This develops most often in people who have underlying disease such as Hodgkin's disease (cancer of the lymph system) or leukemia (cancer of the blood). When these serious disorders already exist, shingles can cause death, but this is rare. A signal that such extreme illness may be present is recurrence of shingles, since the condition seldom occurs more than once.

The most common complication of shingles is a bacteria infection in the rash. Infection can prolong the rash and cause the skin to scar.

Less common complications follow a shingles attack on facial nerves. Eye disorders and Bell's palsy (a disease that temporarily paralyzes one side of the face) can result. Shingles in other parts of the body can cause similar temporary paralysis of the area over the affected nerve.

Since there is no known cure for shingles, treatment focuses on reducing pain. An analgesic, or painkilling drug, may relieve burning. Some physicians prescribe steroid drugs to reduce nerve inflammation in older patients. In order to be effective, steroids must be taken soon after shingles begins. Steroid treatment is not recommended for people with underlying disease because steroids can interfere with natural resistance to infection.

Preventing infection is also important. Baths in warm (not hot) water soothe and clean the skin. For severe itching, patients should cut their fingernails and wear gloves when asleep to control unconscious scratching.

See also Bell's palsy.

Shock

See Emergency first aid section at the end of this book.

Sickle-cell anemia

Sickle-cell anemia is an inherited blood disorder, occurring almost exclusively in blacks, that transforms normally round red blood cells into crescent or sickle shapes. The transformation is caused by defective hemoglobin, the iron-protein substance in the red blood cells that carries oxygen, and it occurs when part or all of the body is not getting enough oxygen. Because of their hooked shapes, the blood cells tend to tangle together and pile up, temporarily clogging tiny blood vessels and slowing circulation. Tissue formerly nourished by the clogged blood vessels dies. Furthermore, the anemia (lack of red blood cells) that results from the breakdown of the cells not only weakens the body but creates more oxygen deficiency, which produces more "sickling" of the cells. The disease is chronic, marked by fatigue, breathing difficulty on exertion, swollen joints, attacks of extreme illness, complications from other diseases, and shortened life. In the past, half of all victims died by the age of 20 and few survived past 40. With new technology and forms of treatment, the outlook is much better, although sickle-cell disease remains a chronic debilitating disease

The disease occurs in about one out of 330 blacks in the United States. About one in ten American blacks is a carrier of the defective gene for sickle-cell anemia but has no symptoms and is not affected by the disease. However, if one carrier marries another, the chance of each child

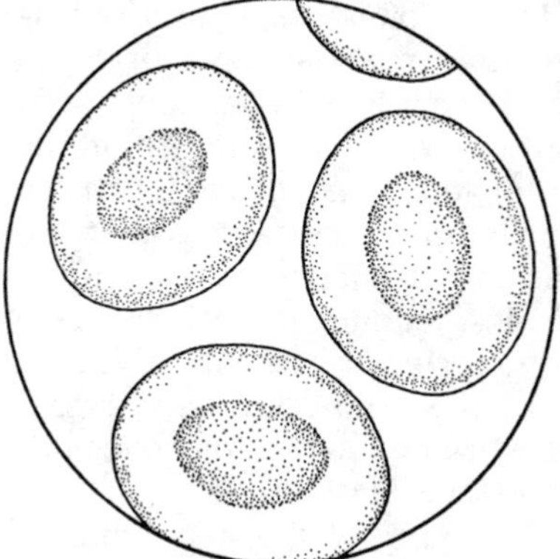

Normal red blood cells

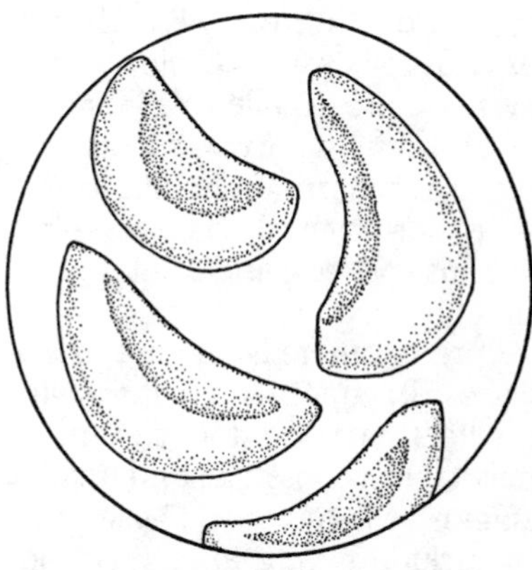

Sickle-shaped blood cells

Sickle-cell anemia is a blood disorder that transforms normally round red blood cells into crescent or sickle shape. Because of their shape, the sickle cells interfere with blood circulation.

being afflicted by the disease is one in four. The chance that the child will also be a carrier is one in two. Both the carrier state and the active state of the disease can be confirmed by a blood test.

Symptoms of sickle-cell anemia in half the victims begin between the ages of six months and two years. Among the first signs is an unusual swelling of the fingers and toes. The bones of the hands and feet thicken, and clumping of sickle cells may affect the bone marrow, where new blood cells are produced. Youngsters are especially subject to "sickle-cell crises," marked by severe pain in the abdomen, joints, bones, and/or muscles. These may last from four days to several weeks, and commonly occur eight to ten times a year before the age of ten. They occur much less often in later years. Signs of a crisis in a sickle-cell anemia patient include pale lips, tongue, and palms; lack of energy; sleepiness with difficulty awakening; irritability; severe pain; and a fever of 104° or one over 100° lasting for at least two days.

Thickening of the heart muscle; enlarged heart, liver, and spleen in children; heart murmurs; and gallstones are common. The heartbeat is usually rapid. Children with the disease are usually small for their age. Those who survive to become adults have narrow shoulders and hips, a barrel chest, curved spine, long arms and legs, and an elongated skull.

At present there is no cure for the disease. Treatment includes giving painkillers, making the patient as comfortable as possible, and treating problems as they occur. These problems include severe anemia, which may require a blood transfusion, and frequent infections that are a result of the body's damaged immunity. Avoiding cold, fatigue, and other stress may help to reduce the number of crises.

Screening programs, some sponsored by public health departments, are available for those who wish to know if they carry the gene for sickle-cell anemia. Those who have the gene can get genetic counseling. There is no risk of disease in the children if only one parent is a carrier, but the children would have a one in two chance of being a carrier.

Sinusitis

Sinusitis is an infection of one or more of the sinuses, usually caused by bacteria and more commonly occurring in adults than in children.

The sinuses are air-filled cavities within the facial bone structure, connected to the nose, and lined with mucous membrane. There are four major groups of sinuses: frontal, ethmoidal, sphenoidal, and maxillary sinuses.

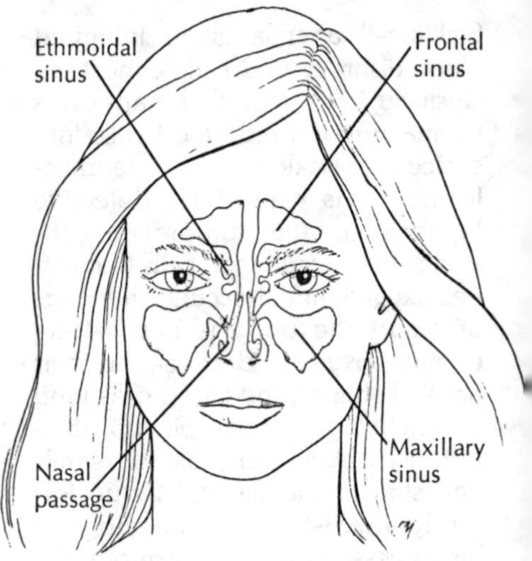

The sinuses are air-filled cavities within the facial bone structure and connected to the nasal passages. The four major groups are the frontal, ethmoidal, sphenoidal, and maxillary. The sphenoidal sinuses are located behind the ethmoidal.

Sinuses are normally kept clear and free when mucus drains through them into the nasal passages. If they are obstructed for any reason, such as from the congestion present during a cold, they are not able to drain properly, and infection of the sinuses can result.

It is rare but possible for long-lasting sinusitis to lead to more serious disorders. A persistent infection may travel to the brain, causing meningitis (inflammation of the membranes surrounding the brain) or to the bone, resulting in osteomyelitis.

A sinus infection can be triggered by anything that prevents the mucus in the sinuses from draining properly into the nasal passages. Possible causes can include swimming and diving, injuries, abnormal structures in the facial bones, congestion from flu or colds, allergies such as hay fever, even an abscess (inflamed pocket of pus) in a tooth, which may penetrate the sinuses and allow bacteria to enter them. Many different bacteria can cause sinusitis, including some of same strains that lead to pneumonia, laryngitis, and middle ear infections.

Sinusitis is characterized by pain and tenderness above the infected sinus, felt in the face, forehead, behind the eyes, in the eyes, near the upper part of the nose, even in the upper teeth (but not in a single tooth). This facial pain may be accompanied by headache, slight fever, chills, sore throat, nasal obstruction, and a pus discharge from the nose.

Sinusitis usually lasts about two weeks, with the pain often subsiding in the morning and worsening as the day goes on, or fluctuating as the patient moves about and changes positions.

Sinuses cannot be seen directly by a doctor, so diagnosis may include X rays to check for fluid present or abnormalities in the sinuses and to identify exactly which sinuses are infected. To identify the bacteria the doctor may need to perform a sinus puncture, in which a needle is inserted into the sinus through the upper jaw above the molar teeth and a sample of the bacteria is removed from the sinuses. This procedure may be necessary because the nasal discharge may contain different bacteria from those in the sinuses.

Sinusitis is treated by draining the sinuses and thereby removing the bacteria that are causing the infection. Nasal decongestants, hot compresses, and dry heat all work to aid sinus drainage. An antibiotic is usually prescribed that will kill one of the two most common bacteria that trigger sinusitis.

If these treatments bring no relief, the doctor may perform a sinus puncture to determine exactly which bacteria are present, then prescribe another antibiotic. In severe cases, codeine may be prescribed to dull the pain, and the doctor may clear the sinuses by injecting a salt water solution through the nose to flush out the bacteria.

In very rare cases, surgery may be necessary to remove a nasal polyp (a mass of swollen tissue), repair abnormal bone structures, or remove infected sinus tissue.

There is some evidence that smokers are more likely to suffer from sinusitis than nonsmokers. In addition, those who frequently have colds are more susceptible to sinusitis. Precautions may be taken along these lines to prevent sinus infections.

Skin

The skin is the outer covering of the body. This waterproof barrier affords protection from invasion of dirt, bacteria, and other harmful substances as well as helping to regulate internal body temperature.

Skin is the body's largest organ. The three layers comprising the skin cover about 18 square feet and weigh about seven pounds in an average adult.

The outermost layer of skin is the epidermis. The epidermis contains pigment cells that determine skin color and shield the skin against damaging sun rays. Specialized cells within this layer manufacture keratin, a tough substance found in hair and nails.

Epidermis cells continually shed and reproduce. This reconstruction is usually invisible, except when skin becomes irritated, such as in psoriasis, a disease that appears as scaly red patches.

Since the outer skin layer repairs itself quickly, any injury to the epidermis rarely causes injury to the body. However, damage which is severe enough to affect the middle layer, or dermis, can affect internal structures.

The dermis is sometimes called the true skin because it contains blood vessels, nerve endings, hair follicles (tubes), sweat glands, and sebaceous (oil) glands. Damage at this level can send infection into the bloodstream and throughout the body.

Within the dermis, blood vessels and sweat glands help the body regulate heat. If the temperature of blood rises, the brain stimulates secretions from the sweat glands. Sweat then flows to the surface of the skin through ducts. Here, the liquid cools the skin by evaporating. Sebaceous glands in the dermis prevent excessive evaporation by coating the surface of the skin with an oily substance called sebum.

The innermost layer, the subcutaneous layer, is the layer in which the sweat glands originate. This layer also stores fat and supports the blood vessels and nerves that supply the outer layer.

Because the dermis and the subcutaneous layer are rich with nerve endings, the skin also serves as a sensory organ. Nerves throughout these layers transmit tactile perceptions to the brain through the nervous system.

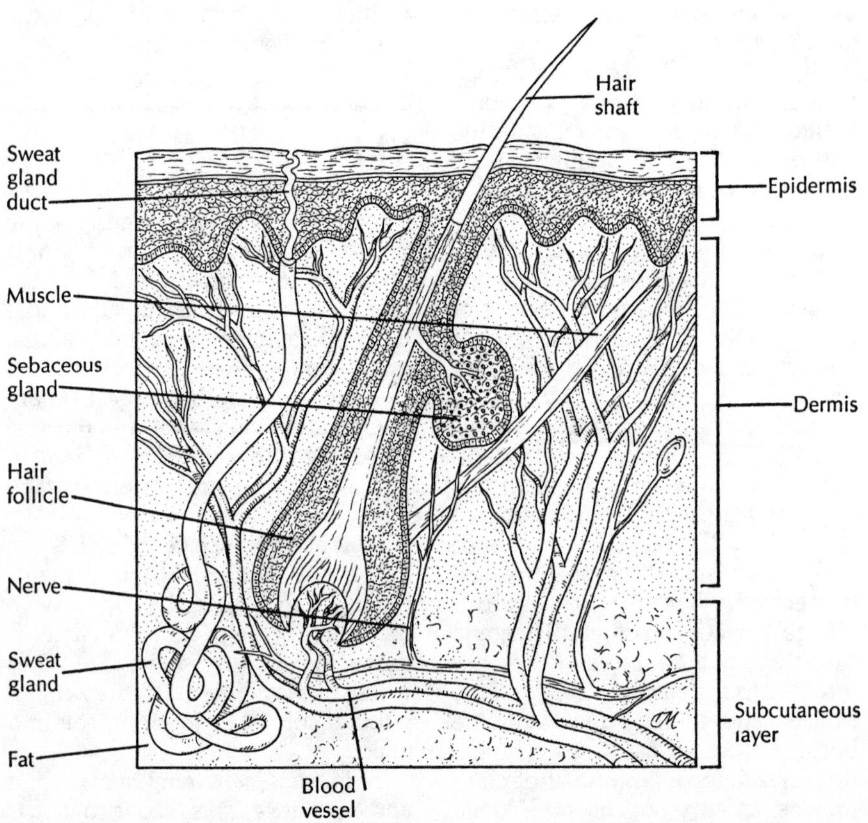

This cross section of skin shows many of its structures.

Slipped disk

A slipped disk is a back problem involving the disks of elastic cartilage tissue located between the vertebrae, the bones of the spine. The bones are loosely strung together by bands of tissue called ligaments that allow the body movement and flexibility. The function of each disk is to cushion any friction between the bones as the body moves.

When this intricate spinal structure experiences strain and overexertion, the rim of the disk weakens and tears, rather than "slips," causing part of the gelatinous center of the disk to be forced out of position. In its new position, the protruding material presses against an adjacent spinal nerve and causes pain along the path of the affected nerve.

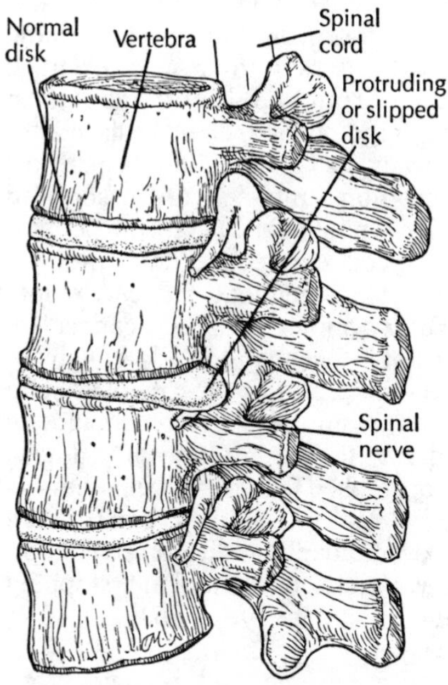

Disks of cartilage lie between the vertebrae to cushion the friction between the bones. If the rim of a disk weakens or tears, part of the jelly-like center becomes pushed out. This protruding material presses on a nearby spinal nerve causing pain along the path of the nerve. This is referred to as a slipped disk.

Most often, a slipped disk occurs when bending and straightening the back to lift heavy objects results in strain or injury. Damage to the disk may not be realized for many months, however. People with the problem frequently have a history of damage to the same area.

Disks also seem to disintegrate with age. They lose some of their fluidity and become more compressed. This form of degeneration usually results in only mild pain with intermittent backache and stiffness.

Symptoms of slipped disk may vary with the location of the disk. The most common slipped disk is the lowest movable disk in the small of the back. Injury to this disk causes pain along the sciatic nerve, a condition called sciatica. Mild or disabling pain and tenderness may result. Any straining, such as coughing or moving, can aggravate the discomfort. Weakness, tingling, or numbness in parts of the arm, leg, or feet may also result from damage to a particular disk.

To determine the source of back pain, a physician requests a current medical history; observes the patient sitting, walking, and bending; and explores for sensitive areas by maneuvering the patient's legs in different positions, checking ankle and knee reflexes and testing muscle strength. If needed, X rays reveal any structural changes in bones, joints, or disks.

For locating particularly problematic disks, or with a recommendation of surgery, special tests are necessary. A myelogram is an X ray taken after dye is injected into the space surrounding the spinal cord and nerve roots. The protruding disk is detected at the point where the flow of dye is interrupted or distorted. Discography gives much the same information; but before this X ray, dye is injected directly into the disks.

The first course of treatment for slipped disk involves complete bed rest on a firm mattress. Rest relieves pressure of the disk on the nerve and may shrink the protruding material. For moving about, some form of back support may improve comfort, but under no circumstances should a patient lift heavy objects.

For severe pain, a physician may prescribe a pain reliever. As pain subsides, an exercise program may be recommended to gradually strengthen muscles.

Most people find partial or complete relief of slipped disk from nonsurgical therapy. However, in some cases, removing the disk surgically provides the only remedy.

There is a new treatment still being investigated that offers the same results of eliminating or reducing the disk without major surgery. With this method, the drug chymopapain is injected into the damaged disk after the patient receives local anesthetic. This drug acts by slowly dissolving the part of the disk that is pressing on a nerve. Treatment is fast and relatively painless, but pain reduction occurs slowly, maybe in a couple weeks, if at all.

See also Sciatica.

Smoking

Smoking usually begins as a social behavior and results in significant physical consequences to the body. Cigarette smoke is much more influential in this regard than pipe or cigar smoke. Cigarette smoking tends to be habit-forming and the accumulated effects increase the risks for development of life-threatening disease.

The chemical makeup of cigarette smoke is complicated and still under scientific investigation. One of the chemicals in tobacco is tar, a powerful cancer-causing agent that is, therefore, called a carcinogen. Another chemical in tobacco, nicotine, produces harmful effects on the nervous system. Other chemicals in tobacco interfere with biochemical changes such as gas exchange and other functions in breathing.

Smoking of cigarettes, pipes, and cigars is linked to oral cancers. The most common oral cancers include those of the mouth, lip, salivary gland, tongue, and throat. Symptoms of oral cancers include a persistent sore, which may be accompanied by bleeding; a thickened area; discoloration; difficulty chewing or swallowing; and/or persistent sore throat. Such symptoms require a physician's attention.

Cigarette smoking is also implicated in lung cancers. Initially, cigarette smoke may destroy tiny hairs which normally function in clearing away mucus in the respiratory tract. The bronchial lining may then undergo changes that result in cancerous cell production. The most common lung cancers associated with smoking are typed the squamous cell carcinoma and undifferentiated small oat cell carcinoma. Early symptoms of lung cancer are variable but may include coughing, wheezing, and/or chest pain. Anyone with a smoking history should be alert to these symptoms. If you have not smoked cigarettes, your chances of developing lung cancer are extraordinarily reduced. If you do have a history of smoking, stopping will decrease your risk for lung cancer.

Emphysema and chronic bronchitis are most often caused by smoking. Both of these diseases are considered chronic obstructive pulmonary diseases in which there is airway blocking. Emphysema and chronic bronchitis frequently coexist. In emphysema, the air sacs of the lungs accumulate abnormal amounts of air. Expiration of air is especially impaired. In chronic bronchitis, the structure and function of the bronchi undergo changes that impede the air flow to the lungs.

The initial symptom of emphysema is shortness of breath. This may or may not be accompanied by a persistent cough. Progression of the disease, usually occurring over a course of years, results in severe difficulty breathing and restriction in activity. In chronic bronchitis, a persistent cough develops initially and is usually accompanied by mucus production. If you experience shortness of breath or develop a persistent cough, consult your physician. Stopping smoking will generally provide the best means of slowing the course of these diseases. Fortunately, emphysema and chronic bronchitis can usually be prevented by avoiding cigarette smoking.

Stopping smoking can also significantly reduce the incidence of arteriosclerosis in which the walls of the arteries thicken and lose elasticity. This is associated with heart attacks and strokes.

Smoking can also produce indirect adverse reactions in the body. Chemicals in smoke can interfere with the action of some medications. These drugs may be altered in absorption rate by the body and in duration of effect. One example of such a drug is a particular type of diuretic prescribed to control fluid retention and high blood pressure. It is prudent to discuss smoking habits with a physician when drugs are prescribed. The physician will then be able to make the proper adjustments in dosage.

Nonsmokers who encounter cigarette smoke of others are known as passive smokers. Research thus far reveals that even a passive smoker can suffer from the body's reaction to cigarette smoke. Passive smokers develop increased heart rates and blood pressure levels, and some people develop constriction of the bronchi in the lungs.

Radioactivity in cigarette smoke is being investigated to determine its effect on the passive smoker. Children are especially vulnerable potential passive smokers. By not smoking in your home, you can reduce your child's risk of developing respiratory disease. Also, unborn babies suffer if their mothers smoke. For example, birth weights tend to be somewhat higher in babies born to mothers who do not smoke compared to mothers who do. Also, stillbirths occur less in women who do not smoke during pregnancy compared to women who do.

In almost every case, stopping smoking is beneficial even if there are no signs of disease. Never starting is even better.

See also Atherosclerosis, Bronchitis, Cancer, and Emphysema.

Sore throat

A sore throat is a painful irritation in the throat, often a symptom of a cold. A sore throat can range from mild scratchiness and dryness to severe pain and difficulty in swallowing.

It is most frequently seen as a symptom of the common cold, when the nasal passages are congested and the person is forced to breath through the mouth, leaving the throat dry and irritated. Coughing may also irritate the throat, as will the secretions that drain into the throat from the back of the nose during a cold.

Irritating environmental substances such as smoke, pollen, pollution, and dust can cause a sore throat when inhaled; also, a sore throat may result when hot liquids or foods are swallowed.

A severe sore throat may be caused by a bacterial (usually strep) infection of the throat, middle ear, nose, or sinuses. Left untreated, strep throat can lead to rheumatic fever, a disease affecting the heart valves.

A sore throat is characterized by dryness and scratchiness in the throat and pain when swallowing. A doctor should be notified if a sore throat lasts more than a week, if it occurs without a cold, or if no obvious irritant can be found, since this type of sore throat may be a symptom of a serious disease, a blood disorder, or a severe infection. If a sore throat is accompanied by fever, achiness, and fatigue, or if the throat and mouth are very red or develop yellow or white spots, a bacterial infection is probably present.

A simple sore throat accompanying a cold is treated by relieving the other cold symptoms. A nasal decongestant may be used if the nose is congested; a cough suppressant may be used if coughing is irritating the throat (although cough suppressants are not always recommended because they allow mucus to accumulate and thus may trigger further complications); sour, hard candy can stimulate saliva production; and gargling with warm salt water every half hour soothes the irritated tissue of the throat.

If a strep infection is the cause of the sore throat, antibiotics are prescribed to prevent rheumatic fever and to fight the infection, as well as aspirin or an aspirin substitute to relieve pain and fever.

See also Rheumatic fever.

Spastic colon

See Irritable bowel syndrome.

Spina bifida

Spina bifida is a congenital (present at birth) defect of development in newborn infants, marked by a defective closure of the bony encasement of the spinal cord, through which the meninges (membranes covering the brain and spinal cord) may or may not protrude as a sac. If they do protrude, the condition is known as spina bifida cystica; if not, it is spina bifida occulta. This defect can range all the way from a form with few visible symptoms to a completely open spine. The cause is unknown.

Spina bifida commonly affects the chest and lower back regions of the spine and extends for three to six vertebral (backbone) segments. The sac, if there is one, may collapse while the child is still in the uterus, but fills with cerebrospinal fluid soon after birth. If the sac is not covered

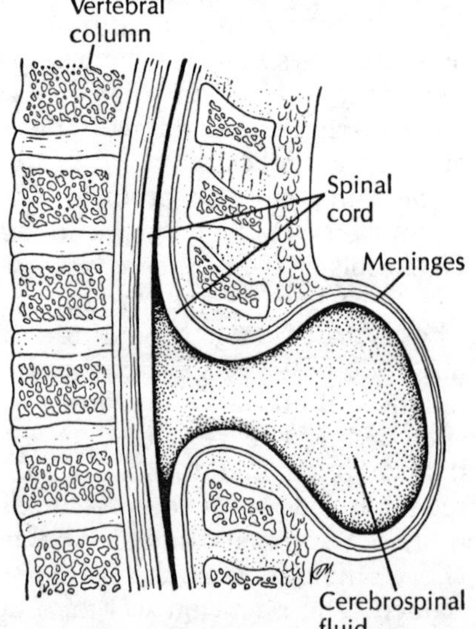

Spina bifida is a defect of development in which there is defective closure of the bony encasement of the spinal cord causing the meninges (membranes surrounding the brain and spinal cord) to protrude as a sac from the opening.

with skin it can rupture and perhaps lead to meningitis (inflammation of the meninges).

Spina bifida can be accompanied by varying degrees of paralysis, depending on involvement of the spinal cord and/or its nerve roots. Since the paralysis is usually present in the fetus, it can lead to problems such as clubfoot or dislocated hip. In addition, the paralysis may affect the sphincters (closure muscles) of the bladder and rectum, resulting in genitourinary disorders and damaged kidneys. An abnormal convex shape to the curve of the spine may occur and can hinder surgical closure. Hydrocephalus (accumulation of cerebrospinal fluid within the skull) also accompanies many cases of spina bifida.

The laboratory analysis of the condition begins with X rays of the spine, skull, hips, and lower extremities, if malformed. Urine tests are also necessary. Further tests depend on the extent of the defect but may include a CAT scan and an evaluation of the cerebrospinal fluid.

Treatment requires an extensive evaluation of the child's condition by neurosurgeons, urologists, orthopedists, pediatricians, and in some cases, social service workers and psychiatrists who work with the parents. Closure of the defect assures a better outcome. Long-term survival and lifestyle depend on the type and extent of the defect to the spine, other defects present, the infant's general health, and treatment resources. It should be remembered that in addition to surgical closure of the spine, the infant may need other more extensive surgery to repair accompanying problems. The most common complications are loss of kidney function, clubfoot, dislocation of the hip joints, scoliosis (curvature of the spine), pressure sores, muscle weakness, and spasm.

There is at this stage no known "prevention" for spina bifida; however, diagnosis through amniocentesis is growing progressively more accurate.

See also Hydrocephalus.

Strabismus

Strabismus is commonly referred to as "squint-eye" or "cross-eye." Technically, the term refers to a deviation of one eye from parallelism with the other.

Amblyopia, or reduced visual sharpness, results from suppressing the image from the deviating eye to avoid confusion. Disuse of one eye, as in cases of severe injury or impaired vision due to disease, may result in this form of strabismus.

Strabismus is usually present at birth (unless, as in the case of amblyopia, it results from later injury to one eye or impaired vision because of disease). The exact cause of congenital strabismus is unknown.

Symptoms include obviously crossed, wandering, or "squinting" eyes, except in some cases in which the lack of parallelism of the eyes is so subtle it cannot be seen.

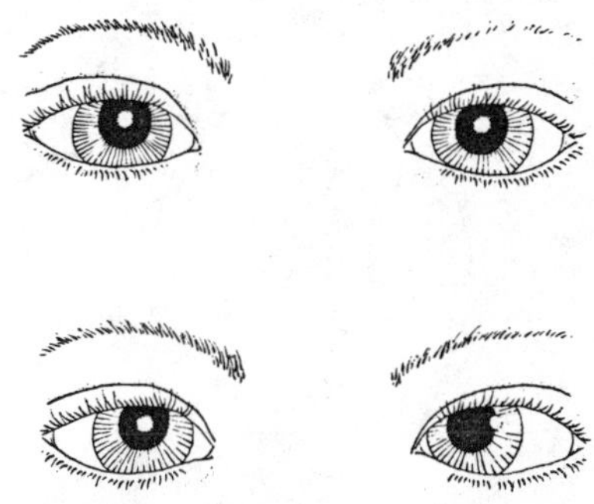

The eyes above are properly aligned while the eyes below are not parallel and, therefore, exhibit strabismus. When a light is shined into the eyes, the highlight should normally be on the same spot in each eye.

Complete evaluation of the eyes is essential to determine if there is involvement of a serious ocular (eye) or neurological (nerve) disorder in strabismus. If muscle imbalance alone is responsible, the strabismus can be treated easily with corrective glasses or contact lenses. Surgical restoration of the muscle balance can be done in more extreme cases. Eye exercises are effective in many less severe cases. Permanent visual loss can result if strabismus is not treated before the child is four to six years old.

See also Amblyopia.

Stroke

Stroke is an interruption of the blood supply to a group of brain cells, damaging those cells and causing malfunction or lack of function in those parts of the body that the damaged cells control. Generally speaking, each side of the brain controls the motor and sensory functions of the opposite side of the body, so damage to cells on the left side of the brain, for instance, will impair function on the right side of the body.

Stroke can have a wide range of consequences; it may, among other conditions, cause temporary or permanent loss of memory and difficulty in speaking, walking, and controlling emotions.

Stroke can be caused by several conditions. One is called cerebrovascular embolism, which occurs when a "wandering" blood clot, formed elsewhere in the body (usually in the heart or in one or both carotid arteries in the neck that carry blood from the heart to the brain), lodges itself in an artery leading to or within the brain. Interruption of blood flow also occurs when a similar clot is formed in the arteries because of the presence of atherosclerosis (a narrowing and clogging of the arteries by various deposits).

Stroke can also be caused by cerebral hemorrhage, in which a diseased artery in the brain bursts, depriving the cells that are normally nourished by that artery, as well as

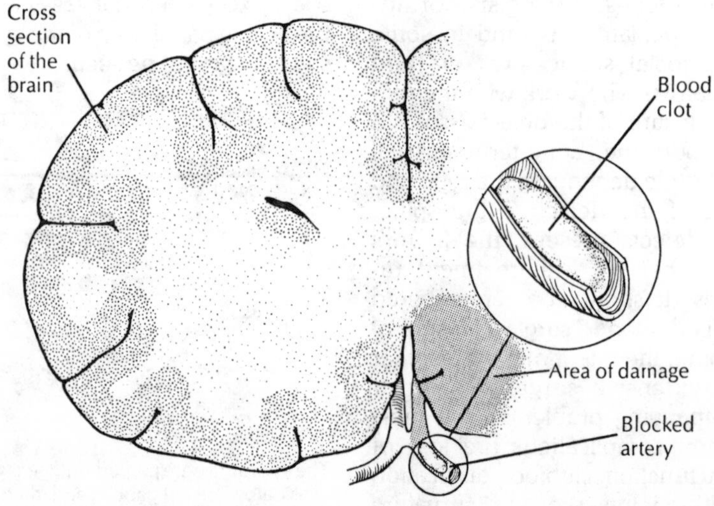

A stroke is damage to brain cells because of an interruption in their blood supply. Some strokes are caused by blood clots blocking an artery leading to the brain.

flooding the surrounding tissue with blood. This accumulation of blood forms a clot which displaces and compresses brain tissue and thus interferes in the brain's functioning. This type of stroke often strikes people who have both hypertension (high blood pressure) and atherosclerosis.

A third condition that can lead to stroke may be an aneurysm (a bulge in an artery because of a defect in its wall) that ruptures and interrupts blood flow to an area of the brain as well as flooding the area with blood. The formation of aneurysms is sometimes associated with hypertension, but is often congenital (present at birth). Thus aneurysms are often the cause of cerebral hemorrhage in young people.

People who have both hypertension and atherosclerosis are the most likely to suffer a stroke, since both diseases weaken and damage the arteries. Hypertension probably encourages hemorrhage. Heredity may play a role in stroke, since the tendencies to develop both hypertension and atherosclerosis appear to be inherited. Black people are more likely candidates for stroke because high blood pressure is at least twice as common among blacks as among whites.

Smoking, diabetes, and high blood cholesterol may also contribute to stroke. Furthermore, stroke is more likely to victimize anyone with a history of mild stroke-like episodes called TIAs (transient ischemic attacks). TIAs are essentially strokes that clear up within 24 hours, that is, an individual may develop total paralysis of one side of the body as in a classic stroke, but the symptoms clear within 24 hours, leaving no residual effects.

A stroke can present itself in many ways, but some of the more common symptoms are a sudden weakness or numbness in the face, arm, and/or leg on one side of the body; loss or slurring of speech or difficulty in understanding others speak; unexplained unsteadiness, and persistent falling to one side. It is possible, however, to suffer a mild stroke and experience minor degrees of these symptoms.

Stroke is diagnosed mostly by the history and physical examination. Sophisticated X ray techniques are also employed. For example, arteriography (the injection of X-ray opaque dye into a main artery) will show damage or clots in the arteries, leading to or within the brain and a computerized axial tomography (CAT) scan produces a cross-sectional picture of the area, which can provide the physician with crucial information such as whether the stroke was caused by a hemorrhage or by blockage of blood flow. Tumors, which can cause symptoms identical to that of stroke, are also frequently diagnosed by these means.

Treatment of stroke begins with immediate hospitalization. Blood pressure is normalized, and drug therapy to prevent future seizures as well as to reduce swelling of the brain tissue is often instituted. Also, depending on the cause of the stroke and other factors, anticoagulants (agents that inhibit the normal clotting of blood) are sometimes administered in the hope of limiting the progress of the stroke or preventing additional strokes. After the acute period, rehabilitation is begun by speech, physical, and occupational therapists who are specially trained in dealing with stroke victims.

For those who have experienced TIAs or other warning signs of stroke, precautions can be taken to prevent an actual stroke. Usually after a TIA, some form of arteriography is performed to locate obstructions or ulcerated areas of the carotid arteries. Depending on the results of the arteriogram along with the general condition of the patient and many other factors, the decision of whether to operate (to "clean out" the arteries) or to treat with anticoagulants is made.

Prevention of stroke mainly involves control of high blood pressure and other risk factors such as smoking and high cholesterol intake.

See also Aneurysm, Atherosclerosis, and Transient ischemic attack.

Sty

A sty is an inflamed or infected swelling of the sebaceous (oil-producing) glands in the eyelid.

The infection is commonly caused by staphylococcus, a type of bacteria. An external sty appears on the surface of the skin at the edge of the eyelid. An internal sty is due to inflammation, infection, or obstruction of a sebaceous gland on the inner surface of the eyelid. This type of sty is often seen as a protrusion or lump on the eyelid without visible pus or redness.

Initially, a sty feels like a foreign object is in the eye. Tearing, redness, swelling, and tenderness in or around a particular area of the eye soon follow. The eye may be sensitive to light and touch. In addition, small, yellow bumps filled with pus may develop. These growths often burst, release the pus, and begin to heal. Once the pressure releases, the pain usually subsides.

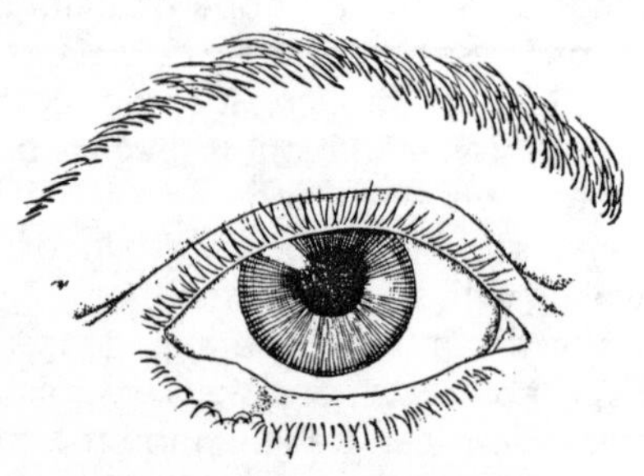

A sty is an inflamed or infected swelling of the oil-producing glands of the eyelid. An external sty appears on the surface of the skin at the edge of the eyelid.

A sty is not usually serious, but it can lead to spread of infection if not properly treated.

Treatment for a sty often involves putting antibiotic eyedrops and/or ointments into the eye. Warm, moist compresses applied to the eye three or four times a day for about ten minutes may encourage the sty to burst. In some cases, particularly in internal sties, surgical opening may be needed to cure the condition. Never should one attempt to open a sty on his or her own, as the risks of spreading and worsening the infection would be quite high.

Sudden infant death syndrome

Sudden infant death syndrome (also called SIDS and crib death) is the unexplained and sudden death of a baby who apparently is perfectly well when put to bed but dies silently in its sleep, often without any signs of a struggle. SIDS is the second leading cause (after accidents) of death in infants from two weeks to one year of age, with 8,000 to 10,000 deaths per year in the United States. Most frequently, deaths occur in the third and fourth month of life, with a higher death rate among boys, children of teenage mothers, infants from poor families, and babies who were premature. There are more deaths in the winter than in the summer. SIDS is a worldwide phenomenon.

SIDS, before it was known by that name, used to be blamed on smothering in the bedding, but this diagnosis is inaccurate. It is also not attributable to vomited food clogging the airways, to bottle feeding, nor to any known cause that parents could prevent. Parents who have lost one child to SIDS are not known to be at higher risk of losing another in the same way.

Some investigators believe a combination of conditions is necessary to trigger SIDS, including a narrowed and inflamed airway, temporary airway obstruction, chronic oxygen deficiency, and irregular breathing, leading to a spasm of the trachea (windpipe) and death. Research is continuing.

Parents who lose a child to SIDS are totally unprepared for the death and usually have overwhelming guilt feelings—that something they did or did not do caused the death of their child. SIDS, however, is not the parents' fault. An autopsy will prove this fact. Doctors and nurses who take the time to discuss the death fully with the parents can be very helpful. So can another parent who has lost a child to SIDS. There are now many local chapters of the National Foundation for Sudden Infant Death Syndrome or the International Guild for Infant Survival, both of which can be valuable counseling and information sources.

Sunburn

Sunburn is an inflammation because of damage to the cells of the skin usually caused by overexposure to sunlight or sunlamps. Sunburn can either be insignificant or serious, depending on the intensity of the sun's rays, the length of exposure, and the susceptibility of the individual to the sun's effects.

Sunburn is caused by prolonged exposure to ultraviolet solar radiation. Certain substances (such as deodorant soaps, perfume ingredients, cosmetics, and certain medications) may produce heightened sensitivity to ultraviolet radiation, with a corresponding increase in the severity of the burn. While light-skinned people usually burn more easily than swarthy or dark-skinned people, skin color is not always a dependable guide to individual susceptibility.

Irritation, a prickling sensation, and skin that is hot to the touch mark the onset of sunburn. Skin capillaries become congested, because of the release of certain inflammatory agents, thus producing the characteristic redness. Oral contraceptive users may develop irregularly shaped dark splotches, and some sensitive individuals may develop allergic reactions in the form of rashes or welts.

As the burn progresses in severity, the skin will feel tight and swollen, dry or brittle, and may become hypersensitive to touch. Overheating and loss of fluids through the damaged skin may also produce dizziness, nausea, vomiting, hyperventilation (rapid breathing causing loss of carbon dioxide from the blood), impaired vision and hearing, irregular heartbeat, and unconsciousness.

The aftermath of severe sunburn often includes blistering and peeling, as well as permanent freckling, splotching, or scarring of the skin. Long-term effects may include premature skin aging, marked by chronic dryness, wrinkling and leathery texture, and loss of elasticity. In some cases, melanomas, or skin cancers may be induced by chronic overexposure to sunlight.

Minor sunburn can be effectively treated by a wide variety of commercially distributed, nonprescription ointments, oils, powders, creams, and sprays that restore fluids and prevent further drying, relieve discomfort, and promote healing. Many over-the-counter medications contain mild anesthetics to relieve stinging and suppress the desire to scratch itching areas. One of the most common complications encountered by sunburn victims is the infection of blistered and peeling areas of the skin. This condition should be treated by a physician.

In the case of severe sunburn, care should be taken not to become overheated or dehydrated (lose too much fluid). Above all, the victim should be taken out of the sun immediately, and placed in a cool, shaded area until a physician can be summoned. Cool, not cold, wet cloths can be applied to the arms, the head, and the legs. Care should be taken not to chill the sufferer. Iced water or other cold drinks may trigger unwanted responses. Commercial mineral and electrolyte mixtures at room temperature will replace lost fluid faster and more safely than water taken alone. If the victim is perspiring profusely, a fan may help evaporate the water on the skin's surface, thus aiding a natural cooling process.

The best prevention of sunburn is simply to avoid prolonged exposure to the direct rays of the sun or a sunlamp. When this is not possible, the first line of defense is to cover the skin completely, preferably with cool, loose-weave, loose-fitting, light-colored clothes. Wide-brimmed hats, long sleeves, white cotton gloves, caps with sun visors, and lightweight scarves for the neck will protect the areas not covered by clothes.

The second line of defense is a sunscreen: an oil, cream, paste, lotion, or liquid. Most sunscreens are intended to block ultraviolet rays. Many common preparations contain para-aminobenzoic acid. This compound may affect some individuals adversely, particularly those with photosensitivity (abnormal sensitivity of the skin to light) because of certain drugs. For these people, opaque (light-blocking) creams, pastes, and lotions are available as well as other chemical sunscreens known as benzophenomes.

Anyone with a question as to possible adverse effects of sunlight with their medication should contact their doctor before exposure to sunlight.

Syphilis

Syphilis is a serious, highly contagious disease spread primarily through direct sexual contact. Syphilis is caused by spiral-shaped bacteria called spirochetes.

Over time, syphilis can affect all parts of the body, the brain, bones, spinal cord, and heart as well as the reproductive organs. If left untreated, blindnesss, brain damage, heart disease, and even death can result. Syphilis can also be passed from a mother to her unborn baby, causing congential syphilis in the child, which may eventually result in blindness and deafness, among other serious consequences. Syphilis in a pregnant woman must be treated prior to the eighteenth week of the pregnancy in order to prevent passage of the disease to the fetus.

Syphilis is a progressive disorder that passes through four stages: primary, secondary, latent, and late or tertiary. Each of the four stages of syphilis is marked by a distinct set (or lack) of symptoms.

Primary syphilis is characterized by the appearance of a painless, open sore (called a chancre) ten to 90 days after exposure to the disease. As a rule, there is usually only one sore (although occasionally there are several), appearing most commonly on the genital organs, but also at times on the rectum, cervix (the opening to the uterus), lips, tongue, fingers, or anywhere that direct contact was made. The chancre first appears as a red bump, sometimes surrounded by a red ring and oozing clear fluid; it soon erodes into a painless ulcer and disappears within several weeks without treatment. Although the chancre is gone, the disease is still active in the body.

Secondary syphilis appears within six weeks to six months of initial contact. Symptoms resembling the flu such as fever, sore throat, headache, fatigue, aching joints, and enlarged lymph nodes are common. Syphilitic meningitis (an infection of the membranes lining the brain and spinal cord) can also be seen in this stage.

Secondary syphilis is also characterized by extremely contagious, grayish-white erosions that can be seen on the lining of the mouth, the penis, the external female sexual organs, the anus, and warm, moist areas such as the underarms; growths resembling warts in the genital area (not to be confused with the more common nonsyphilitic genital warts); and a rash on the palms or soles in the form of round reddish spots that occur in patches and do not itch. These sores, growths, and rashes heal within three to six weeks without treatment, and the disease enters the third stage.

In the latent stage (latent means present but not manifesting itself), all

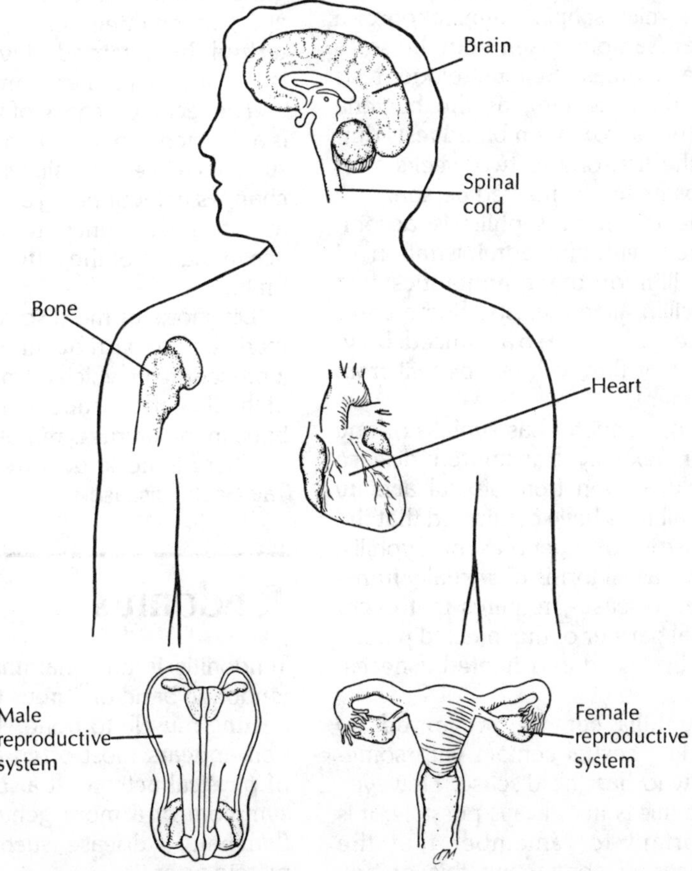

In its final stages, syphilis can seriously damage the brain, spinal cord, bones, heart, and reproductive organs.

symptoms disappear, the patient appears to be healthy, and the disease is probably not contagious (except in the case of pregnant women, who can still pass it on to their offspring). The latent stage can go on indefinitely, but it is estimated that one third of all those with latent syphilis will progress to the final stage of the illness.

By the late or tertiary stage of syphilis, the disease is in all likelihood no longer contagious, but the entire body may come under siege. Late syphilis can damage the brain, bones, spinal cord, and heart, commonly causing blindness, brain damage, heart disease, or even death.

Syphilis is diagnosed with a history and physical exam, blood tests, and a microscopic examination of a smear (sample) taken from the sores or rash areas. Several blood tests may be necessary, as the bacteria may not show up on blood tests during the first one to two weeks after exposure to the infected person.

Treatment of syphilis is accomplished with the administration of penicillin or other antibiotics if a penicillin allergy exists. Some cases of late syphilis are so advanced, however, that they will not benefit from treatment.

A person who has syphilis or any other sexually transmitted disease should abstain from sexual activity until all tests have confirmed that the disease is no longer present. Syphilis, as well as all forms of sexually transmitted diseases, requires that every sexual partner of the infected person also be tested and treated if necessary.

Syphilis can be prevented by avoiding sexual contact with someone who has the disease. However, since this is not always possible, it is important to remember that the chances of contracting this or any other sexually transmitted disease increase with the number of different sexual partners a person has, so limiting the number of partners can be beneficial to some extent in prevention.

T

Tay-Sachs disease

Tay-Sachs disease is an hereditary metabolic disorder chiefly afflicting infants of East European Jewish descent. It is marked by an accumulation of a certain type of fatty acid in the brain. The disease, which is progressive and always fatal (often by age two or three years), is characterized by retarded development, loss of vision, paralysis, and death.

The technical cause of the disease is a deficiency of a certain enzyme (a substance in every cell, which causes changes without being altered itself), and this deficiency results in the accumulation of the fatty acids in the brain.

Diagnosis of the disorder may be made before birth by amniocentesis, a procedure in which a small amount of the fluid in the sac surrounding the baby in the uterus is removed.

There is no known treatment for Tay-Sachs disease.

Tendonitis

Tendonitis is an inflammation of a tendon, a band of fibrous tissue connecting muscle to bone. The condition appears most often as a result of physical activity. It also can be a symptom of a more generalized inflammatory disease such as rheumatoid arthritis.

Improper activity, lack of conditioning, and poor equipment encourage the development of tendonitis. Nonathletes who suddenly begin long distance jogging or other athletic activity or athletes who resume strenuous sports after intervals of passive activity have an increased likelihood of the condition. In addition, people who wear shoes with rundown heels put needless tension on the Achilles tendon, which joins the two major muscles on the back of the legs to the back of the heel bones. Similarly, women who wear high-heel shoes may have problems with inflamed Achilles tendons because the angle created by the shoes considerably shortens the tendons.

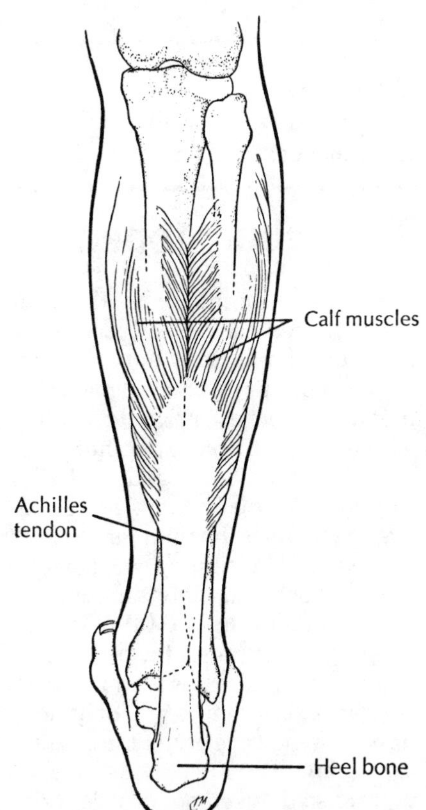

Tendonitis, or inflammation of the tissue connecting muscle to bone, frequently occurs in the Achilles tendon connecting the calf muscles to the heel bone.

A tendonitis attack causes pain in the affected tendon worsened by activity. The tendon may grow thicker than normal and be tender to the touch. Sometimes, the tendon can be very painful. When minor injuries are continually placed under stress, an already inflamed tendon could rupture and become a greater problem.

Physicians diagnose sports-related problems by first acquiring an exercise history to determine the patient's normal activity, and if there have been any changes in routine. A doctor also checks muscle lengths to find unusually short or inflexible muscles which may be producing the problem.

Treatment for tendonitis involves resting the affected area. Pain relievers and anti-inflammatory drugs are used to ease immediate symptoms, but these preparations will not by themselves cure the condition or keep it from recurring.

In rare cases, tendonitis patients may require surgery to remove damaged tendons. Fortunately, surgical procedures have advanced in the past few years. Previously, tendons were replaced with artificial tissues that never assumed the strength and flexibility of natural tissues. Now newer techniques and materials are being developed.

People participating in sports can prevent tendonitis by taking time for warmup prior to exercise. For example, leg and calf muscle stretching before and after running may help prevent inflammation of the Achilles tendon.

Supports in shoes worn during physical activity can correct instability of the foot. Such devices also lessen pain when tendonitis occurs.

Testes, undescended

See Undescended testes.

Tetanus

Tetanus is an acute disease of infectious origin, commonly associated with improperly cleaned deep wounds, that causes severe muscle contraction or tightening.

Tetanus is caused by toxins (poisonous substances) that are produced by the bacteria *Clostridium tetani.* These bacteria usually enter the body through a wound in contact with material such as soil in which bacteria spores are present or by being present on the skin at the time of the injury. Puncture wounds seem especially vulnerable to tetanus infection, since they are, by their nature, difficult to clean and medicate and allow little air to reach the deep tissue (these bacteria cannot live in the air).

Tetanus symptoms are varied, depending on the extent of the infection and the body part that is affected. The most common symptom is called "lockjaw," in which the muscles of the jaw go into severe continuous contraction, thus rendering the jaw immobile. Symptoms also include a bowed or arched body (which is rare), because of contraction of lower back muscles, back muscle spasms, and lethal throat spasms that can cause blockage of the airway. The affected body parts become immobile because of the simultaneous and continuous contraction of opposing muscles.

In severe cases, the contractions affect most of the cells in the affected muscle. The contraction is thus not merely a weak "twitch," but is instead an almost "complete" contraction, similar to what would be required in lifting a heavy weight or marshaling all the potential force of a muscle against a high resistance.

Treatment consists of muscle relaxant drugs such as diazepam to ease the contractions. Antimicrobial drugs such as penicillin are used to fight the infection. Tetanus antitoxin is given intramuscularly in the hope of lessening the severity of the disease. However, the antitoxin does not counteract toxin already in the nervous system nor does it act to relieve symptoms already present.

Immunization beforehand with the tetanus vaccine offers the best preventive against the disease. Also, wounds should be attended to immediately, especially puncture wounds. Tetanus "boosters" should be taken periodically, especially if small skin wounds are a common occurrence in the course of the workday.

Throat

See Ear, nose, and throat.

Thrombocytopenia

Thrombocytopenia is a disorder characterized by a decrease in the number of platelets in the blood. Platelets are tiny components of the blood that act to promote clotting when there is an injury or other problem that requires bleeding to be stopped. Normally there are about five to ten times the number of platelets required for clotting circulating in the bloodstream; this amounts to about 200,000 to 500,000. Thrombocytopenia is present usually when platelet counts are less than 100,000. Abnormal bleeding commonly does not occur, however, until the count is less than 50,000, and serious or unprovoked bleeding usually does not occur with counts above 20,000.

There are basically two mechanisms whereby thrombocytopenia occurs: decreased production and increased destruction of platelets. In the former, the elements in the bone marrow responsible for the production of platelets may be severely diminished (as in aplastic anemia where all of the blood-forming elements are diminished or absent) or may malfunction. Increased destruction of platelets occurs in diseases such as essential or idiopathic (of unknown cause) thrombocytopenia. In this disorder, which is common in children, antibodies are made against the individual's own platelets thereby causing their destruction. Drug-induced thrombocytopenia can be due to this same mechanism or others. Severe, overwhelming infection can also cause increased destruction of platelets. In pregnancy platelets from the fetus can sometimes escape into the circulation of the mother causing antibody formation and the consequent destruction of fetal platelets with abnormal bleeding at birth.

Signs and symptoms of thrombocytopenia include reddish to reddish-purple spots on the skin, seen as a rash. These are due to bleeding within and underneath the skin. Abnormal or easily provoked bleeding is the most dangerous symptom of thrombocytopenia. This bleeding can be minor such as oozing from the gums while brushing the teeth, or bruising caused merely by leaning on or brushing up against something. The bleeding can also be major as in spontaneous internal bleeding that may go unrecognized until shock appears.

Treatment depends on the cause. If infection is present, this must be remedied, and the platelet count will usually return to normal on its own. In essential or idiopathic thrombocytopenia, corticosteroids (cortisone or prednisone) are the first line of treatment. In drug-induced thrombocytopenia, the first move is to discontinue the drug. This will usually result in improvement; if not, corticosteroids may be helpful in some cases. In immune thrombocytopenia of the newborn, if severe, exchange transfusion (where all or most of the blood is exchanged with transfused blood) may be necessary. If the platelet count in any of these conditions is dangerously low (around 20,000), transfusion of platelets until the disease process is controlled is indicated.

Thrombocytopenia may not be preventable in most cases, but early recognition of symptoms and signs such as rash and easy bleeding may lead to prevention of serious complications.

See also Platelets.

Thrombophlebitis

Thrombophlebitis is a condition in which both inflammation and blood clots exist in a vein. This can be caused by a number of factors. Commonly, when a person is immobilized, blood stagnates in the veins of the legs; this induces clotting which in turn prevents blood from returning to the heart. The blood below the clot remains there, causing a buildup of pressure that forces fluid into the tissues thus resulting in swelling. Also, simultaneously, the vein(s) and surrounding area may become quite inflamed and tender. This condition is most often found in the deep veins of the legs, but it can also occur in veins of the pelvis and arms.

Thrombophlebitis itself may not be too serious, but it can lead to a life-threatening condition called pulmonary embolism (a blood clot lodged in the lung). This develops when a clot formed in a deep leg vein breaks loose, travels through the bloodstream, and becomes lodged in the vessels of the lung. A pulmonary embolism can lead to chest pain, shortness of breath, coughing up of blood, and even death.

The development of thrombophlebitis is favored by any condition that inhibits the free flow of blood through the veins. These include prolonged bed rest or inactivity, perhaps following illness or surgery; congestive heart failure, which affects the heart's ability to pump blood throughout the body; and injury or infection that damages a vein. Other factors that may lead to an increased tendency toward thrombophlebitis are the use of birth control pills in susceptible individuals, as well as pregnancy itself; occupations that require long periods of standing or sitting; obesity; old age; and chronic infections. In addition, thrombophlebitis, in some cases, may indicate the presence of a tumor in the pancreas or lung, since these disorders might produce or release a substance that affects blood clotting.

Common symptoms (which often appear only in advanced cases) of deep thrombophlebitis are swelling, aching, and a feeling of heaviness in the leg or affected area; the skin may appear white and will be painful to the touch. If the veins of the leg are affected, the condition is characterized by increased pain when walking or when the foot is flexed backward or forward.

Thrombophlebitis of a surface vein (known as superficial thrombophlebitis) can be diagnosed by a simple physical examination usually revealing a red, warm, tender cordlike vein. Superficial thrombophlebitis rarely, if ever, leads to pulmonary embolism.

Diagnostic tests for thrombophlebitis include the Doppler (a technique used to detect obstructions by changes in sounds made by flowing blood), nuclear scans, a test to measure the resistance to flow in the veins, and venography. Venography involves the insertion of X-ray contrast dye into the veins so that the X ray will visualize a clot. This is the most sensitive and specific test for thrombophlebitis.

Treatment of superficial thrombophlebitis consists of bed rest with elevation of the leg. Warm compresses are also helpful as are anti-inflammatory drugs.

Deep vein thrombophlebitis, because of the potential for pulmonary embolism, is treated much more aggressively. The patient is usually hospitalized and put on bed rest with

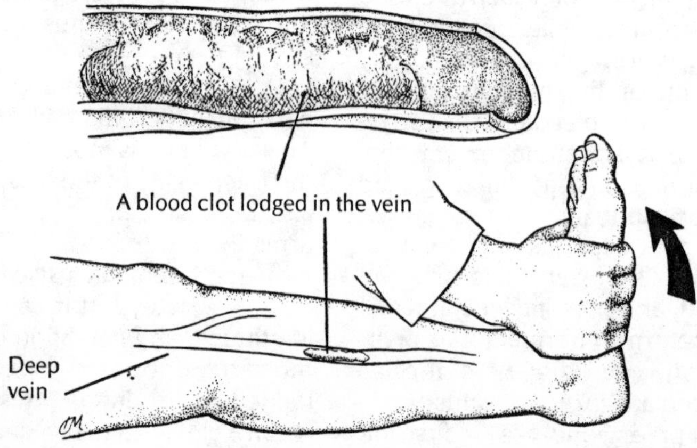

Thrombophlebitis, or inflammation of a vein accompanied by the formation of a blood clot, often occurs in the deep veins of the legs. Thrombophlebitis is suspected if moving the foot forward or backward causes pain.

the leg elevated. The anticoagulant (an anticoagulant is an agent that inhibits the normal clotting mechanisms of the blood) heparin is given intravenously, usually for about seven days and up to ten days if pulmonary embolism has occurred. The patient is also usually placed on the oral anticoagulant warfarin for about six weeks or three to six months if pulmonary embolism has occurred. It is important to note that these drugs do not dissolve an existing clot, but serve to prevent new clots from forming while the old ones are resolving. Newer drugs do dissolve clots, but are still used only in special situations.

Prevention of thrombophlebitis is a controversial subject. In hospitalized patients who are immobilized for long periods or about to undergo major surgery, leg exercises along with long support stockings and increased activity as soon as feasible may be helpful. So-called "mini-heparin" (low doses of heparin given by injection under the skin two to three times a day) has also been beneficial in preventing deep vein thrombophlebitis in certain patients. For nonhospitalized patients who are susceptible to this condition, regular exercise of the legs along with elevation of legs when lying down and support hose are probably helpful. Self-injected heparin and warfarin are also used.

See also Pulmonary Embolism.

Tic

A tic is a spasmodic movement or twitching that is usually a brief, repetitive, purposeless, semi- or involuntary muscle contraction, most commonly seen in the face, shoulders, or arms. A typical "nervous tic" is a twitching of the corner of the eye or the mouth, grimacing, blinking, or making repetitive motions with the arms or shoulders.

Tics in children often occur between the ages of five to ten years and may gradually disappear as the child grows older; however, they can also persist into adulthood. Nervous tics, when they first arise, can usually be voluntarily controlled, but persistent tics often become automatic after a period of time.

Some tics are associated with nerve or brain damage. However, most tics are of unknown origin.

With the exception of the tics that develop as a result of other conditions, the physiological basis of ordinary tics is largely unknown. They often, but not always, accompany tension, emotional upset, or some hidden psychological problem. Such conditions as hereditary tremors and organic disorders such as Parkinson's disease also often worsen with emotional stress.

There are several different kinds of specific tics: *facial tic,* or spasms of the facial muscles, and *Gilles de la Tourette's syndrome,* a childhood disorder marked by multiple tics and compulsive use of profane language are two examples.

Facial tic, the simplest, is marked by simple spasms of the facial muscles. These may be simple twitches, such as twitching of the corner of the eye, twisting or grimacing of the mouth, or raising of an eyebrow.

Gilles de la Tourette's syndrome, the most complicated of the types of tics, may be marked by single or multiple tics (blinking, grimacing, shrugging of the shoulders, repetitive arm movements) that gradually worsen in extent, severity, and frequency. In many patients, vocal tics such as sniffling, grunting, shouting, or barking noises also occur. About half of all patients develop coprolalia, or compulsive swearing.

Tourette's syndrome is the only type of tic associated with a definite syndrome. The other tics are at the beginning hard to distinguish from many neurologically-based illnesses.

For mild childhood or adult tics, minor tranquilizers or muscle relaxants may be prescribed. Tourette's syndrome has been known to respond to the major tranquilizer, haloperidol. Psychotherapy as treatment for tics may be ineffective, but it may help to relieve some of the emotional stress that precipitates attacks or intensifies symptoms.

No preventive measures for tics are known at present.

See also Gilles de la Tourette's syndrome.

Tonsillitis

Tonsillitis is an infection and often enlargement of the tonsils, occurring most commonly in children ages five to 15 years, and rarely in those under the age of two.

The tonsils are two small, almond-shaped lumps of tissue located in the throat at the back of the mouth. They are barely visible in infants, increase in size during the preschool and early school years, and shrink by adulthood.

The function of the tonsils has not been exactly pinpointed, but scientists believe that they perform at least two vital jobs: they release an antibody, or protective agent, into the throat to prevent infection from spreading into the lungs (a useful service to children, who are highly susceptible to ear, nose, and throat infections); and they attract bacterial infection and thereby stimulate the production of antibodies, which accumulate in the body in order to prevent future, and much more serious, infections. Antibodies normally do not develop unless infection is present.

If the tonsils do indeed perform these two functions, then each attack of tonsillitis may help immunize a child from disease, and once this resistance is developed, the function of the tonsils is complete.

There are two types of tonsillitis: acute tonsillitis, in which the infection flares up, then disappears in a short time; and chronic tonsillitis, in which the tonsils seem to be permanently engorged and have abscesses (pus-filled cavities) on them.

Complications resulting from tonsillitis seldom occur today because of effective and fast-acting antibiotics, but rare cases of rheumatic fever (a disease affecting the heart valves) and infections of the sinuses, ears, or kidneys are possible.

Tonsillitis is caused by many different infectious agents, both viral and bacterial, the most common bacteria being streptococcus bacteria. Acute tonsillitis is usually a "strep" infection. Chronic tonsillitis, however, is more of a mystery; it is not known why chronic tonsillitis occurs in certain people or what causes it.

The symptoms of acute tonsillitis are a sore throat, fever up to about 101°F, chills, headache, and muscle aches. These symptoms worsen for one to three days, then subside. In addition, nausea, vomiting, stomach ache, and swelling of glands located in the neck may also occur and may last for about a week.

The symptoms of chronic tonsillitis include a persistent or recurrent sore throat, difficulty in swallowing or breathing, and foul breath.

Tonsillitis is diagnosed by an examination of the tonsils, to check for redness, swelling, and a gray or yellow infectious material deposited on them. The doctor will take a sample of this material with a cotton swab in order to identify the bacteria causing the infection.

Bed rest or reduced activity and the use of antibiotics, often penicillin, are recommended to treat tonsillitis if the inflammation is due to bacteria.

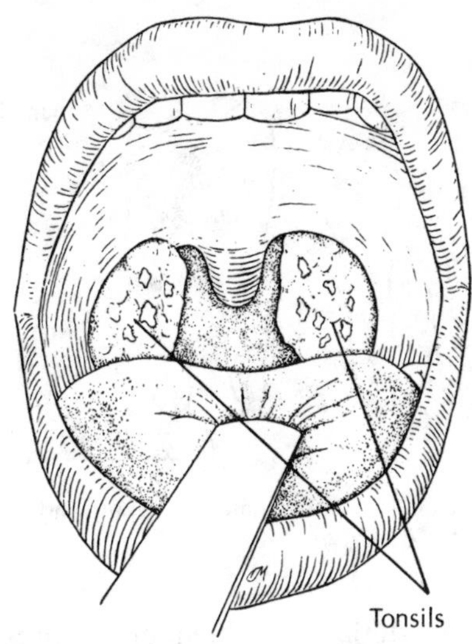

Infected tonsils, such as these, are inflamed and sometimes display gray or yellow patches on their surface.

Gargling with warm salt water can help relieve sore throat.

Surgical removal of the tonsils (called a tonsillectomy) is performed only if the tonsils are abscessed (filled with pus) or greatly enlarged, thus blocking the air passages. Tonsillectomies are seldom performed today, because research has found that even when tonsils are enlarged, they almost always shrink over time. Furthermore, removing the tonsils does not necessarily prevent recurrent sore throats or colds, as was once believed.

Since it is not known why some people suffer from chronic tonsillitis, preventive measures are also uncertain. Because episodes of acute tonsillitis may help build up immunities in the body, prevention of such episodes may not be of vital importance until more research is completed in this area.

Tooth decay

Tooth decay (or dental cavities or caries) is the gradual destruction and loss of minerals in the enamel (outer layer) and dentin (the bony second layer) of a portion of a tooth, which causes it to become soft, discolored, and porous.

A combination of factors causes tooth decay. The actual destruction is probably done by bacteria and by-products of their metabolism such as acid. These bacteria feed on sugars and starches that cling to the teeth. They live and multiply to become dental plaque. The plaque is made up of sugars, starches, bacteria, and proteins, and builds up on dental surfaces, especially near the gums and in other hard-to-clean areas. Here the production of acid is concentrated. The plaque prevents the saliva from performing its natural protective function.

When the cavity has progressed into the dentin or begins on the surface of an exposed root, the tooth becomes sensitive to touch and to rapid temperature changes. Sweet foods can cause pain as dissolved sugar enters the cavity. Bacteria may pass through tiny tubes in the dentin and inflame the pulp, which contains blood vessels and nervous tissue, producing toothache. The cavity reveals itself to the examining dentist as a darkened area or as a softness that "gives" when probed with a sharp instrument. It is also detected by X rays.

Cavities are treated by drilling out the decayed material and replacing it with a filling. In front teeth, where appearance is important, the filling may be of porcelain cement or a plastic resin (which is also used to fill pits and tiny cracks in the enamel). In other teeth the filling is usually silver-colored or an alloy of gold, which is the most durable material. Where a tooth is badly damaged with involvement of the root canal, the dentist removes all decay, fills the cavity and/or root canal with cement, then grinds and tapers the outer surfaces and covers them with what is

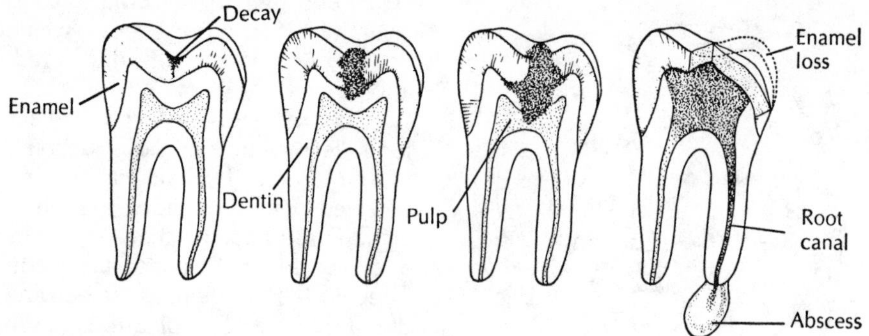

Tooth decay, if untreated, can progress from the surface enamel to the dentin to the pulp and finally through the root canal to form an abscess (pus-filled cavity).

known as a gold crown. On teeth toward the front, the gold crown is overlaid with porcelain to provide a natural appearance.

To prevent decay, teeth should be cleaned daily with a soft-bristled brush, preferably after each meal, to remove food particles and plaque. Equally important is the use of dental floss to remove debris between the teeth. Avoiding sweet, sticky foods, or at least rinsing or brushing shortly after eating them, may also help prevent decay. A child's teeth will be more resistant to decay if the child drinks water containing the proper amount of fluoride in the first 12 years while the teeth are developing. If the water supply is not fluoridated, a vitamin supplement containing fluoride can be taken daily. Adults and children alike can benefit by using a fluoride-containing toothpaste or mouthwash.

See also Fluorides and Periodontal disease.

Toxemia of pregnancy

Toxemia of pregnancy is a severe condition which sometimes occurs in the latter stages of pregnancy and is characterized by high blood pressure; swelling of the feet, hands, and other extremities; and an excessive amount of protein in the urine. If allowed to worsen, convulsions and coma may set in. Toxemia of pregnancy is actually a misnomer from the days when it was thought that the condition was caused by toxic (poisonous) substances in the blood. The illness is more accurately called preeclampsia before the convulsive stage and eclampsia afterward.

The causes of toxemia in pregnancy are not clearly understood. It tends to develop more often among mothers from lower socioeconomic status. One theory is that dietary deficiencies may be at the roots of some cases. Also, there is the possibility that some types of toxemia are the result of uterine ischemia (deficiency of blood flow in the uterus, or womb).

Toxemia is divided into three stages, each progressively more serious and leading, ultimately, to eclampsia if not treated.

- *Mild preeclampsia symptoms:* swelling, high blood pressure, and protein in the urine;
- *Severe preeclampsia symptoms:* headache, dizziness, fever, drowsiness, tachycardia (interruption of natural heart rhythm), *tinnitus* (noise in the ears), double vision, nausea, vomiting, and abnormal urine production;

- *Eclampsia:* convulsions, coma, death.

Toxemia in pregnancy cannot be completely cured until the pregnancy is over. Until that time, treatment includes stimulation of kidney functions, control of high blood pressure, control of convulsions, and, in severe cases, early delivery of the infant to insure the survival of the mother.

There is no known preventive for toxemia of pregnancy. The first line of defense is the monitoring of all bodily functions in order to spot any preeclampsia symptoms as they first begin to appear.

Toxic shock syndrome

Toxic shock syndrome (TSS) is a rare, sometimes fatal disease that develops very suddenly and progresses rapidly when the *Staphylococcus aureus* bacterium enters the bloodstream. TSS was first defined in 1975, when its link to the use of tampons was suspected. Since then, almost 90 percent of all reported cases have occurred in menstruating women under the age of 30 who use tampons. About three in 100,000 menstruating women have contracted toxic shock syndrome. Five to 15 percent of these cases have been fatal.

Toxic shock syndrome occurs when the bacterium enters the bloodstream and produces a toxin (poison) that causes leaks in cell walls allowing blood to seep into the tissues. This results in a sudden, very dangerous drop in blood pressure, shock (collapse of circulation), and sometimes death.

In serious cases, the low blood pressure and the weakened cell walls (which allow foreign bodies to enter) can leave the victim susceptible to further complications, such as heart and liver damage. Often the body does not produce enough antibodies (protective substances) to fight off this invasion, so TSS can easily reoccur.

This disorder is caused by a toxin which is produced by a bacterium, but the identity of this toxin and why it is produced in certain cases remain a mystery. Moreover, the bacterium can be present in the body without producing the toxin.

The exact link between toxic shock syndrome and the use of tampons also remains somewhat vague. Although their use is considered to be a definite risk factor, tampons do not actually cause the disease, but they may promote the growth of bacteria that leads to it.

Researchers now theorize that the new "superabsorbent" tampons as well as tampon applicators may be responsible for triggering TSS. The superabsorbent tampons may swell so much that they entirely fill the vagina, totally blocking the elimination of blood and creating a breeding ground for infection; also, these tampons tend to be left in the vagina hours longer than the less absorbent varieties, again increasing the chances for infection. Tampon applicators, moreover, may accidentally scratch the walls of the vagina, allowing bacteria to enter.

However, since 10 percent of all cases occur in men and nonmenstruating women, the bacteria can apparently enter the body in ways other than through the vagina. Toxic shock in these cases often occurs when the body has been weakened by major surgery, severe burns, or cases of boils or abscesses. Also, women who have recently given birth are at a higher risk of developing TSS because the vagina (or birth canal) is more susceptible to the invasion of bacteria at this time.

The symptoms of toxic shock syndrome are high fever, vomiting, diarrhea, a rash that looks like sunburn, peeling of skin on the soles and palms, blurred vision, and disorientation.

Immediate emergency medical treatment should be sought by anyone noticing the symptoms of TSS. This will almost certainly mean hospitalization, during which the patient will be given therapy similar to that administered to poison victims. Fluids or whole blood transfusions are given to raise blood pressure, an ice blanket is used to reduce fever, and antibiotics are administered to fight the infection.

The best precaution that can be taken to prevent toxic shock syndrome is probably to discontinue or limit the use of tampons, especially the superabsorbent variety. Tampons can still be safely worn, but they should be changed every three to four hours and alternated with sanitary napkins as often as possible, especially before going to bed, as they tend to remain inserted for much longer periods of time during sleep.

Transient ischemic attacks (TIA)

Transient ischemic attacks (TIA) are sudden, neurologic deficits (such as loss of vision in one eye, inability to speak, paralysis, or weakness of one side of the body) that last for less than 24 hours. Although they are similar in appearance to minor strokes, they do no discernible lasting damage to the brain's functions.

TIAs are probably due to an interruption in blood flow to an area of the brain. They can be caused by a narrowing in the carotid arteries (the arteries in the neck that supply the brain with oxygenated blood). This narrowing is usually due to the presence of atherosclerosis. Blood vessel spasms and showers of tiny emboli (clots that travel to the brain) are also possible causes of TIAs.

The symptoms of transient ischemic attacks are both varied and frightening to the victim. They can include weakness of the side of the face; numbness in various parts of the body; blindness in one eye; weakness in the arms or legs on one side; difficulty in speaking and/or understanding speech; and prickling or "pins and needles" sensation in parts of the body. Vertigo (sensation of spinning) combined with any of these symptoms and others can also be due to TIAs. Fainting spells alone and dizziness (light-headedness) are usually not due to TIAs.

The major importance of transient ischemic attacks is their use in the diagnosis of stroke. Any such attack may be a predictor of stroke. Often, when a person describes a "light stroke," he or she is really talking about a transient ischemic attack. If left unattended, TIAs can indeed lead to major strokes, with permanent damage to all parts affected, as well as to the possibility of sudden death.

The first line of attack in diagnosis is a complete examination, including history and physical, neurological, and eye exam. "Bruits," noises caused by narrowing in an artery, are heard in the carotid artery(ies). Detailed testing, commonly with arteriography (injection of X-ray contrast into the artery with subsequent X-ray pictures taken), is performed to determine the problem.

Treatment of TIAs is basically aimed at preventing stroke. There are two basic methods of treatment: medical with anticoagulant drugs, and surgical with the opening and "cleaning out" of the carotid(s).

Which one of these methods is more effective in preventing further TIAs and /or stroke is dependent on many factors and is presently a subject of considerable controversy. TIAs can be an indication of serious problems and, if experienced, must be brought to the attention of a physician immediately.

See also Atherosclerosis and Stroke.

Trichinosis

Trichinosis is a condition caused by the parasitic infestation of the body by the *Trichinella spiralis,* a worm commonly found in pork.

Trichinosis is most commonly caused by eating pork that has not been cooked for a sufficient length of time or at a sufficiently high temperature to kill the *Trichinella spiralis* worms. The worms are encapsulated in the meat itself. When the meat is eaten the worms emerge from it and begin their life cycle in the human host. This begins in the small intestine, where the worms' larvae mature within two days after they emerge from the meat. The adults breed, the males die, and the females give birth to other larvae that invade the tissues of the bowel and are then dispersed to the body's muscles where they lodge.

The muscles around the eyes, the tongue, the diaphragm (the muscle separating the chest cavity from the abdomen), and the muscles between the ribs are the most common sites of larvae attachments. Quite often, the infested patient is entirely unaware of the presence of trichinosis. When large infestations do occur, however, they are accompanied by symptoms. Soon (one to two days) after consumption of the contaminated meat, a severe flu-like illness consisting of fever, nausea, vomiting, diarrhea, and abdominal pain occurs. After about a week, severe symptoms such as rash, swelling of the eyelids, and neurologic disorders may develop. Myocarditis (inflammation of the heart muscle) can also be seen in this stage. Eventually the larvae in the muscles die and become calcified; tenderness and swelling around the muscle tissue are quite common.

Since there is no way to get the larvae out of the muscle tissue, treatment is aimed at relief of discomfort. Analgesics, such as aspirin, are administered for pain, and anti-inflammatory steroids (cortisone drugs such as prednisone) are administered for allergic symptoms, myocarditis, and/or central nervous system involvement. Thiabendazole (which tends to kill worms, such as the trichinella) is often given with good results. A close watch is kept for drug fever, abdominal pain, vomiting, and dermatitis (inflammation and/or rash of the skin).

The only real preventatives are keeping the hogs from becoming infected by thoroughly cooking their food and making sure that pork is sufficiently cooked to kill the larvae (30 minutes for each pound of meat, to an internal temperature of at least 185°F).

Tuberculosis

Tuberculosis is an infection that causes small nodules called tubercles to break down healthy tissue and form pus. Tuberculosis usually affects the lungs, but it can travel to other parts of the body, such as the spine, kidneys, digestive tract, and lining of the heart. It also may be complicated by a streptococcal (a type of bacteria) infection.

Eighty percent of all people who

contract tuberculosis will never experience its symptoms. This happens because the tuberculosis bacteria usually lie dormant in the body, never developing into an active disease; instead, the body surrounds the offending bacteria with closed sacs, or cysts. This acts to contain the bacteria and prevent the spread of infection; however, the body cannot kill the bacteria, but only contain them.

Of the remaining 20 percent who do develop an active case of tuberculosis, only half of them will become sick within three months of contracting the infection, and the other half will suffer from the disease some time in their lives, perhaps years later. The bacteria often lie inactive until some other disease weakens the body's defenses.

Tuberculosis is contracted when a person breathes in droplets containing bacteria, called *Mycobacterium tuberculosis,* that have been coughed or sneezed into the air by an infected person. Tuberculosis can be contagious, especially for people living in crowded conditions. Also highly susceptible to this disease are those who are undernourished, in poor health, living in poor urban areas, as well as the very young and very old, and people in the medical professions. Anyone who has been in close contact with a tuberculosis patient should be tested for the disease.

The symptoms of tuberculosis are similar to those of many other diseases, and its true symptoms do not appear until the disease is in its advanced stages. For these reasons, coupled with the fact that the incidence of tuberculosis has been declining in recent years in the United States, this disorder often remains untreated or misdiagnosed for some time before the patient is finally tested for it.

Early signs include fever, particularly in the afternoon, as well as fatigue, loss of appetite, and weight loss. Its later signs include coughing up of a blood-tinged discharge called sputum, chest pain, and shortness of breath.

Patients can be tested for tuberculosis with a tuberculin skin test. If the bacteria are present, whether active or inactive, the patch of skin that has been treated with dead tuberculosis bacteria will swell. Chest X rays or an analysis of the patient's sputum may also help to pinpoint the infection.

Tuberculosis is treated with a variety of antibacterial drugs simultaneously so that the body will not become immune to one particular medication. The drugs are usually prescribed for a long period of time, perhaps nine to 18 months, but after two weeks the patient is no longer contagious and can resume normal activities. With this type of treatment, the disease is rarely fatal any longer, and the biggest problem with such drug programs is that the patient discontinues the medication too soon. Also, severe side effects, such as liver or hearing damage, can result from some antituberculosis drugs.

An active case of tuberculosis can be prevented in some persons who are considered to be high risks by the administration of certain antituberculosis drugs, but these are likely to have undesirable side effects. (High risk cases include persons under the age of 35, especially children, who have been exposed to the disease, as well as those with chronic diseases that may weaken their respiratory systems enough to make them more likely candidates for the disease.) Liver damage from the drugs is more likely to occur in those over the age of 35, so people in this age group seldom receive these drugs.

Regardless of age or physical condition, anyone who has been in close contact with a person with active tuberculosis should be tested for the disease.

U

Ulcer

An ulcer is an open sore or erosion on the surface of an organ or tissue. The most common ulcers erupt in the digestive tract, in which case they are known as peptic ulcers. Peptic ulcers can appear in the lining of the esophagus (tube leading to the stomach), stomach, or duodenum (beginning of the small intestine).

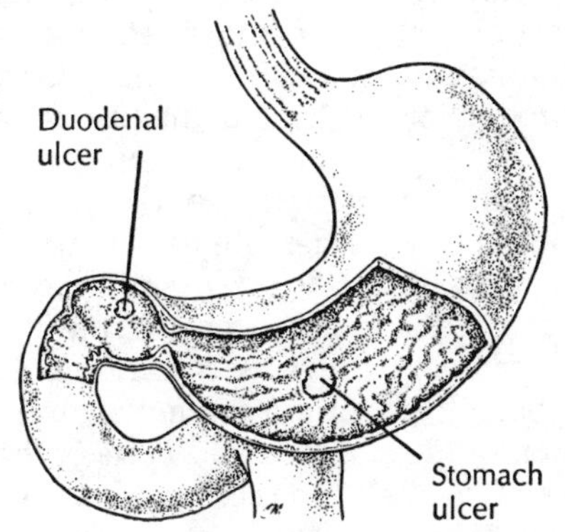

The most common ulcers are those that affect the stomach or the duodenum, the beginning section of the small intestine.

Although the cause of a peptic ulcer is unconfirmed, scientists believe that the more common duodenal ulcers may result from excessive amounts of digestive juices produced by the stomach. The stomach may increase acidic secretions after coffee, alcohol, aspirin, and other painkillers are consumed, or after cigarettes are smoked. Therefore, these substances are thought to contribute to ulcers.

The less common stomach ulcers may be due to an inherent weakness in the wall of the stomach. However, this weakness may result from the same environmental conditions that aggravate duodenal ulcers.

Emotional stress may play a role in ulcer development. However, physicians distinguish between stress as a factor by itself and the way certain people deal with stress that would make them susceptible to ulcers.

Heredity plays an important role in contributing to ulcers since people who have a history of ulcers in their family seem to have a greater likelihood of acquiring the condition. Furthermore, for unknown reasons, people with type O blood are more likely to develop ulcers. In addition, liver disease, rheumatoid arthritis (inflammation of connective tissue), and emphysema (overinflation of the lungs' air sacs) may increase vulnerability to ulcers.

Ulcers can produce mild symptoms resembling heartburn or indigestion, or severe pain radiating throughout the upper portion of the body. The most common discomfort of ulcers is a burning in the abdomen above the navel that may feel like hunger pangs. Pain comes about 30 to 120 minutes after eating or in the middle of the night when the stomach is empty. At this time, the stomach's acidic juices are more apt to irritate the unprotected nerve endings in the exposed ulcer. Usually, pain subsides after eating or drinking something or taking an antacid to neutralize stomach acid.

Some people experience nausea, vomiting and constipation. Blood in feces (discoloring it black), blood in vomit, extreme weakness, fainting, and excessive thirst are all signs of internal bleeding, and may appear with more advanced ulcers.

While ulcers are not life-threatening, they can cause serious damage if left untreated. Ulcers may corrode nearby blood vessels and cause internal seepage of blood or massive internal bleeding (hemorrhage). A perforated ulcer may penetrate an adjoining organ, causing infection. In addition, scar tissue growing around the ulcer may lead to an intestinal obstruction.

Physicians diagnose peptic ulcers primarily by X ray. The patient swallows barium, a chalky substance, and stands in front of a fluorescent screen. As the X-ray tube moves down from the shoulder, the barium shows an opaque outline of the digestive tract that allows the doctor a view of any abnormalities.

When an X ray is inconclusive, the doctor inserts a gastroscope (long, flexible lighted tube) through the mouth and down the esophagus to see the ulcer. Stomach ulcers require a gastroscopic examination and a biopsy (removal of tissue sample for analysis) to confirm that the ulcer is not actually a cancer showing up as an ulcer on the X ray.

Treatment for ulcers involves relieving the irritation so healing progresses naturally. Over-the-counter antacids counteract stomach acid and relieve symptoms; but they can cause complications. For example, sodium bicarbonate, a primary antacid ingredient, contains large amounts of sodium (salt) that can aggravate kidney disease or high blood pressure.

For more problematic ulcers, a physician may prescribe other preparations to promote healing. Anticholinergic drugs delay emptying of the stomach and keep the lining cushioned against acidity. Antispasmodic drugs relax digestive tract muscles and relieve tension if stress is a contributing factor to a particular ulcer case. Various new medications either form a protective coating against the acid in the stomach (sucralfate) or inhibit gastric acid secretion (cimetidine and ranitidine). With any drug, caution is suggested as side effects can outweigh their benefits.

Although recent studies have shown that a bland diet is unnecessary for ulcer management, a mild diet may be recommended until acute symptoms disappear. Thereafter, many doctors suggest avoiding only those foods known to cause stomach distress.

The effects of milk on ulcers is also questionable. Its neutralizing action on stomach acid is mild and temporary at best. Nevertheless, people who substitute milk for proven irritants, such as alcohol or caffeine, are less likely to stimulate their ulcers.

Most ulcers heal within two to six weeks after treatment begins. To prevent recurrence patients should still refrain from cigarettes, caffeine, alcohol, or other known stimulants that would stimulate stomach acid production or irritate the digestive tract lining.

When drug therapy and diet cannot cure an ulcer, surgical removal may be necessary. Surgery follows repeated ulcers or ulcers that are life-threatening, such as a perforation. Sometimes, surgeons remove a portion of the stomach and parts of the vagus nerve (which controls digestive secretions) to reduce stomach acid production. Usually, ulcers do not reappear after surgery.

Ulcerative colitis

Ulcerative colitis is a chronic, inflammatory disease of the colon (the latter section of the large intestine), characterized by bloody diarrhea. The lining of the colon becomes ulcerated—exhibiting open erosions.

Although there is a familial tendency to develop ulcerative colitis, the cause of the disorder is unknown. Any age group may be affected, but it tends to begin in persons between the ages of 15 and 40.

Among possible contributing fac-

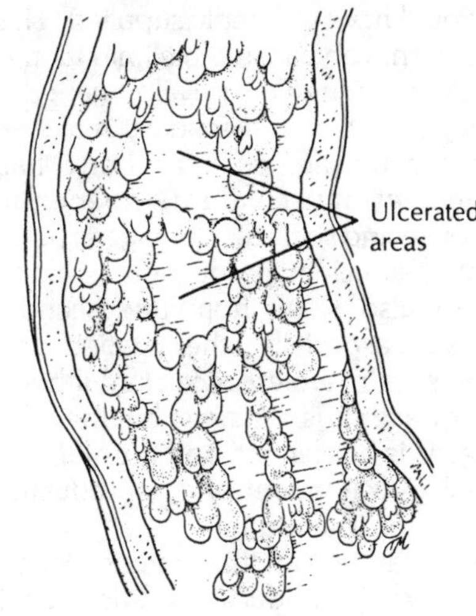

Ulcerative colitis is a chronic, inflammatory disease characterized by bloody diarrhea and ulcerated areas in the lining of the colon.

tors are infection, immunological derangement (some breakdown in the patient's protective system), lack of protective elements in the bowel wall, either nervous or psychological disturbances, and alterations in the nature of the connective tissue in the colon. However, the best clue as to cause is the strikingly higher proportions of the disease in certain families.

The first sign of ulcerative colitis is usually a series of attacks of bloody diarrhea. The attacks can vary in intensity and duration, and are usually interspersed with normal periods. The onset of the attacks may be severe, with sudden violent diarrhea, high fever, symptoms of abdominal inflammation, and bacterial invasions. Often, an attack will be preceded by mild lower abdominal cramps and the appearance of small amounts of blood or mucus in the feces.

If ulceration is confined to the rectum and terminal portion of the colon, the bowel movements may be normal or very hard and dry, with discharges of mucus full of red and white blood cells between stools. If the disorder extends to other portions of the colon, however, stools become looser and more frequent (perhaps 10 to 20 per day), and the patient suffers severe cramps, watery stools, fever, anemia (iron-deficient blood), and loss of appetite.

If the condition persists in this severe form, hemorrhage (internal bleeding) is the most common complication. In toxic colitis, a serious complication, the colon loses muscular tone and dilates almost completely, resulting in perforations of the organ. The risk of colon cancer and cancer of the bile ducts is also increased in patients with ulcerative colitis.

Ulcerative colitis is diagnosed through medical history, a stool examination, and sigmoidoscopy (in which a lighted, flexible tube is inserted into the colon for a visual examination of the interior). X ray studies with a barium enema are indicated except in cases where risk of perforation makes the barium enema procedure an active danger for the patient.

Mild cases of ulcerative colitis can be managed by adequate physical and mental relaxation, since the disease appears to be stress-related in some patients; a normal diet low in high-fiber fruits and vegetables and possibly milk; and anti-diarrheal medication. More severe cases may respond to a drug known as sulfasalazine. In cases that do not respond to sulfasalazine therapy, hydrocortisone (artificial hormones) may be given by enema injection once or twice a day.

Unconsciousness

See Emergency first aid section at the end of this book.

Undescended testes

Undescended testes is a condition in which one or both of the testes (male gonadal or sex glands) do not descend into the scrotum (a small sac located between the legs), but remain in the abdomen, where they have developed before birth. This condition is also called cryptorchidism or cryptorchism and is not uncommon.

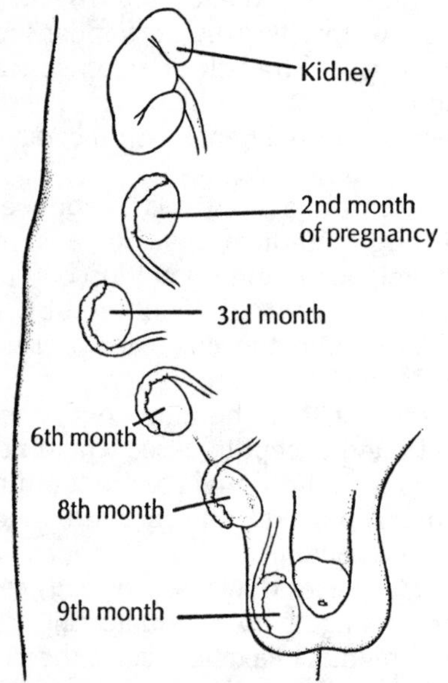

The male sex glands, the testes, develop in the abdomen and gradually descend downward into the scrotum before birth. Occasionally this progression does not occur, and the child is born with undescended testes.

The causes of this condition are not clearly understood. It is conjectured that perhaps a membrane in the abdomen gets in the way. If only one testis is undescended, the problem is most likely mechanical; if both are involved, the underlying cause may well be hormonal.

If the testes do not descend, they often degenerate or atrophy (shrink), and thus do not secrete into the system the male sex hormones that they would have ordinarily supplied. This, in turn, can cause the elimination or suppression of the development during puberty of secondary male sex characteristics such as body hair, heavier musculature, deepening voice, and so forth. Damaged sperm, or insufficient production of them, can also result from undescended testes, especially if the situation is still present in adolescence or adulthood. If one testis is damaged but the other testis is descended and normal, sexual development and reproduction function are normal.

Treatment for this condition is controversial. In deciding upon treatment, three important considerations must be kept in mind: the potential fertility of the testes, even if they do not descend; the probability (or lack of probability) that they will descend without intervention; and the chances of the undescended testes becoming malignant (cancerous). Hormone therapy is sometimes effective, but in many cases where it is successfully applied, it is thought by some doctors that the testes would probably have descended by themselves anyway. Surgery to bring the testes into the scrotum is usually a successful treatment if done before the age of five years. Sometimes, the testes can be made to descend by manipulation of the tissues around them.

There is no known preventive for undescended testes.

Urinary system

The urinary system are those organs of the body that produce and eliminate urine, a combination of water and waste products passing out of the body as fluid. By controlling urine flow, the system maintains proper water balance throughout the body. Individual parts of the urinary system monitor concentration of salts and other nutrients necessary for good physical health.

The organs responsible for control of nutrients in the blood are the two kidneys. Kidneys are the bean-shaped structures located in the back of the abdomen. Their chief functions are to filter waste from the blood and insure reabsorption of essential nutrients back into the bloodstream. In the kidney, waste products combine with water to form urine.

Urine passes from each kidney into the bladder through tubes called ureters. The bladder stores the urine prior to elimination from the body. A muscle around the exit from the bladder prevents urine from escaping. When the bladder is about half full, the body feels an urge to empty the organ. At this time, the muscle relaxes to release the urine through the urethra.

The urethra is a tube that conveys urine from the bladder to the exterior of the body. The female urethra is about an inch and a half long and is enclosed within the body. The male urethra passes through the penis and is approximately nine inches long. For the male, the urethra serves the dual function of transporting urine and semen (fluid from male reproductive organs). Semen is ejaculated during sexual intercourse, an occurrence during which urine is automatically blocked from leaving the bladder.

Changes in urine and urinary habits that do not seem to have an obvious cause, such as drinking more liquids than usual, may be symptoms of disease.

Some symptoms requiring medical attention—if they last for more than a day or two—are changes in frequency, timing, control, quantity, and color, as well as accompanying pain.

A doctor should be contacted immediately if there is extreme pain while urinating; blood in the urine; a noticeable decrease in frequency (a symptom of kidney failure); or strong color changes or cloudiness, often accompanied by pain or fever.

Changes in urine or urinary habits may be caused by a variety of dis-

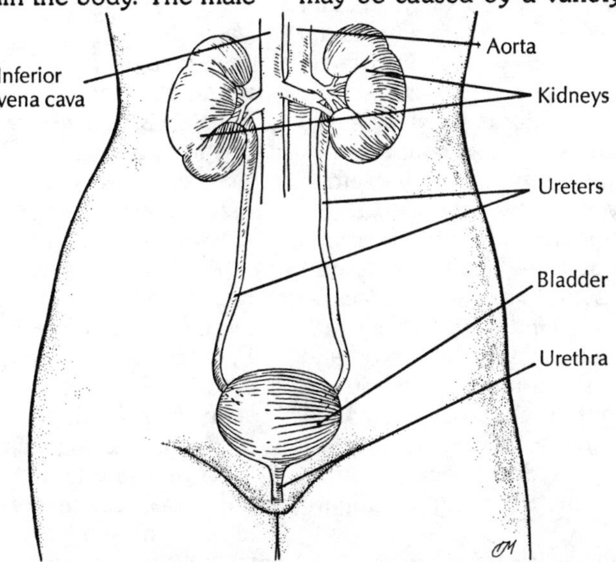

This drawing shows the urinary system of a female. The blood is filtered through the kidneys, and the waste products, plus excess body water, are sent as urine through the system for excretion.

orders involving the kidneys, urinary tract, bladder, and prostate (a doughnut-shaped gland surrounding the male urethra), among others. The exact cause of a urinary problem is often related to the type of symptom displayed.

Increased frequency may be caused by inflammation of the kidneys, bladder, or urethra; diabetes (an imbalance in blood sugar level); or an enlarged prostate.

A change in timing of urination, usually in the form of very frequent nighttime awakenings accompanied by the urge to urinate (called nocturia) is often coupled with painful urination, a poor stream, or difficulty in starting. These may be symptoms of an inflammatory or infectious disease within the urinary tract, as well as tumors or other disorders that result in increased pressure on the bladder.

Difficulty in controlling, starting, and maintaining the flow may also be symptoms of an inflammation of the prostate gland. Inability to hold back urine is a common problem of elderly people as their control of the bladder muscle weakens. Also affected by this problem are women in the late stages of pregnancy. In this case, the weight of the uterus presses heavily on the bladder without letup.

Changes in the quantity of urine normally produced can also signal disease. Producing an excessive amount of urine (called polyuria) may be a symptom of kidney disease, diabetes, or glandular disorders.

Slight changes in the color and clarity of the urine day to day are normal, but strong color changes and extreme cloudiness may signal infection, tumors, kidney stones, prostate problems, or cysts along the urinary tract.

Pain while urinating, most commonly in the form of a burning sensation felt along the urethra, may be a sign of a lower urinary tract infection. Excruciating pain across the abdomen or the back may signal the presence of kidney stones.

Treatment of urinary problems usually involves treating the underlying cause of the sudden change, which can range from mild infections to very serious diseases. An accurate diagnosis by a physician is the first step to proper treatment of these disorders.

See also Cystitis and Prostatitis.

Urinary tract infection

See Cystitis.

V

Vaginitis

Vaginitis is any one of a number of bacterial or fungal infections and inflammations of the vagina (the female passageway from the uterus to the outside of the body), usually marked by burning and itching of the external genital organs. A discharge may or may not be present.

An untreated infection can become chronic (recurring) or can lead to a urinary tract infection. Pregnant women, as well as those who have diabetes or gonorrhea (a sexually transmitted disease) are at a higher risk for vaginitis.

Vaginal infections can be transmitted to male sexual partners, but usually with no serious results. However, vaginitis is not considered a sexually transmitted disease, since it is not contracted or transmitted only by direct sexual contact.

Vaginitis is caused by an imbalance of the microorganisms normally present in the vagina, resulting when some outside factor causes one of the strains to reproduce more quickly than the others. Possible causes include birth control pills, which, because of their high estrogen (a female hormone) content, cause the vaginal lining to change in such a way that it is more likely to nourish microorganisms that cause infection; certain antibiotics, which may kill bacteria that normally help to maintain the microorganism balance in the vagina; a warm, moist, environment, often caused by tight pants or pantyhose, nylon underwear, or a wet bathing suit, which creates a breeding ground for infection; and the chemical irritation arising from the excessive use of douches, feminine hygiene sprays, bubble baths, talcum powder, and scented or colored toilet paper.

Vaginitis tends to occur more often in the summer, because of the fact that excessive heat and moisture are known to trigger the infection.

One variety of the disease, called nonspecific, noninfectious vaginitis, is not caused by this overproduction of microorganisms, but rather by an irritation from some outside source. However, vaginitis is most commonly caused by one of three microorganisms: *Candida albicans,* or monilia (a fungus); *Hemophilus vaginalis* (a bacterium); or *Trichomonas vaginalis* (a protozoan, or one-celled organism). Each type displays a slightly different set of symptoms and requires a specific method of treatment.

The fungus *Candida albicans,* or monilia, results in severe itching of the external genital organs and pain during intercourse. A thick, white discharge from the vagina, resembling cottage cheese in texture and having a "yeasty" odor, is the reason why this condition is more commonly known as a yeast infection. This is the most frequently contracted variety of vaginitis by diabetic and pregnant women.

The bacterium *Hemophilus vaginalis* causes a creamy white or

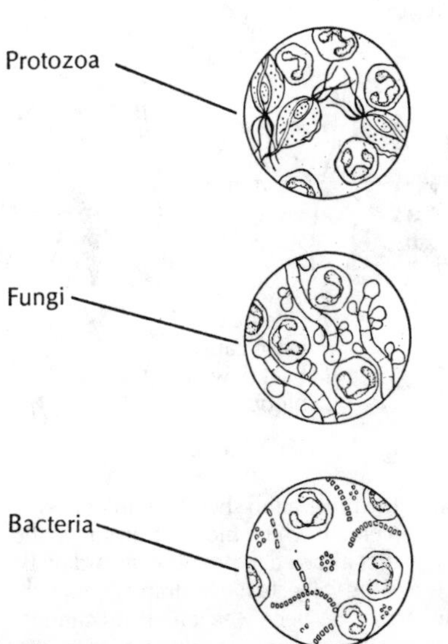

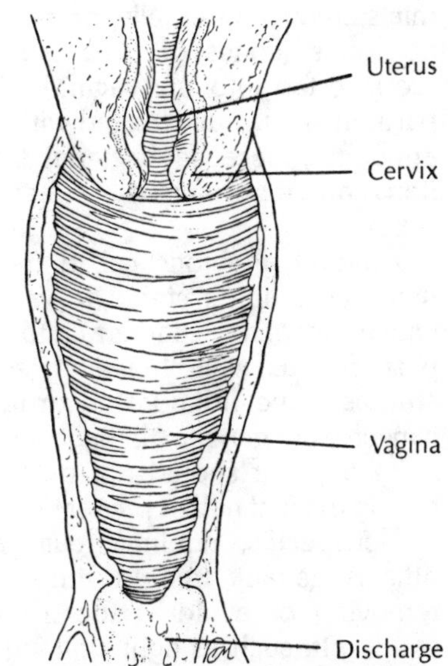

Vaginitis is an infection or often inflammation of the vagina, characterized by a discharge from the vagina. It is commonly caused by a protozoan, a fungus, or a bacterium, each of which is shown here as it would appear under a microscope.

grayish, foul-smelling discharge. The presence of the protozoan *Trichomonas vaginalis,* also marked by itching and burning as well as a greenish-white discharge and foul odor, is more likely to appear during or immediately following menstruation.

Noninfectious, nonspecific vaginitis is characterized only by irritation and dryness, usually with no discharge.

Men can be infected by the bacterium or protozoan varieties during sexual contact, but they usually display no symptoms.

Vaginitis is diagnosed by determining which of the three microorganisms is causing the infection by examining a smear of vaginal discharge under a microscope.

Treatment will vary somewhat according to the type of microorganism that has been causing the problem. Those infections caused by a fungus are treated with antifungal cream which is applied directly to the vagina.

Bacterial infections are treated with sulfa drugs or antibiotics, administered either orally or as suppositories (cones of medicine that are inserted into the vagina). Both partners are usually treated with oral antibiotics because bacterial infections can be transferred between the sexes.

An oral antibiotic called metronidazole is administered to women with protozoan infections and to their partners, as well; however, some studies have linked this drug to cancer and genetic damage in lab animals, so it should not be taken during the first half of pregnancy.

Nonspecific, noninfectious vaginitis is usually treated simply by removing or avoiding the irritants causing it, such as tight clothing, or perfumed soaps, chemical sprays, or scented tissues.

Some types of vaginitis can probably be prevented by using only nonscented, white toilet paper; wearing cotton underwear and loose-fitting pants; and avoiding the overuse of douches, feminine hygiene sprays, and scented toiletries.

Varicose veins

Varicose veins are swollen, stretched veins in the legs, close to the surface of the skin, caused by pooling of blood.

Blood from the legs needs to return uphill, against the force of gravity, to the heart, so the veins in the leg

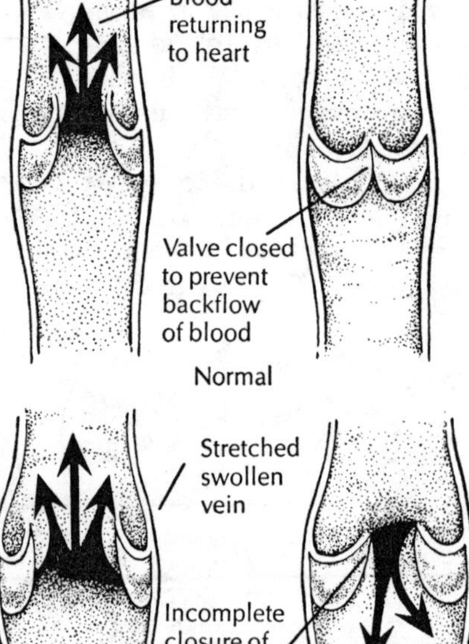

At top, the illustration shows the interior of a normal vein, in which blood returning to the heart is not allowed to drop downward by the action of the valve. In the bottom drawing, the vein's valve has been weakened and cannot completely close, thus resulting in an accumulation of excess blood in the vein. The result is a varicose vein.

are lined with one-way valves to prevent blood from flowing back down toward the feet. When pressure on the veins stretches them, the valves cannot close properly, and some blood travels back down. This blood accumulates in pools, which stretch the veins even more. The result is varicose veins, highly visible bluish lines that bulge from the legs and that can be very painful.

Varicose veins alone are not too serious, but they may lead to other conditions: a leg ulcer (an eroded patch on the skin); phlebitis (an inflamed vein); or a blood clot (a thrombus).

Varicose veins are caused by a number of factors that put excess pressure on the veins in the legs: prolonged standing; prolonged sitting, especially with the legs crossed; lack of exercise; confining clothes; a diet low in fiber (hard stools and the pressure needed to excrete them put extra stress on the veins); obesity (which puts excess pressure on the legs and contributes to the muscles' inability to push blood upward); heredity (a tendency toward weak vein walls and valves seems to be inherited); and even height (tall people may be more likely to develop this conditon because their blood needs to travel farther in its return trip to the heart).

Pregnancy greatly contributes to the development of varicose veins because female hormones, especially those released at this time, tend to relax the walls of the veins. Thus, the condition is more commonly seen in women than in men. Varicose veins often appear during the last few months of pregnancy due to the increased strain from the weight of the growing uterus. These veins may recede, however, after the baby is born.

Varicose veins are very noticeable since they form close to the skin.

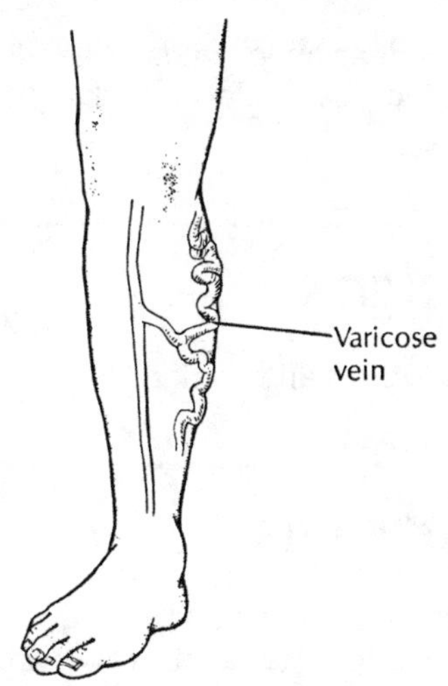

Because varicose veins are close to the surface, they are very visible.

They appear as bulging, bluish, cordlike lines running down the legs. Symptoms that accompany varicose veins are feelings of achiness, heaviness, and fatigue in the legs, especially at the end of the day; itchy, scaly skin covering the affected areas; and, in advanced cases, swollen ankles, pain shooting down the leg, and leg cramps at night.

Varicose veins are usually treated by wearing elastic stockings, which act like muscles to help push the blood upward. Severe cases may require a surgical procedure called vein stripping, in which the afflicted veins are tied off and removed; other healthy veins in the area will take over the job of pushing blood toward the heart. A chemical can also be injected into the veins, closing them off and forcing the blood to find other channels to the heart. However, this procedure can cause more complications, so it is not performed as often as surgery.

Those with varicose veins may need to lose weight, increase the fiber in their diets, exercise regularly, and stretch their legs or put their feet up whenever possible. Exercises that improve the circulation in the legs, such as deep knee bends or standing on tiptoe, may help to relieve pressure.

Vertigo

See Dizziness and vertigo.

Vital signs

Vital signs is a term used in diagnostic medicine to include four observable phenomena in patients: temperature, pulse, respiration rate, and blood pressure. These four items are all important indicators of disease and are easily obtainable information for the physician. Separately or together, they offer important clues to the patient's physical condition and may point toward other tests or diagnostic procedures that need to be performed.

Temperature is a useful index to a patient's condition, since a fever, or an abnormal rise in body temperature, is usually a significant indicator of disease. Fever is generally a sign of infection, but it can be present whenever there is tissue destruction —from a severe sunburn, for example, or when large amounts of tissue deteriorate for lack of blood supply.

The *pulse rate* is another easily obtainable and important piece of information about a patient's condition. The heart rate varies with a person's level of physical activity. For example, it beats faster during exercise and more slowly during rest. An inappropriate heart rate, or pulse, may indicate disease. A feverish patient will show an increased heart rate, while a weak but rapid pulse is characteristic of severe blood loss or diseases of the heart itself. Irregular pulse (arrhythmia) also suggests conditions ranging from malfunction of the heart to stress, anxiety, or over-consumption of caffeine.

Respiratory rate, or rate of breathing, is a vital sign that changes with disease. Patients with fever show an increased respiratory rate (hyperventilation) which lowers body temperature. Hyperventilation is also a common response to pain or stress. Also, any condition which leads to acidosis, or higher acid levels in the body than basic levels, similarly drives the respiratory rate upward. Diseases of the lungs, with simultaneous inability to oxygenate the blood, also increase respiratory rate.

The fourth vital sign, *blood pressure*, is equally significant. It indicates to the physician the amount of blood in circulation. A decrease in circulating blood volume, as is true in cases of severe bleeding, lowers blood pressure and deprives the body tissues of adequate blood flow. Reflexes then are initiated that compensate in part for the reduced blood volume and pressure. For example, the heart rate increases and compensates partially for the sudden reduction in blood volume. Also, peripheral blood vessels in areas such as the abdomen constrict, thus diverting the remaining blood to vital areas such as the brain. And finally, unusual elevation of blood pressure constitutes a disorder in its own right: *hypertension*.

While the observation of the vital signs does not always provide a clear diagnosis of a patient's condition, these four items taken together do serve as important indicators of the presence of disease or injury. They are often the first step in a sophisticated, comprehensive program of testing and observation that will lead to a precise diagnosis of the patient's condition.

Vitamins

A vitamin is any of a large group of unrelated organic substances often identified as "enzyme components," which are found in many foods in small amounts and are necessary for normal body functioning. Many vitamins help to regulate the rate at which chemical reactions take place in the body.

The main vitamins necessary for human beings are discussed here.

Vitamin A. Vitamin A is found in fish liver oils, liver, butter, egg yolks, cheese, and yellow vegetables and fruits. Deficiency of this vitamin in the diet causes inadequate production of rhodopsin, or "visual purple," a substance important in the retina's functioning, resulting in night blindness. Vitamin A deficiency can also result in epithelial (surface) tissue disorders and generally lessened resistance to infection.

Vitamin B. The name Vitamin B may refer to any member of the Vitamin B complex, including thiamine, riboflavin, niacin, niacinamide, the B_6 group, biotin, pantothenic acid, folic acid, para-aminobenzoic acid, inositol, cyanocobalamin (or Vitamin B_{12}) and choline.

Vitamin B_1, or *thiamine,* is found in whole wheat, enriched flour, meat, and fish. A deficiency can result in beriberi, a disease characterized by abnormal heart functions, swelling, and inflammation of the nerves.

Vitamin B_2, *riboflavin,* is found in milk, organ meats (liver, kidneys, brains), eggs, malt, and various algae. It acts as a catalyst in bodily processes that involve oxidation (the body's use of oxygen). Dietary deficiencies may result in stomatitis (inflammation of the mucous tissue in the mouth), cheilitis (inflammation of the lips), eye-related malfunctions, and dermatitis (skin inflammation).

Vitamin B_6 is a group of substances (including pyridoxine, pyridoxal and pyridoxamine) widely distributed in animal and plant tissues. These substances are involved in amino acid (a building block of protein) metabolism and in the breakdown of glycogen (a stored sugar). Vitamin B_6 appears in wheat, bran, yeast, seeds, and corn. A deficiency can result in functional disturbances of the nervous system.

Vitamin B_{12}, *cyanocobalamin,* affects the formation of red blood cells and is found in all animal products, especially liver, fish meal, and eggs. When Vitamin B_{12} is absent from the diet or is not absorbed by the body, anemia (red cell deficiency in the blood) may result.

Vitamin C. Vitamin C, or *ascorbic acid,* is found in many vegetables and fruits, especially such green vegetables as green peppers and most citrus fruits. It is an essential element in the human diet. A deficiency may result in a disease called scurvy, in which the victim suffers anemia, spongy gums, bleeding, and hardening of the leg muscles. An overdose of Vitamin C is potentially dangerous and may result in diarrhea, kidney stones, decreased fertility for both men and women, spontaneous abortion in women, liver damage, bone fractures, drug interactions, a B_{12} deficiency and iron poisoning.

Vitamin D. Vitamin D includes any of several related anti-rickets compounds. These compounds are present in fish liver oils, in butter, egg yolks, fortified milk, and are also produced in the body on exposure to sunlight. A Vitamin D deficiency may cause rickets in children and *osteomalacia* (softening of the bones) or *osteoporosis* (decreased bone mass) in adults.

Vitamin E. Vitamin E is necessary in human diets for normal muscular and reproductive functioning and development, normal red blood cell functions, and other necessary biochemical processes. Vitamin E is found in milk, wheat germ oils, cereals, egg yolks, beef liver, muscle meats, leafy green vegetables, and other foods.

Vitamin H. Vitamin H is also listed as *biotin* under Vitamin B.

Vitamin K. Vitamin K is a group of vitamins found in their natural state in alfalfa, spinach, cabbage, and other green, leafy vegetables; also in hog-liver fat, egg yolk, putrefied fish meal, and hemp seed. These vitamins promote clotting of the blood by increasing the production of prothrombin, the blood's clotting agent. A deficiency can result in blood coagulation abnormalities.

Vitamin M. Vitamin M is also listed as *folic acid* under Vitamin B.

Vitamin supplementation. Vitamins are not themselves direct sources of energy. As enzyme components, they can act only in the presence of food-contained nutrients. Hence, taking massive doses of vitamin supplements without eating food is useless and may even be dangerous.

In general, vitamin megadoses (abnormally large doses far beyond daily requirements) are not needed. Many reputable nutritional guides suggest that for restricted-calorie diets below 1000 to 1200 calories daily, a multivitamin preparation may be useful, but higher potency or "therapeutic" formulas are not generally necessary. The prescribed multivitamin dosage is based on amounts of individual vitamins equal to the recommended daily allowances.

Recommended dietary allowances. A table, compiled by the Food and Drug Administration is issued periodically as "United States Recommended Daily Allowances" (USRDA). This latter table suggests the following daily vitamin dosages for adults and children four years and older: Vitamin A, 5,000 international units; B_1, 1.5 milligrams; B_2, 1.7 milligrams; B_6, 2 milligrams; folacin, 0.4 milligrams; biotin, 0.3 milligrams; niacin, 20 milligrams; pantothenic acid, 10 milligrams; ascorbic acid, 60 milligrams; Vitamin D, 400 international units; and Vitamin E, 30 international units.

See also Minerals.

W

Warts

Warts are infectious swellings or tumors in the outer layer of skin. Because they are contagious, they can spread from person to person or from one site to another on the same person. Most frequently, warts appear on hands, fingers, and soles of feet. However, they can emerge anywhere on the skin, including the genital and anal areas.

Common warts are caused by exposure to a virus called the human papilloma virus. The virus can remain inactive for up to six months after contact before erupting into abnormal skin masses.

The virus transfers to another person or another site on the body by direct contact. For example, brushing or combing the hair can spread the virus from a wart on the scalp. Shaving or scratching a given area on the body and then touching another spot will also carry the virus. In addition, moist parts of the body, such as the soles of the feet, provide a breeding ground for growth of the wart virus.

As people become older they

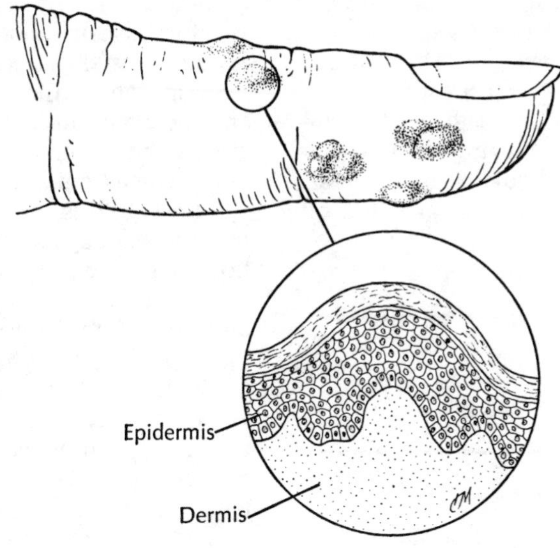

Warts, infectious swellings or tumors in the outer layer of skin, are caused by a virus.

seem to develop an immunity or resistance to wart virus. For this reason, children acquire warts more frequently than adults. Nevertheless, warts can occur at any age.

Usually, warts appear as firm gray masses that feel tender or itchy. Their size and shape vary depending upon the location and severity of the virus. Children develop flat warts most often, particularly on the face. This variety looks smooth, flat, and yellow-brown.

Plantar warts grow on the soles of the feet, where they can become as large as two inches in diameter. These warts cause considerable pain because the tissue swelling pushes inward with the pressure from walking. Discomfort from plantar warts feels like stepping on a pebble in the shoe.

Most warts are not health threatening. However, they can be so extensive in number as to cause extreme sensitivity or pain.

Studies report that two out of every three warts disappear on their own within two years. Consequently, physicians usually recommend leaving warts alone unless they cause discomfort or obstruction.

Sometimes, doctors treat one or two warts and find that other warts on the same person also clear up. In this situation the original treatment stimulates manufacture of antibodies (protective substances) that fight the virus in other warts.

There are over-the-counter preparations to aid removal of warts. Most of these remedies contain a form of acid, which is dangerous if not used according to directions. Although some of these drugs are effective, only a doctor should remove a wart. Home care could scar tender skin by pulling or cutting.

Physicians may try a variety of topical preparations to loosen the warts. A solution containing cantharidin, a substance that causes blistering, may be applied directly on the wart. About one week after application, the doctor should be able to remove the wart with a knife or scissors. Corn plasters with salicylic acid placed over the tissue softens the wart so it can be scraped away.

When a wart persists, physicians may advise surgery to remove affected tissue. Electrosurgery dissolves wart tissue with electric current. Cryotherapy freezes the area with dry ice or liquid nitrogen. Freezing allows the wart to be lifted off easily.

Z

Zygote

When a female sex cell (an ovum or egg) is fertilized by a male sex cell (a gamete or sperm), the two fuse together to form a single cell called a zygote. This single cell contains genetic information in the form of 46 chromosomes (microscopic chemical strings made up of genes), 23 of which come from each parent.

The zygote is the first stage of a process that begins with the fertilization of the egg and ends with the birth of a fully-formed infant. Within a few days after fertilization, the second stage begins, as the zygote starts to divide into a multiple-celled body. About three days later, a spherically-shaped structure called a morula is formed, consisting of many cells all joined together.

The word *zygote* applies only to the single cell that is formed by fertilization.

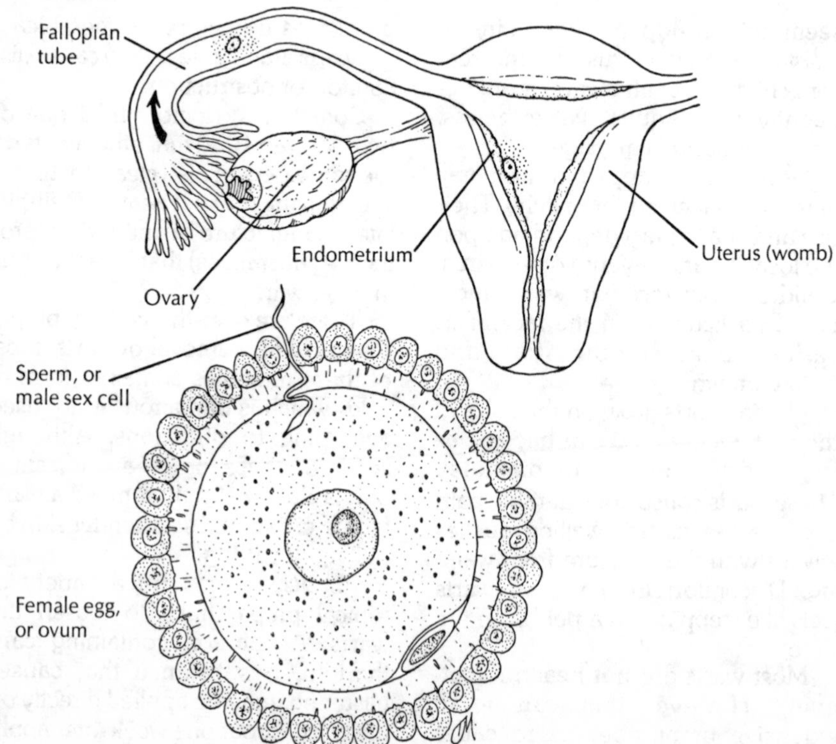

Under normal circumstances, a ripe egg cell, or ovum, is expelled once a month from the ovary to travel up the fallopian tube. If it is fertilized by the male sex cell, or gamete, the two together form a zygote that travels to the endometrium, the lining of the uterus, where it embeds itself and begins to form an embryo, the first stage of human life.

Emergency first aid action guide

Emergency first aid action guide

Handling an emergency successfully takes training, nerve, a calm hand, and the ability to work effectively under pressure. Nobody has an instinctive knowledge of what to do during a medical emergency. If you do not know what to do, you will assuredly do more harm than good. The purpose of this section is to acquaint you with the basic types of emergencies you may someday face and teach you the accepted procedures for handling those emergencies.

This section is not intended as a substitute for professional medical care. Instead, it is just what it says it is: a guide that will tell you what you can do during an emergency to keep a victim alive until the professionals arrive. It is arranged in alphabetical order for fast reference except for the section on Unconsciousness and cardiopulmonary resuscitation. This section appears first because the technique is vital to almost every first aid emergency and it must be mastered first. Read this section thoroughly, and discuss it with your family and friends. Someday, your life or theirs may depend on what you learned as you read this section. The approach is simple and step-by-step. The emphasis is on *how to do what needs to be done*.

Before learning about specific emergency procedures, you should know some facts about emergency situations themselves, regardless of what the particular emergency may be. Imagine that you have just walked into an emergency situation. A victim needs help. What do you do first? And what do you do next? Here are the first steps to follow in an emergency situation.

Make certain that the environment poses no threat to you or to the victim.

Take a few seconds to look around for safety hazards. If the emergency is an auto accident, is the victim still in the car? Is there leaking gasoline? Are power lines down? Is the car on fire? Are other cars bearing down on you? Do you have lighting equipment to warn other drivers? If you get into the victim's car to try to get him or her out, will the car then roll off the edge of the cliff? Many would-be rescuers have wound up being rescued themselves (or killed) when they did not assess the situation in terms of hazards.

Check the victim to see if he or she is breathing.

Sometimes a victim will have a blocked airway (the passage through which air goes through the mouth, down the throat, and into the windpipe is called the "airway"). This means that he or she cannot breathe even if nothing else is wrong. Look to see if the victim is breathing or not. If not, then immediately check the airway to see if it is blocked by food, broken teeth, tissue, blood, or any other obstruction. If the airway is blocked, remove the obstruction. Use your fingers. In case of food choking, you may want to perform chest compression techniques such as the Heimlich maneuver (see the section on Choking). The main objective is to *clear the airway* so the victim can breathe. If the victim cannot breathe, then he or she has only a few minutes to live. And you have only a few seconds to do something about the problem so that the victim will not die. If the airway is not blocked, or if you have unblocked it, proceed to the next step.

Make certain that the victim is now breathing.

Do not assume that the victim will start breathing just because you have unblocked the airway. Absence of breathing can be due to conditions other than a blocked airway. If the airway is not blocked and the victim is still not breathing and is unconscious, it is time to begin CPR—cardiopulmonary resuscitation (see the section on CPR). If you do not succeed in getting the victim breathing in a few seconds, it may be too late.

Check to see if the heart is beating.

Absence of heartbeat can be the result of a number of circumstances, ranging from cardiac arrest (sudden halt of heartbeat) to a heart attack to an interruption in the heart's electrical impulses because of electrical shock (such as in accidental electrocution). The task here is to get the heart beating again as soon as possible.

If the victim is not breathing and has no heartbeat, seconds count. If the airway is blocked, the victim will not be able to breathe. If the victim cannot breathe, it will do no good to restart the heart: there will be no way that the blood pumped into the lungs by the heart can be oxygenated if there is no oxygen in the lungs.

By the same token, if the airway is clear and the victim's breathing cycle is restarted by forcing breaths down his or her throat, without the heartbeat the blood will not go into the lungs to become oxygenated. Restoring breathing without restoring the heartbeat or restoring a heartbeat without restoring breathing is useless. This is why the fundamental victim-revival technique is called *cardiopulmonary* resuscitation; "cardio" refers to the heart and "pulmonary" refers to the lungs. Life depends on both of them.

In addition to breathing and heartbeat, you should look for other problems.

Check for heavy bleeding.

While heavy bleeding will not lead to death immediately, left unattended it will assuredly cause death in a short time. Furthermore, some people are more prone to shock than others, and even a small drop in blood pressure caused by bleeding will put them into shock (see the section on Shock). Once you have made certain that the victim both is breathing and has a pulse, attend to any heavy bleeding (see the section on Bleeding). If you cannot completely stop the bleeding, you can at least slow it down so that the natural clotting mechanisms in the blood can begin their work.

There is one more important objective:

Do no harm to the victim.

Your task is to save, not harm, the victim. If you are not sure about what to do, find somebody who does know what to do to take over. If there is no such person available, then call medical professionals immediately and try to prevent further injury to the victim until they arrive.

In order to be fully prepared for an emergency, you should *have emergency telephone numbers at your fingertips at all times.*

Basically, these are the numbers you should have:

Police
Fire department
Poison Control Center
The nearest hospital
The nearest ambulance service (especially if the hospital or fire department in your area has no ambulances)
Your own physician.

This information should be posted by every telephone in your home and at your place of work. You should also carry this list in your purse or wallet.

You now have the framework within which you can act decisively and effectively during an emergency. The next step is to learn first aid techniques for specific problems. The following sections will instruct you about particular emergencies, beginning with cardiopulmonary resuscitation—the most important procedure you can learn.

Cardiopulmonary resuscitation (**CPR**) is the fundamental victim revival technique. Without both heartbeat and breathing, no victim can survive. Regardless of the cause, if a victim is not breathing and there is no heartbeat, CPR will mean the difference between life and death. You will have only a few seconds to act.

You cannot learn CPR by reading about it alone.

CPR involves not only knowing why certain actions are taken and how they should be done, but it involves *actually doing* them as well.

For this reason, it is *strongly* recommended that you attend one of the CPR courses that are offered at almost every hospital in the country as a public service. You will be taught by professionals, and you will get a certificate that shows that you have developed some skill in performing the technique. You might also check the fire department, the ambulance companies, and your local college or university if your hospital does not offer the courses.

When you sign up for the course, you should look for the following to make certain that you are enrolling in a legitimate program of study and practice:

- How long is the program? (It should last for at least six hours.)

- How much time will you spend actually working with the simulation mannikin? (You should spend at least two hours with the mannikin so that you will "get the feel" of how to apply the various techniques.)

- Does the course teach how to clear a blocked airway? (If it doesn't, then you won't be able to learn the first step to follow if the victim you try to help has a blocked airway.)

- What is the size of each class unit? (Classes with more than six participants are not recommended by the professionals.)

- Do you get a certificate or a card from the Heart Association if you successfully complete the course? (If you do not receive some kind of certificate or card from either the Heart Association or the Red Cross the course may not be up to their minimum standards—which means that it should not be up to your minimum standards either.)

In the next few pages, you are going to learn what to do when you must revive an unconscious victim. Remember that CPR is a skill that has to be learned, and it is the only way that you can keep a victim alive when he or she has suffered a cessation of breathing or heartbeat.

Unconsciousness

1. Try to get the victim to respond.

- Prod the victim or pinch his or her shoulder or another spot on the body near the head.
- Shout in the victim's ear. If you know the victim's name, shout it.
- **Warning:** Do not shake or roll the victim suddenly or vigorously. There may be a back, head, or neck injury that would be aggravated by such a move.

2. If there is no response, call for help.

3. Gently place the victim on his or her back.

- **Do not** let the victim's head hit the ground.
- **Do not** let the victim's neck bend or twist.
- **Do not** give the victim anything to drink or eat.

4. Open the victim's airway.

- Place your hand under the victim's neck and gently lift it up until the neck is straight.
- As you lift the neck, push back and down on the victim's forehead.

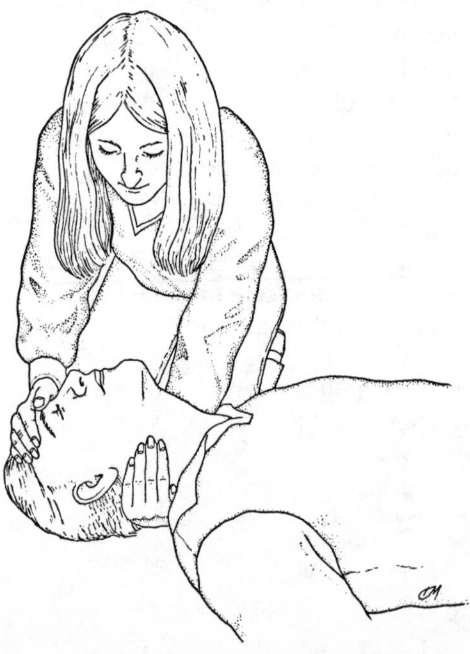

Step 4. Lift neck and push back on forehead.

5. Check to see if the victim is breathing.

- Lean over the victim's face and listen for breathing sounds.
- Place your cheek close enough to the victim's mouth to feel breathing exhalations.
- Watch the chest to see if it rises and falls with breathing movements.

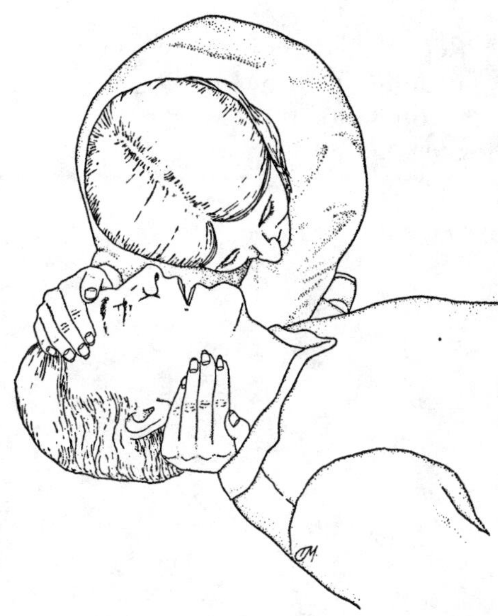

Step 5. Listen, look, and feel for breathing.

- **Warning:** Take about 5 seconds for these three actions.

6. If breathing is absent, give 4 quick breaths.

- Pinch the victim's nose between your thumb and fingers.
- Take a deep breath and fill your lungs with air.
- Cover the victim's open mouth with your mouth.
- Blow in a quick breath, then take your mouth away immediately.
- Repeat this 3 more times, taking your mouth away from the victim's mouth between each breath.

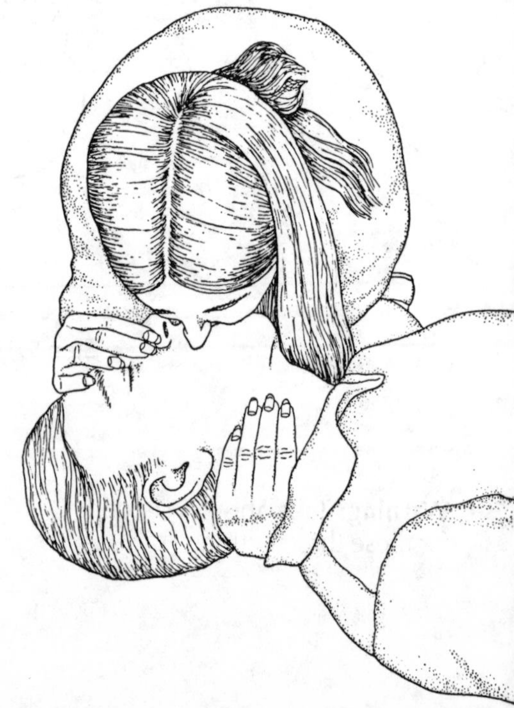

Step 6. Pinch victim's nose and give breaths.

7. **Check for a pulse.**

- Keep one hand on the victim's forehead and put the fingers of the other hand on the victim's Adam's apple.
- Slide your fingers from the Adam's apple to the side groove.
- Feel with your fingertips for a pulse. Feel for about 10 seconds. Move to the next step quickly.

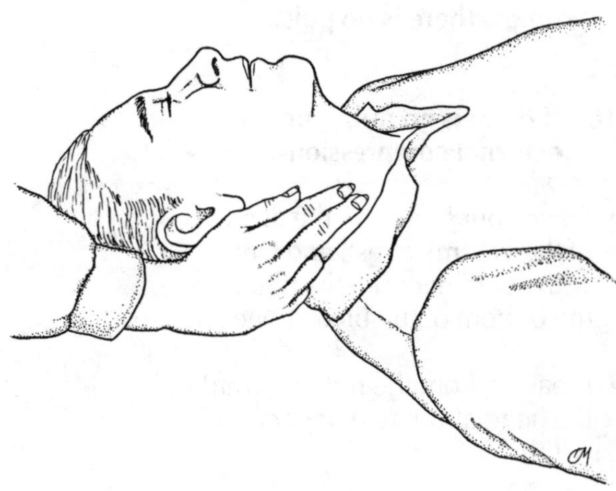

Step 7. Feel for pulse.

8. **If there is a pulse, blow in a breath every 5 seconds.**

- Pinch the victim's nose between your thumb and fingers.
- Take a deep breath and fill your lungs with air.
- Cover the victim's mouth. Blow a short, deep breath into victim's lungs.

- Between each breath, take your mouth off the victim's mouth and watch for a natural rise and fall of the victim's chest.

- Repeat this procedure every 5 seconds.

- Check the pulse periodically as you keep up the breathing cycle.

9. Continue giving breaths until the victim can breathe alone unless there is no pulse.

10. If there is no pulse, begin external compressions:

- Place your hands on the center of the victim's chest, and feel with your fingers for the notch at the bottom of the breastbone.

- Measure from the notch toward the head about two fingers width.

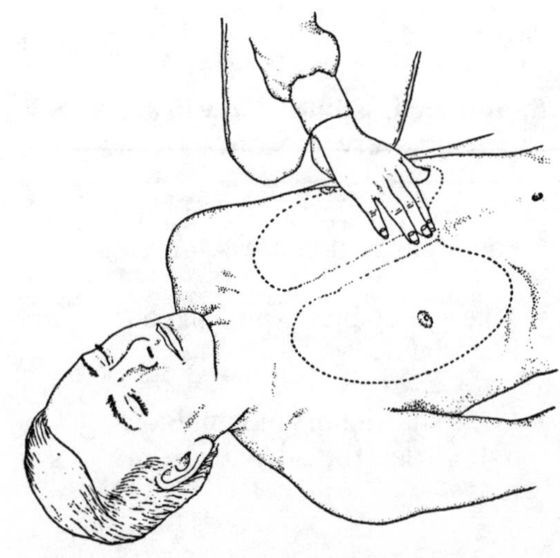

Step 10. Find notch at tip of breastbone.

- Place the heel of your hand on the lower breastbone above your fingers.

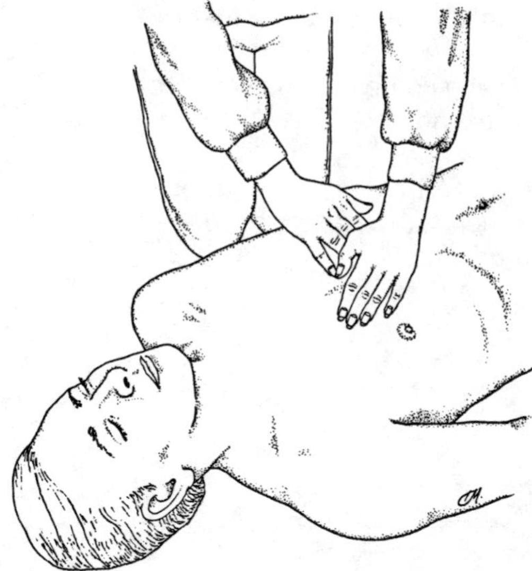

Step 10. Place heel of hand on lower breastbone above your fingers.

- Place the other hand on top.

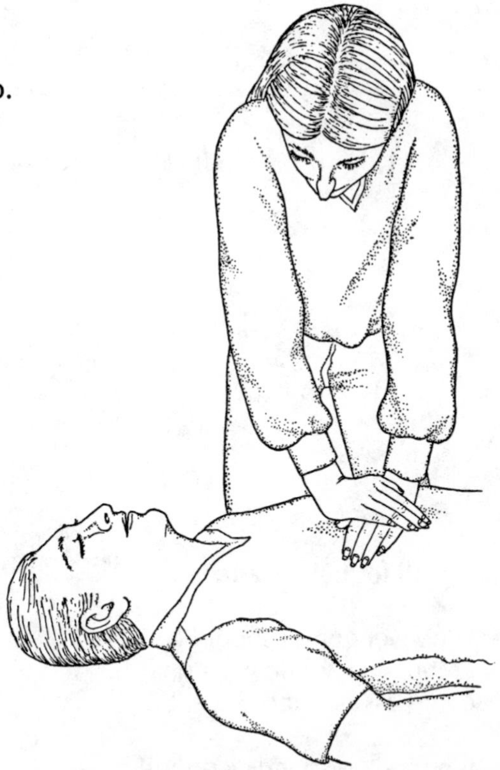

Step 10. Place other hand on top.

- Straighten your arms and press straight down to compress (push in) the chest 1½ to 2 inches.
- Each compression takes ¾ of a second.
- Make 15 compression movements, then give 2 short, deep breaths.

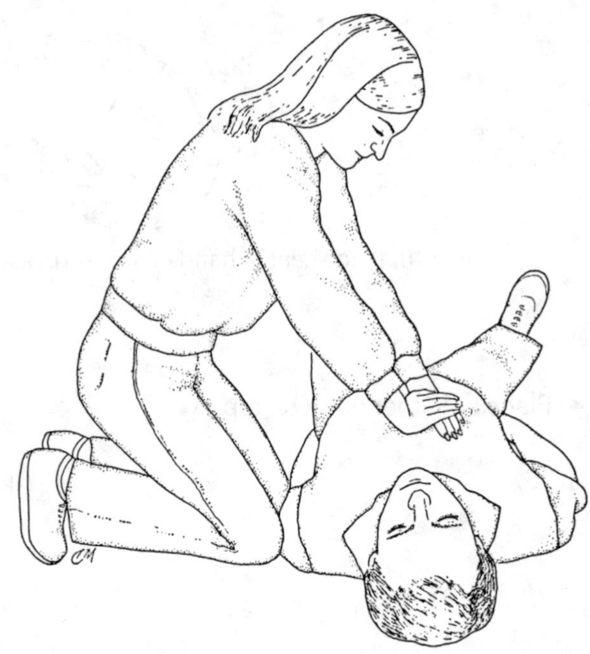

Step 10. Compress chest 1½ to 2 inches.

11. Call for help again.

- Whoever comes should call an ambulance while you continue compressions and breaths.
- If nobody responds, continue CPR for about 5 minutes.

12. Call the ambulance or rescue squad yourself.

- Tell the person who answers:
  Address
  Telephone number from which you are calling
  That the victim is unconscious

13. Restart CPR.

- Continue CPR until either the victim's pulse and breathing return.
- Or the ambulance or rescue squad arrives.

14. If victim is breathing and there is a pulse, keep the airway open.

15. Look for medical identification.

A bracelet
A necklace
A card in the victim's purse or wallet

16. If the victim is diabetic, place one of the following under the victim's tongue:

A cube of sugar
½ teaspoon of granulated sugar
A piece of candy (not sugar-free)

- **Do not** pour liquids in the victim's mouth!
- Keep the airway open while you are giving the sugar.
- Stay with the victim for about 5 minutes until you see some improvement. Then, call the ambulance.
- If somebody else is there, have him or her call the ambulance while you stay with the victim and watch for signs of improvement.

17. If the victim is not a diabetic, check the skin to see if it:

- Looks red.
- Feels very hot.
- Is dry, even under the arms.

18. If these skin conditions exist, move the victim to a cooler place.

- See the section on Heatstroke for treatment procedures.

19. Periodically check the pulse and breathing.

Reasons for your actions: Unconsciousness

Your main objective is *to keep the brain alive and undamaged.*

You are trying to prevent

a. insufficient oxygen to the brain (from absence of a heartbeat and insufficient breathing)
b. very low blood sugar levels that can lead to brain injury (in the case of a diabetic)
c. very high temperature (over 105°F.) that can injure the brain.

All of the steps of CPR are directed toward achieving that goal.

The "pinch, prod, and shout" technique is done to see if the victim is really unconscious. You should never start CPR on somebody whose heart is beating or who is breathing, because you may upset the heartbeat or breathing cycle if you administer CPR. In short, you may do more harm than good.

When you roll the victim over onto his or her back to begin CPR, make sure that there are no injuries that could be worsened by such a movement.

Since the victim cannot survive without oxygen, you must first make sure that the victim *can* breathe. This means that you must inspect the airway and see if it is blocked. It will do no good to initiate mouth-to-mouth resuscitation techniques if the airway is obstructed.

If the airway is clear, then the victim can breathe. If he or she is not breathing, mouth-to-mouth resuscitation is started. Mouth-to-mouth technique is the most effective method known.

If the airway is clear and the breathing has begun, blood still has to be pumped through the lungs so that it can be oxygenated. Oxygenated blood is then taken back to the heart, to be pumped to the rest of the body. See if you can detect a heartbeat (feel for a pulse with your fingers). It is absolutely imperative that you know for sure that the heart is not beating before you commence CPR. Feel for at least 10 seconds. If you definitely have felt no pulse, then begin CPR.

The chest compressions squeeze the heart between the breastbone and spine. This helps the heart begin pumping again.

CPR is about 30 percent as effective in getting blood through the heart as a normal heartbeat would be. There is about 16 percent oxygen in the air that you breathe into the victim's lungs. However, this 16 percent of oxygen per volume of air and 30 percent efficiency in heart action is enough to keep a victim alive and enough to keep the brain from being damaged.

In the case of the diabetic who has lost consciousness, there may be both a heartbeat and breathing. The diabetic victim is unconscious for either of two reasons: diabetic coma or insulin shock. If he or she is in diabetic coma, then blood sugar levels are too high. If he or she is in insulin shock, it is because blood sugar levels are too low. Since it is impossible for you to discern which is the cause, you should give the sugar cube under the tongue. If the problem is insulin shock, the sugar may bring the victim out of it. If the cause is diabetic coma, one lump or a ½ teaspoon of sugar will not make that much difference.

Whatever the causes of unconsciousness, you should stay with the victim until professional help arrives. If you have restarted the victim's breathing and heartbeat, watch him or her carefully in case they stop again. The causes of unconsciousness discussed here are the most dangerous ones: the ones where a few seconds mean the difference between life and death. Read the 19 steps that should be followed in cases of unconsciousness over and over until you are familiar enough with them to perform the procedures without having to look them up.

Bleeding

In the case of bleeding, minutes count (unless the person has been bleeding for some time in which case seconds count). Further, some people are more susceptible to shock from loss of blood than other people, so you must never assume that bleeding is unimportant.

1. Apply pressure to the wound.

- Cover the wound with some kind of bandage material:
  A cloth
  A paper napkin
  A piece of torn clothing
  A handkerchief
  A sterile dressing if you have one
  A sanitary napkin
- Place your hand over the bandage and press down firmly.
- Keep the pressure applied until the bleeding stops or slows.
- **Do not** remove a bandage. If the bandage becomes soaked, place another one on top of it and keep the pressure on the wound.

2. Raise the bleeding part of the body (unless it is broken) so that it is higher than the level of the heart.

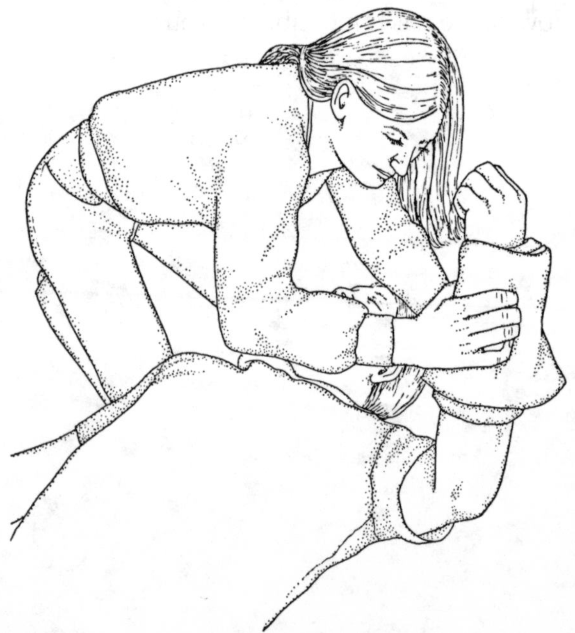

Step 2. Elevate wound above heart.

3. **Do not allow the victim to move the wounded part.**

4. **Do not pour antiseptics on or into the wound.**

5. **If the bleeding does not stop under pressure within 5 minutes, do the following:**

- Apply pressure to a pressure point between the wound and the heart.
- **Arm wound**—press your fingers into the groove between the two big muscles on the inside of the arm.

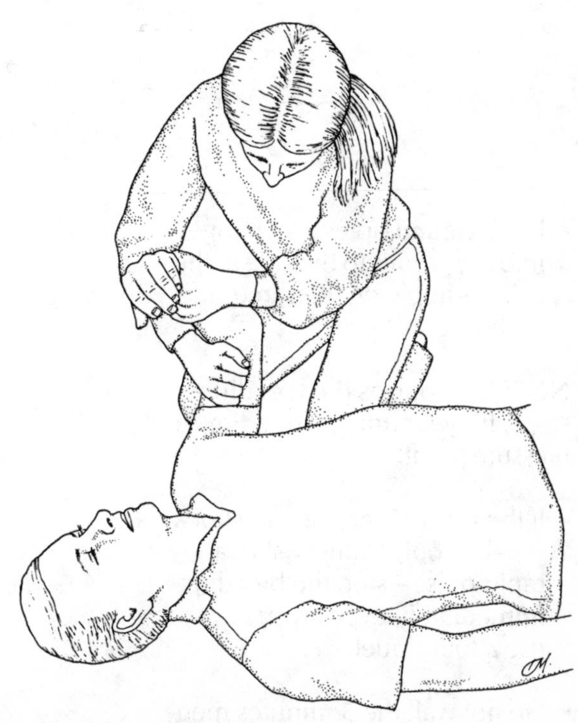

Step 5. Pressure point for arm wound.

- **Leg wound**—press your fingers into the middle of the crease where the thigh joins to the body at the groin.

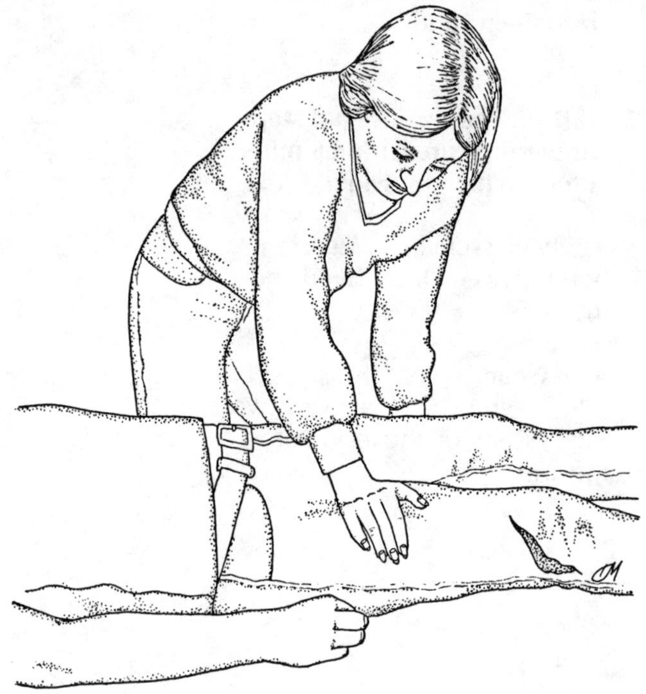

Step 5. Pressure point for leg wound.

- **Neck wound**—press your fingers into the groove to the side of the Adam's apple on the same side as the wound.

NOTE: As soon as the bleeding stops, lift your fingers from the pressure point.

- If the victim is going into shock—pale, cool, clammy skin and rapid pulse—stop the bleeding **immediately,** even if you have to use a tourniquet.

- Do not wait the 5 minutes mentioned above.

6. If the victim has suffered an amputation or is going into shock, do the following:

- Use material—cloth, bandage, tie, belt, sock—at least 1½ inches wide. Do not use a rope, a piece of string or twine, or a piece of wire!

- Position the tourniquet above and near to, but not on, the wound.

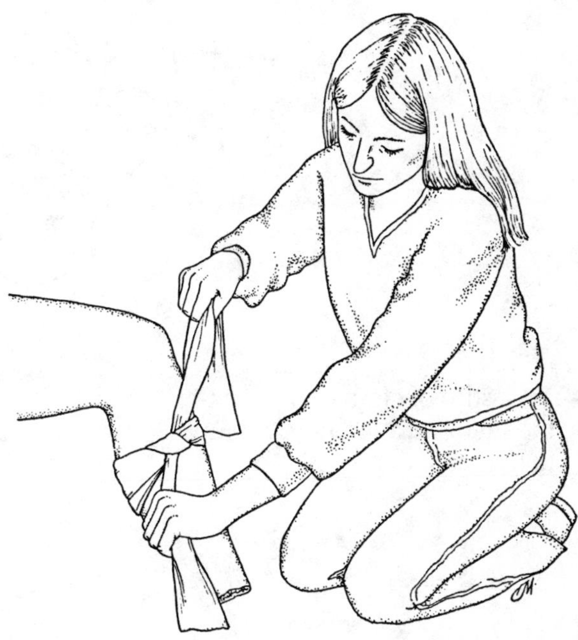

Step 6. Use a cloth for a tourniquet.

- Tie a small stick to the tourniquet with a single knot.

- Twist the stick until the bleeding stops, but no tighter.

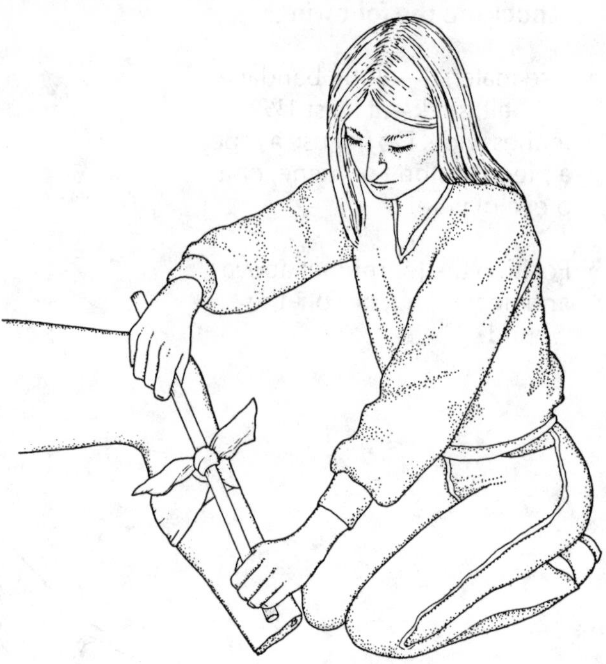

Step 6. Tighten the tourniquet with a stick.

- Tie a strip of cloth to one end of the stick and attach stick to limb to maintain tightness.

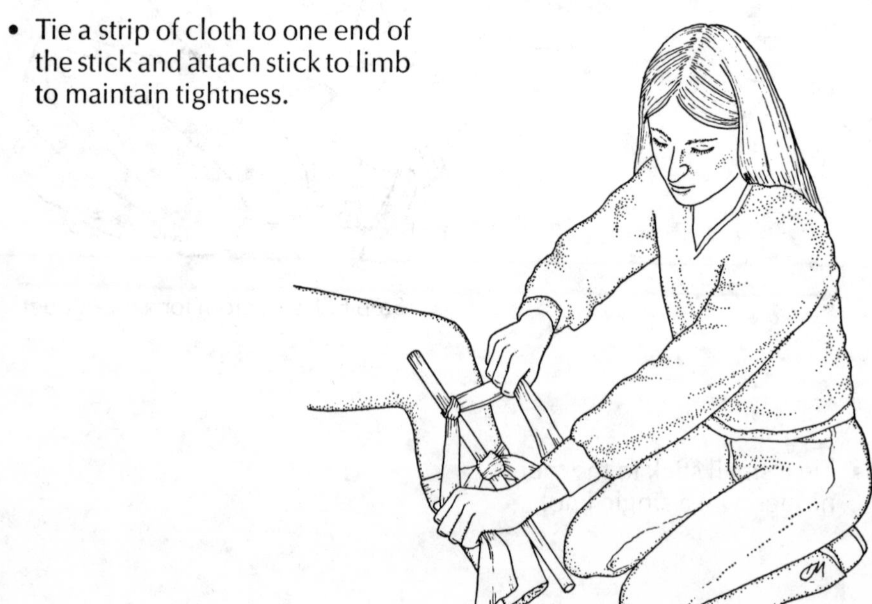

Step 6. Attach stick to limb.

- Note the exact time that you apply the tourniquet.
- Once you put the tourniquet on, do not take it off.
- Use a tourniquet only as a last resort when all other methods of stopping the bleeding have failed.

7. Treat for shock.

- Lay victim down.
- Prop up legs (12 inches) but not if you suspect head injury or broken leg.
- Cover victim with blanket or coat.
- Do not move victim.
- Do not give victim anything to eat or drink.

8. Call ambulance.

Reasons for your actions: Bleeding

Your main objective is to stop the blood loss at once.

The major risk in heavy bleeding is that the victim's circulation will decrease to a point where insufficient oxygen (which is carried in the blood) will reach the brain.

In most cases, you can stop bleeding by applying direct pressure to the wound. You should put on plenty of bandage material and apply pressure on top of the wound.

Do not take off the soaked bandages. This can break up the clots that have already formed to slow the bleeding, thus making the treatment ineffective. Apply clean bandages on top of the soaked ones.

If the wound is in the arm or leg, you should raise it above the level of the heart to help the blood in the limb flow back toward the body and slow the bleeding even more Keep the wounded limb immobile to slow the bleeding even further and prevent the breakage of the blood clots.

An antiseptic is not needed. Some antiseptics can actually damage healthy tissues. You do not need to worry about infection at this point. Your main job now is to stop the bleeding.

Sometimes you will need to shut off the blood supply to an area in order to stop the bleeding. That is what happens when you push on a pressure point. However, this procedure can be dangerous since all the tissues beyond that point also need blood. You might cause permanent damage to a limb or other body area by using pressure points to stop bleeding, but you should do it if necessary to save the victim's life. To minimize the risk of this kind of damage, release the pressure on the point as soon as the bleeding stops. Push on it when the bleeding starts again. This will help stop the bleeding while doing the minimum damage to the rest of the area. If you keep up this off-on pressure, usually the bleeding will stop in a few minutes.

In rare instances, neither direct pressure nor pressure on pressure points will stop the bleeding. Then you may want to use a tourniquet to save the victim from bleeding to death. Tourniquets are very dangerous and should be used only as a last resort. Use a tourniquet only in cases of amputation, where part of a limb has already been lost, or when shock occurs and the bleeding has not been stopped by other measures.

Do not loosen or remove a tourniquet if you put one on. Poisons from the crushed tissue under the tourniquet can return to the body via the bloodstream and cause shock.

If a great deal of blood has been lost, the victim should be treated for shock. In this case, remember to keep the blood flowing back to the brain. Elevate the victim's legs, if possible, to help the blood flow back to the body (trunk) and brain. The only exceptions are in the case of a head injury (you want to avoid increasing the pressure and swelling in the victim's brain) and in the case of a broken leg.

Broken bones

Broken bones can be dangerous, not only in terms of the bones themselves, but in terms of the damage that sharp bone edges can do to blood vessels and nerves around the area of the break. When you treat a victim with broken bones, keep in mind that the sharp end of a broken bone can be as destructive as a knife.

1. Check that the airway is clear.

- If the victim is unconscious, do not lift the neck or bend it.
- Open the mouth by pulling the jaw down or forward.

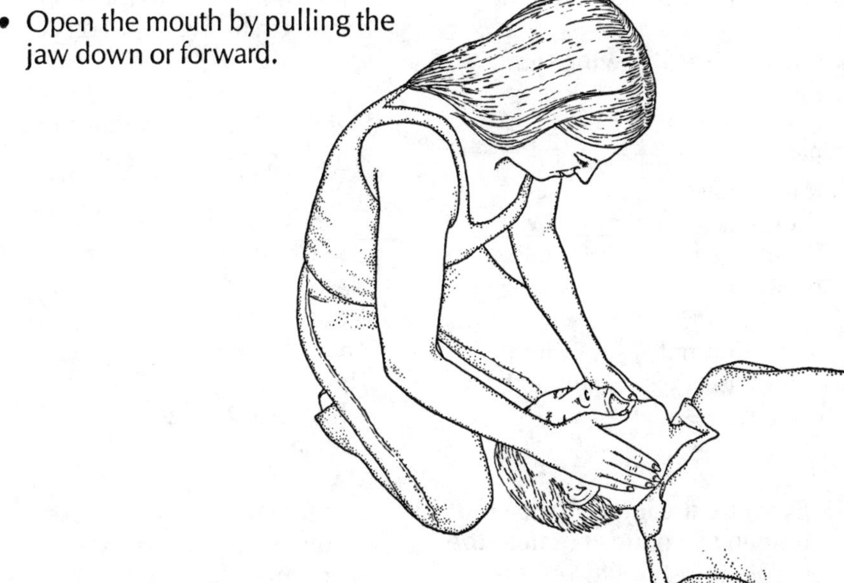

Step 1. Lift jaw and tongue to check airway.

- Clear the mouth and throat of any broken teeth, bones, or other debris.

2. Control any heavy bleeding.

- Cover the bleeding area or wound with one of the following:

  A sterile bandage
  A piece of cloth or clothing
  A sanitary napkin or a handkerchief

- Press on bandage until the bleeding stops.

- Do not cause movement or pain if you can help it.

- Refer to the section on Bleeding.

3. Examine the victim for shock.

- Look for the following symptoms:

  Pale, cool, clammy skin
  Rapid pulse
  Victim is restless or drowsy
  Pulse rate is over 100 beats per minute

- If the victim displays shock symptoms, refer to the section on Shock.

4. Examine the injury to see if it is open (a wound at or near the break point) or closed (no break in the skin).

- If the break is *open,* cover the wound with a clean cloth, a bandage, a sanitary napkin, or a handkerchief.

- Do not try to clean the wound.

- Check the pulse and the skin color on the limb on the side of the break farthest away from the heart.

- See if the victim can feel you touch the skin on either side of the break.

5. Immobilize the broken bone.

- First: Immobilize the joint above and the joint below the break so that they cannot move.

- Second: Do not try to straighten bent arms or legs at their joints.

- Third: Do not try to move the bone(s) in trying to put on a splint.

- Here is a list of materials from which splints can be made.

  Pillows
  Boards
  Newspapers
  A baseball bat
  An umbrella
  The other leg
  A light barbell bar
  Blankets
  Magazines
  Cardboard
  A golf club
  A broomstick
  A hockey stick

- To tie the splint on, here is a list of things you can use:

  A belt
  Masking tape
  Adhesive tape
  A shirt sleeve
  A tie
  Electrical tape
  Duct tape
  A pair of pants
  A scarf
  A curtain sash
  A curtain

- In the case of broken fingers, you can splint with the following:

  A small stick
  A tableknife
  A cigarette holder
  A tongue depresser
  A pencil or pen
  A watercolor brush

- In the case of a hand, wrist, or forearm, apply the splint as follows:

  Run splints up both sides of the forearm, from the wrist to the elbow.

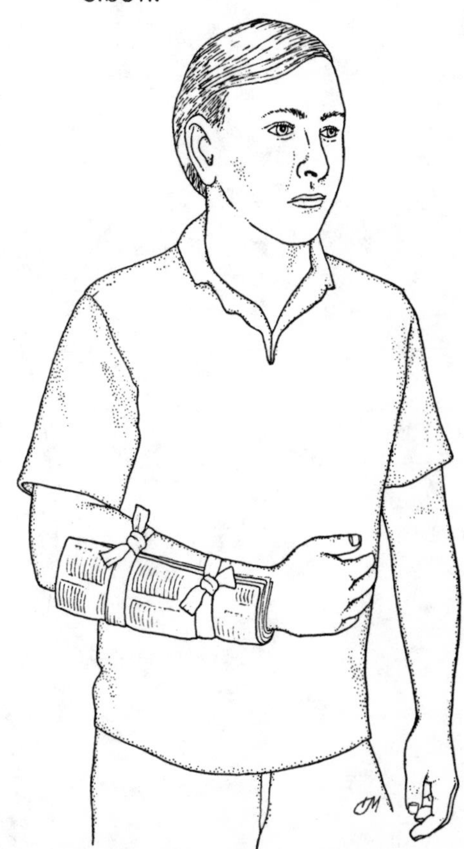

Step 5. Splint forearm from elbow to wrist.

Position the arm so that the thumb points up, and put it into a sling that wraps around the arm, then loops around the neck.

- In the case of an upper arm, collarbone, shoulder, or elbow break in which the elbow is bent, do the following:

  Use a sling to immobilize the arm and support its weight. Loop this sling around the neck.

  Tie another sling so that it wraps around the chest, bringing the arm close to the body.

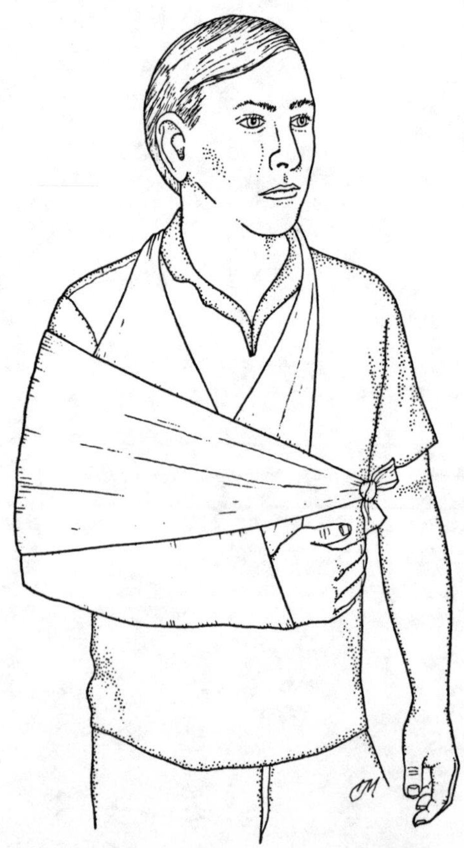

Step 5. For upper arm injury, tie sling to chest.

- In the case of a broken elbow that is straight, do the following:

  Use a splint that reaches from the armpit all the way to the wrist. Wrap the arm so that the elbow does not shift from side to side or off the splint.

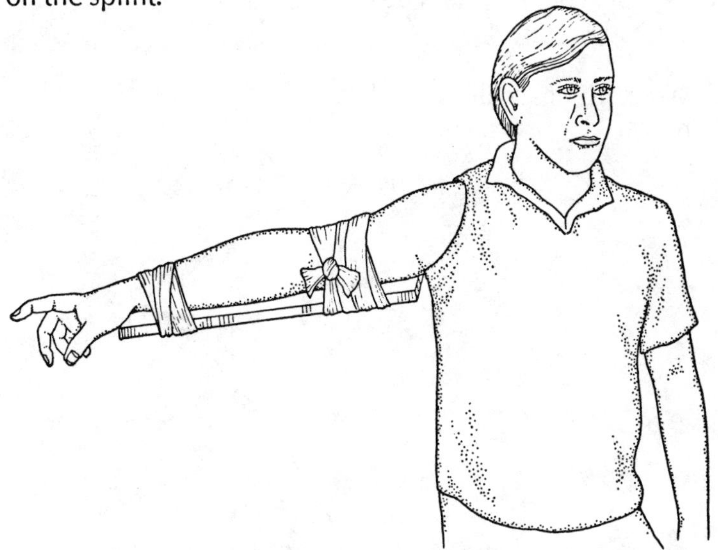

Step 5. For elbow injury, use splint from armpit to wrist.

- In the case of a broken pelvis, do the following:

  Keep the victim still, and tie his or her legs together to keep them from moving.

  Do not move the victim unless it is absolutely necessary!

  Examine the victim and treat for shock if necessary.

- In the case of a broken leg, do the following:

  Place some padding between the legs, and tie them together.

  Use a single splint between the legs or a splint on the side of each leg.

  Wrap the legs so that they do not move.

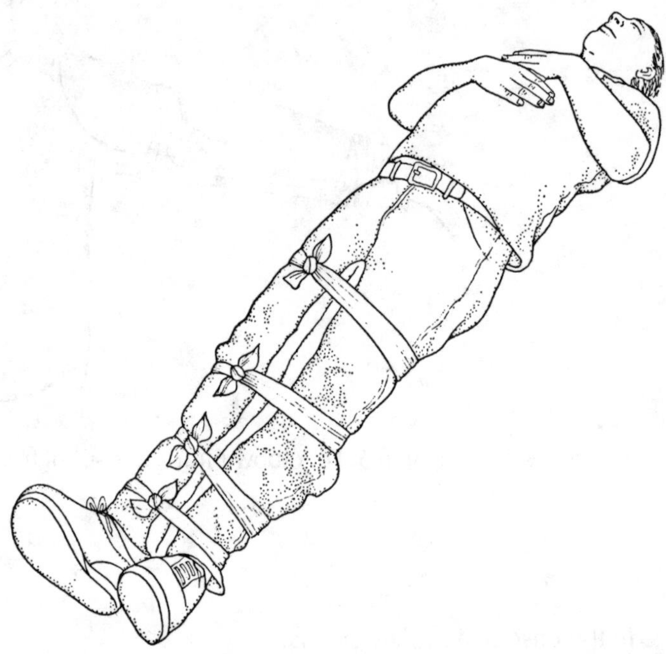

Step 5. For leg or pelvis injury, tie legs together.

- In the case of a broken and bent knee, do the following:

  Keep the knee bent, and use a splint between the upper and lower leg that will keep the knee from moving from a bent position.

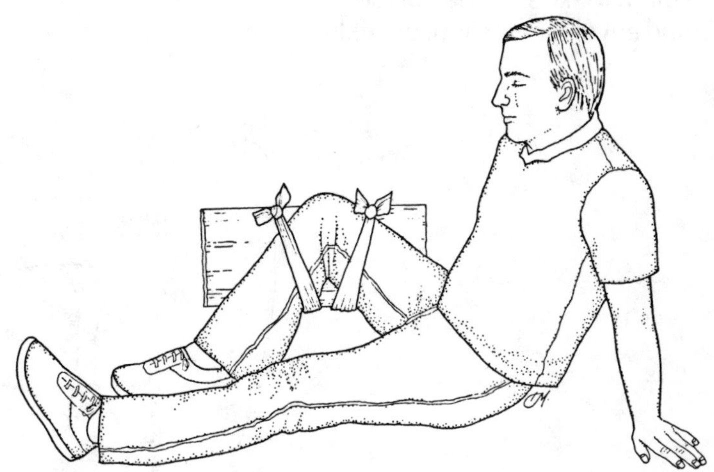

Step 5. For knee injury, keep knee bent and splint between upper and lower leg.

- In the case of a broken foot or ankle, do the following:

  Remove the victim's shoe or boot carefully. Cut it off if necessary.

  Use a pillow or a blanket for the splint. Make sure that it is soft, and envelopes the foot or ankle.

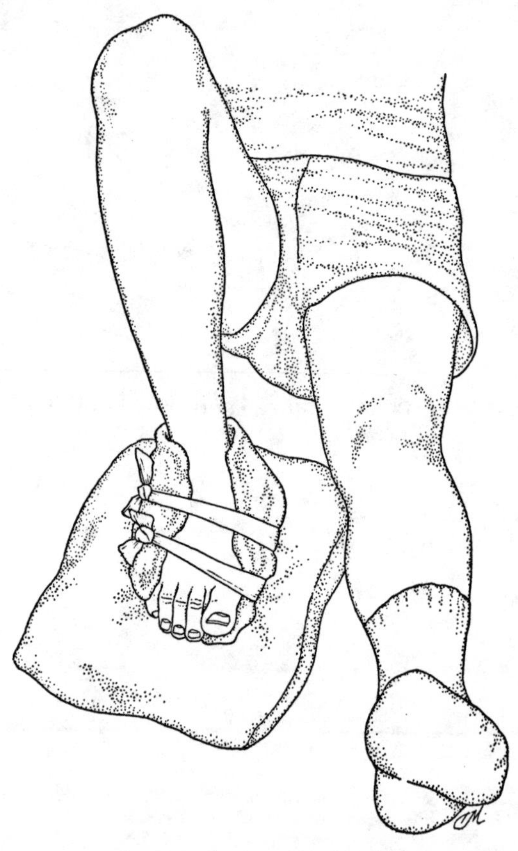

Step 5. Use thick, soft splint for foot injury.

6. Call an ambulance.

7. Make periodic checks of the splinted part.

- Watch for the following symptoms:

  An increase in pain
  Decreased feeling on the skin in the area
  Lack of pulse in the affected area
  Paleness or blueness of the skin.

8. If any of the symptoms described in Step 7 are noted, do the following:

- Check to see if the ties holding the splints are too tight.
- Check to see if an unbroken joint is bent to the extent that the normal circulation is impaired.
- If either of these problems exists, loosen and/or reset the ties or wraps. Be careful not to disturb the injured area.

Reasons for your actions: Broken bones

Your objectives are to
a. stop blood loss
b. keep blood flowing to the brain
c. prevent further damage
d. prevent infection
e. reduce pain.

Broken bones themselves are not fatal and need not be serious. However, they can do a great deal of damage with jagged edges (which can cut muscles and veins and can also cause bleeding in the area of the break). The edge of the break can often cut nerves and major blood vessels, especially in the case of breaks near joints such as the elbow and knee. Here, the edges can poke through the skin (this is called an open break rather than a closed break that does not penetrate the skin). Bacteria then enter the area and cause infection. However, in either an open or closed break, the edges of the bone will grind against one another, causing intense pain.

The break itself is not the major concern. Instead, first concern yourself about the more life-threatening problems: blocked airways, lack of breathing or pulse, and bleeding.

Your first step is to make certain that the airway is open and that the victim is breathing. Your next step is to control any bleeding that is taking place. Do this with the pressure bandage method. Use a sterile bandage, a piece of cloth, a strip of clothing, a sanitary napkin, and/or a handkerchief.

If the broken bones are large, or there are several breaks, there may be enough internal bleeding to cause shock. Therefore, you should examine the patient and treat for shock, if necessary, to keep oxygen flowing to the brain. (Review section on Shock, if necessary.)

After you have taken care of bleeding and determined that the victim is not in shock, you should next examine the victim to see if any nerves are damaged. If this is the case, the skin area below the break will be numb. Also look to see if any large blood vessels have been cut. In this case, there may be no pulse beneath the break and skin color will be abnormal.

If you can immobilize the broken bone(s), this will prevent damage. Thus, the jagged edges of the bone will not be moving around and slicing the tissue. This will also reduce pain since the edges will not grind together. To immobilize the break successfully, you will have to keep both the joint above and the joint below from moving.

Do not try to straighten broken or displaced bones. If you do, this could cause more slicing of tissue or nerves when you move the bone. Put the splint on the limb in the position you find it (especially in the case of the elbow and knee where nerves and blood vessels are close to the bone).

If the break is open, cover it. Do not try to clean the wound; you might force germs and dirt in more deeply.

Make sure an ambulance is called The victim will need to have the broken bone(s) set as soon as possible.

Burns

Burns are frightening and painful injuries, especially in severe cases. The first step to take is to reassure the victim and try to keep him or her calm. Move swiftly and decisively.

1. Determine the severity of the burn.

- *First degree burn:* The skin will be red and painful (as in a sunburn).
- *Second degree burn:* The affected area will be red, painful, and will have blisters.
- *Third degree burn:* The affected area may be black, white, or painless.

2. Treatment for first degree burns.

- Place the burned body part in cold water (**do not** put salt or ice in the water).
- If you cannot immerse the burned body part, put cold water on it by gently pouring the water or by soaking and squeezing a sponge over the burn.

3. Treatment for second degree burns.

- Place the burned body part in cold water (**do not** put salt or ice in the water).
- Place cold, wet dressings on the burn. Use only clean cloths (freshly ironed sheets, for example) or sterile bandages (preferably).
- Call a doctor or an emergency room.
- Do not break blisters.
- Do not put oil, butter, or ointments on the burned area.
- Do not remove burned or blistered skin.

4. Treatment for third degree burns.

- Do not remove burned clothes. Leave them on the skin.
- If the victim's face is burned, keep him or her sitting upright.
- Make sure that the airway is kept open. Tilt the head back if necessary.
- Call an ambulance or rescue squad.

- If the victim is awake, and there will be no medical help for an hour or more, you may give the victim the following to drink: 1 quart of water, with 1 tsp. salt and ½ tsp. baking soda added. Give ½ glass every 15 minutes. If water is all that is available, give the same amounts of water.

- Keep the burned areas higher than the heart: elevate arms, hands, feet, legs.

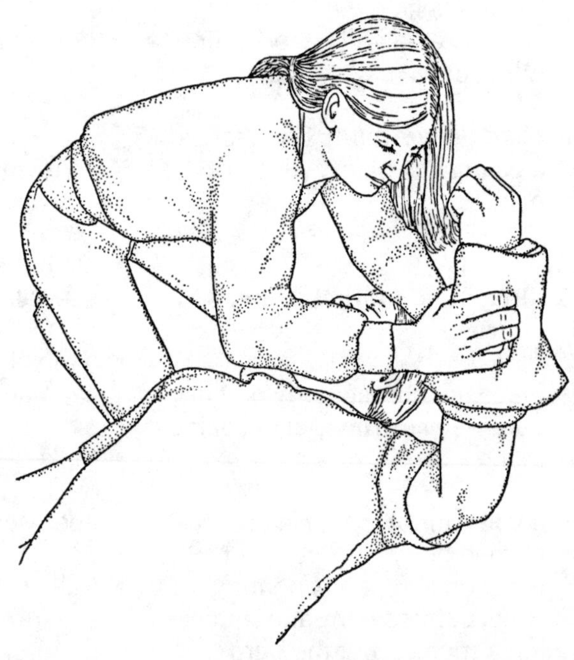

Step 4. Keep the burned area higher than the heart.

Reasons for your actions: Burns

Your main objectives are

a. for first-degree burns: relieve pain
b. for second-degree burns: prevent infection and relieve pain
c. for third-degree burns: keep oxygen flowing to the brain, prevent infection, and reduce swelling.

Many first-degree burns can be treated at home. In these instances, your chief goal is to relieve pain. These burns are not severe and will generally heal rapidly once the pain subsides.

In second-degree burns, the skin is damaged to the point of risking infection. The blisters at the site of the burn are potential areas of infection. The blisters should not be broken; if they are not, there is no danger of infection. However, if they are, often the tissue beneath becomes infected and is severely scarred later on. Do not use butter and ointments since they may carry bacteria and may actually cause infection. The best treatment is to use freshly ironed cloths, which will be nearly sterile, and will not be a source of infection. You can then treat the pain with cold water.

If you use salt and ice together in the water the water temperature could be lowered enough to increase damage to the tissues. It is better to use plain cold water.

Third-degree burns signal extensive damage to the skin and to other tissues, including blood vessels (hence the white or pale skin) and nerves (there will be no pain—in this case, absence of pain is worse than pain).

Remember that with a third-degree burn or burns, your goals are to keep oxygen flowing to the brain, to prevent infection, and reduce swelling.

If the victim's face is burned, the hairs in his or her nose are singed, the mouth cavity is black or dark, or there is a deep cough, suspect burns to the lungs and airway. This may cause the airway to swell shut, so check frequently to see that the airway is still open. Also, remember that burned lungs collect fluid and shortness of breath will result. It may be easier to keep a victim with burned lungs breathing if he or she remains sitting up.

Serious burns can cause a tremendous fluid loss from the bloodstream. Even when there is no apparent bleeding, the victim may be in shock. Treat as for blood loss shock, since the problems are the same: low blood pressure and low blood supply to the brain.

Most burn victims in shock should have nothing to drink, since vomiting may be a problem in severe burn cases. However, if medical help is late in coming or is not available, give salt water solution in very small amounts to restore some fluid to the victim's bloodstream.

Occasionally, clothing will be burned directly onto the skin. Removing the clothing or fabric could cause more damage by opening up infection-prone tissue. However, you should remove any clothing or fabric that is actually smoldering or still burning.

If you can elevate arms or legs that are burned, this will reduce swelling, which might increase the tissue damage. Medical attention is especially important if the burned area involves face, hands, feet, and/or genitals.

Chemicals in the eyes

Eye tissues are extremely delicate. A few seconds can mean permanent loss or impairment of sight if the victim is not properly treated. You will have to take charge immediately.

1. Take over the victim's actions. Do not let the victim rub his or her eyes.

- Do not let the victim keep his or her eyes closed.
- Assure the victim that you are going to help, that you know what you are doing, and that you are going to do it immediately.

2. Rinse the eye with clean water for 15 minutes. Do not use hot water.

- Have the victim lie down near a source of water (a bathtub or a sink).
- Hold the victim's eyelids open. Do not touch the eyeball.
- Pour water slowly over the eyeball. Do not pour it directly on the eyeball, but at the inner corner of the eye instead.
- Let the water flow across the eye from the inner corner and out at the outer corner.
- Keep pouring clean water for 15 minutes by the clock.

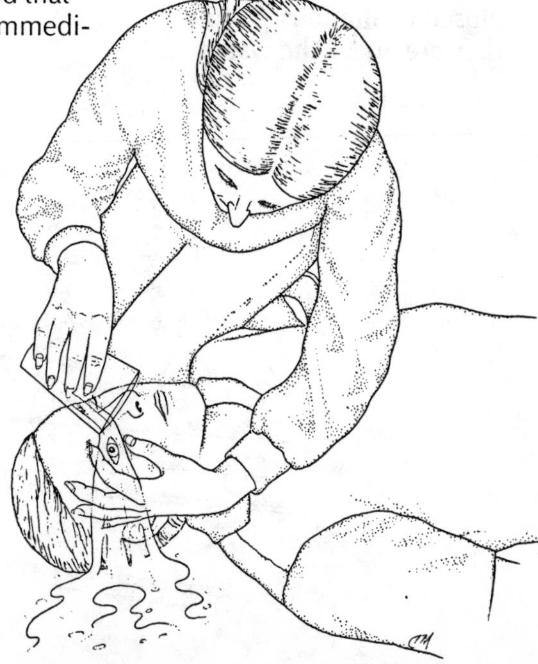

Step 2. Rinse eye with clean water for 15 minutes.

3. **Do not use antidotes or other chemicals such as vinegar unless a doctor tells you to do so.**

4. **Take victim to emergency room or doctor's office.**

NOTE: Someday, you might be the victim, and if you are alone, it will be up to you to save your eyes. Read this section thoroughly, and learn it well enough to be able to help yourself without looking at the guide. Remember: you will not be able to read this if you are the victim.

1. **Get to a source of water. Fill a deep bowl or the sink with water and put your face into it. Blink your eyes open and closed continuously while they are under the water.**

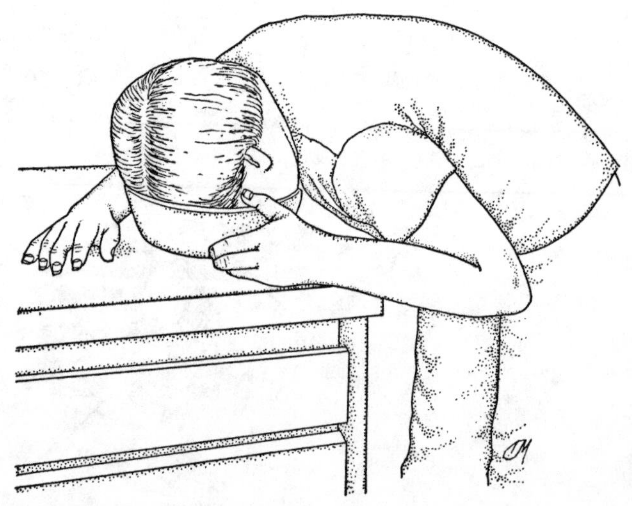

Step 1. If you are alone, place face in water and blink eyes continuously.

2. Change the water every 3 to 5 minutes for 15 minutes.

3. If only one eye is involved, do the following:

- If you have a sink with a faucet that you can get your head under, set the flow at a gentle stream and put your head under the faucet. Position your head so that the water flows from the inner corner of your eye at the nose over the eyeball and runs down your cheek. If you cannot put your head under the faucet, use the bowl or sink but keep the unaffected eye tightly clenched shut to make sure that none of the chemical gets into the unaffected eye.

4. Do not use antidotes or other chemicals such as vinegar unless on the orders of a physician.

5. Have someone take you to an emergency room or a doctor's office as soon as you have rinsed the affected eye(s) for 15 minutes.

Reasons for your actions: Chemicals in the eyes

Your main objective is to remove the chemical as quickly as possible.

Some chemicals are extremely harmful to eyes and can cause permanent scars and damage to the eyeball of the victim. This can lead to partial or total blindness if the chemicals are not removed at once.

Time is important. Do not waste time. Start rinsing the eyes immediately, before the damage is done. Remember that you must rinse the eyeball itself and not just the outside of the eyelids.

It helps to have the victim lie down near a source of water, such as a bathtub or sink. The victim may be in so much pain that he or she resists opening the eyes, but you must force the eye open. If necessary, hold the eyelids open yourself. Be careful not to touch the eyeball if you can avoid it.

The water should not be poured directly on the eyeball but at the inner corner of the eye instead. Let the water flow from inner to outer corner for more complete cleansing. In order to get all the chemicals out, continue to rinse for a full 15 minutes.

When you are through rinsing, even if the victim says that his or her eyes feel fine, make certain they are checked by a doctor. Sometimes scarring of the eyes can take place and the doctor needs to examine the eyes and treat the victim accordingly.

If you are victim yourself, try to immerse your upper face in water from a sink, pan, or deep bowl. Or place your eye under a running faucet. If none of these is available, cup your hand, fill it with water, and immerse the affected eye in it. Blink the eyes continuously while they are under the water. When you have rinsed the eye(s) thoroughly for 15 minutes, be certain you have someone take you to a doctor or hospital to have your eyes checked.

Choking

When a person is choking, a few seconds can mean the difference between life or death. You must act quickly.

1. **Ask the victim if he or she can talk.**

2. **If the victim can speak, wheeze, or moan, the following applies:**

- Stay with the victim and tell him or her to try to cough out whatever is stuck in the throat.

- **Do not** slap the person's back.

3. **If the victim cannot make any sounds, do the following:**

- Stand behind the victim and hold his or her chest with one hand.

- Give the victim 4 quick slaps on the back (between the shoulder blades) with the palm of your hand.

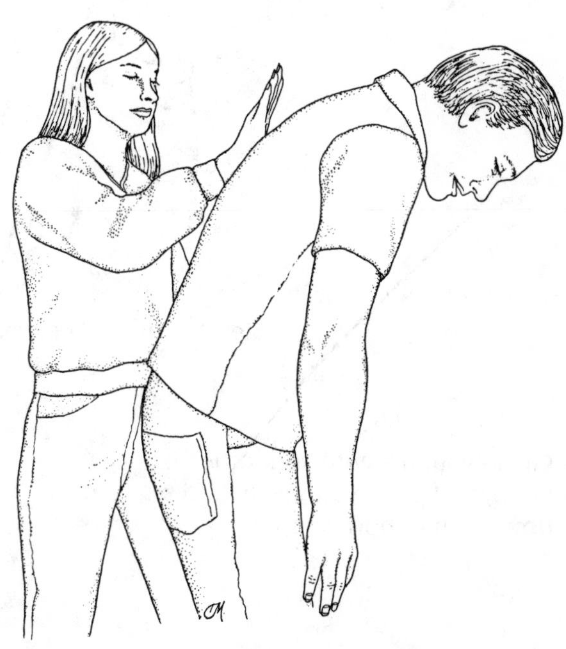

Step 3. If victim makes no sounds, give back blows.

4. Reach around the person's waist with your arms, and do the following:

- Find the spot halfway between the navel and the breastbone.

- Place thumb side of other fist in that spot.

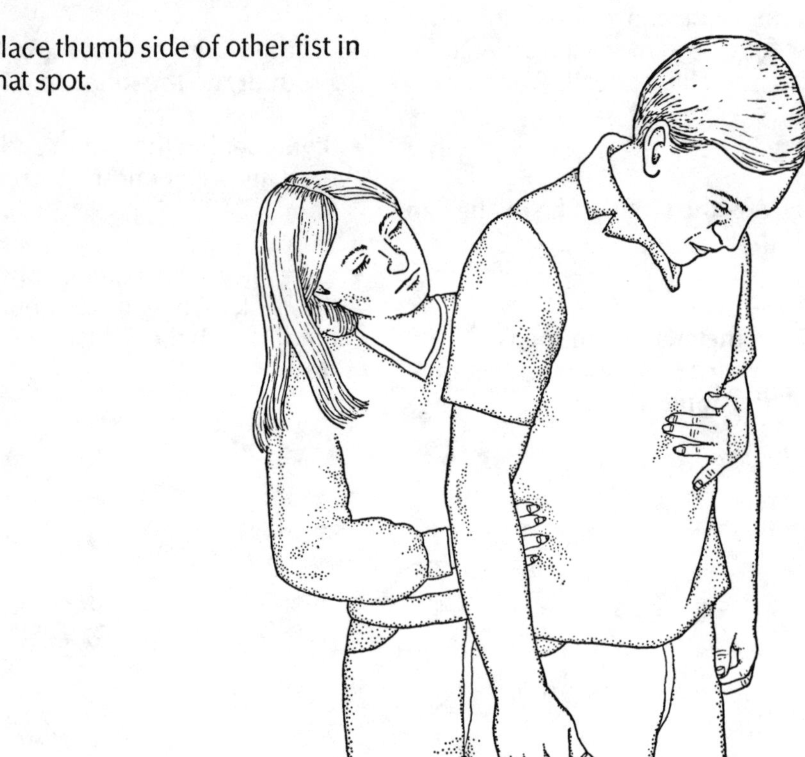

Step 4. Find spot between breastbone and navel.

- Grasp your fist with your other hand, and press your fist in and upward in a short, snappy movement.

- Repeat the movement 4 times.

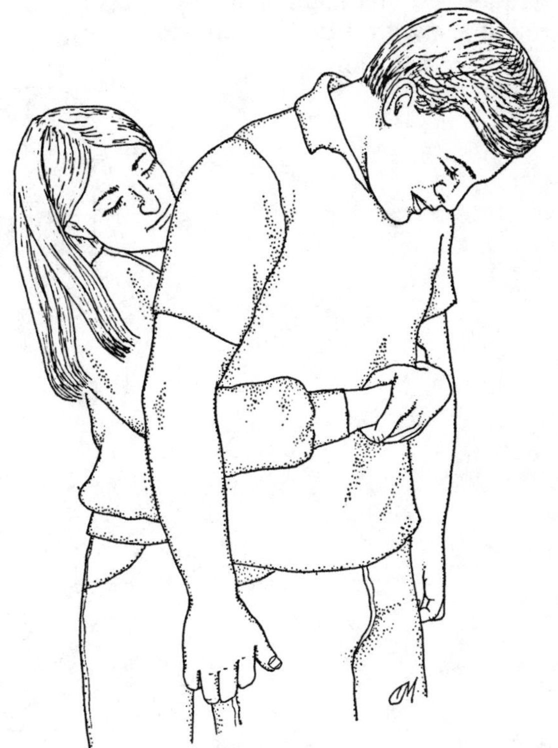

Step 4. Press fist in and upward.

NOTE: If the victim is pregnant or very fat, do the following:

- Stand behind the victim and reach around under his or her armpits and position your hands in the middle of the breastbone (not at the bottom tip). If the victim is a woman, be careful not to injure her breasts.
- Place the thumb of your left fist against the middle of the breastbone and grasp your fist with your right hand.

- Squeeze the victim's chest 4 times with short, snappy squeezes. Make sure that you squeeze with sufficient force to compress the chest.

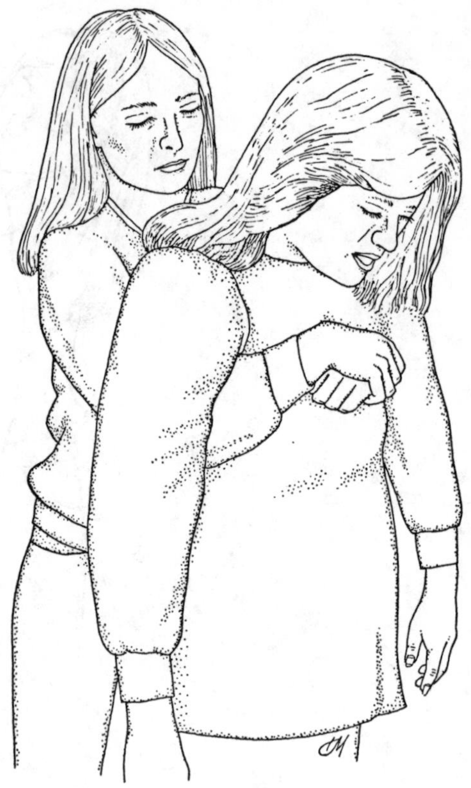

Step 4. If victim is pregnant, give chest squeezes.

5. Repeat the following:

- 4 blows to the back.
- 4 upward and inward presses of the fist in the abdomen.
- If the victim is pregnant or very fat, give 4 quick chest squeezes with the fist at the middle of the breastbone.
- Try to remove the object that is causing the choking.

6. If the victim becomes unconscious, do the following:

- Lower the victim to the floor on his or her back.
- Do not let the victim's head hit the floor.

7. Open the airway and try to give a forced breath.

- Place your hand under the victim's neck and gently lift it up until the neck is straight.
- Push back on the victim's forehead and pinch the nose between your thumb and fingers.
- Take a deep breath, cover the victim's mouth with yours, and blow air in forcefully.

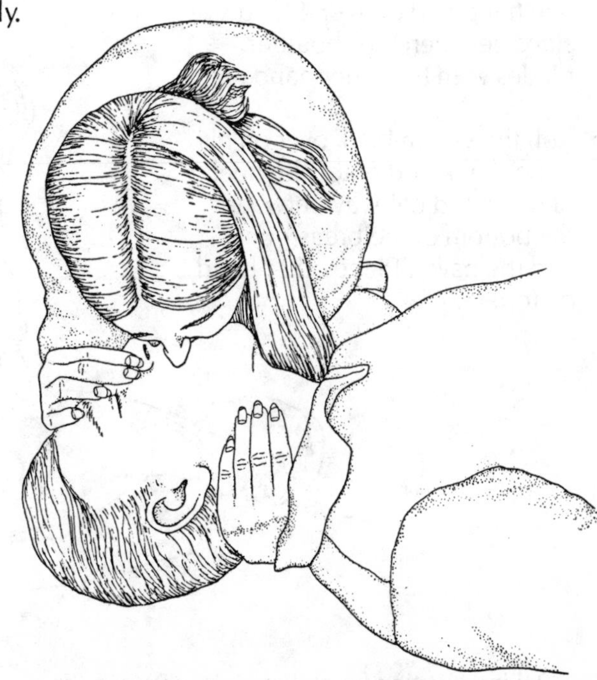

Step 7. Pinch victim's nose and give breaths.

- Check to see if the chest is rising.

8. If the air goes into the victim's lungs and the chest rises, do the following:

- Give the victim another forced breath every 5 seconds.
- Take your mouth away from the victim's mouth between breaths.

9. If no air goes into the victim's lungs during Step 7, do the following:

- Roll the victim toward you and lean him or her against your thigh (you are on your knees).
- Hold the victim's shoulder with one hand and deliver 4 hard slaps between the shoulder blades with the other hand.
- Roll the victim back over on his or her back and place the heel of one hand halfway between the bottom of the breastbone and the navel. Place other hand on top.

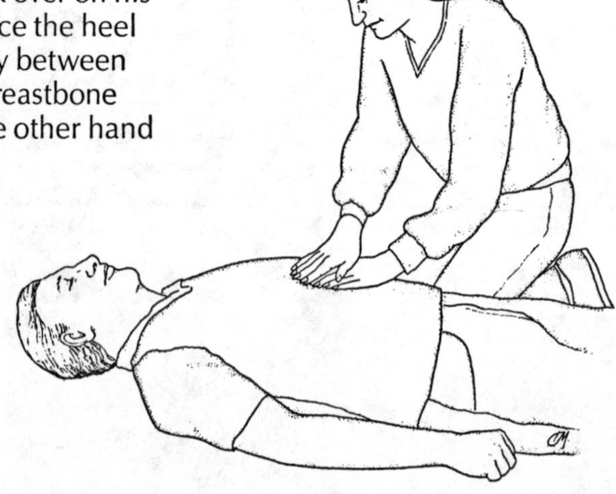

Step 9. Find position for abdominal thrust midway between breastbone and navel.

- Push inward and upward toward the upper part of the abdomen with 4 quick thrusts.

NOTE: If the victim is pregnant or very fat, do the following:

- Place the heel of one hand (with the other hand on top of it) on a spot in the middle of the breastbone (not at the bottom tip).

- Push straight down quickly and forcefully 4 times. Use enough force to compress the chest 1 to 2 inches. Start with the arms almost straight.

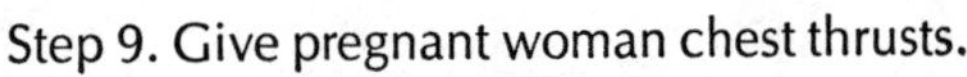

Step 9. Give pregnant woman chest thrusts.

10. Try to remove the object that is causing the choking.

- Turn the victim's head to one side.

- Open the victim's mouth and pull the jaw down so that you can get your hand into the victim's mouth.

- Lift the tongue out of the way and sweep deeply into the back of the mouth with a hooked finger.

11. Try to give another breath.

12. Repeat the following:

- 4 back blows.
- 4 abdominal thrusts (or 4 chest thrusts if the victim is pregnant or very fat).
- Try to remove the object.
- Try to give a breath.

13. Final advice:

- Do not leave the victim until he or she is breathing.
- Do not begin heart compressions.
- Do not give any other first aid.

Reasons for your actions: Choking

Your main objectives are to

a. decide if the blockage causing the choking is complete or partial

b. watch to see that a partial blockage does not become complete

c. if the blockage is complete, get air into the victim somehow.

In the step-by-step emergency procedure above, you are reminded in Step 1 to ascertain whether or not the victim can talk. Remember that so long as he or she can talk or make any noises at all—even if the words are not distinct—it is a sign that air is moving from the lungs. In this case, do not slap the victim's back or you may cause the blockage to move down the airway, blocking it completely. Thus, as long as the person is able to talk or make noises, try to encourage him or her to cough up whatever object or bit of food is causing the blockage.

If the blockage is complete, the victim will be unable to make any sound at all. You must then try to "blow" out the chunk of food or the object by forcing air out of the lungs—an action very similar to the way a pea shooter works. As Step 3 in the procedure indicates, you should stand behind the victim and hold his or her chest with one hand. Then, to force the air out, give the victim 4 quick slaps on the back between the shoulder blades, using the palm of your hand. Follow this with 4 upward abdominal thrusts directed toward the spot just between the navel and the breastbone.

The reason for the last procedure is simple: when the abdomen is squeezed it will push up the diaphragm, the muscle between the abdomen and chest, and thus will force the air out of the chest.

The procedure differs somewhat for a pregnant woman or a very fat person. The abdominal thrust could be dangerous to a pregnant woman and might be impossible to use with an obese person, so you vary the technique and use a chest thrust. The results are the same, but you do not run the risk of injuring the patient.

If the victim becomes unconscious, you must try to get air into him or her before death occurs. You must try to give a breath, following the procedure in Step 7. You always run a slight risk of blowing the chunk of food or the object down farther, but you might also manage to open up one lung for the victim to use in breathing.

If no air goes into the victim even by using this procedure, then repeat the sequence of 4 back blows, 4 abdominal thrusts, and then another attempt to give a breath. Keep repeating this sequence until the airway clears enough for the victim to breathe on his or her own.

Even if the victim's heart stops, there is no value to any other kind of first aid until you clear the airway and the person can get some breaths.

Remember: The first step in any emergency is always to open the airway and allow the victim to breathe. Do not move on to another emergency procedure until that is done and the person is breathing again.

Convulsions

Some people are so startled by a person having convulsions they are practically useless when it comes to giving first aid. What is required of someone giving first aid is calmness, decisiveness, and quick action.

1. If the victim is still standing, gently ease him or her to the floor or ground.

2. Hold onto the victim firmly, but gently.

- **Do not** allow the victim's head to strike the floor or ground.
- **Do not** allow the victim to hurt himself or herself.

3. Do not try to open the victim's mouth (it will probably be clenched shut).

- **Do not** put your fingers in the victim's mouth.
- **Do not** insert any object into the victim's mouth.

4. Place the victim on his or her side.

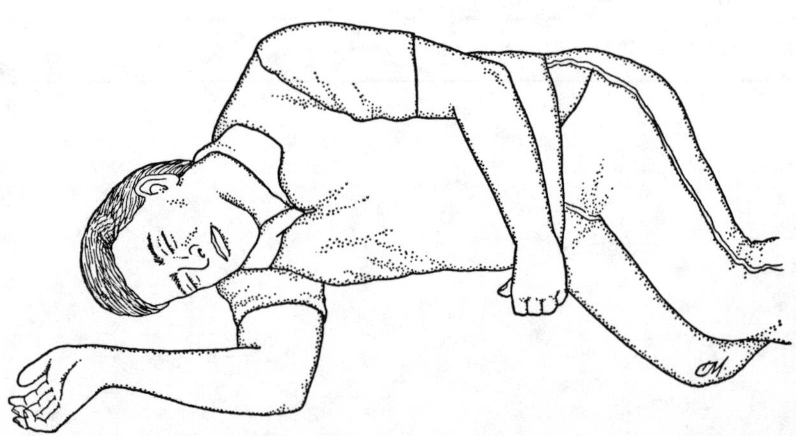

Step 4. Place victim on his side.

5. Stay with the victim until the seizure is over.

6. When the seizure is over, do the following:

- Make sure that the airway is open.
- Roll the victim over on his or her back.
- Lift the neck with your hand.
- Push back on the forehead until the neck is straight.
- Check for easy, regular breathing.

7. Call an ambulance and tell them the following:

- What has happened and where you and the victim are located.
- A telephone number where you can be reached.

8. Do not let the victim stand, walk, drive, or otherwise exert himself or herself after the convulsion has ended.

9. Do not give the victim anything to drink or eat.

10. If the victim is a child with a high temperature, do the following:

- Remove the child's clothes and place cold, wet towels on his or her body until the fever comes down.
- Give a child's dose of aspirin if the child is awake.
- Call an ambulance.

Reasons for your actions: Convulsions

Your main objective is to protect the victim.

Two ideas should be dismissed at the beginning: a person having a seizure or convulsion is not to be feared nor is he or she to be treated with force. What such a person needs is to be protected from hurting himself or herself during the seizure.

A convulsion is actually a massive electrical stimulation to the brain. It will cause all the muscles to become stiff, causing the victim to twitch and temporarily stop breathing. There is nothing that you can do to stop this process.

You can protect the victim by keeping him or her from falling on sharp objects, knocking head on the floor, or striking furniture with arms and legs. Move any heavy or sharp objects or furniture away from the victim. If you need to hold or restrain the victim, do so gently.

Do not try to pry the mouth open nor insert any object into the mouth. If the victim bites the tongue, it will heal.

After the seizure is over, the victim may be groggy and disoriented. Protect the victim from having vomitus inhaled into airways and lungs by placing him or her on side. Also avoid giving food or drink that might cause vomiting and thus endanger the open airway.

Stay with the victim until the seizure is completely over. Call an ambulance and return to the victim: another seizure may occur.

Remember that in small children, a high fever can actually cause convulsions even if the child is not epileptic. In a case such as this, first aid can prevent a seizure from occurring by lowering body temperature (see instructions in Heatstroke section).

Drowning

Drowning can result from a variety of mishaps. If the victim is still in the water, you must be careful not to become a victim yourself. If the victim has been in the water for five minutes or more, there is little reason to risk your life. On the other hand, if you have arrived immediately after the mishap, there is much that you can do.

1. Do not become a victim, too.

- Throw the victim a life preserver, a float, a rope, or an inner tube.
- Reach out to the victim with a pole.
- Row out to the victim in a boat.
- Swim out only as last resort.
- Watch out for rocks, reefs, submerged trees, snakes, or sharks.

2. If the victim is still in the water, but is not breathing, do the following:

- Turn the victim's face up out of the water.

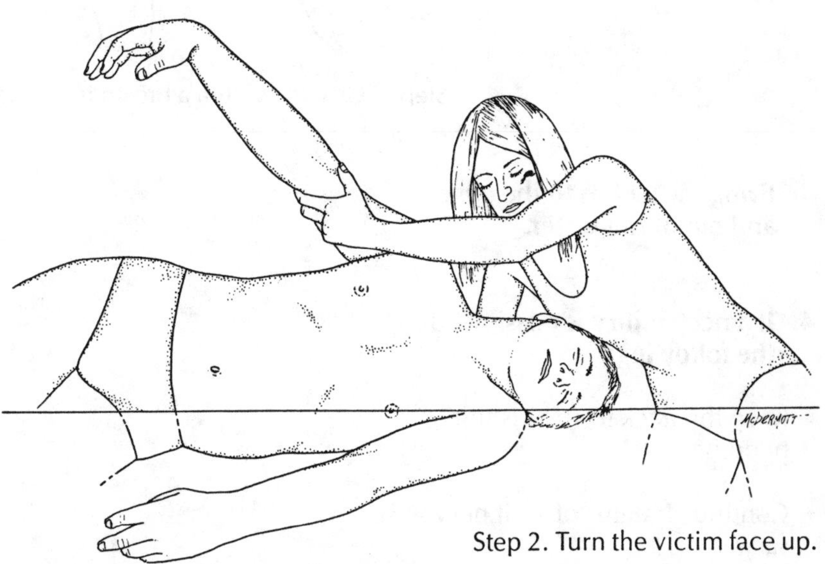

Step 2. Turn the victim face up.

- Keep the victim's neck straight.
- Pinch the victim's nose between your thumb and fingers.
- Take a deep breath.
- Cover the victim's mouth with your own, and blow 1 quick, deep puff of air into his or her mouth every 5 seconds.

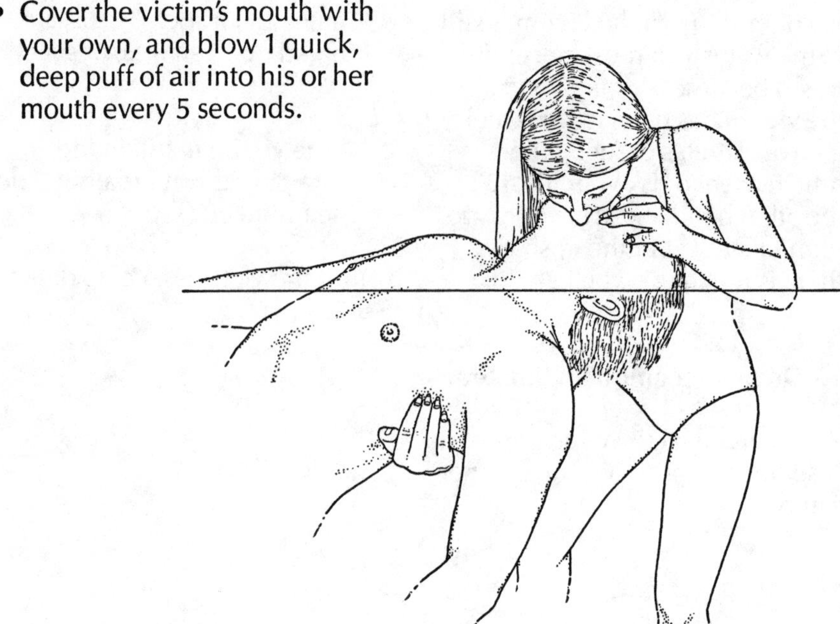

Step 2. Give the victim a breath in the water.

3. Bring the victim to the edge and out of the water.

4. If a neck injury is possible, do the following:

- Keep the neck from twisting or bending.
- Continue breaths of air if necessary.

- Get help and place a board (surfboard, wood) under the victim.
- Raise the board until the victim's body is supported.
- Carry the victim on the board to a safe place.

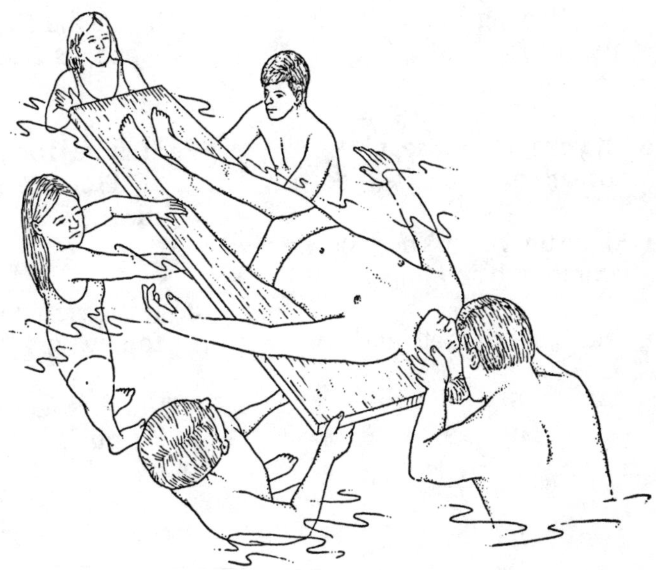

Step 4. Carry a victim with a neck injury to shore on a board.

- Continue to give the breaths of air.
- Do not bend the victim's neck nor let head roll from side to side.

5. Check the victim's pulse.

- Place your other hand on the victim's neck.
- Slide the fingers from the Adam's apple to the side groove in the neck.
- Feel for a pulse.
- Keep feeling for a pulse for about 10 seconds.

6. If you feel a pulse, give 1 breath of air every 5 seconds.

- Pinch the victim's nose between your thumb and fingers.
- Take a deep breath and hold it.
- Cover the victim's mouth with your own and blow forcefully into the victim's mouth.
- Take your mouth off of the victim's mouth between each puff of air.
- Watch the chest to see if it is rising and falling.
- Repeat the puffs of air every 5 seconds.

7. If there is no pulse, refer to the first section on Unconsciousness.

8. If the victim vomits, do the following:

- Turn the victim's head to the side quickly.

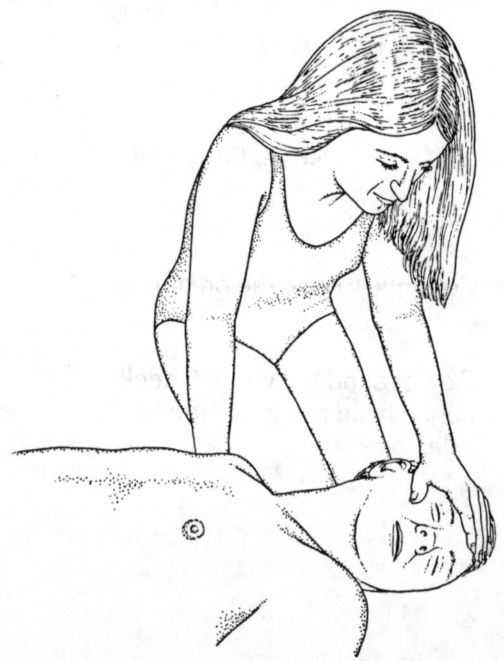

Step 8. If victim vomits, turn head.

- If you suspect a neck injury, keep the neck straight and turn the whole body to the side.

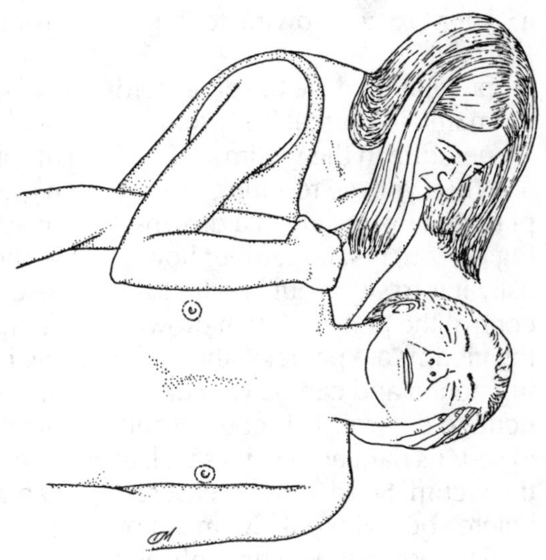

Step 8. If victim with neck injury vomits, turn entire body to the side.

- Clean out the victim's mouth.
- Continue breaths and compressions immediately.

9. When the victim recovers, cover him or her with a blanket, towels, or a jacket.

10. Call an ambulance or rescue squad.

- Tell them your location.
- Tell them that CPR is in progress.
- Tell them if you suspect a neck injury.

Reasons for your actions: Drowning

Your main objectives are to

a. keep oxygen flowing to the brain
b. prevent damage to spinal cord
c. maintain normal body temperature in the victim.

When you are rescuing or planning the rescue of a drowning person, first remember how risky it is to swim out and try to control the person. Often drowning victims are panicky and frightened and can be very difficult to control. This could result in serious danger to you as well as the victim. So try other measures before you swim out. Swim out or dive to rescue the victim only as a last resort.

The major problems in drowning cases are suffocation and low body temperature. Sometimes, however, a victim who hits bottom with his or her head can suffer a neck injury. So remember that your major objectives are to keep oxygen flowing to the brain, to prevent damage to the spinal cord if the neck is injured, and to maintain normal body temperature.

As soon as you have reached the victim, try to correct any breathing problems. If you are a particularly strong swimmer, you may be able to start some artificial respiration before you reach the shore. Certainly you can do so if the victim is rescued in a boat. But do not become overtired and risk your own life.

If CPR is needed, begin it regardless of how long the victim has been underwater. If the victim is still in the water but not breathing, follow the procedure in Step 2 using artificial breaths to start him or her breathing again.

There is always danger of a neck injury and consequent risk of spinal injury in drowning cases. If there is a neck injury, you will need help in getting the victim out without further injury. During the rescue effort, try to keep the neck straight and immobile by supporting it with your hand or a flat surface (surfboard, piece of wood, life preserver).

Also, watch for vomiting. You can save the victim's life with CPR but if the vomit flows down into his or her lungs, there's little chance of survival. Watch and make sure that the vomit does not go down the airway.

If the victim needs CPR but you suspect neck injury, make certain to administer CPR without bending the neck.

Remember that a drowning victim has suffered severe exposure and is in danger of severely lowered body temperature. Cover him or her with a blanket, towels, jacket, beach gear, or tent cover in order to increase body temperature. Make certain that an ambulance or rescue squad is called as soon as possible.

Heart attack

Most sudden deaths from heart attacks occur in the first two hours after the pain starts. Fast action is essential.

NOTE: If the victim is conscious, go directly to Step 11.

1. If the victim is unconscious, lay the victim on his or her back on the floor, the ground, or a bed.

2. Check that the airway is open.

- Place your hand under the victim's neck and lift upward.
- Push back on the forehead so that the neck straightens.

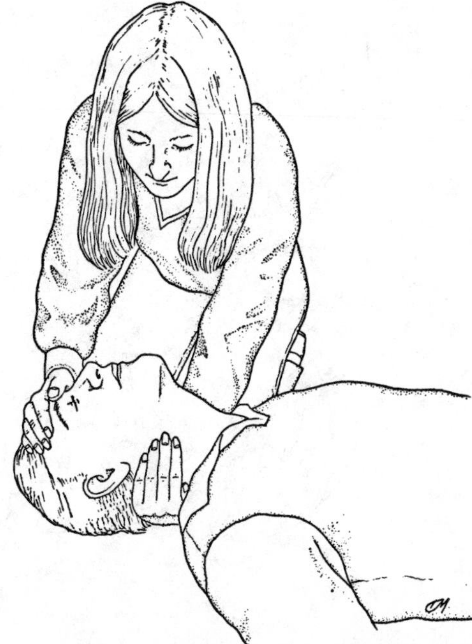

Step 2. Lift neck and push back on forehead.

3. Check that the victim is breathing.

- Look at the chest to see if it is rising or falling.
- Lean over the victim's face and listen for breathing sounds.
- Place your cheek next to the victim's mouth or nose and see if you can feel breaths of air.
- Do these steps for 5 seconds.

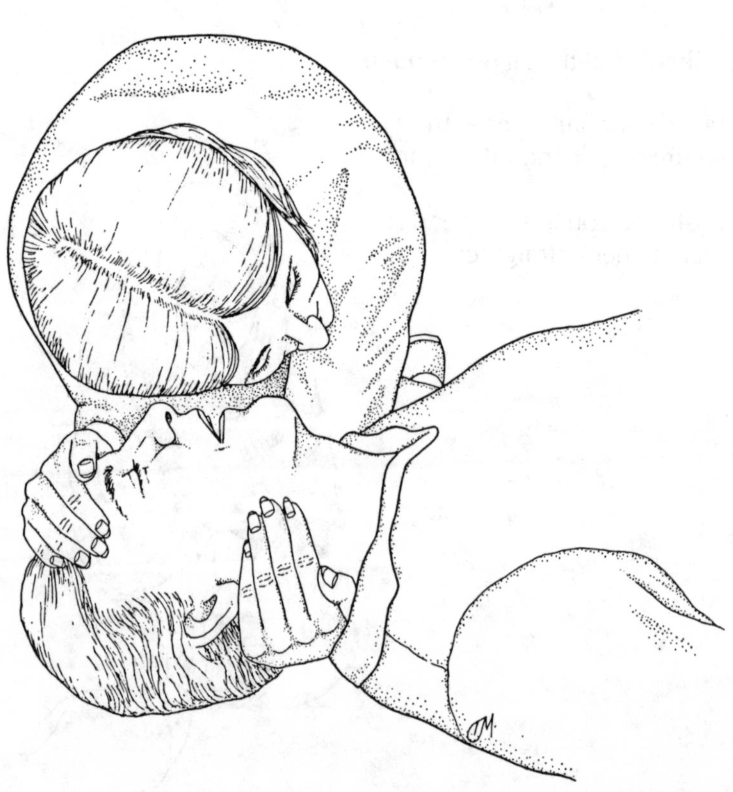

Step 3. Look, listen, and feel for breathing.

4. If the victim is not breathing, start CPR.

- Pinch the victim's nose between your thumb and fingers.
- Take a deep breath and hold it.
- Cover the victim's mouth with your mouth.
- Blow 4 quick, deep breaths into the victim's mouth.
- Take your mouth away from the victim's mouth after each breath.

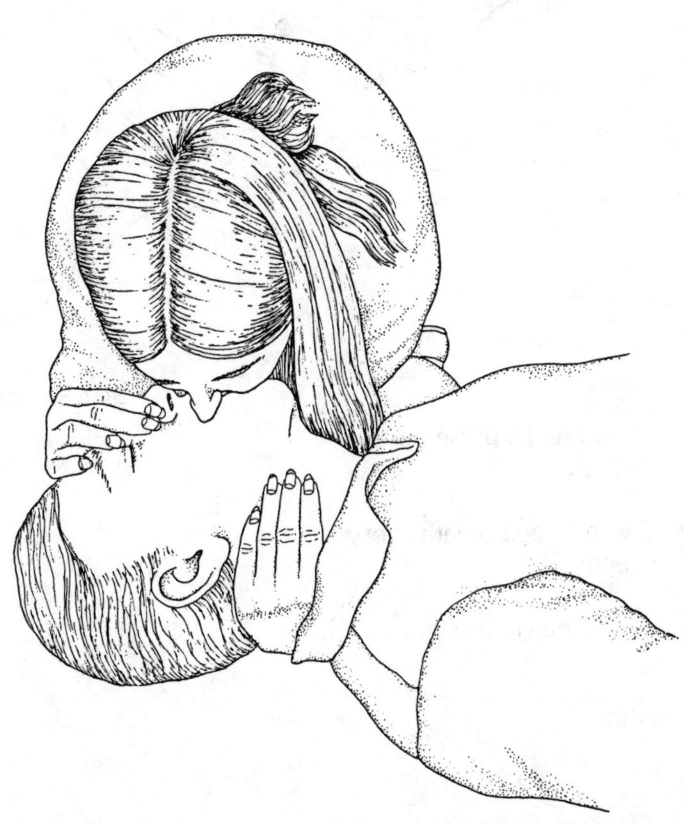

Step 4. Pinch victim's nose and give breaths.

5. Check the victim's pulse.

- Place your fingers on the victim's Adam's apple, and then slide them to one side into the neck groove.
- Feel gently for a pulse.
- Keep feeling for a pulse for 10 seconds.

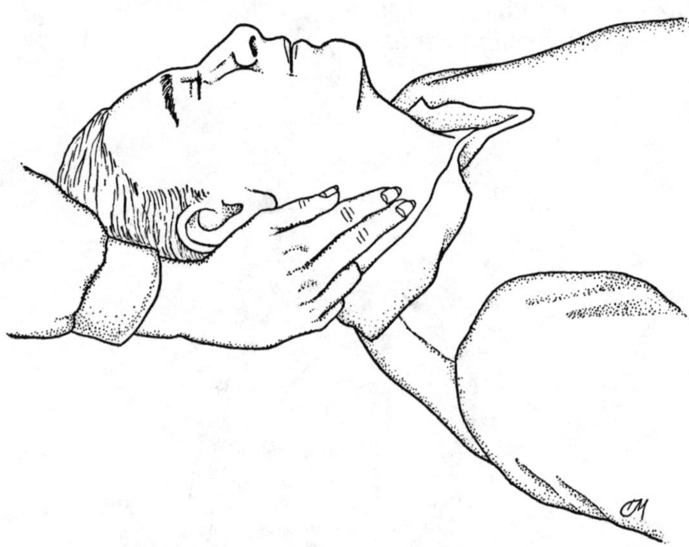

Step 5. Feel for pulse.

6. If you feel a pulse, give breaths.

- Give a forced breath every 5 seconds.
- Check the victim's pulse periodically.

7. If you do not feel a pulse begin compressions.

- Find notch at tip of the breastbone.
- Measure toward the head two fingers' width.

Step 7. Find notch at tip of breastbone.

- Place the heel of your hand on this spot on the lower half of the breastbone.

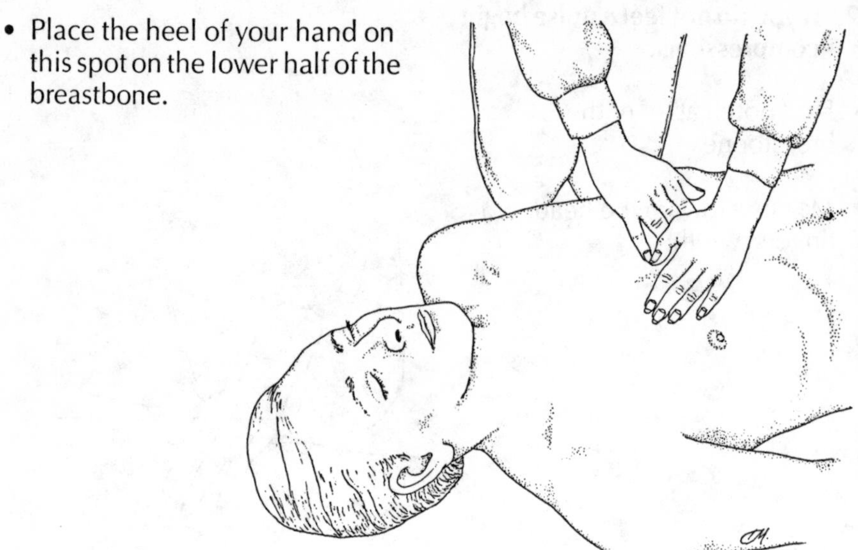

Step 7. Place heel of hand on lower breastbone above your fingers.

- Place your other hand on top and straighten your arms.

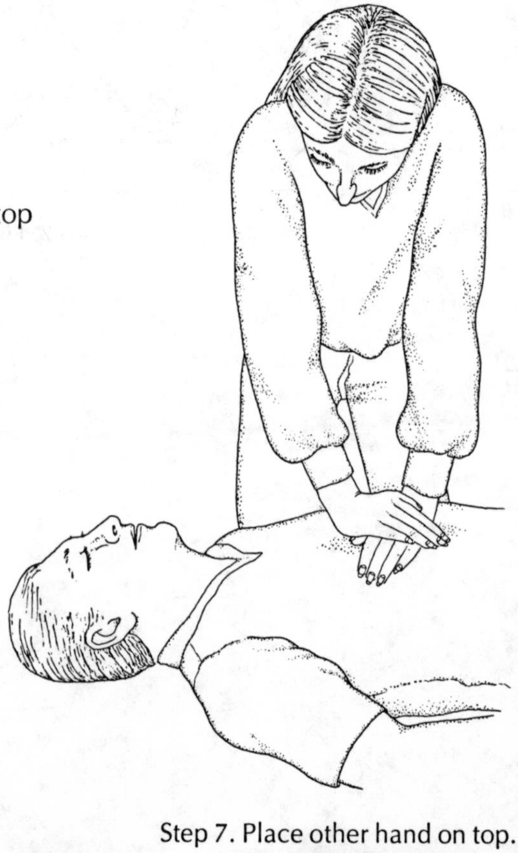

Step 7. Place other hand on top.

- Press straight downward to compress chest inward about 1 to 1½ inches.
- Each compression of the chest should last about ¾ of a second.

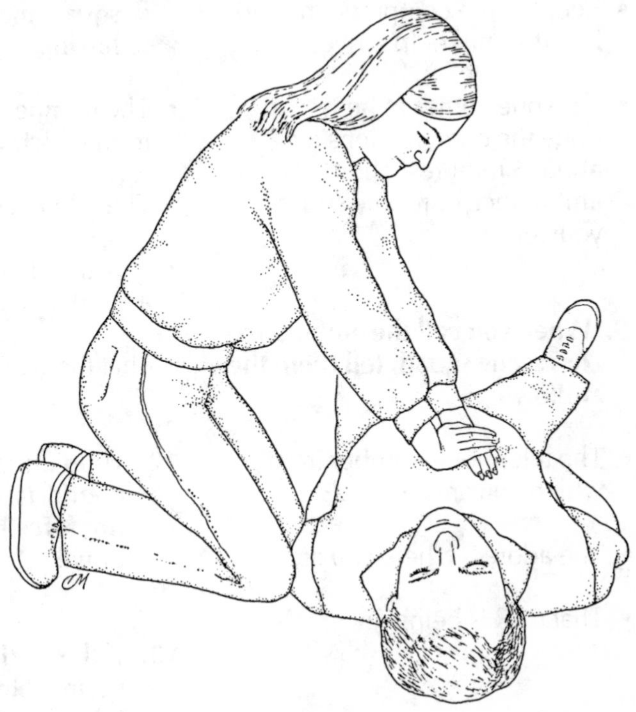

Step 7. Compress chest 1½ to 2 inches.

- After 15 compressions, give 2 quick, deep breaths. Then repeat the compressions. Continue until you get a heartbeat.

8. Call for help.

- If someone responds to your call, tell them to call an ambulance or a rescue squad.
- Keep up the compressions and breaths until help arrives.
- If no one comes to help, continue the compressions for about 5 minutes. Then, call an ambulance or rescue squad yourself.

9. When you call the ambulance or rescue squad, tell them the following:

- The telephone number from which you are calling.
- The address where you are.
- That CPR is being given.

10. Return to the victim immediately and restart CPR.

11. If the victim is conscious, call an ambulance or rescue squad and tell them the following:

- The number of the telephone from which you are calling.
- The address where you are.
- That the victim has possibly had a heart attack.
- That the victim is conscious.

12. Help the victim to get into a comfortable position, but do not force him or her to lie down.

13. If the victim has nitroglycerin tablets, let him or her take them as prescribed.

14. Stay with the victim until the ambulance or rescue squad arrives, and do the following:

- Be alert for a sudden lapse into unconsciousness or a sudden cessation of heartbeat and/or breathing.

- Be prepared to give CPR instantly if the symptoms indicate it.

15. Do not take the victim to the hospital yourself unless there is no ambulance or rescue squad available.

16. Do not allow the victim to refuse to go to the hospital.

Reasons for your actions: Heart attack

Your main objectives are to
a. recognize a heart attack immediately
b. bring medical care to the victim at once
c. be prepared to treat sudden heart stoppage
d. keep oxygen flowing to the brain, if the heart stops.

At any minute during the first two hours after a heart attack, the victim's heart could suddenly stop. CPR (including artificial breathing and external compressions) must be started immediately if the victim is to survive. If CPR is started at once and is done well, the victim's chances for survival are generally good.

The first symptom of a heart attack is usually chest pain, described as a feeling of "heavy pressure" or a sense of indigestion-like burning over the breastbone. The pain may extend all the way to the jaw and arms (usually to the left arm and left side of the body). Other signs include shortness of breath, fear, sweating, pale or bluish skin, and nausea.

If the victim is already a heart patient and has nitroglycerin pills for the heart pain (angina pectoris), he or she may take the medication as prescribed. But if the pain does not subside once the pills are taken, you should suspect heart attack rather than simple angina pains.

If you suspect a heart attack, do not drive the victim to the hospital or clinic. If you are the victim yourself, do not attempt to drive. If the victim's heart suddenly stops while you are in the car, there will be no one and no room to give CPR, which is the only way to save his or her life. Instead, call an ambulance. The ambulance or emergency unit will be equipped, staffed, and otherwise prepared to deal with heart stoppage if it occurs. Therefore your first priority is to call the ambulance yourself or have some trustworthy person call it.

Do not waste time in "waiting to see what happens." The greatest risk period is the first two hours, and during this time the patient should be in the hospital, or at least in an ambulance where lifesaving equipment and professionals are at hand. While you are waiting for the ambulance, however, be sure to stay with the victim and watch for sudden heart stoppage so that you can start CPR and continue it until the ambulance comes.

Ask the victim how he or she feels most comfortable and put him or her in that position. Often if the heart is weak, the patient's shortness of breath will be worse lying down.

If the victim suddenly becomes unconscious, go through the CPR procedure step by step. Do not interrupt CPR, once you have started the procedure, for more than five seconds.

If there is no one else available to make the call to the ambulance and you have not called before starting CPR, you may have to leave in order to call. But make sure you continue the CPR for at least five minutes before making the call. You can then make the call quickly and return to continue CPR until the ambulance arrives.

Heatstroke

Heatstroke can result in brain damage if the victim does not receive competent care. Seconds count.

1. Decide if it is heatstroke.

- Observe the victim and see if these conditions exist:

  The skin is red instead of pale.

  The skin is hot to the touch instead of cool.

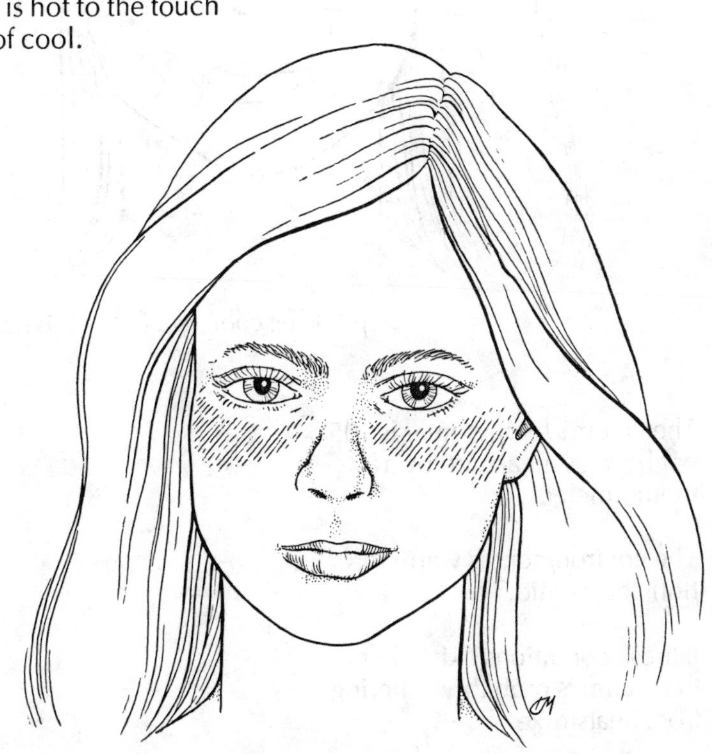

Step 1. Red, dry, and hot skin is heatstroke.

The skin is dry instead of wet or clammy.

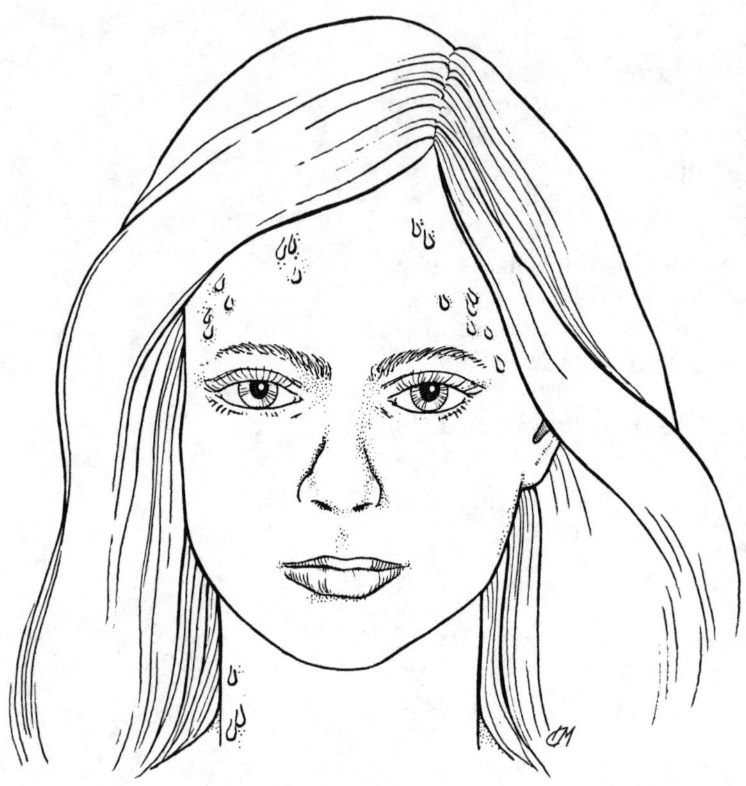

Step 1. Pale, cool, and wet skin is *not* heatstroke.

The victim's temperature is 105° or above as measured by a thermometer.

The environment is warm (or hot) and humid.

- If these conditions exist, then the victim is probably suffering from heatstroke.

2. Do not give the victim anything to eat or drink.

3. Move the victim into a cooler environment.

- An air conditioned home or building.
- An air conditioned automobile or bus.
- A shady place with a breeze.

4. Remove almost all of the victim's clothing.

5. Cover the victim's body with wet, cold cloths.

- Use towels, washcloths, tablecloths, or even cloth-like paper towels.
- Change the cloths as soon as they begin to get warm, and replace them with cool ones.

6. Fan the victim.

7. If possible, immerse the victim in cold water.

A bathtub
A creek or stream
A pond or cool inlet of a lake
A calm section of beach water if you are near the ocean

NOTE: Do not use ice. Keep the victim's head above the water!

8. Recheck the victim's temperature periodically.

- Feel the victim's skin if you have no thermometer.
- Take the victim's temperature with a thermometer.

9. Call an ambulance when the victim's temperature is almost normal (98.6°F).

- Do not stop treatment to call an ambulance until the victim's temperature is almost normal.
- Do not leave the victim alone until his or her temperature is at a safe level.

10. Final note: From time to time, check the victim's pulse and breathing.

Reasons for your actions: Heatstroke

Your main objective is to lower the body temperature fast.

Heatstroke is a critical condition and is very common in the summertime, especially in very hot or very humid climates. Occasionally the part of the brain that controls the body's temperature fails for various reasons and heatstroke can occur. In drier climates the risk is less; it is much higher for hot, very humid environments, especially when the person has been working or exercising vigorously.

In heatstroke, the skin does not sweat or cool the body by evaporation of sweat, and the body temperature climbs higher. Blood vessels in the skin will swell to give off heat, and the person's skin will look red. The body's temperature will continue to rise, while sweating still does not occur. The condition is serious because permanent brain damage can result if the body temperature remains high for too long a time.

Remember that your main goal is to reduce body temperature as quickly as possible. The best way to do this is to put the victim in a cold shower or tub of water. If this is not possible, cold, wet towels or cloths will do. The most important fact to remember is that fast action is essential.

Poison swallowed

The first rule is always to keep poisons out of the reach of children or people who do not know their dangers. This goes for many cleaning preparations, as well as medications. Above all, stay calm: fewer than 20 percent of all suspected poisonings actually require hospital treatment.

1. **Look immediately for the poison's container, or look for signs of the poison itself (powder or liquid on the floor).**

2. **Call the nearest Poison Control Center, hospital, or emergency room and tell them the following:**

- Who and where you are
- A telephone number where you can be reached
- The name of the poison and the ingredients as they are described on the label of the container
- The amount of poison you think was swallowed.

3. **Follow the instructions they give you.**

4. **Do not give antidotes! Do not induce vomiting unless you are directed to do so by the Poison Control Center, hospital, or emergency room.**

5. **Do not give any (salt) solutions.**

6. **Take the poison container to the hospital or emergency room with the patient.**

Reasons for your actions: Poison swallowed

Your main objectives are to
a. find out exactly what poison was swallowed
b. call for help.

Since there are so many Poison Control Centers and emergency rooms throughout the country, you do not need to take any emergency measure without guidance. If you can find out exactly what poison was swallowed, you are well on your way toward getting that help.

The important thing is to call a Poison Control Center (PCC) at once with the information you have obtained. Then do exactly what you are told to do.

Although inducing vomiting is the right measure in many cases, it is not necessarily so in all cases. For example, when acid, lye, or other corrosives or petroleum products such as lighter fluid are swallowed, vomiting could cause more harm than good. Also, some solutions that induce vomiting can be hazardous (for instance, salt).

Remember that diluting the poison by giving lots of milk or water may make things worse, since this increases the speed at which the poison is absorbed throughout the system.

This is a case where the cardinal rule of first aid applies in every instance: *do no harm*. The main task is to identify the poison accurately and quickly and then call the PCC. Do exactly what the Poison Control Center tells you to do.

Shock

Quick attention is necessary when a victim goes into shock. No visible wounds are necessary for a person to go into shock.

1. **Examine the victim for shock symptoms.**

- Pale skin
- Cool, clammy, and sweating skin
- Restlessness or drowsiness
- Thirst
- Rapid pulse (over 100 beats per minute)
- Rapid and weak breathing
- Dilated (enlarged) pupils

2. **If any or all of these symptoms are present, lay the victim down immediately and do not let him or her walk, sit, or stand.**

3. **Prop the victim's legs up (about 12 inches high) unless you suspect a head injury or a broken leg.**

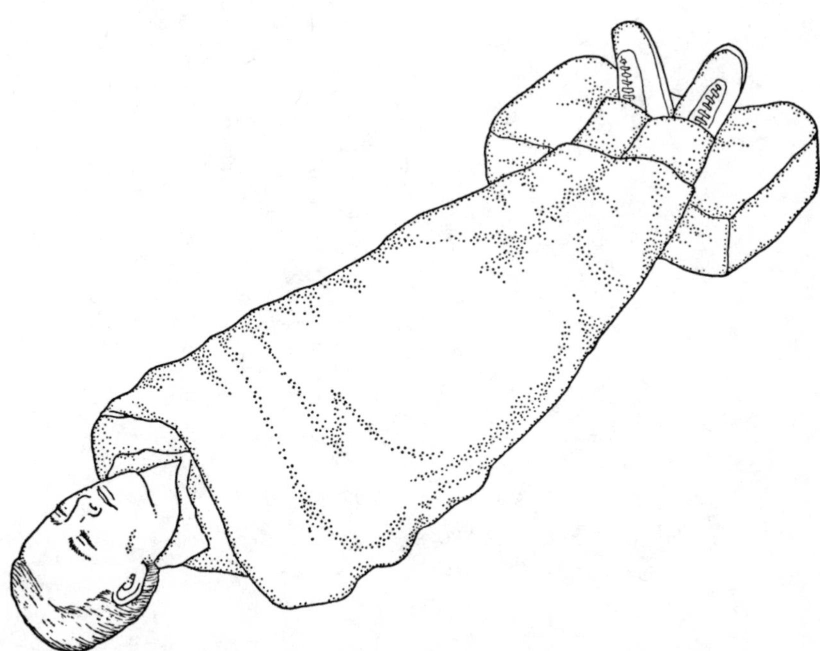

Step 3. Prop victim's feet up about 12 inches. Cover with a blanket.

4. Stop any bleeding.

- Cover the wound with one of the following:
  A sterile dressing or bandage
  A clean cloth
  Some piece of clothing
  A sanitary napkin

- Place the material over the wound, and then place your hands on the bandage and press down or against the wound firmly.

- If the bleeding does not slow or stop immediately, apply pressure to the appropriate pressure point:

Arm wound—place your fingers in the groove between the two large muscles on the inside of the upper arm.

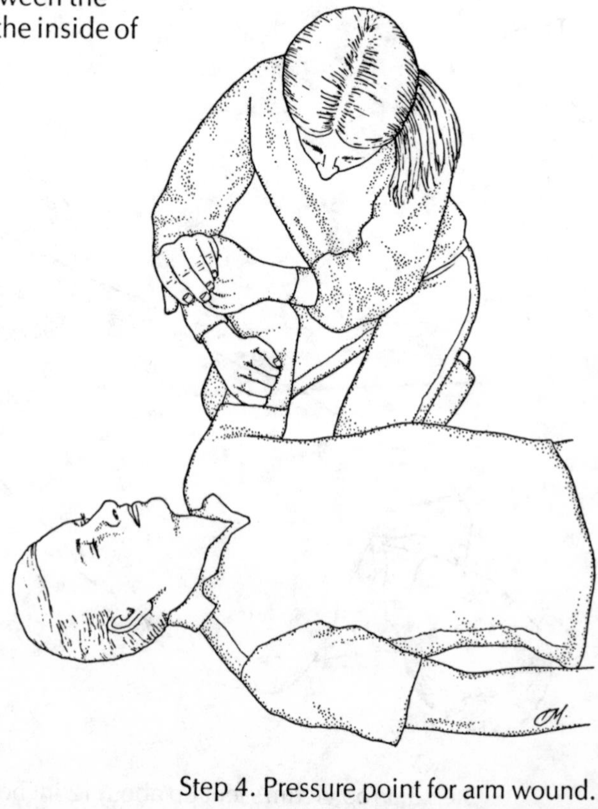

Step 4. Pressure point for arm wound.

Leg wound—place fingers in the crease where the thigh joins to the torso at the groin.

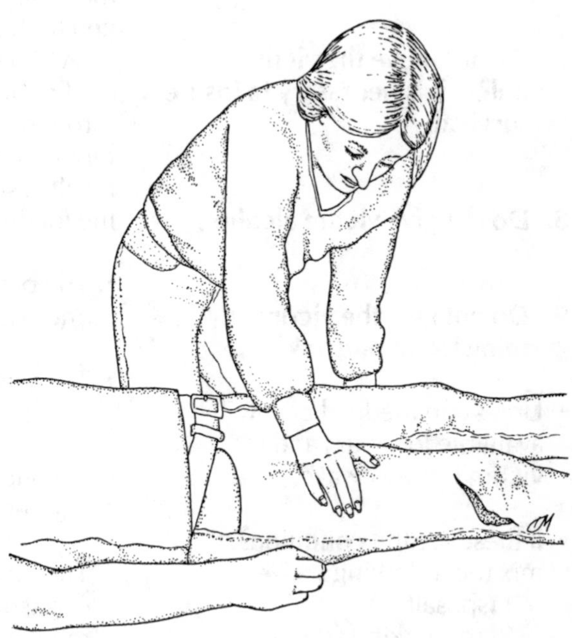

Step 4. Pressure point for leg wound.

Neck wound—place the fingers in the groove at the side of the Adam's apple on the side of the neck that is bleeding.

- When the bleeding stops, ease up on the pressure point. If the bleeding starts again, apply pressure again.
- If you are dealing with an amputation victim, if the bleeding does not stop in 2 to 3 minutes, use a tourniquet. Refer to the section on Bleeding for directions.

5. Keep the victim warm by covering with a blanket or a piece of clothing.

6. Call an ambulance.

7. Do not move the victim unless it is necessary to insure survival.

8. Do not give victim alcohol.

9. Do not give the victim anything to eat or drink.

- Unless no medical care will be available for hours and the victim is fully awake.
- If these are the conditions, then mix the following:
  1 tsp. salt
  ½ tsp. baking soda
  1 quart of water
- Give the victim a half a glass of this mixture every 15 minutes.
- If water is all that you have, give the patient a half a glass of water every 15 minutes.

Reasons for your actions: Shock

Your main objective is to keep as much blood as possible flowing to the brain, in order to supply oxygen to the brain.

When there has been a great deal of bleeding, or fluid loss through burns in burn cases, the blood pressure goes down. The result is shock. In cases of shock, the following happens:

- The brain is "starved" for blood and oxygen.
- The victim is thirsty because of loss of fluid in the body.
- The victim becomes drowsy and restless at the same time.
- The victim will breathe rapidly or gasp for breath to draw in more oxygen.
- The victim has a rapid pulse, because the heart beats faster to keep the blood pressure up.
- The blood vessels in the skin narrow to divert blood from the skin to the brain, and the victim's skin becomes pale and cool to the touch.

The best treatment, of course, is to give oxygen, blood transfusions, and fluids into the veins. That raises the oxygen level and blood pressure. That is exactly what a physician, paramedic, or hospital staff does for a person in shock. However, until a victim receives such medical help, you simply must try to stop further blood loss, if possible, and also try to divert blood from the legs and extremities toward the brain. To do this, you lay the patient down. Raise the legs about 12 inches high to send blood toward the brain—unless, of course, you suspect a head injury. Then, you want to avoid increasing pressure and swelling in the brain, so keep the victim lying flat. Also, if a leg is broken, moving the broken limb will only increase the damage and bleeding. In this case it is best simply to keep the victim lying flat.

You can control external bleeding by using the usual techniques: direct pressure, then pressure points, then a tourniquet as a last resort. Stop the bleeding as quickly as you can. Go directly to using a tourniquet if the blood flow is heavy. The victim who is in shock is already very near death and cannot afford to lose any more blood.

The shock victim is losing body heat, so cover with blankets or warm clothing to protect against loss of more body heat.

Since shock victims will often go directly into surgery once they are in the hospital, it is advisable to give them nothing to eat or drink. Especially do not give alcohol, which could be dangerous in this situation.

If help is far away and it may be some time before an ambulance or emergency unit can be dispatched, you should consider giving small amounts of water with salt. This helps to replace some of the blood fluids lost. Do not give large amounts or the victim may vomit. Give very small amounts of the fluid, but give them often.

Spinal injury

Spinal injuries can result in permanent paralysis of a portion or all of the body. Consequently, you should proceed with extreme caution any time that you treat a victim who has or is suspected to have a spinal injury. The basic rule is, "Always assume spinal injury in accident cases." If you follow this rule, you will avoid possible additional injury to the victim.

1. The following situations may indicate that a spinal injury has occurred:

- An accident victim is unconscious.
- The victim is unconscious and has bruises or cuts on his or her head.
- The accident victim is awake, but is not moving.
- The accident victim complains of pain in the back of the neck.

NOTE: In each of these cases, spinal injury may be present. Always treat victims who show these symptoms as if they have spinal injuries until you know for sure that they do not.

2. Check the victim's airway to see if it is clear of obstruction.

- **Do not bend the neck or lift the neck** as you would if the victim were not a spinal injury case!
- Look at the chest to see if it is rising and falling.
- Lean over the victim and listen for breathing sounds.
- Place your cheek near the victim's mouth and see if you can feel breaths of air.

- If the victim has breathing difficulty, do the following:

  Pull the mouth open by grasping the jaw.

  Lift the tongue out of the way. If the jaw will not hinge downward, try to pull it forward without shifting the position of the neck.

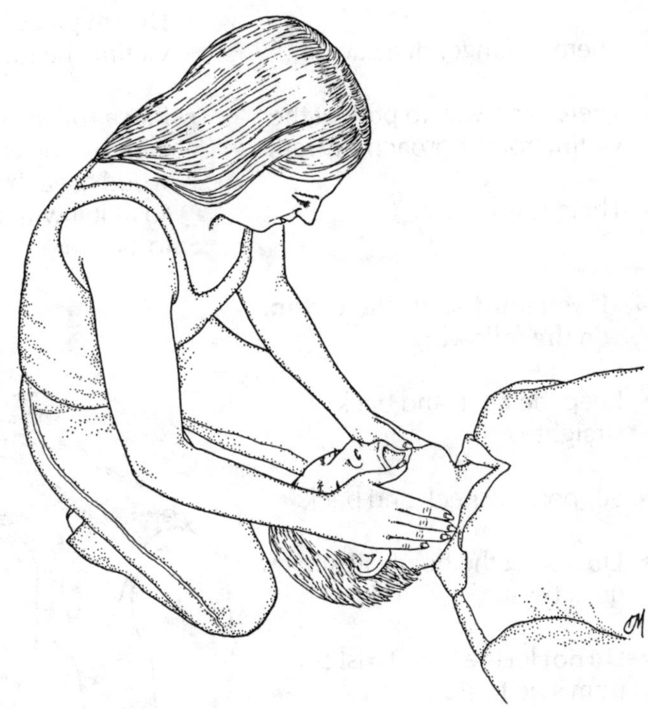

Step 2. Pull the mouth open by grasping the jaw to check airway.

Warning: Do not move the neck unless you absolutely cannot open the mouth otherwise.

3. Do not move the victim unless the victim's life is in danger.

- Move the victim only under the following circumstances:

  There is a fire.

  There is danger of an explosion.

  There is danger of drowning.

  There is danger of a cave-in.

  There is no way to protect the victim from approaching traffic.

  There is no pulse.

4. If you must move the victim, do the following:

- Keep the neck and back straight.
- Support the neck and back.
- **Do not** let the head fall and the neck twist.
- **Do not** let the back twist or arch from side to side.

5. If the victim is conscious, instruct the victim to stay still and not move the back or neck.

6. If the victim is lying down, do the following:

- Support the spine so that it will not move.
- **Do not** place a pillow under the victim's head.
- Place rolled-up blankets, clothes, rocks, or pieces of wood at each side of the head so that it will not roll from side to side.

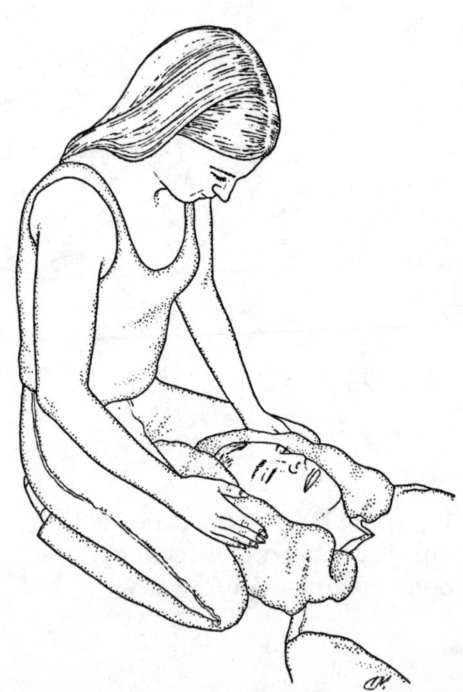

Step 6. Place rolled-up blankets or clothes on either side of the head to immobilize the head.

- If the neck is bent at an odd angle, **do not** try to straighten it. Prop the head on either side to keep the neck in the position that you found it.

- Call an ambulance.

7. If the victim is in a sitting position, do the following:

- Support the victim's head so that it will not move:

- Get behind the victim.

- Place your hands at the sides of the victim's head and support the head.

- Keep supporting the victim's head until someone comes who can call an ambulance.

NOTE: In all cases of spinal injury, whether of the neck, or the upper, middle, or lower back, the key step is to prevent movement.

Reasons for your actions: Spinal injury

Your main objective is to prevent damage to the spinal cord by preventing movement of the broken or shifted vertebrae (backbones).

Sometimes when an accident occurs, one or several of the bones in the victim's spine (vertebrae) will be broken or caused to shift. While this condition is painful, it seldom causes any permanent damage—unless the broken or shifted vertebrae damage the spinal cord, which is encircled by the vertebral bones. Thus your main objective as a first-aider is to prevent damage to the spinal cord.

This is an important "prime directive" for any person practicing first aid or emergency procedures. All too often, well-meaning people try to "help" a victim of an accident by pulling or dragging the individual from a wrecked car and placing him or her somewhere else. Remember that if the victim's spinal cord is damaged by any twisting or bending movements, he or she could become paralyzed. Therefore, do not move any person you suspect of having a spinal injury unless absolutely necessary to avoid traffic, fire, or water.

If the victim is unconscious when you arrive on the scene, assume that he or she has a spinal injury and act accordingly. If there is an injury to the head or neck, a spinal injury can be considered likely.

If the victim is awake and conscious, ask him or her if there is any neck or back pain. If the victim appears dazed or uncertain, treat for spinal injuries anyway and tell the person to remain as is.

The first step, as always, is to make sure the airway is open. If you need to open the airway, do so without bending the neck. Do not lift the neck and push back the forehead as you would do in cases without spinal injury. Instead, keep the neck still and lift the victim's jaw. Or pull forward from the angles of the jaw. You can even give forced breaths using this technique.

If it is a case of risking death or risking moving the patient, you must try to save the victim's life. Check Step 4 if you must move a patient in order to minimize damage. Similarly, if the patient is not breathing and there is no airway open, do what is necessary to give breaths—but again, minimize the risk of paralysis as much as possible.

If cardiopulmonary resuscitation (CPR) is needed (in cases where there is no pulse) you may have to move the victim in order to get him or her on a solid surface for the CPR. Also, if the victim is in a car that is burning, about to explode, or sinking in water, and the victim must be moved, do so; however, try to minimize risk by keeping the neck and shoulders immobilized as much as possible. Check Steps 4 and 6 for pointers.

To prevent accidental spinal cord damage while you wait for the ambulance, keep the neck stable by holding the head of a sitting victim or immobilizing the head, neck, and spine of a victim who is lying down. This will keep the spinal bones in line so that the spinal cord does not kink. Maintain this immobilization until the ambulance crew or paramedics have attached the necessary splints and tell you that it is all right to let go.

Home first aid kit

The following items should be in every home first aid kit.

Syrup of ipecac. You should have enough for 1 ounce for each member of the family. You should get syrup of ipecac, not the fluid extract.

Epsom salts

A roll of 1-inch adhesive tape

A roll of 2-inch duct tape (for splints)

The following supply of sterile bandages:
- A dozen 4-inch by 4-inch
- A dozen 3-inch by 3-inch
- A dozen 2-inch by 2-inch

Sterile vaseline gauze

Two 4-inch elastic bandages

Two 2½-inch elastic bandages

A bottle of hydrogen peroxide

Scissors

Tweezers

One insect sting kit (if a member of the family has insect sting allergies)

Aspirin (with child-proof cap)

Two thermometers (one rectal, one oral)

Cotton-tipped swabs

One triangle bandage

Anesthetic ointment

Antibacterial ointment

One roll of 1-inch-wide gauze bandage

One roll of 4-inch-wide gauze bandage

Assorted adhesive bandages

Family medical history

Detailed family medical records are helpful in diagnosing and treating potential health problems, especially those that tend to reoccur in some families. To help your doctor become fully informed about your family's medical history, note any serious diseases in your family. The list below should be consulted when filling out the form. In addition to listing diseases that have occurred in the family, be prepared to discuss with your doctor your personal habits and lifestyle (diet, exercise, smoking, and so forth), any medications you take on a regular basis, and your past health history (hospitalizations, operations, illnesses).

Is there any history in your family of:

Allergies
Arthritis
Cancer
Cystic fibrosis
Diabetes
Epilepsy
Hearing defects
Heart defects
Hemophilia
Huntington's chorea
Hypertension
Mental disorders
Mental retardation
Muscular dystrophy
Sickle-cell anemia
Stroke
Tay-Sachs disease
Visual defects
Other recurring family diseases

Name	Birth date	Blood type and Rh	Allergy and disease history
Mother			
Her mother Her father			
Father			
His mother His father			
Child			
Child			
Child			

Emergency telephone numbers

Poison Control Center ________________

Paramedics ________________

Doctor ________________

Doctor ________________

Doctor ________________

Hospital emergency room ________________

Fire department ________________

Police department ________________

Ambulance ________________

Work phone numbers ________________

Local pharmacy ________________

24-hour pharmacy ________________

Dentist ________________

Neighbor ________________

Relative ________________

Your address and phone number (for babysitters and visitors)

____

____

Index

A

B

C

D

E

F

G

H

I

J

K

L

M

N

O

P

Q

R

S

T

U